SCUBA DIVING

MALTA | GOZO | COMINO

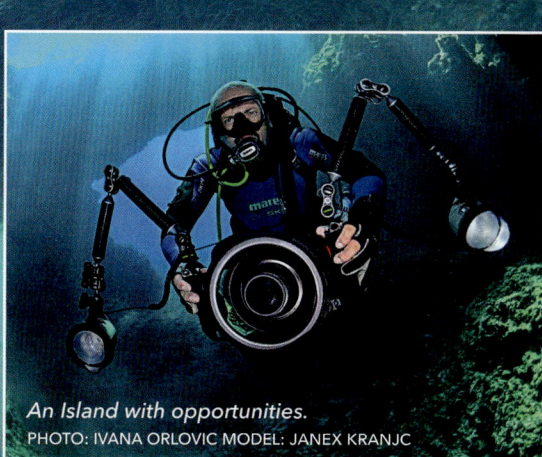

An Island with opportunities.
PHOTO: IVANA ORLOVIC MODEL: JANEX KRANJC

FIFTH EDITION **PETER G. LEMON**

Main photo: A very good friend enjoying the West reef at Wied iz-Zurrieq not far from possibly the best wreck shore dive in the Mediterranean Sea, the MV Um el Faroud.

All rights reserved. No part of this publication may be reproduced, stored in any retrieval system or transmitted in any form or by any means, mechanical, electronic, recording or otherwise, without the prior written permission of the Publisher, Peter G. Lemon.

All requests for permission should be addressed in writing to Peter G. Lemon.

Although every care has been taken in compiling this book, using the latest information available at the time of going to press, some details are liable to change and cannot therefore be guaranteed. The Publisher/Author does not accept any liability whatsoever arising from errors or omissions, however, caused.

Would readers please note that the illustrations of the underwater plans and road maps to be found in the following pages have been made as accurate as possible. They are to compass bearings but not to scale, information for distance and time can be found within the text. The author accepts no responsibility for the loss, injury or inconvenience sustained by any person using these illustrations.

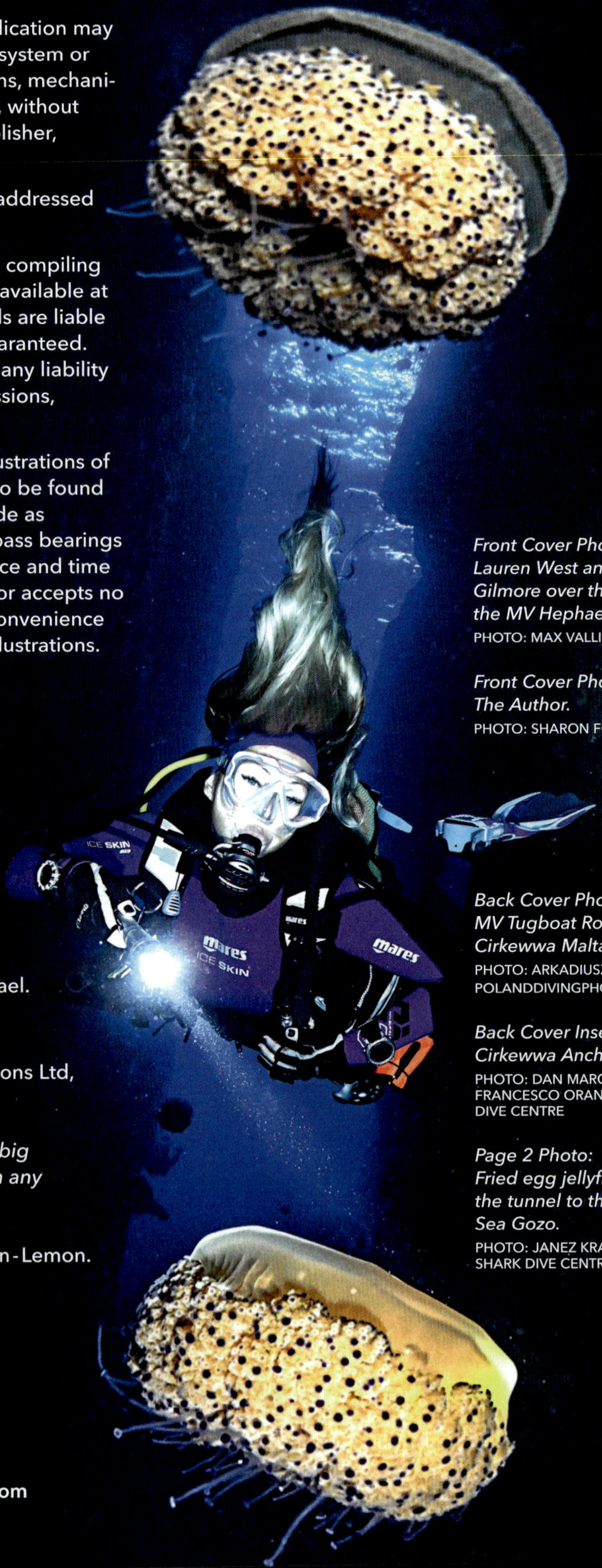

Front Cover Photo right:
Lauren West and Paddy Gilmore over the bridge of the MV Hephaestus.
PHOTO: MAX VALLI

Front Cover Photo top left:
The Author.
PHOTO: SHARON FORDER

PUBLISHER Peter G. Lemon.

PROJECT MANAGER Sue Lemon.

DESIGN / ARTWORK
SMK Sean King, SMK Graphic Design.

ARTWORK UPDATES Wade Carmichael.

PRINTED BY
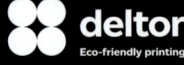 Deltor Communications Ltd, Cornwall.

Back Cover Photo:
MV Tugboat Rozi off Cirkewwa Malta.
PHOTO: ARKADIUSZ SREBNIK
POLANDDIVINGPHOTO

Back Cover Insert:
Cirkewwa Anchor.
PHOTO: DAN MARCELLO Di
FRANCESCO ORANGE SHARK
DIVE CENTRE

Page 2 Photo:
Fried egg jellyfish inside the tunnel to the Inland Sea Gozo.
PHOTO: JANEZ KRANJC ORANGE
SHARK DIVE CENTRE

Peter and Sue would like to say a very big thank you to all persons who helped in any way to produce this book.

WEBSITE Designed by Chris Appleton-Lemon.

PLANNED AND PRODUCED BY
Peter G. Lemon and Sue Lemon
7 Earls Hill Gardens, Royston,
Herts SG8 9DA.

www.scubadivingmalta.co.uk
www.scubadivinggozo.co.uk
www.scubadivingmaltagozocomino.com

Copyright © Peter G. Lemon.

ISBN 978-0-9541789-4-9

Contents

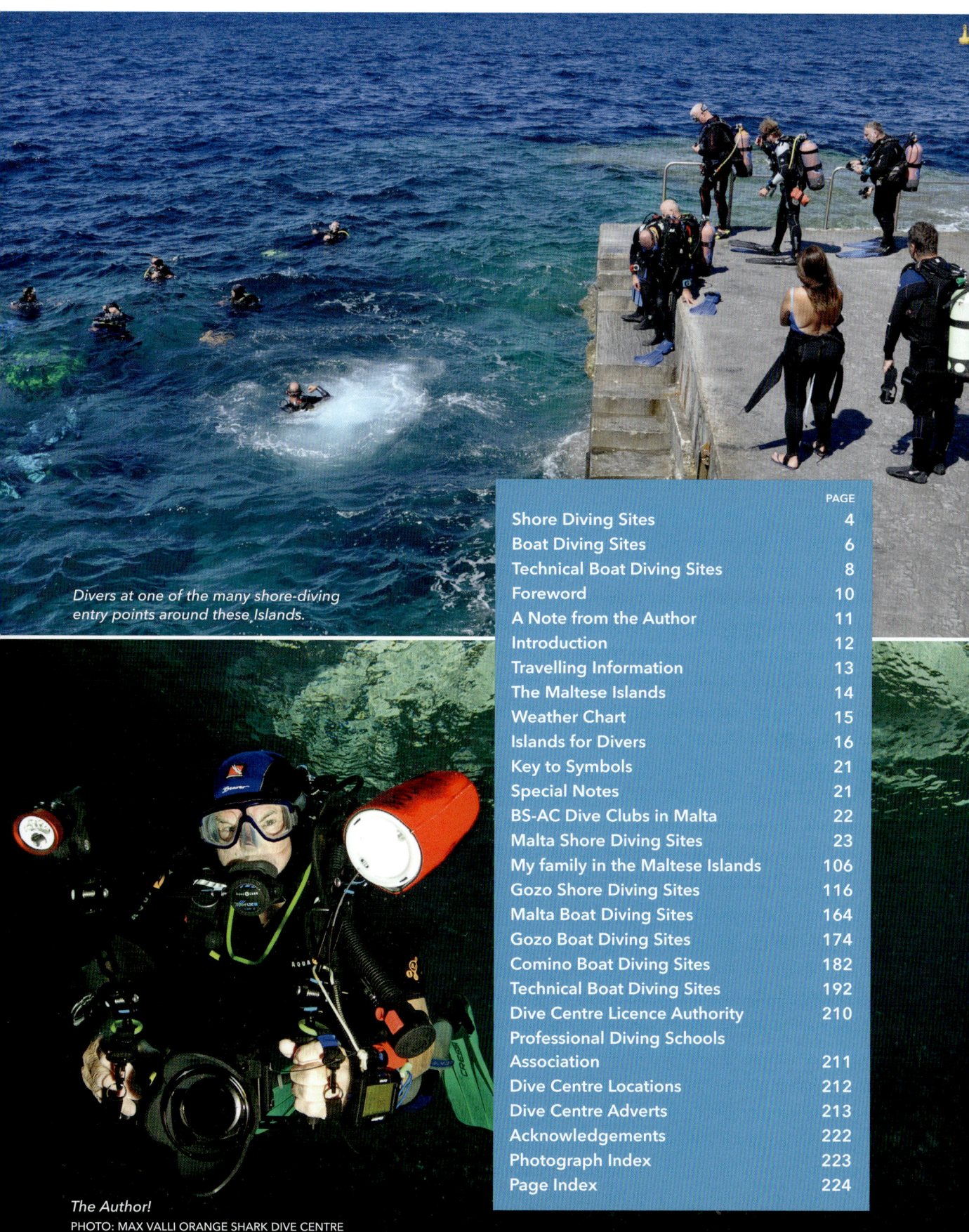

Divers at one of the many shore-diving entry points around these Islands.

The Author!
PHOTO: MAX VALLI ORANGE SHARK DIVE CENTRE

	PAGE
Shore Diving Sites	4
Boat Diving Sites	6
Technical Boat Diving Sites	8
Foreword	10
A Note from the Author	11
Introduction	12
Travelling Information	13
The Maltese Islands	14
Weather Chart	15
Islands for Divers	16
Key to Symbols	21
Special Notes	21
BS-AC Dive Clubs in Malta	22
Malta Shore Diving Sites	23
My family in the Maltese Islands	106
Gozo Shore Diving Sites	116
Malta Boat Diving Sites	164
Gozo Boat Diving Sites	174
Comino Boat Diving Sites	182
Technical Boat Diving Sites	192
Dive Centre Licence Authority	210
Professional Diving Schools Association	211
Dive Centre Locations	212
Dive Centre Adverts	213
Acknowledgements	222
Photograph Index	223
Page Index	224

Shore Diving Site Locations

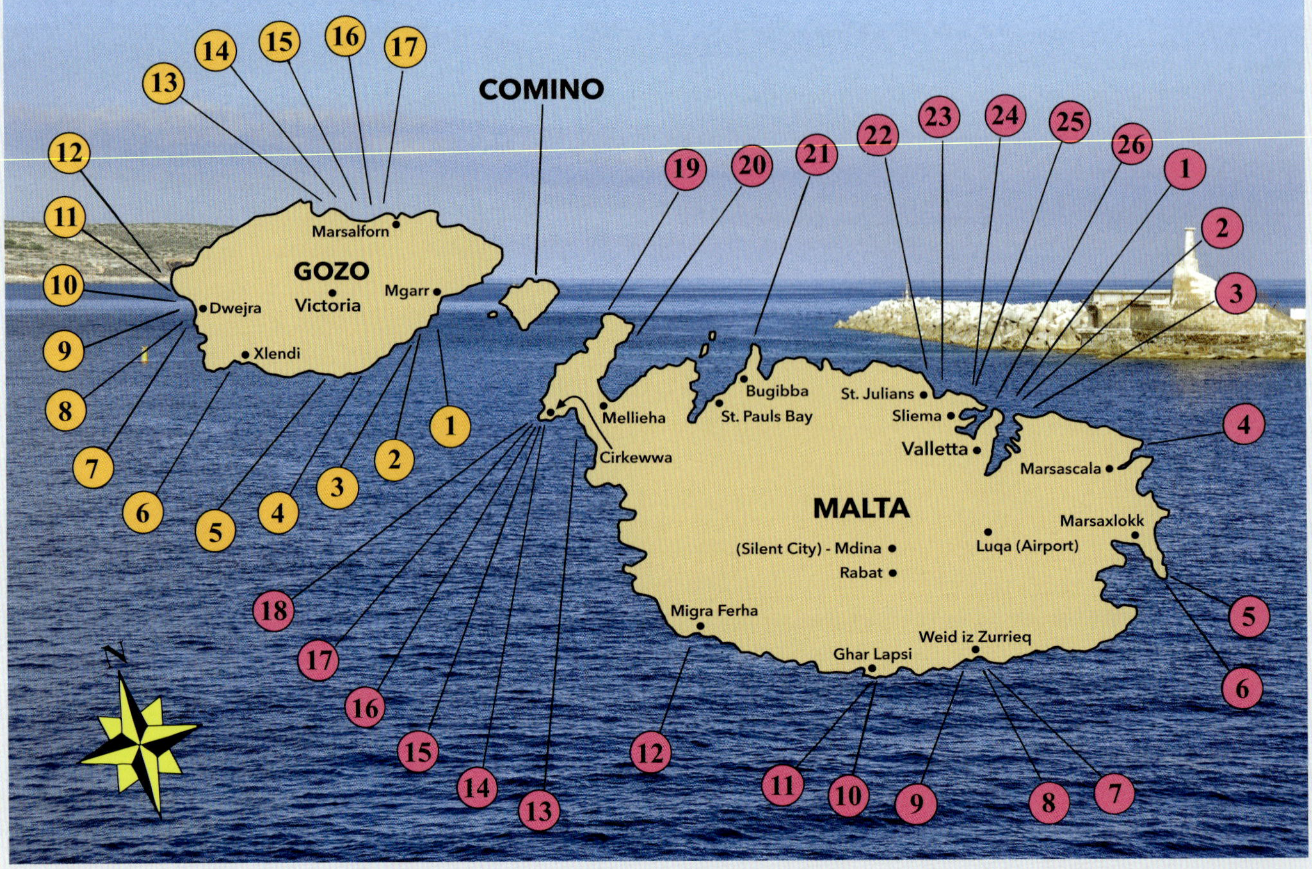

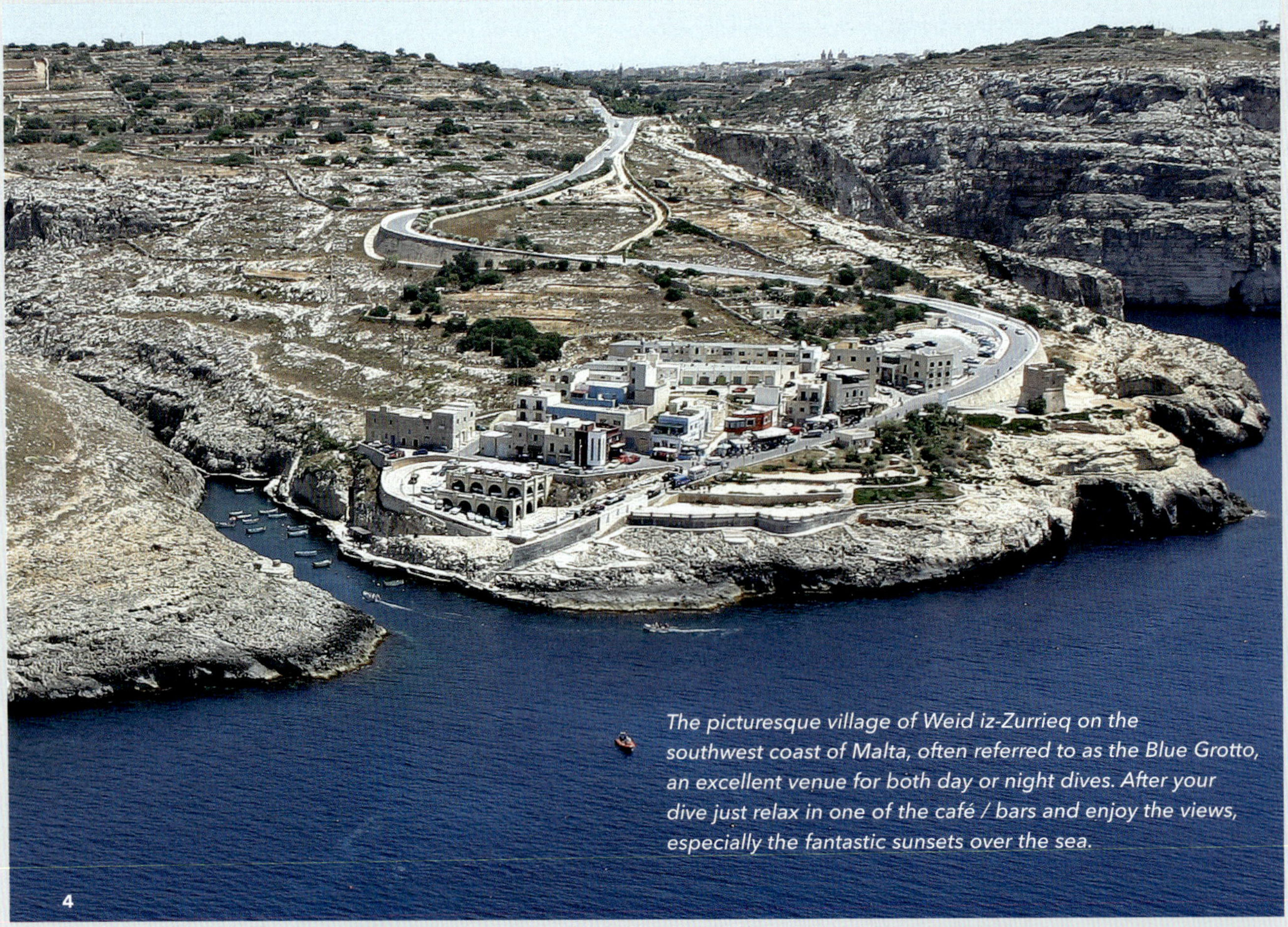

The picturesque village of Weid iz-Zurrieq on the southwest coast of Malta, often referred to as the Blue Grotto, an excellent venue for both day or night dives. After your dive just relax in one of the café / bars and enjoy the views, especially the fantastic sunsets over the sea.

Shore Diving Site Index

Malta Dive Sites

#	Site	Page	Description
1	St Elmo Bay - HMS *Maori*	23	Interesting wreck 10m - 14m - lots of marine life
2	Valletta - Fort St Elmo	28	A good rummage & reef dive - 20m drop off down to a maximum depth of 35m
3	Kalkara Creek - SS *Margit*	30	WW2 Wreck - good dive in right conditions 22m
4	Marsascala - Zonqor Point	36	Tugboat St. Michael - Tugboat 10 - Wreckage of P33 all at 22m - Gently sloping intresting reef 3m - 22m
5	Delimara Point - East Reef	40	Long walk - well worth the effort 3m - 34m
6	Delimara Point - South Reef	44	Long walk - the reefs are excellent 3m - 30m
7	Wied iz Zurrieq - East reef	54	Visibility here can be excellent 40m plus
8	Wied iz Zurrieq - West Reef	52	Drop-offs, ledges, gullies & caves 4m - 28m
9	Wied iz Zurrieq - Um el Faroud	46	Large wreck possibly the best in the Mediterranean Sea - Depths on the wreck range from 20m - 35m
10	Ghar Lapsi - Finger reef & Crib	60	Reef, crib & cave - a long dive 0m - 22m
11	Ghar Lapsi - Black John	56	Difficult walk out of the way dive 3m - 38m
12	Migra Ferha	64	Only for the fit - 90 steps- excellent reef 14m - 45m +
13	Anchor Bay	68	Reef & cave dive - good training area 2m- 21m
13	Cirkewwa / Marine Park	72	Malta's most popular diving area
14	Cirkewwa - Paradise Bay	86	Variable depths around the headland 0m - 33m
15	Cirkewwa - Patrol Boat *P29*	83	Scuttled in 2007 on the seabed at 38m
16	Cirkewwa - Sugar Loaf & Madonna	80	The Madonna stands silently in a recess 0m - 28m
17	Cirkewwa - Tug boat *Rozi*	77	Possibly the best known tug boat in Europe 5m - 35m
18	Cirkewwa - Cirkewwa Arch	74	Great photographic opportunities found here 4m - 20m
19	L-Ahrax Point - Inland Sea & Tunnel	89	Reef tunnel & Inland Sea a unique dive 2m - 28m
20	Slugs Bay	92	The name does not do this dive site justice 1m - 10m
21	Qawra Point - Reef & Cave	94	Good dive for experienced & novice divers 1m - 12m
21	Qawra Point - North Reef	96	A deeper dive for experienced divers 0m - 35m
22	St Julians - Mercanti Reef	99	Navigate yourself to this excellent reef 2m - 12m
23	Sliema - Exiles - Tug boat *2* & Reef	102	A nice wreck at 22m with a reef to enjoy 0m - 22m
24	Sliema - Fortizza	107	Good dive with small tunnels & arches 4m - 15m
25	Sliema - Coral Gardens	110	Unique limestone rocks - a very pretty dive 4m - 14m
26	Manoel Island - Lighter *X127*	112	This WW1 barge makes a good dive 4m - 23m

Gozo Dive Sites

#	Site	Page	Description
1	Xatt l'Ahmar - Red Bay	124	A quiet dive site with an excellent reef 0m - 35m +
2	MV *Karwela*	120	Scuttled in 2006 upright on seabed at 42m
2	MV *Cominoland*	122	Scuttled in 2006 upright on seabed at 42m
3	MV *Xlendi*	117	This up-turned wreck still offers a good dive 42m
4	Ras iL-Hobz Middle Finger	130	A unique dive only metres from the shore 0m - 50m +
5	Mgarr ix Xini	132	Great place for a night or second dive 0m - 16m
6	Xlendi - Reef & Tunnel	134	A 70 metre tunnel & a reef to explore 3m - 25m
6	Dwejra Inland Sea / Blue Hole	138	Gozo's most popular diving area
7	Dwejra - Little Bear / Crocodile Rock	140	Excellent reef with 25m drop offs 5m - 34m +
8	Dwejra - Big Bear / Coral Gardens	142	Good reef & cave dive 1m - 45m +
9	Dwejra - Blue Hole / Coral Gardens	144	Underwater headland with drop offs of 40m +
10	Dwejra - Azure Reef / Blue Hole	146	Unique rock formation Blue Hole & window 15m - 38m
11	Dwejra - Inland Sea to Blue Hole	148	Inland Sea to Blue Hole via tunnel 3m - 45m +
12	Dwejra - Inland Sea / Tunnel	154	70 metre Tunnel & reef dive 3m - 45m +
13	Ghasri Valley Cathedral Cave	161	100 Steps - Ladder - Boat, worth the effort 0m - 36m
14	Marsalforn - Billinghurst Cave	160	This is a fantastic cave dive! 70 metres in length, with a minimum depth 20m. Always take an experienced guide.
15	Marsalforn - Reqqa Point	158	Possibly the best! But its only my opinion 2m - 45m +
16	Marsalforn - Anchor Reef	156	Excellent reef an abundance of marine life 9m - 50m +
17	Marsalforn - Double Arch	152	Spectacular dive great for photography 0m - 45m

Boat Diving Site Locations

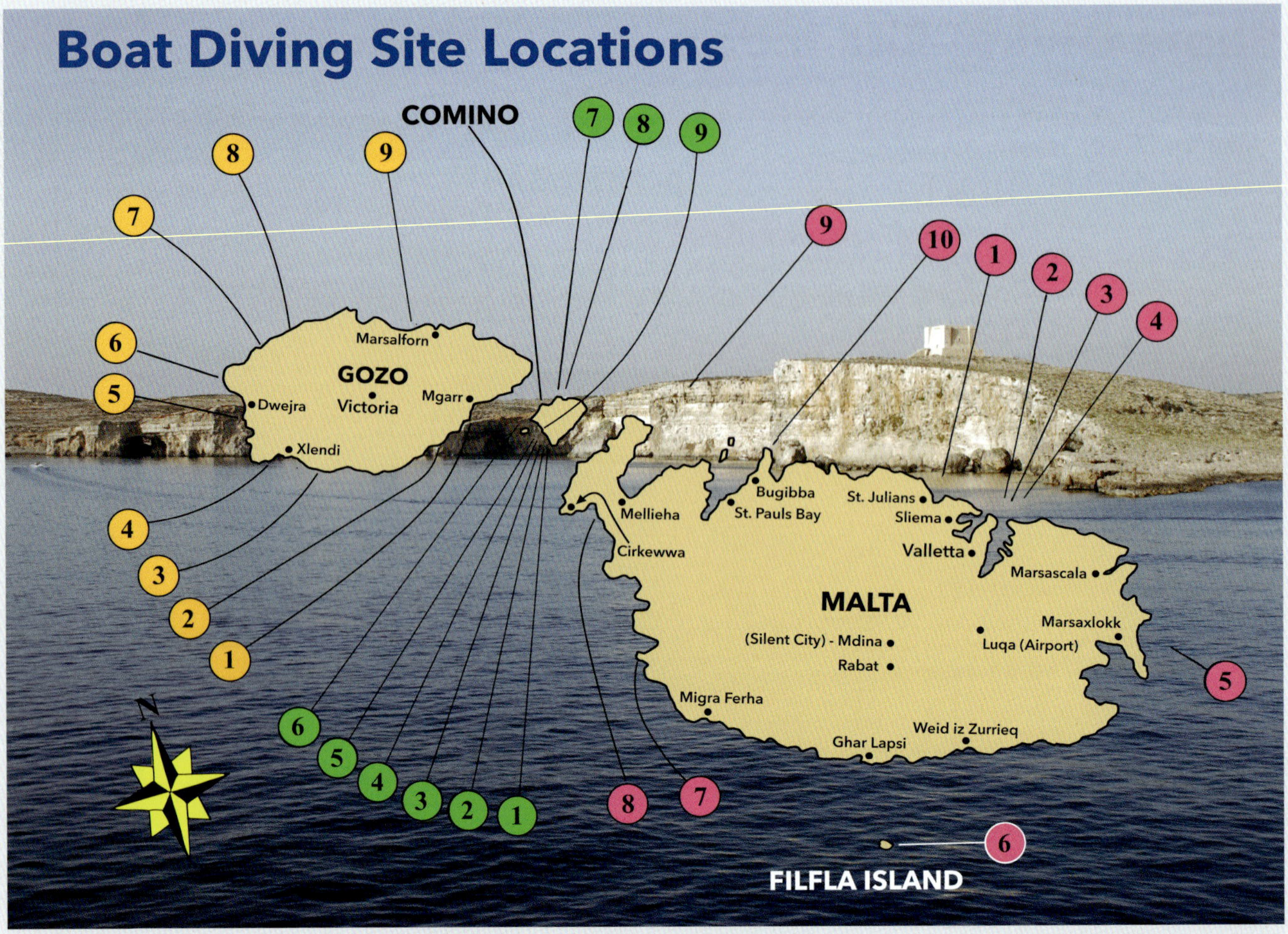

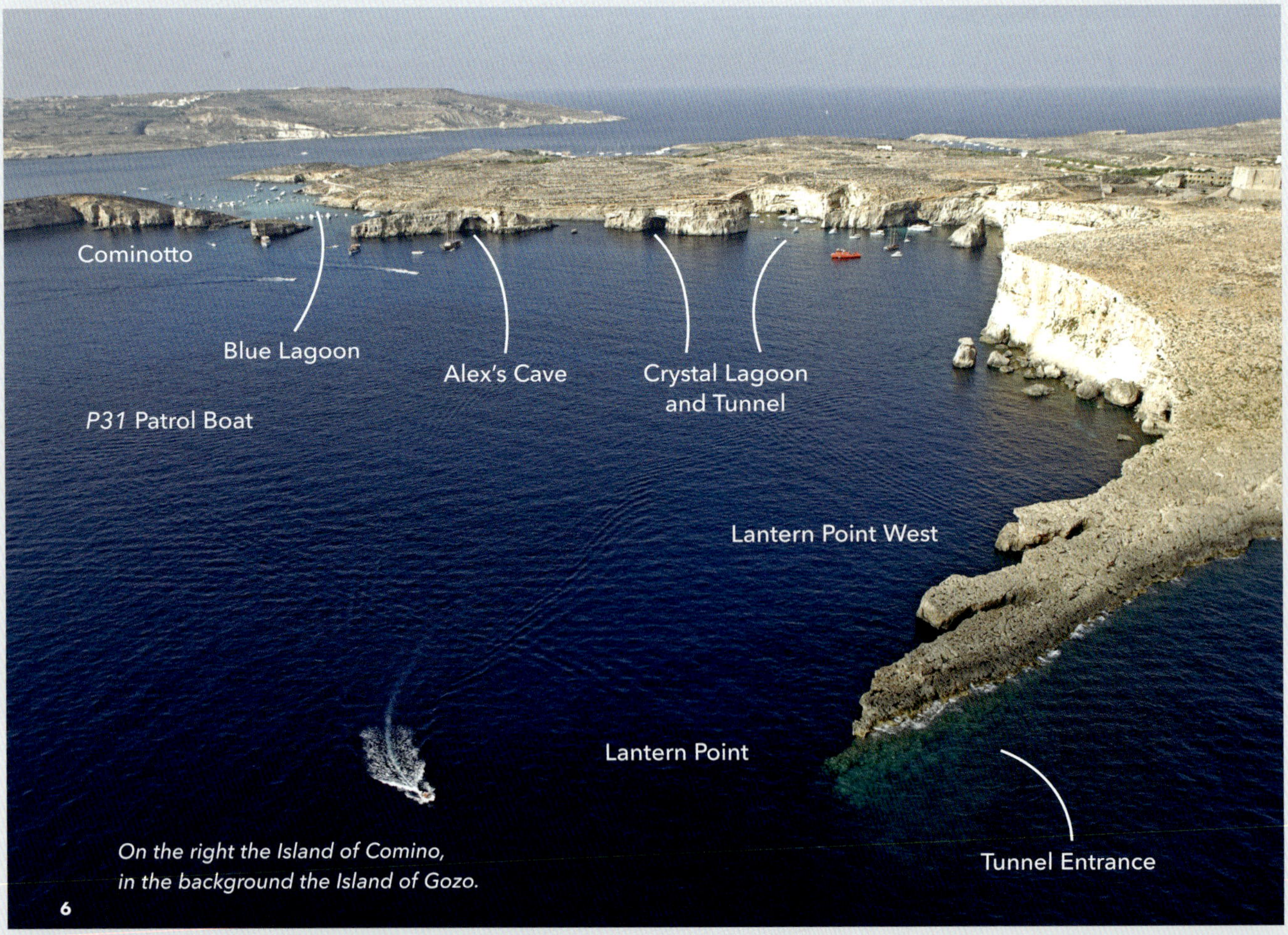

COMINO

GOZO
- Marsalforn
- Dwejra
- Victoria
- Mgarr
- Xlendi

MALTA
- Mellieha
- Cirkewwa
- Bugibba
- St. Pauls Bay
- St. Julians
- Sliema
- Valletta
- (Silent City) - Mdina
- Rabat
- Marsascala
- Marsaxlokk
- Luqa (Airport)
- Migra Ferha
- Ghar Lapsi
- Weid iz Zurrieq

FILFLA ISLAND

- Cominotto
- Blue Lagoon
- P31 Patrol Boat
- Alex's Cave
- Crystal Lagoon and Tunnel
- Lantern Point West
- Lantern Point
- Tunnel Entrance

On the right the Island of Comino, in the background the Island of Gozo.

Boat Diving Site Index

Malta Dive Sites

#	Site	Page	Description
1	The Bristol Beaufighter	164	The upturned wreckage of this WW2 plane is almost intact on a sandy seabed at a depth of 38m
2	HMS *Hellespont*	165	Stunning wreck which is remakably intact 45m
3	HM *Drifter Eddy*	165	Carried out duties in WW1 & WW2 56m
4	HMS *St Angelo*	166	Sunk in 1942 now upright on the seabed at 55m
5	Bristol Blenheim	166	A highly rated dive of this WW2 aircraft upright on a sandy rocky seabed at 42m, largely intact, an excellent dive
6	Filfla Island	168	This island, now a protected nature reserve, has to be booked in advanced by your dive centre
7	Ras ir-Raheb	168	The wreck of a mystery yacht upright on the sand, next to the cliff face reef at 32m, excellent reef with cave
8	*Scotscraig*	169	Started life as passenger ferry in UK 21m
9	HMS *Stubborn*	170	Fanastic dive, intact, almost upright on the seabed at 57m scuttled in 1946 as an Asdic target, two miles off Qawra
10	MV *Imperial Eagle*	172	Scuttled in 1999 as a diver attraction sitting upright on the sand close to a reef, near by is the statue of Christ

Gozo Dive Sites

#	Site	Page	Description
1	MV *Hephaestus*	174	This wreck washed ashore at Qawra Point Malta in 2018 Scuttled off Xatt L-Ahmar in 2022, she is the largest of four wrecks in this area, upright on the sandy seabed at 45m
2	Fesse Rock	176	An abundance of marine life can be found here 45m +
3	Dawra Tas-Sanap and Cave	176	This is a great dive with much to explore 45m
4	Zurzieb Cavern and reef	177	The rock formation here is quite spectacular 45m
5	Fungus Rock	177	Originally named 'The Generals Rock' - good dive 45m
6	San Dimitri Point	178	Gozo's most westerly point, great visablity, look out into the blue for barracuda, dentex and tuna, great dive 50m +
7	Ta'Camma - Gudja Cave	179	There are 5 caverns / caves in this dramatic reef 30m +
8	Wied Il-Meilah - Valley of Salt	180	Dive below the arch, take your camera and enjoy, 30m
9	Calypso Tunnel/Cave	181	A very impressive and interesting dive 35m, after the tunnel look back and see the face

Comino Dive Sites

#	Site	Page	Description
1	Lantern Point	182	Good reef & chimney tunnel - an excellent dive 3m - 45m +
2	Lantern Point West	183	Sometimes referred to as inner Lantern Point 30m
3	Crystal Lagoon	184	The lagoon is a nursey for young fish 3m - 14m
4	Patrol boat P31	185	Scuttled in 2009 as a diver attraction 22m
5	Alex's Cave	188	Popular second dive - suitable for all levels of diver 12m
6	Comino's Blue Lagoon	191	Possibly your mooring place during your surface interval 6m
7	Cominotto Reef (Anchor reef)	189	Normal depth for this dive 25m - WW2 anchor at 35m
8	Santa Marija Reef	189	Gullies, caverns, swim-throughs and caves 10m - 22m
9	Santa Marija Caves	189	Almost the perfect dive? 9m - 16m

Shore diving plays an important part of the attraction of diving Malta & Gozo. The entry points do vary, some are reasonably easy, others are more difficult, these can sometimes be reached by boat, it is really down to personal choice. Gozo dive centres will sometimes boat dive some of the dives I have listed on Malta as shore dives, likewise, Malta dive centres will sometimes boat dive some of the Gozo dive sites listed as shore dives.

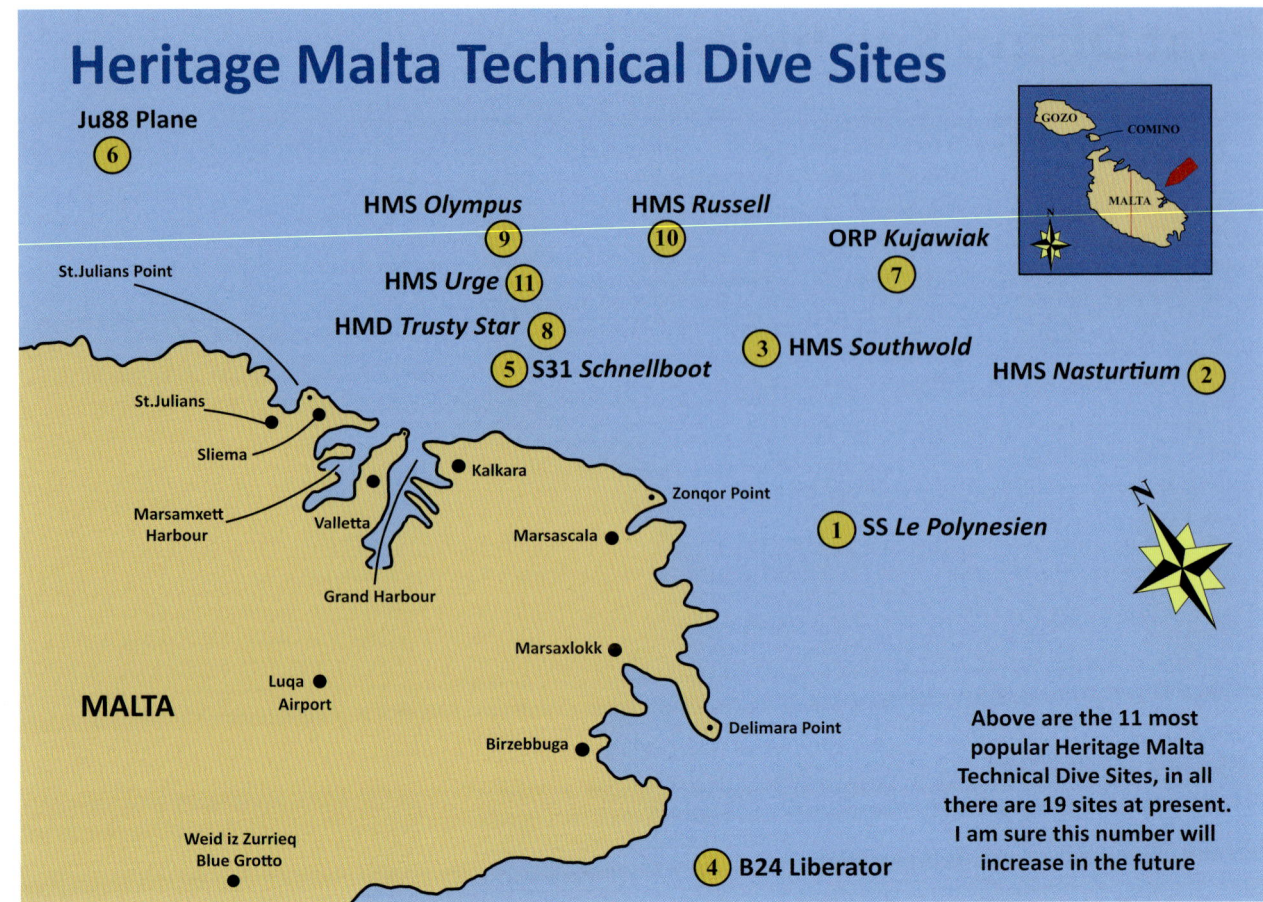

Heritage Malta Gozo Technical Diving Sites Index   • War Graves

		Page		
1	SS *Le Polynesien*	192	•	French luxury cruise liner 6659 tons - 1914 troop carrier - depth 65m
2	HMS *Nasturtium*	194		Built 1915 - Arabis Flower class ship - 1250 tons - depth 67m
3	HMS *Southwold* L10 Bow	196	•	Built 1941 - Hunts Class Destroyer - 1050 tons bow section - depth 67m
3	HMS *Southwold* L10 Stern	198	•	The stern section lies 300 metres away from the bow - depth 74m
4	B24 Liberator	189	•	American heavy bomber crash landed in the sea May 1943 - depth 58m
5	Ju88 aircraft	201		German twin engine multirole combat aircraft - depth 55m
6	S31 Schnellboot	202	•	German fast motor torpedo boat - 100 tons - depth 70m
7	ORP *Kujawiak* L72	204	•	Hunts-type ll Class Destroyer - transferred to the Polish Navy - depth 97m
8	HMD *Trusty Star*	206		Built 1919 - Royal Naval drifter, minesweeper 1939 - depth 90m
9	HMS *Olympus*	207	•	Odin-class submarine -launched 1928 - intresting history - depth 115m
10	HMS *Russell*	208	•	Built 1902 - A Ducan-class Dreadnaught battleship - 1500 tons - depth 115m
11	HMS *Urge*	209	•	U-class training submarine 630 tons - made fully operational -depth 130m
12	Fairey Swordfish Biplane			Swordfish torpedo bomber - nicknamed "stringbag" - depth 65m
13	Ju88 aircraft south			Found in 2019 this Junker considered to be good condition - depth 106m
14	Supermarine Spitfire Mk		•	From the 308th Fighter Squadron - took part in Operation Husky - depth 70m
15	SS *Luciston*			Known as the *Luciston Collier* - length 98 metres - 2948 tons - depth 95m
16	Maryland Bomber Mk1			Martin Maryland light bomber 167 - reconnaissance aircraft - depth 70m
17	Douglas A-1 Skyraider			American single-seat attack aircraft - depth 96m
18	Xlendi Underwater Archaeological Park			Both 18 and 19 are parts of the Xlendi Underwater Archaeological Park
19	Phoenician Ship Wreck			3rd and 7th century amphora - sandy, small rocky sea bed - depths 60-105m

For further information on all sites visit: www.underwatermalta.org

Heritage Malta

In accordance with Malta's Cultural Heritage Act, declared protected sites are Archaeological Zones at Sea, access is managed by the Underwater Cultural Heritage Unit (UCHU) within Heritage Malta.

The Maltese Islands are in the centre of the Central Mediterranean, a location that has created an inextricable link between the history of Malta and maritime activity of the Mediterranean. Millennia of history is reflected on the archaeologically rich seabed surrounding Malta and Gozo. A long-term project surveying the seabed of the Maltese Islands has been ongoing for several years. The aim is to map the entirety of Malta's territorial seabed, and during this project, important cultural remains have been discovered, mapped and studied. Wreck sites vary from a 2700-year-old Phoenician shipwreck, the oldest in the central Mediterranean, to shipwrecks from the two world wars, including many aircraft crash sites, some of which date to the Cold War.

The need for controlled monitoring of these sites and appropriate heritage legislation was already identified in the early 1960s, since terrestrial heritage sites have had legal protection since the late 19th century. The recognition of responsibility towards properly managing and protecting Malta's underwater cultural heritage, resulted in the decision to create a platform for the protection, valorisation, management, and public outreach of Malta's diverse underwater cultural resources. This platform took shape in the form of UCHU, set up within Heritage Malta.

The public access system implemented by the UCHU is based on the principle of ticketed access to underwater sites. This follows the same principles as purchasing tickets to terrestrial sites. Prior to this, divers visiting underwater sites were not regulated, resulting in a situation whereby cultural material could easily be looted, sites damaged, and delicate marine flora disturbed. A system of registration for local dive centers, clubs, and dive vessels, was also introduced.

This registration requires the acceptance of terms and conditions that govern access, and it is only through those registered dive centers, clubs and vessels that divers can visit Malta's managed underwater sites.

On an annual basis, between one and three historic sites are opened to the diving public, and the creation of new accessible sites is giving added value to Malta's deep-water technical diving repertoire.

Instructions for boat skippers
Do not anchor on shipwrecks.
Use moorings wherever possible.
Locate the wreck using a depth sounder.

Instructions for dive leaders
Respect measures that protect sites.
Do not tie marker buoys or access lines directly to a wreck.
Keep divers in small groups.
Observe the group at all times during the dive.
Be a role model and stay safe.
Strictly respect the rules of no contact with wreck.
No penetration inside the wreck.

Instruction for divers
Obey legal rules that protect archaeological sites.
Do not touch or penetrate the wreck.
Keep your dive kit trimmed, beware of snags on the wreck.
Good buoyancy and be aware of marine life and wreckage.
Avoid contact with the wreck and stay safe.

Heritage Malta monitors these historic wrecks by:
Spot checks at departure points of dive boats.
Spot checks at sea by UCHU personnel.
Spot checks at sea by AFM, TM, and Fisheries personnel.
Use of drones for offshore patrols.
Installation of CCTV in key areas.

For further information contact:
uchu@heritagemalta.org   www.underwatermalta.org

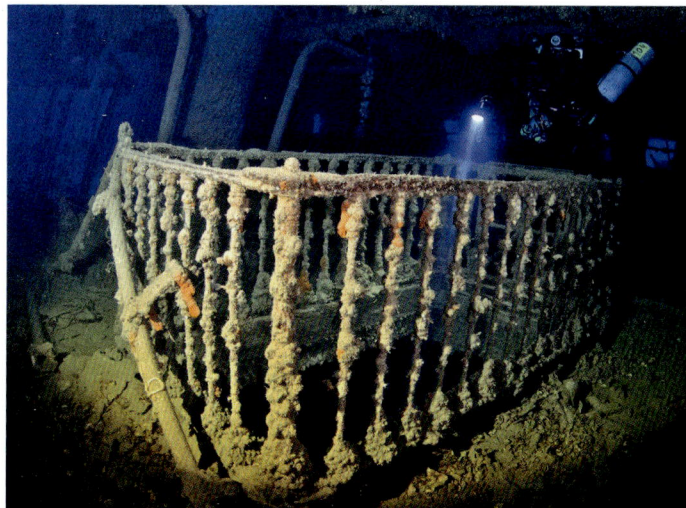
One of the staircases on this luxury liner SS Le Polynesien
PHOTOS: STEVEN GALICIA www.galicia.be

The sea has turned this warship into a coral garden.

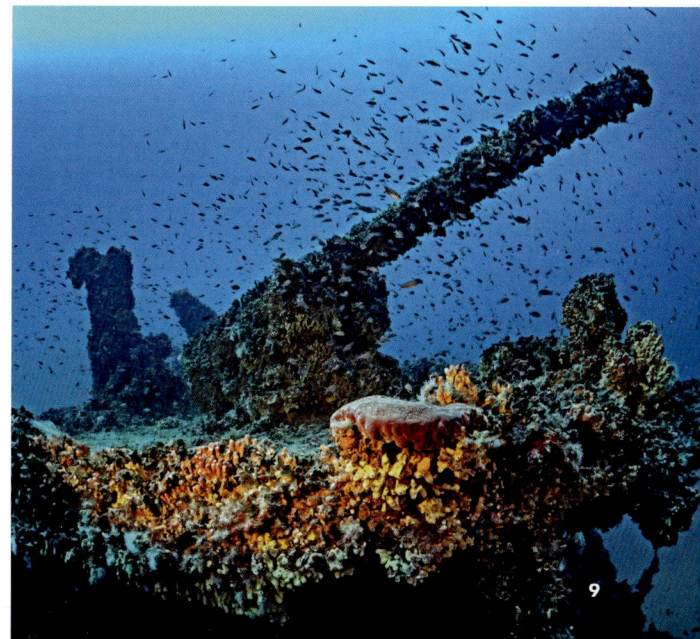

Foreword

It is not usual for the wife of the author to write the Foreword of a book, but this is not a 'usual' book. Peter is still as enthusiastic about the Maltese Islands and diving there, as he was when he first visited them forty years ago. I think in the following pages the reader will find all the information one would need to safely enjoy the beautiful underwater world of the Maltese Islands.

In the early days Peter used to complete his log book, not only with what he had seen on the dive, but with a small sketch of the underwater terrain, a cave, fish and wrecks. His dive buddy, Chris, suggested he should maybe make this into a book... Hence in 2002 A Guide to Shore Diving the Maltese Islands was created followed by Scuba diving Malta Gozo Comino and the rest is history. Many hours of hand drawing each dive site featured, depth, routes, and aerial photographs above each drawing, a description of what may be seen on each individual dive featured within the following pages. Also included are many lovely underwater photographs, taken by Peter and also many of which have been donated too.

After a career of 37 years in the Fire Service, scuba diving became more or less another career, Peter's enthusiasm has rubbed off on many divers and he has encouraged the most nervous of us to complete diving training and join him in many explorations underwater. We used the lump sum Peter received on retirement from the Fire Service to publish the first book, no sooner was it in print we saw that it needed improvement! This, I believe has been achieved over the years with the subsequent editions. We feel that this, the fifth and final edition, is the best one. It has taken much longer to produce than expected, but life gets in the way sometimes!

Over the years of visiting the Maltese Islands we have both enjoyed the hospitality of the residents of the islands and receive a warm welcome whenever we return. We have many fond memories from our visits, I think at the top of Peter's list would be that he managed to dive with our son and at various times, three of our grandchildren, all of whom enjoyed the experience.

I hope that you enjoy what you find within the following pages, it has been put together with love, care and attention to detail by Peter, with a little help from yours truly, also many others, too many to mention by name, but they know who they are!

Thank you, Sue Lemon

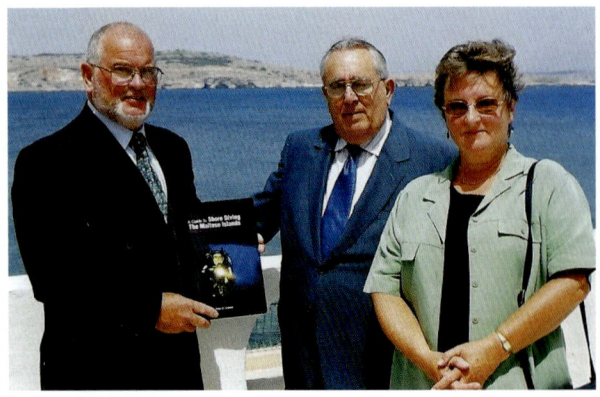

The launch of our first book in 2002 Peter and Sue pictured with Dr Michael Refalo, KOM, BA(Hons, LLD, FRSA Minister of Tourism 1987-1994 1998-2003.

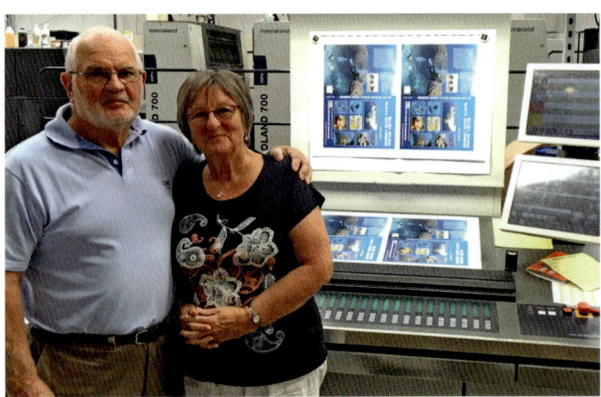

Peter and Sue at the premises of Deltor, in Saltash, Cornwall, for the printing of our fourth edition.

A note from the Author

It was in 1983 when I first visited the Maltese Islands and enjoyed my first dive in the warm clear waters around these islands at the pretty little inlet known as the Blue Grotto, at Wied iz-Zurrieq. Just before Christmas in 2001 we, my wife Sue and I, released our first diving guide for the Maltese Islands, now in 2024 after over 110 visits we have completed the fifth and final edition. None of these editions would have been possible without the help of many individuals, with a special mention of Bent and Chris my main dive buddies and Bent's wife Marthese. The Dive Centres and their staff, both Maltese and visiting photographers generously donating their photos for use in these guides, the Armed Forces of Malta. So, I would like to say a huge thank you to all that made it possible to complete these scuba diving guides.

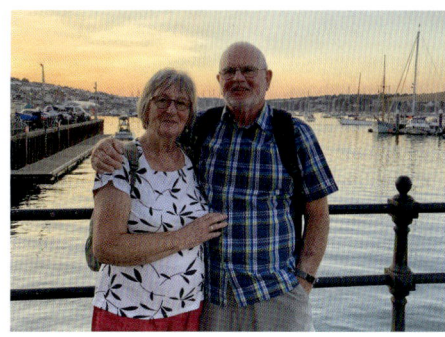

It has not been a good couple of years health wise for myself, which has ended my diving career after 40 years. My problems started just after Covid lock down with arthritis in my right knee and hip, this was followed by a heart attack and having a stent fitted, almost at the same time I was diagnosed with prostate cancer which was treated with radiotherapy. In January 2024 another illness started which I was diagnosed in March with Mesothelioma, there is treatment but no cure. With all this going on it has made it much harder to complete this final edition.

Peter and Sue enjoying the sea.

From the first time I set foot on these islands, it changed my life for ever, the warm clear blue waters that surround these islands, the friendly people and the way of life, I just loved it, and returned again and again. And to the many good people we meet during our visits, thank you for your friendship and hospitality. Then came the book, from firefighter to author, not an easy task to start with, but I think we have improved the book with each edition, this has been a labour of love which I have enjoyed so very much, and for anyone who thinks it's not a labour of love, may I suggest you try it!

I would like to dedicate this, my fifth book, to my wife Sue.

Peter G. Lemon

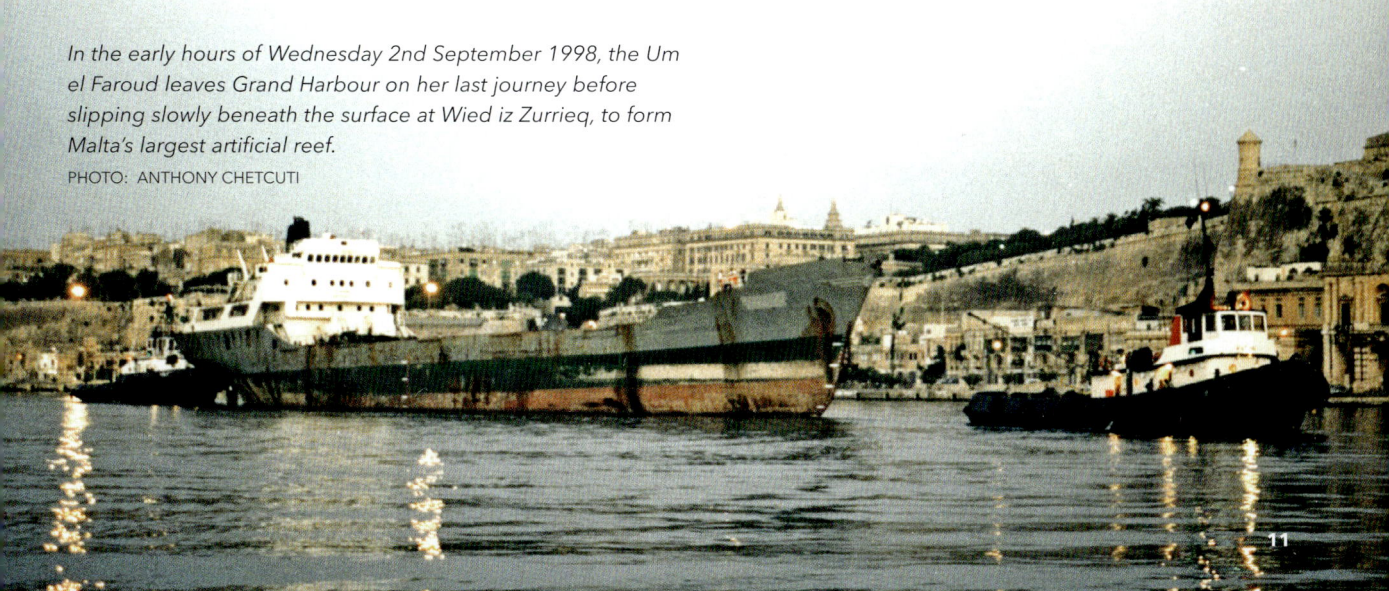

In the early hours of Wednesday 2nd September 1998, the Um el Faroud leaves Grand Harbour on her last journey before slipping slowly beneath the surface at Wied iz Zurrieq, to form Malta's largest artificial reef.
PHOTO: ANTHONY CHETCUTI

Introduction

This guide has been written by a diver for divers, who wish to explore the underwater world of the Maltese Islands. Your dive centre will offer dive guiding and transport to the dive site, this I would recommend, at least for your first visit and use this book for information, or as a souvenir of the places visited. If you do hire a car, you could find navigating your way to some of the dive sites difficult, even with a road map, so confirm your route with the dive centre before you leave.

Each dive location begins with a short text giving you basic information on how to arrive at your chosen destination; there is a local map of the area. These road maps have been surveyed and drawn by myself, they are not to scale, but you will find details of times and distances within the text. They show details of parking, entry/exit points and amenities, **it should be noted that at some dive sites, mobile phones do not work.**

There is also a brief description given on the area of the dive site, for the experienced diver with the correct qualifications you can follow my dive plan, with a suggested minimum dive time. It is important before making your dive plan, that you read and understand the text.

There is an aerial photograph for each shore dive site and underneath an underwater dive plan, both will show your entry/exit points which will enable you to relate one to the other. I feel sure all experienced divers would check the immediate coastline for entry/exit points to be used other than those identified.

These underwater dive plans, are to compass bearings and not to scale, they have also been surveyed and drawn by myself; you will find details of times taken to cover distances within the text of each dive location. They are based on my average speed under the water which is, whilst exploring and moving slowly, is 10/12 metres per minute.

Although every effort has been made to obtain the correct depths, you may find that they may vary by one or two metres. This is due to the undulating seabed and of course you could be slightly off the position of the depth marked on the plan.

There are four more sections in this book for boat diving, Malta, Gozo, Comino and Technical Diving. My selection on each, of possibly the most popular, are just a few of the sites available, there are also two location maps.

If you have not chosen or pre-booked your dive centre and wish to find the nearest one to your accommodation, refer to the dive centre location map. For further information and details enquire at your chosen dive centre, an index can be found at the back of this book.

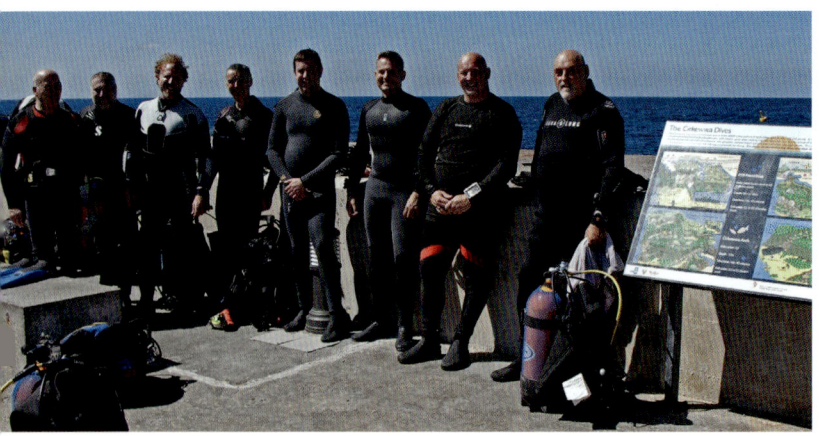
Members of Mid Herts Divers at Cirkewwa's Marine Park enjoying their trip to the Maltese Islands.

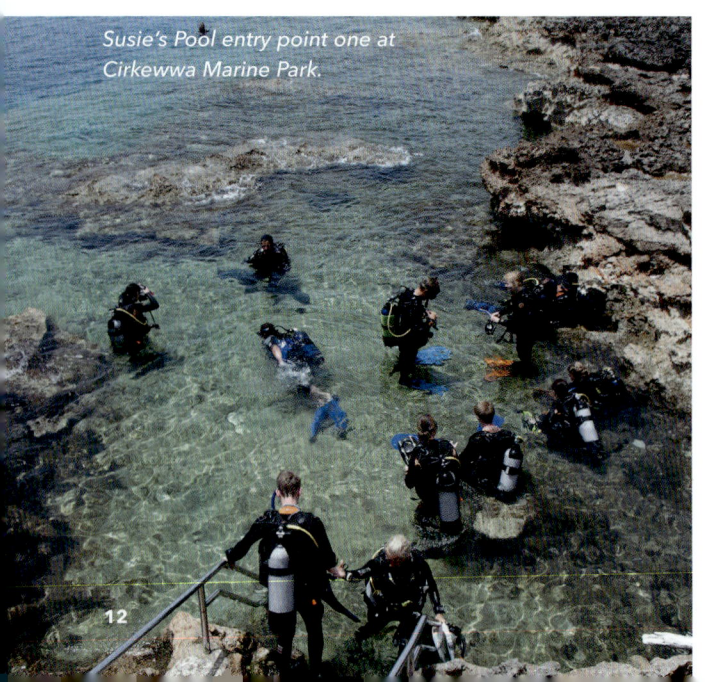
Susie's Pool entry point one at Cirkewwa Marine Park.

EMERGENCY TELEPHONE NUMBERS
Police - Fire - Ambulance   112
Nature Trust - Marine Rescue   99999505

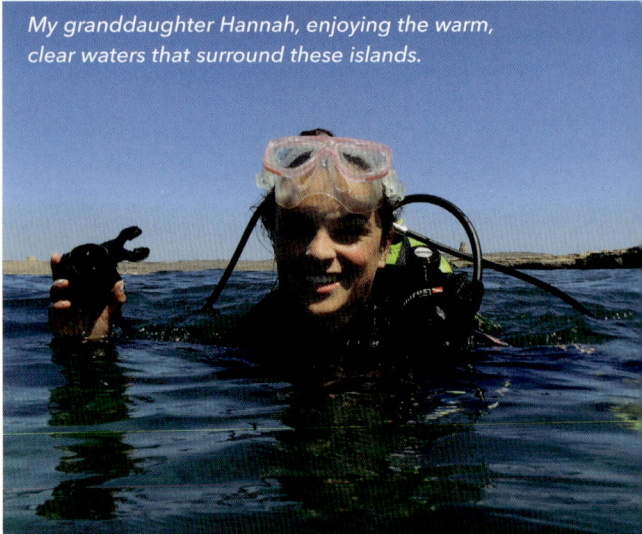
My granddaughter Hannah, enjoying the warm, clear waters that surround these islands.

Travel Information

To the Maltese Islands Luqa is Malta's International Airport; it is very modern with all amenities. A number of major international airlines operate scheduled services from most major European cities, some of these services are not available in the winter months. Flying time is approximately 3 hours, Malta time is 1 hour ahead of GMT. Air Malta, now KM Malta Airlines will recognise the needs of scuba divers and their equipment; extra weight allowance should be available at reasonable charges.

Passport and Visa regulations all visitors to the Maltese Islands require a full passport; it must have at least 3 months to run before expiry. Visitors from the UK, Australia, Canada and America do not require a visa, others should check with the immigration authorities.

Ferry Service - Malta Gozo there is a 24-hour passenger car ferry service between Cirkewwa, Malta and Mgarr Gozo, the sea journey takes approximately 30 minutes. During public holidays and summer weekends extra trips are run, often on a shuttle basis. Very reasonable fares for both passengers and cars.

Public Transport - Buses - Taxis Malta and Gozo's public transport systems offer a very reasonable and efficient way of getting around the Islands. The main bus terminus in Malta is Valletta and Victoria, in Gozo from where the buses operate to all parts of the islands. A Hop On, Hop Off, bus service operates on both Malta and Gozo enabling visitors to see and experience the delights of the Maltese islands.

Taxis are available in most towns and villages as well as the airport, it is possible to hire these for sightseeing trips. I recommend you discuss and agree a price before your journey.

Car Hire and Traffic Laws car hire can be booked with some dive centres, at the Airport and private companies, minimum age of 25, if the driver is over 70 a medical from a doctor is required. Remember to take your driving license and passport when hiring a car; they drive on the left and the laws are similar to those in the UK. **Apart from if you are unfortunate enough to be involved in an accident, vehicles must not be moved until the Police or Traffic Warden arrive even if there are no injuries. Do not park within 5 metres of a corner and do not cross a single white line even to park on the opposite side of the road, these actions could result in receiving a fine.**

If requested to produce your license by either the Police or a Traffic Warden, you have 48 hours to present it at the nearest Police Station.

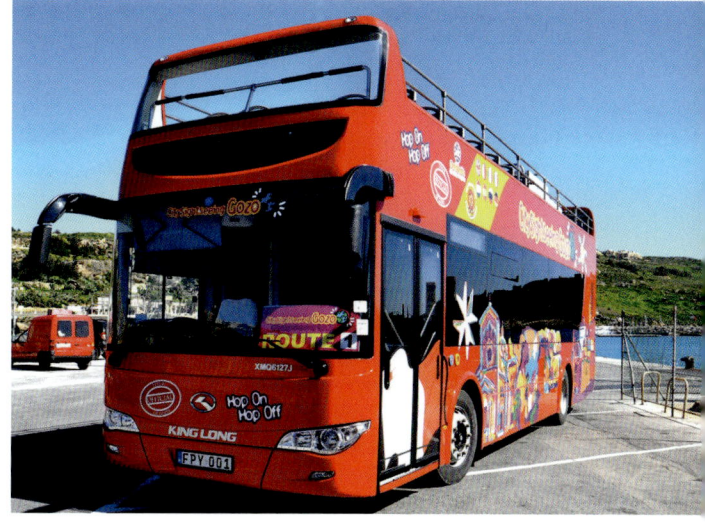

The red Hop On, Hop Off bus meeting passengers at Mgarr Quay side for sightseeing trips around Gozo.

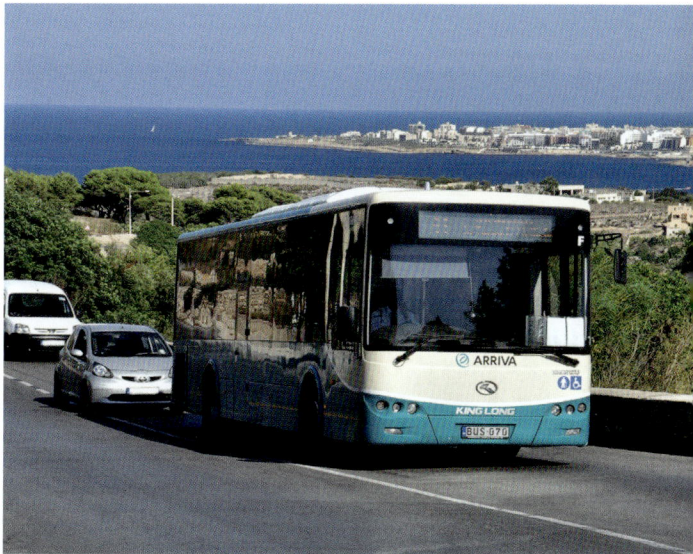

The local bus service is good and reasonable.

Below: Enjoy this journey between the two islands, this trip passes the smaller islands of Comino and Cominotto.

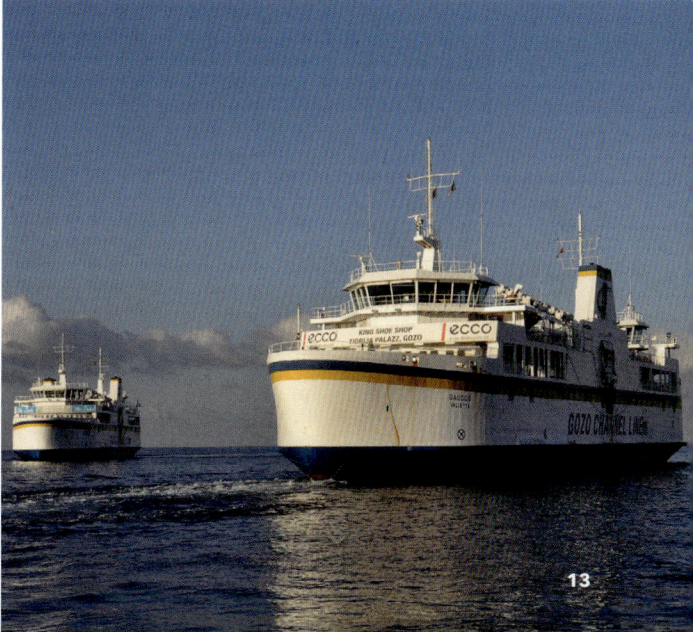

The Maltese Islands

You or your group will not be the first to visit these Mediterranean Islands, it all started some 6000 years ago. Throughout history, they have been at the heart of many world events, they have been a safe haven, a battleground, and visited by many famous figures through various episodes of European history.

The Maltese archipelago consists of three inhabited islands in the middle of the Mediterranean Sea. They lie approximately 93 km south of Sicily and 200 km north of the port of Tripoli in Libya, North Africa. Malta, is the largest of the three with a total land area of 246 square km. Gozo is smaller with a land area of 67 square km. Comino, which lies between the two and has a land area of 2.7 square km. There are also a number of small un-inhabited islands, such as Filfla; Cominetto and the most well chronicled St. Paul's Islands where the Apostle Paul was shipwrecked in AD 60.

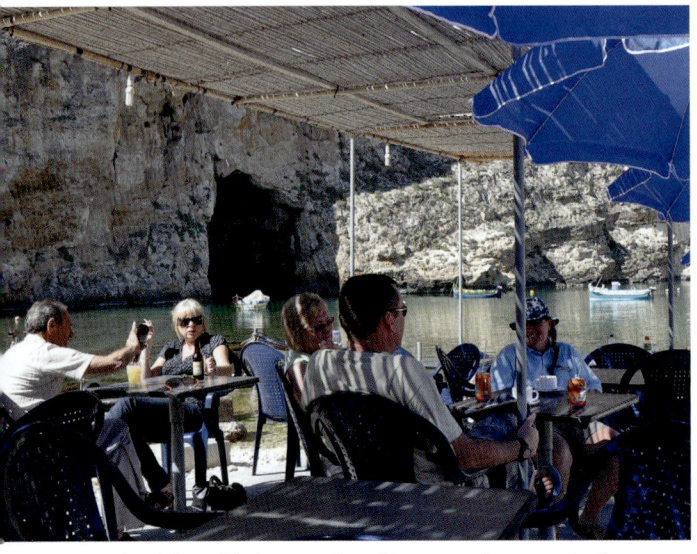

Inland Sea, this is one of my favourite places to sit after a dive and enjoy refreshments at this local run café.

Below: Dockyard Creek, and Malta's Naval Museum.

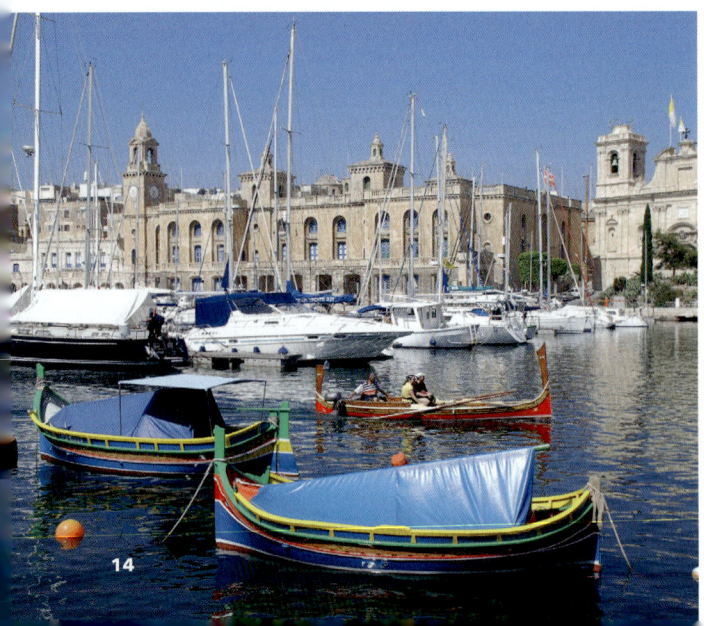

The People of Malta and Gozo have a rare sense of hospitality and friendliness to visitors to their Islands. They enjoy life and find great strength and unity in their common language, religion and strong family ties. Many Maltese like to travel so they take an interest in what is happening to the rest of the world, and with their flair for languages, makes communication with their visitors so easy, it is often said that many lasting friendships are made and many of the visitors return again and again.

They are proud of their independence, having one of the highest electoral turnouts in the world. Their patriotism was at its most evident during World War II, when they stood up so bravely against the enemy in that in 1942 King George V1 awarded the Maltese Islands the highest award for civil bravery, The George Cross.

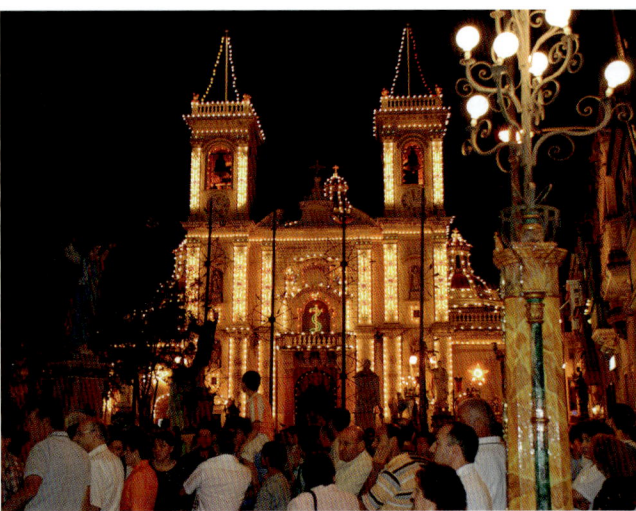

The church of St Philip in the village of Zebbug is lit up by hundreds of multi coloured bulbs for the festa.

The Islanders love festivals and between May and October nearly every town and village in Malta and Gozo celebrates their feast day or 'festa' of its patron saint. The festa is an important event for each village's annual calendar and they eagerly look forward to this special day. The village church will be decorated with beautiful flowers, all its gold and silver treasures are put on display thus creating a fitting setting for the statue of the patron saint. The outside of the church will be illuminated with hundreds of multicoloured bulbs, over the streets, suspended drapes and on buildings huge flags of the village colours, are flown from the rooftops.

On the festa day, as the statues are carried along the streets of their village, church bells ring and bands march in the procession.

The nougat and candy floss stands do excellent business whilst the crowds look on. The noise reaches a crescendo, as the statue is about to re-enter the church; at this point there is normally a fireworks display. During the summer season there is a festa practically every weekend and no holidaymaker should leave the Islands without visiting one.

Language the local language is Maltese, but, English and Italian are widely spoken by most of the population.

Medical Care, the Maltese people enjoy a high standard of medical care. There is a large General Hospital; Mater Dei in Malta, The Craig Hospital, Victoria in Gozo, both have hyperbaric units, there are also government health clinics in various towns and villages. British nationals holidaying on the islands are entitled to one month's free medical and hospital care in Malta and Gozo. **You should carry the UK Global Health Insurance (GHIC or EHIC) Card.** Persons who are receiving medical treatment and who may need to carry medicine into the Maltese Islands or purchase fresh supplies locally would be well advised to carry a letter of introduction from their family doctor.

Sport being an island swimming and the sea plays a large part in the Maltese social life especially in the summer months by just cooling off in the sea.

Football is a favourite sport, and their National Stadium is at Ta'Qali Malta. There is strong support for world and European football especially the English and Italian Premier Leagues and there are a number of supporter clubs.

Shops most open early and close late in the evening, during the summer period they will have a siesta break at mid-day early afternoon. Half the joy of planning a day out in Malta or Gozo is that it is easy to combine both sightseeing and shopping; there are many bargains to be had. You may be able to pick up a painting by one of the many local artists or find an unusual piece of jewellery, made from gold or silver and very reasonably priced. Maltese lace can be bought in the form of shawls, soft furnishings or trimmings. Hand knitted woollens and Arran styles can be purchased and are of exceptional value and anyone who is fond of glass or pottery is spoiled for choice. If you want to get all your shopping out of the way in one go, visit the Crafts Village at Ta'Qali in Malta or the Craft Village near San Lawrenz in Gozo. At both these villages you can watch potters, glassblowers, and filigree craftsmen at work.

Religion The Maltese people are predominantly Roman Catholic, but the Constitution guarantees freedom of worship. I have been informed, but not checked, that there are 365 churches on the Maltese Islands one for every day of the year.

Currency can be exchanged in banks and some shops. Major credit cards, travellers' cheques are accepted at most leading shops and restaurants.

Electricity supply is 240 volts, single phase, 50 cycles. The square fitting standard three-pin British plugs and sockets are used.

The weather climate is warm and healthy. There are no biting winds, fog, snow or frost, normally. Rain falls for only short periods which can be heavy at times, mostly during the late autumn and mid-winter, During the summer the average temperature can be 32°C occasionally higher, with the sun shining for an average of 10/11 hours each day. The hottest period being from mid-July to mid-September, when the temperature will not normally rise above 37°C, even in the height of the summer.

A Maltese annual average weather chart.

Month	Daily Sunshine hours	Monthly Rainfall mm	Air Temp. °C	Sea Temp. °C
January	7	95	13	17
February	8	63	13	16
March	9	37	14	16
April	11	26	16	17
May	12	9	20	19
June	13	5	23	22
July	14	0	27	26
August	13	6	27	27
September	10	67	25	26
October	9	77	21	24
November	8	109	17	22
December	7	108	14	19

Tap Water is safe to drink, but I would recommend that you use bottled water for drinking, which is reasonably priced and can be purchased almost anywhere.

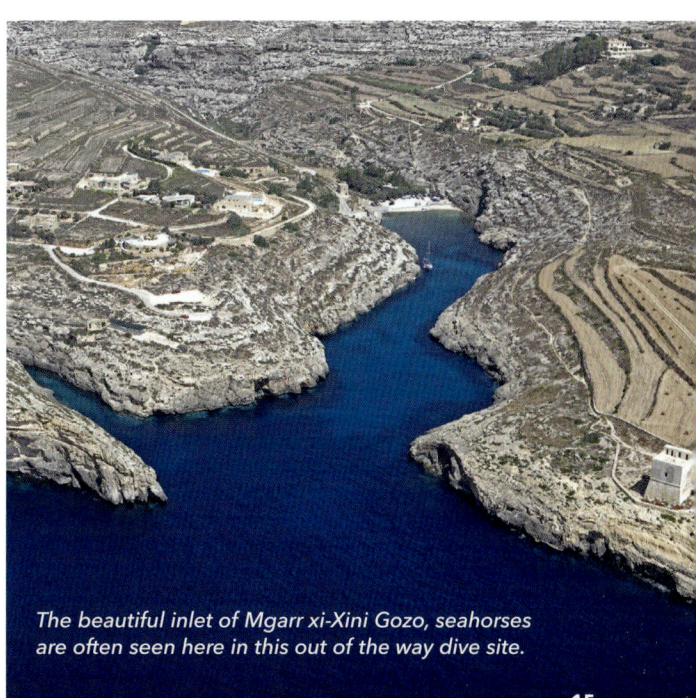

The beautiful inlet of Mgarr xi-Xini Gozo, seahorses are often seen here in this out of the way dive site.

Islands for Divers

The Maltese Archipelago is made up of three inhabited Islands Malta, Gozo, Comino and the smaller islands of Filfla, Cominotto and St. Pauls. There are also a number of islets and rocks which rise out of these clear blue waters.

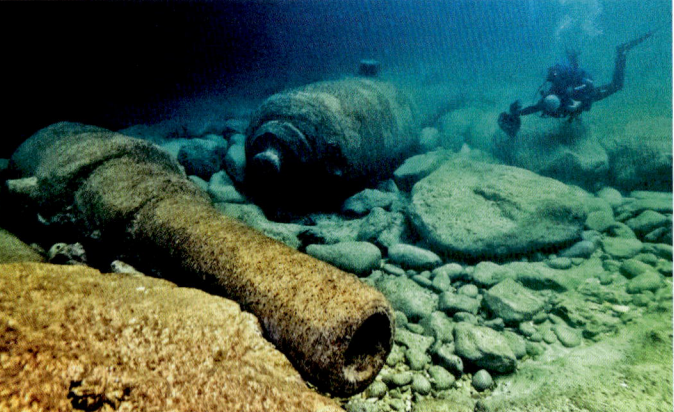

The history of these islands below the surface.
ARKADIUSZ SREBNIK POLANDDIVINGPHOTO

In the summer the sea temperatures can rise to 26°C, even remaining high as 22°C during November then gradually reducing in February and March to 16°C The climate and duration of sunshine at this time of year is similar to an average North European summer. This makes the Maltese Islands an all the year-round destination for divers. During inclement weather, these Islands still have a sufficient number of sheltered interesting dive sites.

Surrounded by blue seas, with rugged and beautiful coastlines, makes these islands a real paradise for divers and snorklers.

My grandson Ben's first dive in these warm waters.

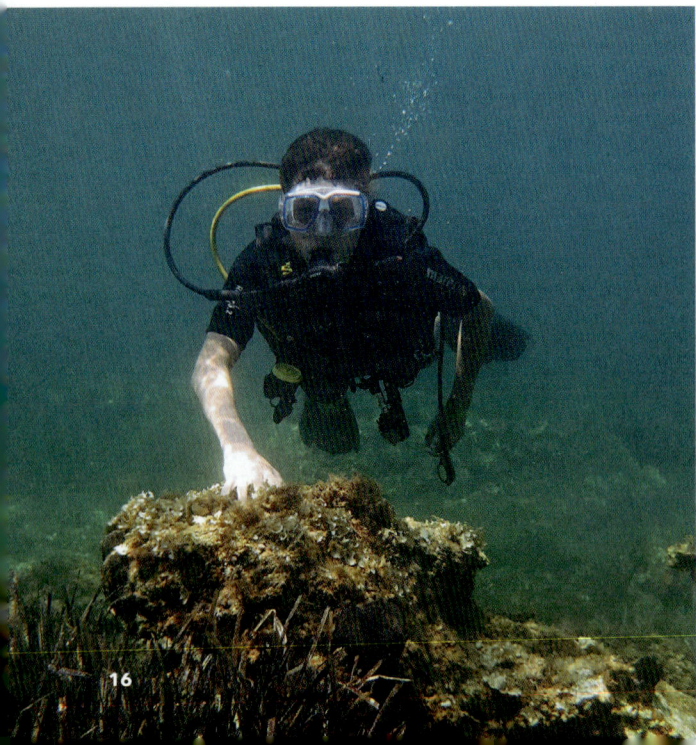

Government Regulation for Divers the object of these is to ensure that all divers, diving in Maltese waters enjoy their experience with safety in mind, following the three headings below.

1. Safety Standards for Diving.
2. Protection of finds of cultural value.
3. Protection of the sea, its flora and fauna.

These regulations aim to maintain and improve the high level of care already administered by the dive centres. Licenses are issued by the Malta Tourism Authority who will define the standards for facilities, equipment and service. Only licensed dive centre will be allowed to provide diving services to the public. A number of conservation areas have been established along these coastlines which include areas where the wrecks are located, these areas are considered **"No stopping area"** apart from dive boats, they may anchor. It is unlawful to fish from boats or spear fish in these areas. Spear fishing is allowed if you have a license, without aqua lung and not in the conservation areas.

Boat traffic becomes increasingly busy in the summer season, it is mandatory for dive boats to fly the 'A' flag when divers are in the water.

Removal and non-reporting of any cultural finds is unlawful. It is a criminal act, which will lead to prosecution. Do not let temptation spoil your holiday, report any such findings to the officials directly or to your dive centre.

These guidelines are in the diver's main interest and are practically self-evident to any responsible diver and are in harmony with regulations of other international diving clubs and centres. All of which will help to protect the sea, its fauna and flora, for future generations of divers.

www.visitmalta.com   www.pdsa.org.mt

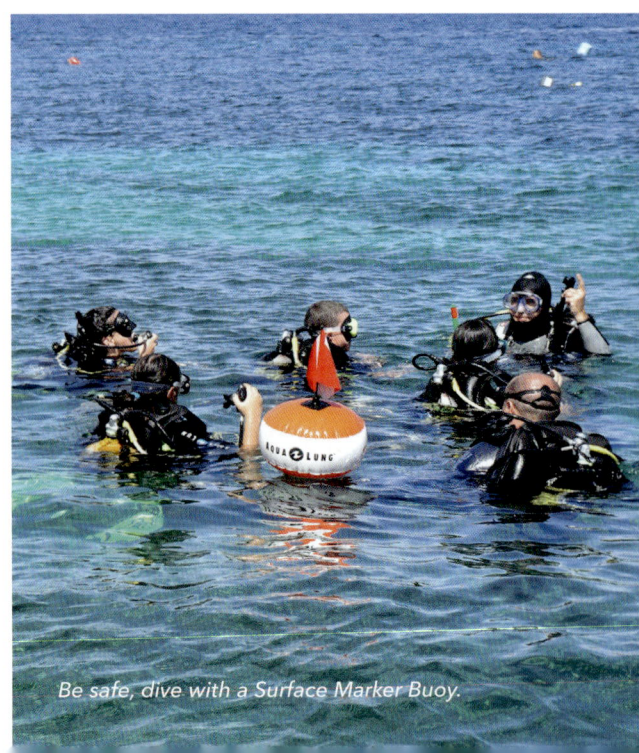

Be safe, dive with a Surface Marker Buoy.

The sea around the Maltese Islands is virtually tideless; however sometimes there are underwater currents even when the sea is calm. At times these underwater currents will travel in the opposite direction to the wind and the surface sea conditions.

The individual diving sites and the weather conditions influence the underwater visibility, but thanks to the mostly rocky coastline and the unpolluted waters the visibility is normally very good 25 metres plus, but this can be affected by the short periods of heavy rain during the winter months, then followed by sunshine.

The rather strong topographic structures of the Maltese Islands continue beneath the surface. In this most bizarre underwater landscape of the Mediterranean, you will find many caves, some large enough for a double decker bus to enter, arches, grotto's, crevices and undulating reefs with their magnificent and dramatic drop-offs, all these areas are home to many species of fish and an abundance of rich marine life.

All divers will be required to complete a self-certificated medical form, any queries arising from completing this form could require a doctor's medical, the dive centres have the right to request you to have a doctor's medical, the cost of this is minimal, this also applies to non-divers who wish to undertake diver training.

During recent years the Maltese Tourism Authority and the Professional Diving Schools Association has arranged for twelve boats/ships, to be made environmentally safe and then scuttled. These have become artificial reefs/diver attractions and now conger, moray eels, groupers and a multitude of other marine life live and hide within these wrecks. Add these to the number of existing wrecks and the variety of reefs and caves; it is no wonder these islands are a mecca for divers.

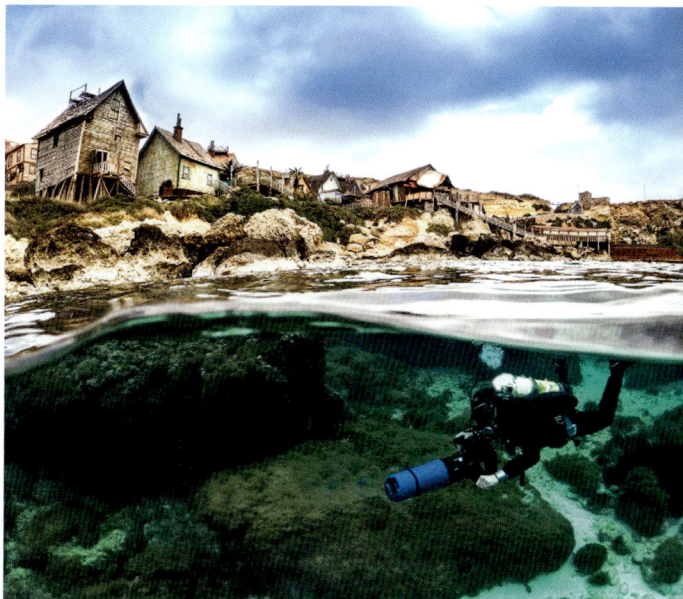

DPV's are available to hire from many dive centres.
ARKADIUSZ SREBNIK POLANDDIVINGPHOTO

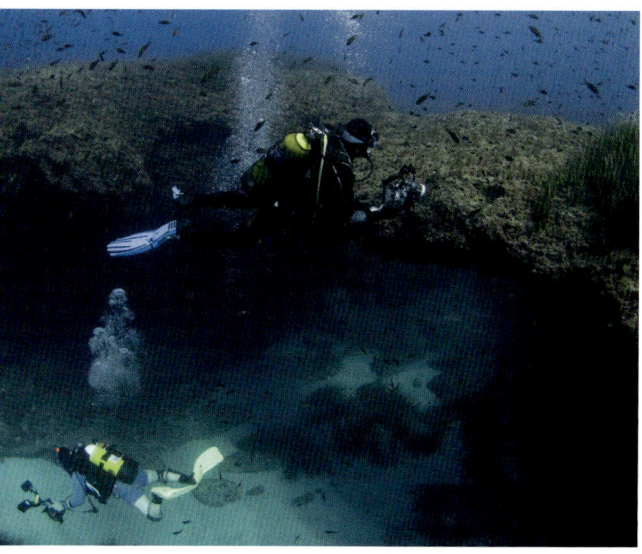

Cirkewwa Arch part of the underwater landscape.

Diving Centres / Schools offer many options for the visiting diver, The Professional Diving Schools Association has been formed to promote diving within the regulations, making diver safety their prime concern. These dive centres offer dive guiding, courses leading to international dive qualifications which can be undertaken with a majority of dive centres, all your equipment can be hired at very favourable rates. Beginners and advanced divers will receive all help and assistance from the centres to ensure that their diving holiday is trouble-free and enjoyable.

The Government have official inspectors who regularly check the centres and their equipment.

The diver who wishes to dive independently and hire equipment, has to present a qualification certificate to the chosen dive centre, they must be qualified to dive to 30m or deeper, or be accompanied by a Certified Diving Instructor.

The stern of the MV Um el Faroud scuttled on the 02-09-1998.
PHOTO: JON BORG www.jonborg.com

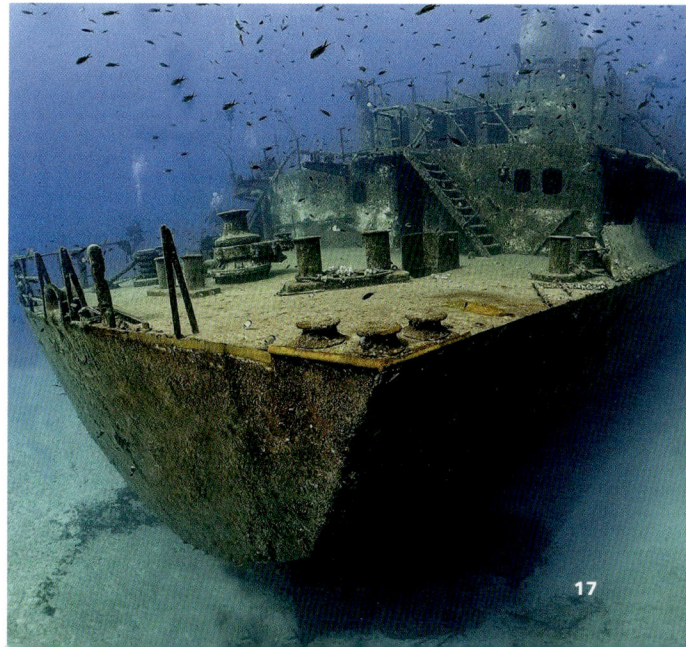

ISLAND FOR DIVERS

Marine life it would be difficult to list and comment on the many various species of fauna and flora to be found in the waters around these islands. The chance of seeing 'Big Game' fish or certain species of shark which maybe dangerous to man, is unlikely, also spotting underwater, tuna, dolphins or turtles is rare as they seldom come close to shore. Species which the diver will find around the Maltese Islands are barracuda, groupers, amberjacks, various bream, wrasse, damsel fish, octopus, squid, flying gurnard, stingrays, meagre, bogue, red mullet, painted combers, cardinal fish, parrot fish and sea hares to name but a few, the structure of the coast and the rocks seem to offer ideal living conditions for them.

John Dory can be found, mostly during wintertime as they normally spend their time at greater depths. Sea horses are here too, possibly the best time to see them is July and August, but they are so small and very well camouflaged, you have to be very careful and patient to find them.

There are a few sea animals, which are beautiful to watch but dangerous to touch; they are not deadly but could be very painful. These include scorpion fish, jellyfish, the bristle worm, the weaver and the stingray.

Giving the Marine life a helping hand

Nature Trust Malta operate the Wildlife Rehab Centre Project. Like us dolphins, whales, sharks, turtles and other marine life sometimes need help and Nature Trust Malta is providing this through its wildlife rescue team. This is a group of volunteers which offer a twenty-four-hour rescue service for wildlife. They are a Non-Government Organisation (NGO). Nature Trust Malta was founded on the 12th December 1962 as Natural History Society of Malta and in 1999 became as it known today. The trust is very active in environment education to create awareness of nature conservation, they are also carrying out projects to protect habitats and the creation of marine protected areas. On arrival at the rescue site volunteers assist the animals as much as possible, take details and photos, treat and remove any visible obstructions. Some of the rescued marine life are taken to San Lucjan's rehab centre to be treated by a vet, cared for over time and eventually released back to the wild whenever possible.

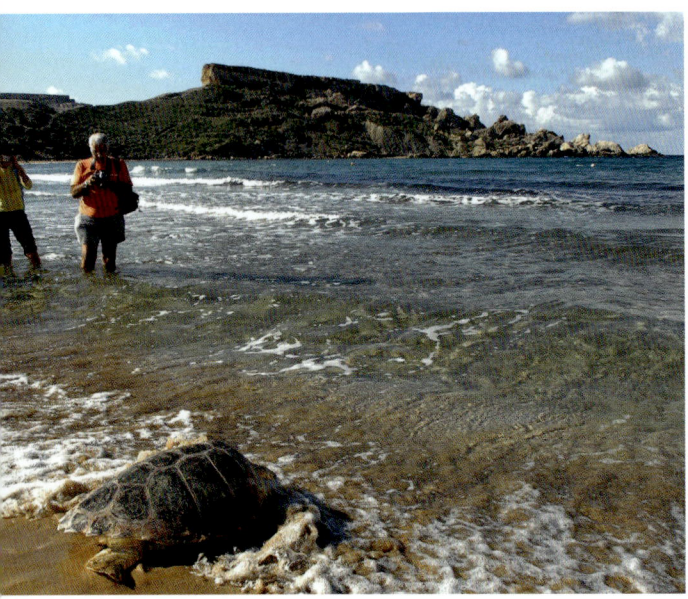

Turtle release at Ghajn Tuffieha Bay Malta.

Malta's National Aquarium on the front at Qwara, the roof designed in the shape of a starfish.

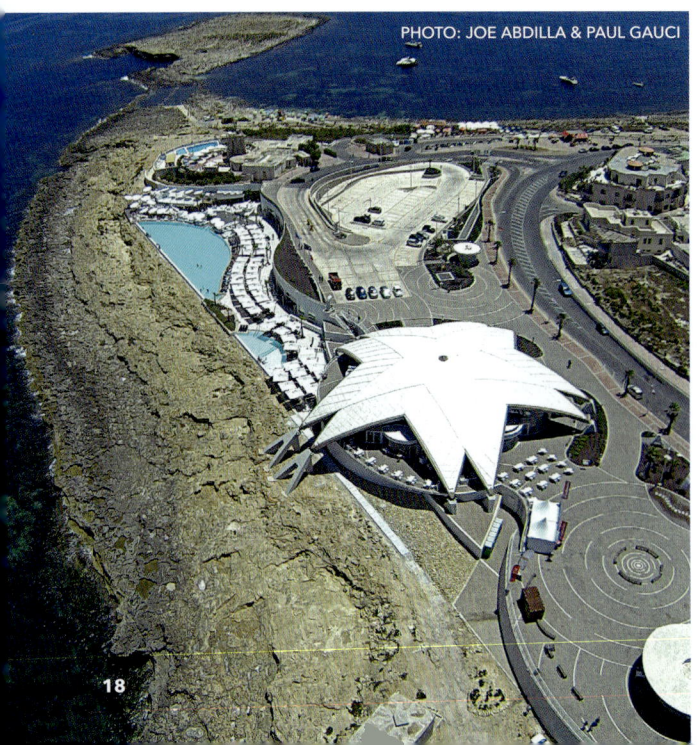

PHOTO: JOE ABDILLA & PAUL GAUCI

A number of turtles released from Mellieha Bay.

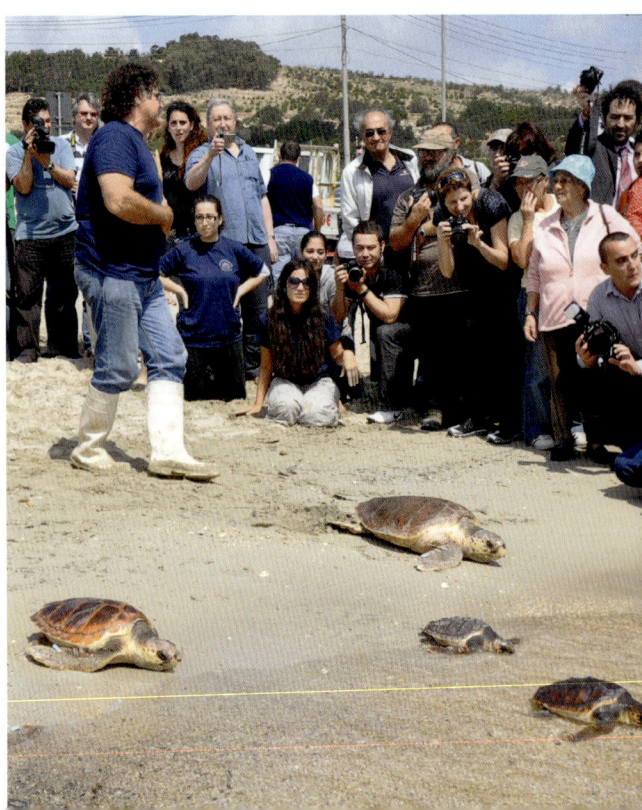

Sharklab Malta is an NGO dedicated to protecting sharks, rays and skates through research and public education around the Maltese Islands. They identify species which live in or travel through local waters and those species that need better protection and management. They make a difference by recovering eggs from female dead species, the Malta National Aquarium nurtures them until they hatch. Sharklab Malta work in conjunction with the Aquarium and have a release programme for the lesser spotted cat shark and nursehound sharks which are tagged before release. This happens normally when they are two years old. To date they have released 350 species. They promote a better understanding of all sharks, rays and skates and their habitats, engaging with schools, communities and the media. If, whilst diving you see a shark or ray, please tell Sharklab about it, you can easily identify these using their guide and report them through their website and sightings page.
www.sharklab-malta.org

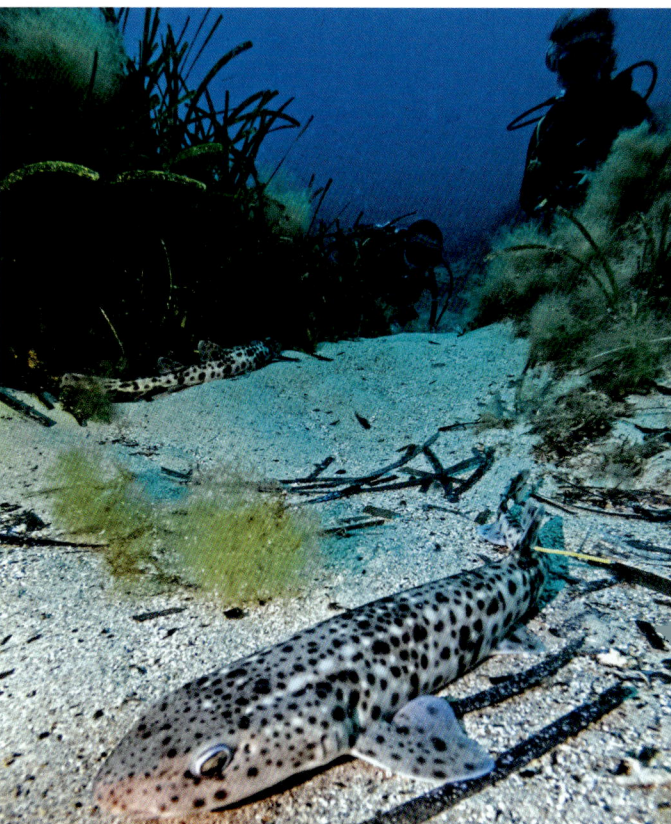

These small sharks are exploring their new world.
PHOTO: ARKADIUSZ SREBNIK POLANDDIVINGPHOTO

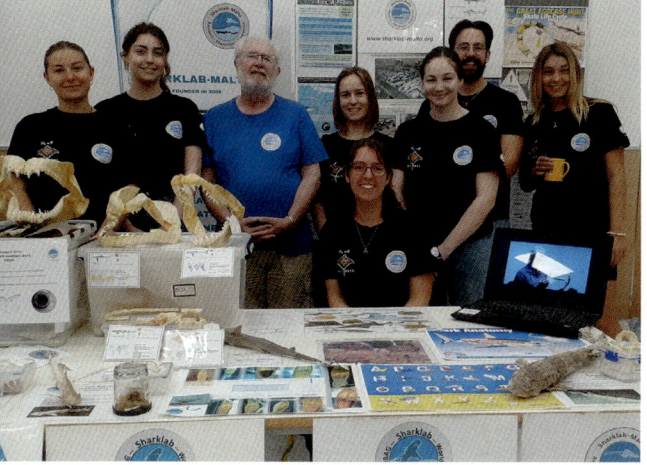

The team's stall promoting Sharklab.   PHOTO: PAM MASON

Zibel Malta this group is a registered voluntary organisation (NGO) their aim is the reducing overall generated waste on the Maltese Islands and restoring the land and sea bed back to its natural state. Zibel was founded in 2017 and since then has grown and grown with the helpful hands of its volunteers. Their motto is 'It starts with you' and their goal is simple, to make the Islands and sea free from waste and spread awareness about the situation so that we can all appreciate a cleaner environment.
www.zibel.org

After a hard mornings work this happy and friendly team of Zibel volunteers pose for a photo.

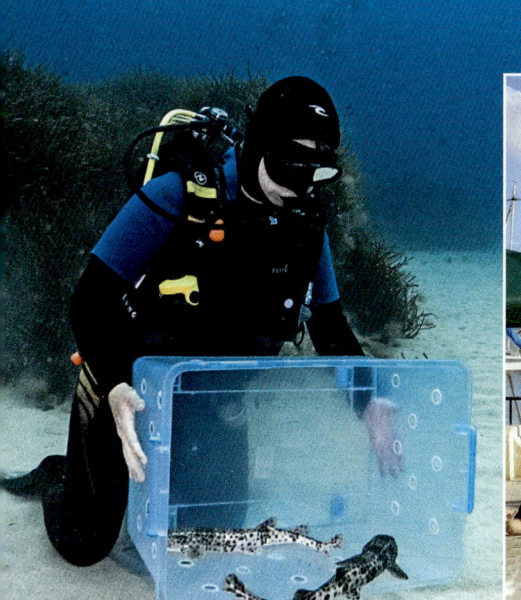

Two, two-year-old nursehound sharks being released.
PHOTO: ARKADIUSZ SERBNIK POLANDDIVINGPHOTO

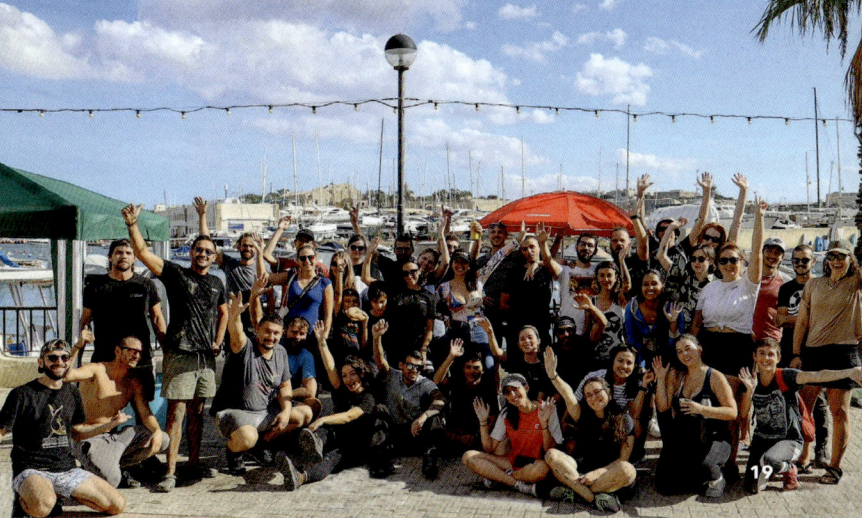

ISLAND FOR DIVERS

Dive Centres and Club Members from both Malta and Gozo also organize clean ups on dive sites. Making it environmentally friendly not only for divers, snorkelers and swimmers but also for the marine life, by removing hazards such as discarded fishing nets, plastic and general waste from the sea bed.

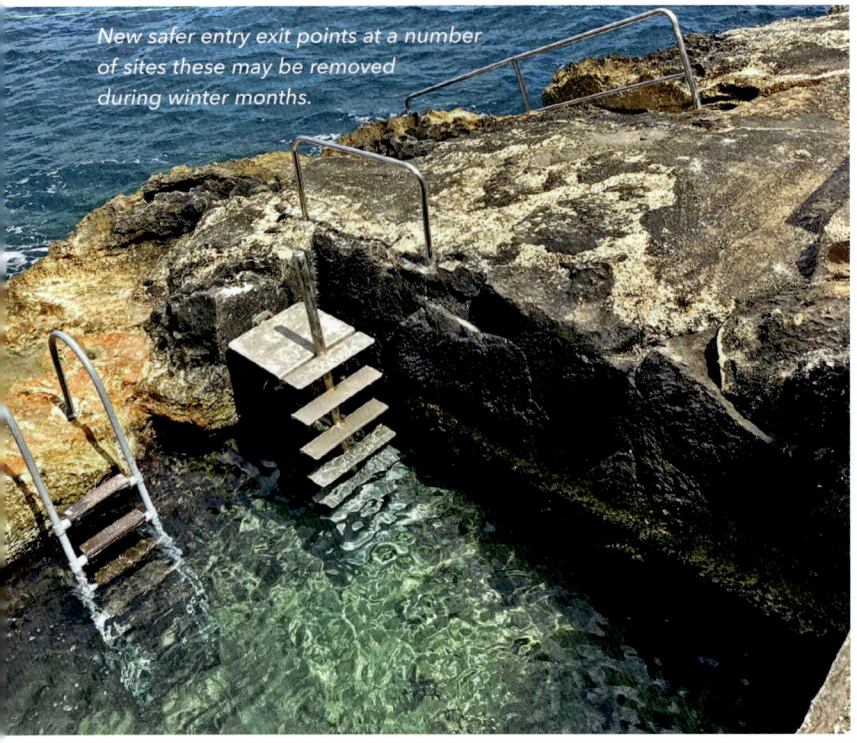

New safer entry exit points at a number of sites these may be removed during winter months.

Underwater Photography Maybe it's the crystal blue waters of the Mediterranean and the visibility below the surface that entices divers to the shores of the Maltese Islands, bringing with them their cameras to capture the delights of this underwater world.

You will need a buddy with good buoyancy skills and the patience to match. He needs to be a hunter to find some of the elusive marine life, gently persuading it towards the waiting camera, and in the meantime keeping himself as part of the backdrop if required.

Around the islands' coastline, there is a variety of underwater landscapes, areas of sand, fields of sea grass tall and green, shallow reefs where the marine growth sparkles in the rays of the sun to the dramatic sheer drop-offs that disappear into the abyss. There is a kaleidoscope of colour to be found amongst the corals and marine life. Here the coral is not of gigantic size, sometimes small can be beautiful, with the vivid red and orange colours of the soft coral and sponges together with the not so colourful hard coral you just need a torch. Together with the many species of tubeworm gently swaying to catch their prey, and many other wonderful sights, all this adds up to the underwater photographer's paradise.

Diving for the disabled The International Association for Disabled Divers is an association who promote, develop and conduct programmes for the training of the physically disabled in scuba diving. Since its introduction in 1993 the IAHD has conducted professional programmes around the world. There are a number of centres in Malta who offer introductory dives and diver training for the disabled.

One of the easy entry points around these islands.

Night Diving opens a whole new dimension for the experienced diver, and Malta is ideally suited for this kind of diving. At night the diver will see an entirely different variety of fish and the colours seen are more vibrant under a diver's torch. Most dive centres have night diving within their dive packages and with the right conditions a night dive is an enjoyable experience.

Fireworms on a feeding fenzy DO NOT TOUCH.

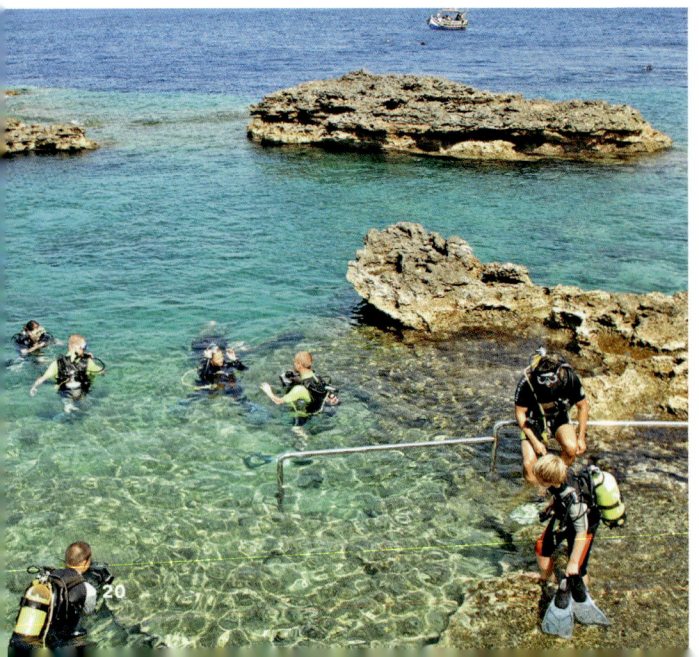

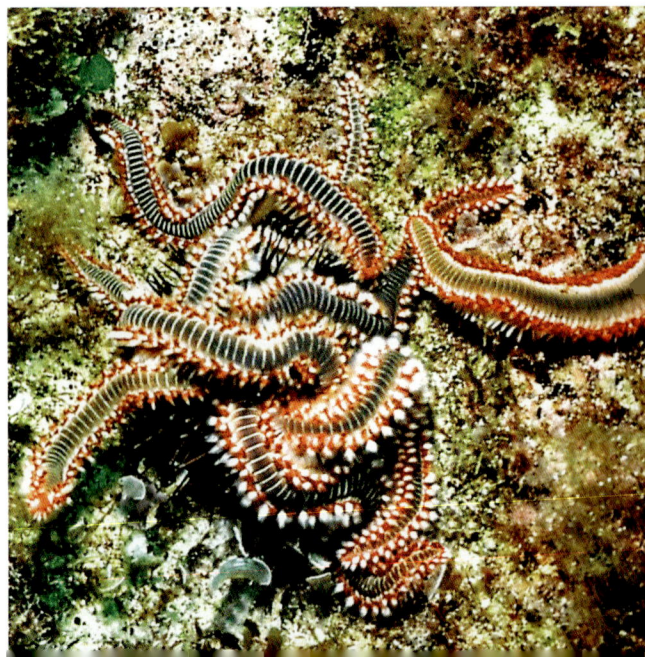

ISLAND FOR DIVERS

The variety of this fantastic underwater world

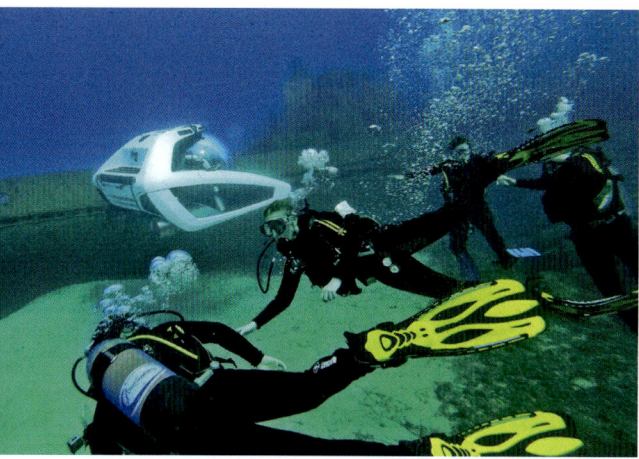

These divers are surprised by a visitor to Tugboat 2.
PHOTO: SERGEY MARKOV DIVE SYSTEMS

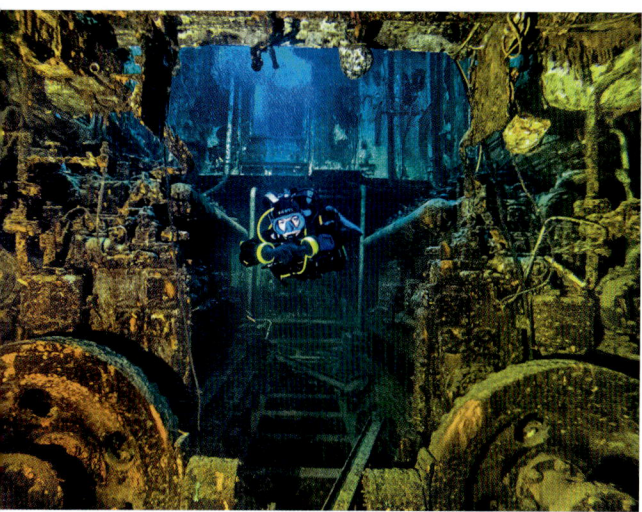

Exploring the engine room of the MV Karwela
PHOTO: ARKADIUSZ SREBNIK POLANDDIVINGPHOTO

This large shoal of fish heading towards Tugboat Rozi.
PHOTO: JON BORG www.jonborg.com

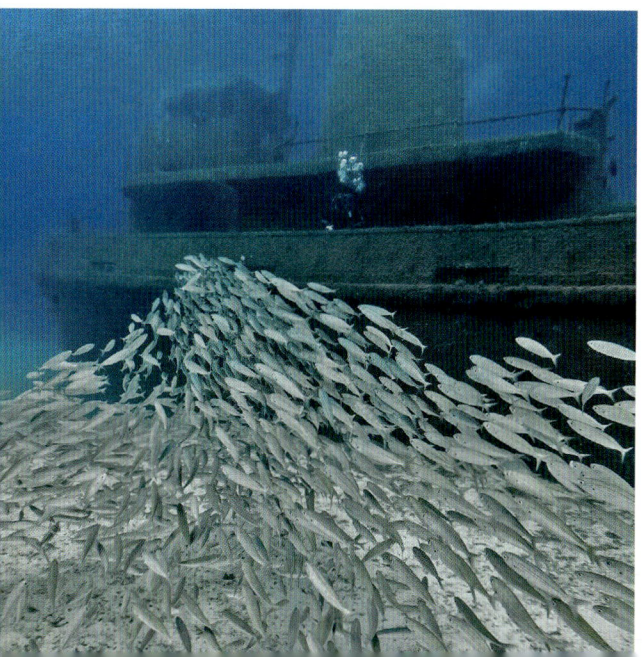

Key to Symbols Chart

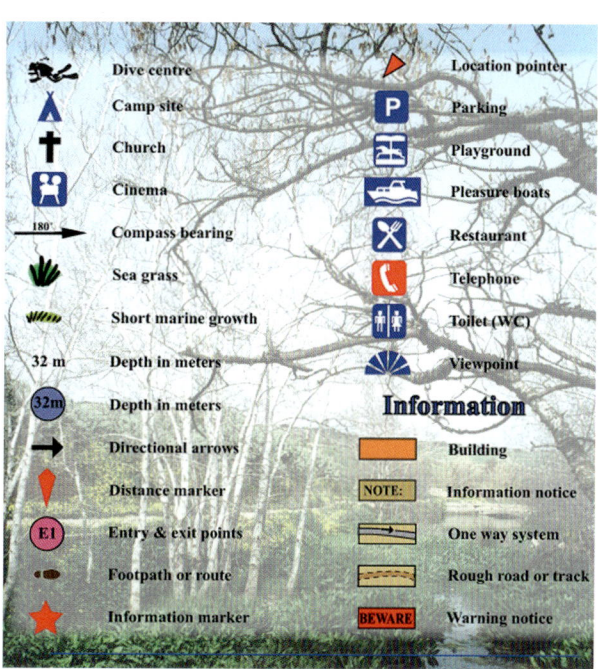

Special Notes

If this is your first visit to the Maltese Islands or you have any doubts in your dive planning or navigational skills, I would strongly recommend that you ask your chosen dive centre for an orientation dive or dive guiding. You will find that they are friendly and only too pleased to assist you in any way they can.

It is a requirement of Maltese law that a Surface Marker Buoy should be used when diving in a harbour and in some cases, permission must be granted from the Harbour Master to dive there. I would also strongly recommend when your dive plan takes you away from the reef into open sea that you carry a DSMB

Would readers please note that the illustrations of the underwater plans and road maps to be found in the following pages have been made as accurate as possible. They are to compass bearings: but not to scale, information for distance and time can be found within the text.
  Although every effort to ensure that the information given on the dive sites was as accurate as possible, other information given in this book was correct at the time of going to press, the author accepts no responsibility for any loss, injury or inconvenience sustained by any person using this book.

Further information on diving the Maltese Islands go to **divinginfo.mt**

BS-AC Scuba Dive Clubs in Malta

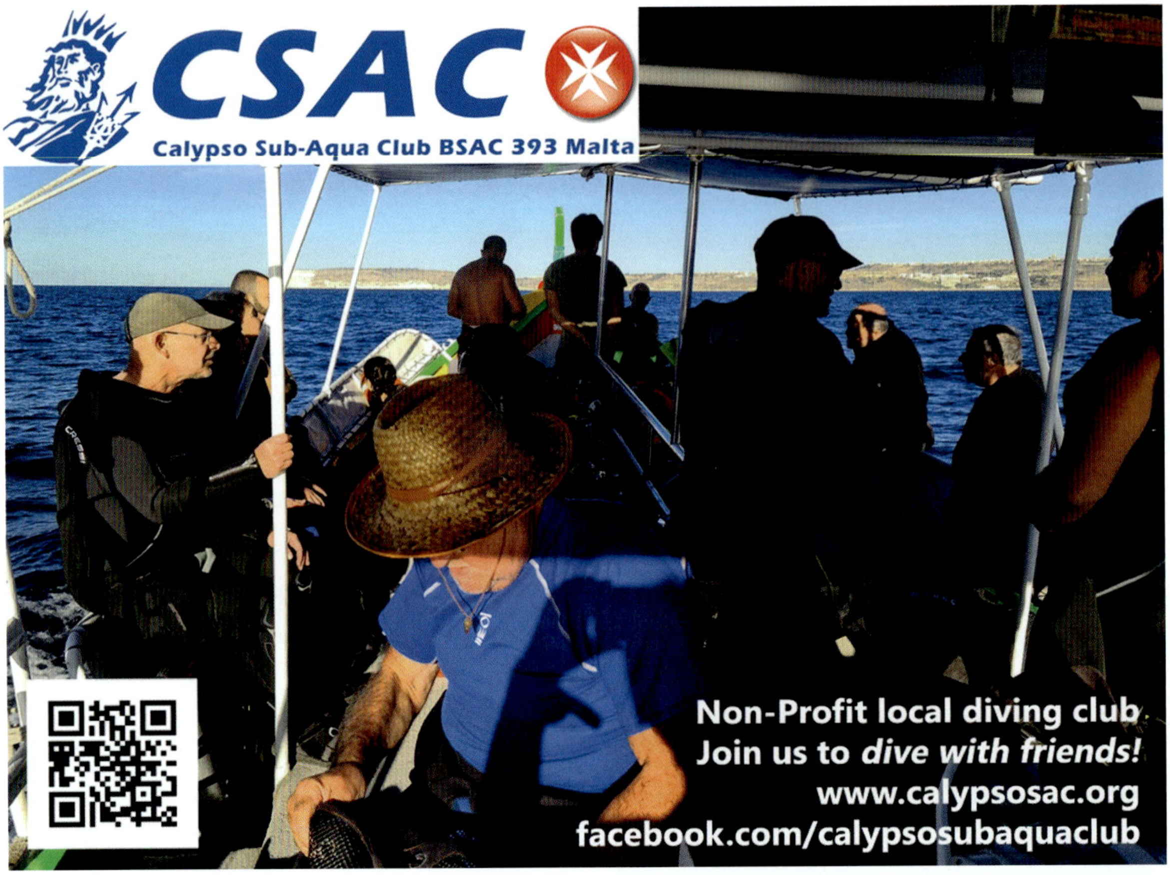

CSAC
Calypso Sub-Aqua Club BSAC 393 Malta

Non-Profit local diving club.
Join us to *dive with friends!*
www.calypsosac.org
facebook.com/calypsosubaquaclub

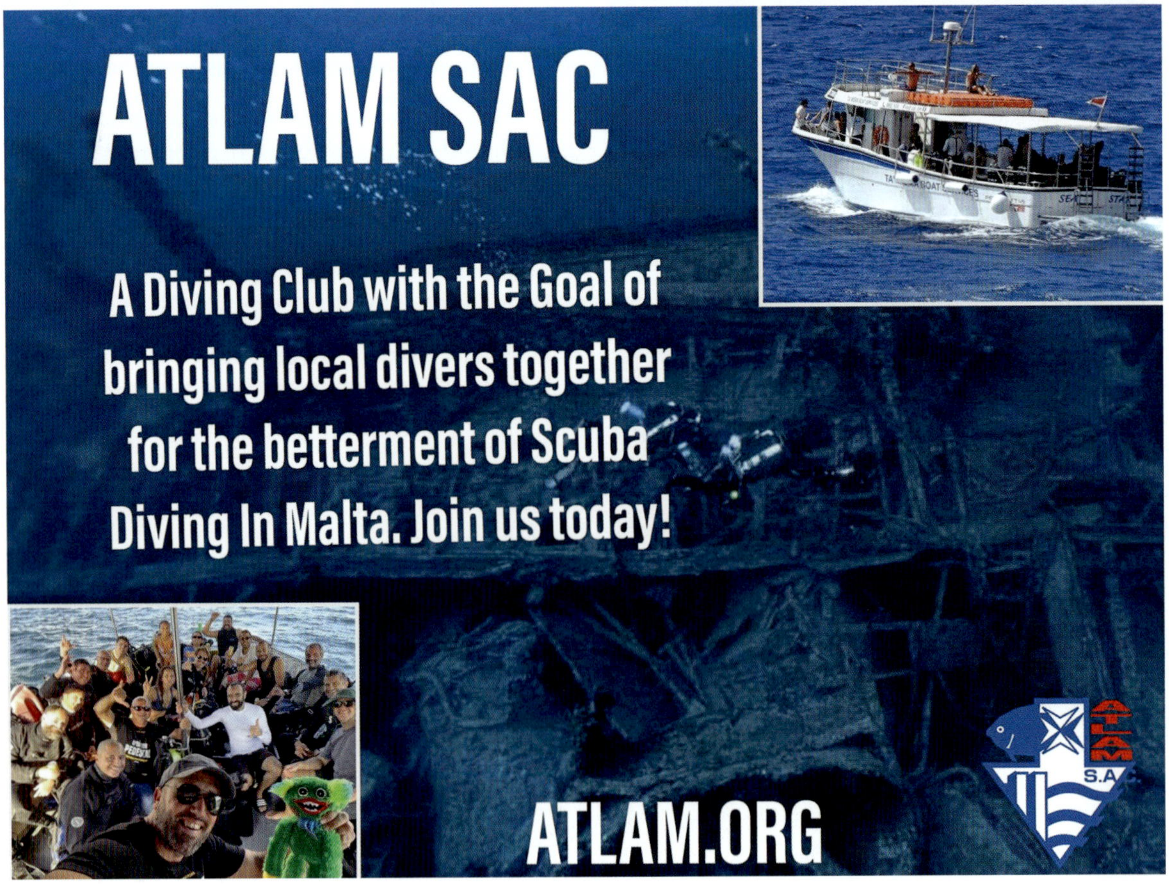

ATLAM SAC

A Diving Club with the Goal of bringing local divers together for the betterment of Scuba Diving In Malta. Join us today!

ATLAM.ORG

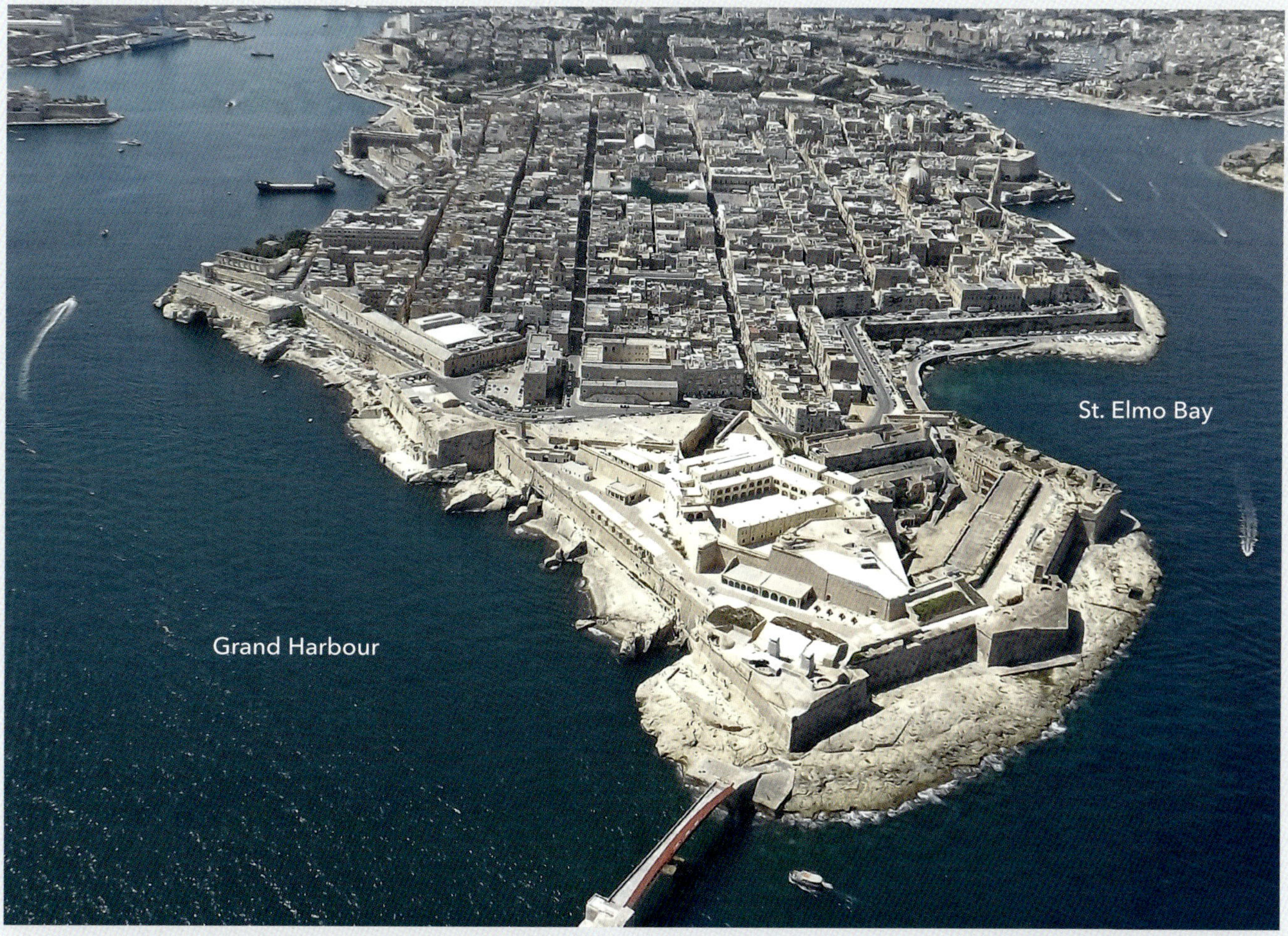

VALLETTA - ST. ELMO BAY

Grand Harbour
St. Elmo Bay

PHOTO: JOE ABDILLA & PAUL GAUCI

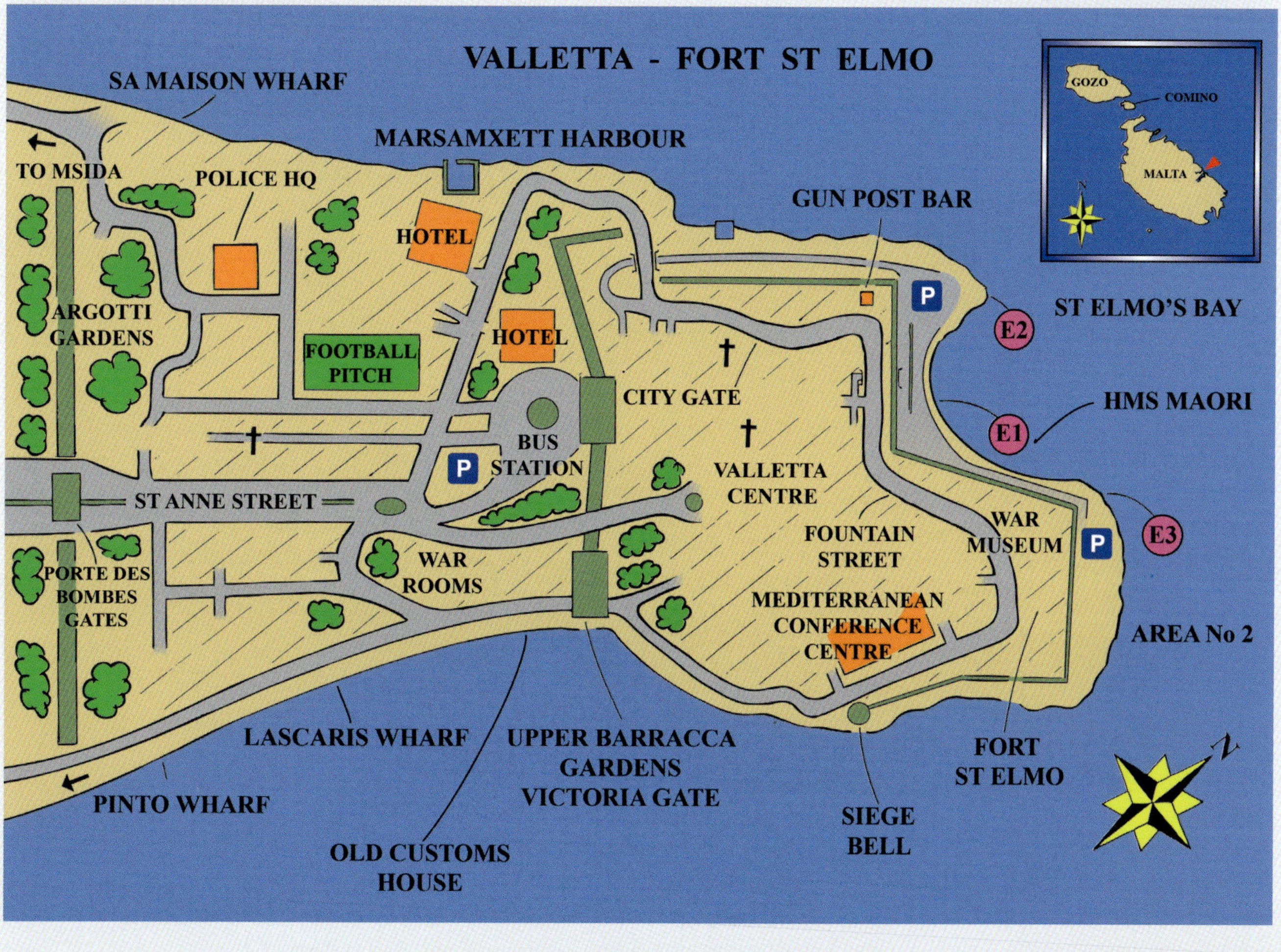

VALLETTA - FORT ST ELMO

- SA MAISON WHARF
- TO MSIDA
- POLICE HQ
- MARSAMXETT HARBOUR
- GUN POST BAR
- HOTEL
- ST ELMO'S BAY
- ARGOTTI GARDENS
- FOOTBALL PITCH
- HOTEL
- E2
- CITY GATE
- HMS MAORI
- E1
- BUS STATION
- VALLETTA CENTRE
- ST ANNE STREET
- FOUNTAIN STREET
- WAR MUSEUM
- E3
- PORTE DES BOMBES GATES
- WAR ROOMS
- MEDITERRANEAN CONFERENCE CENTRE
- AREA No 2
- LASCARIS WHARF
- UPPER BARRACCA GARDENS VICTORIA GATE
- FORT ST ELMO
- PINTO WHARF
- OLD CUSTOMS HOUSE
- SIEGE BELL

(Inset: GOZO, COMINO, MALTA)

HMS *MAORI*

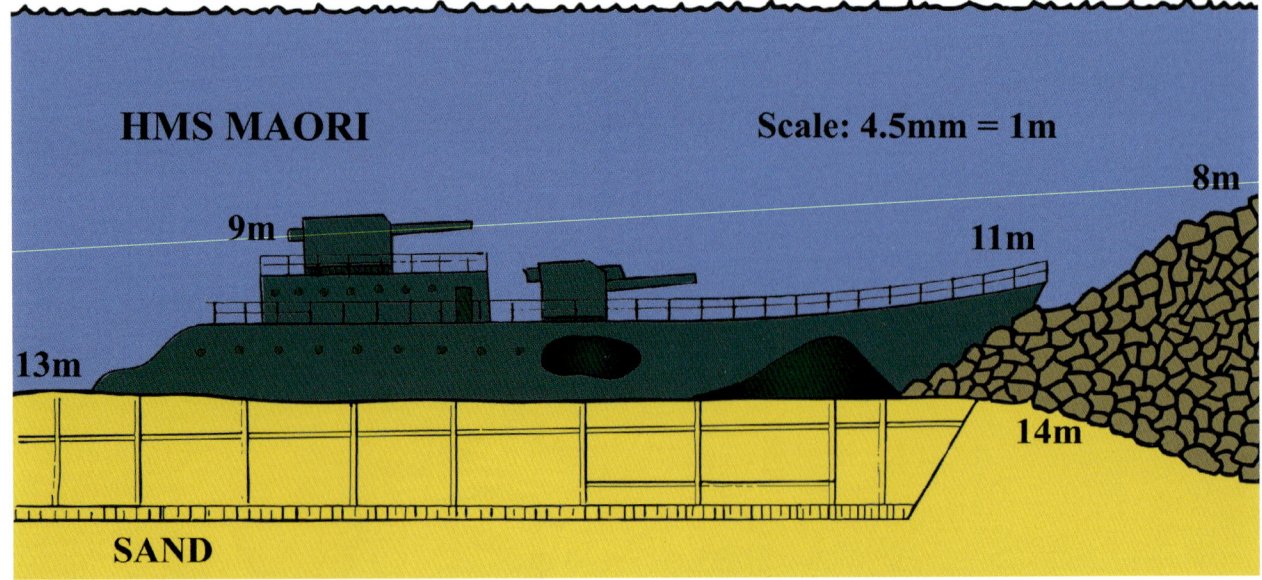

Details of HMS Maori under the water showing the wreckage which is above and below the seabed.
The two guns shown in the diagram were removed and used as shore batteries.

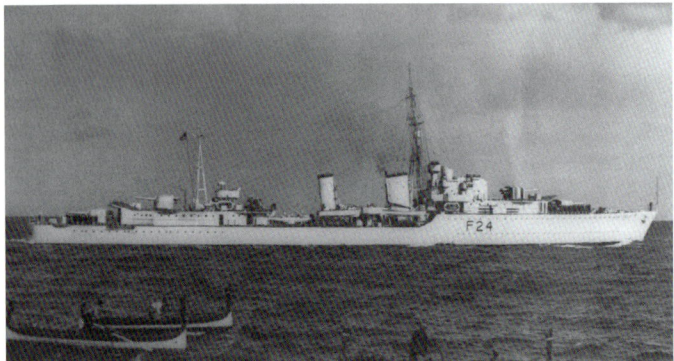

HMS Maori outside Grand Harbour and in the foreground two Maltese gondolas.
PHOTO: by kind permission of Joseph Bonnici, AUTHOR OF "A Century of the Royal Navy in Malta".

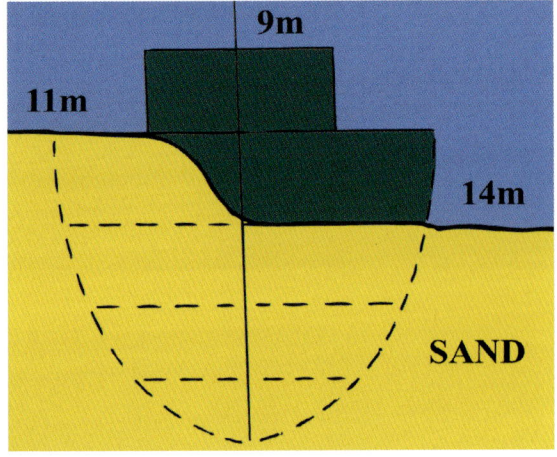

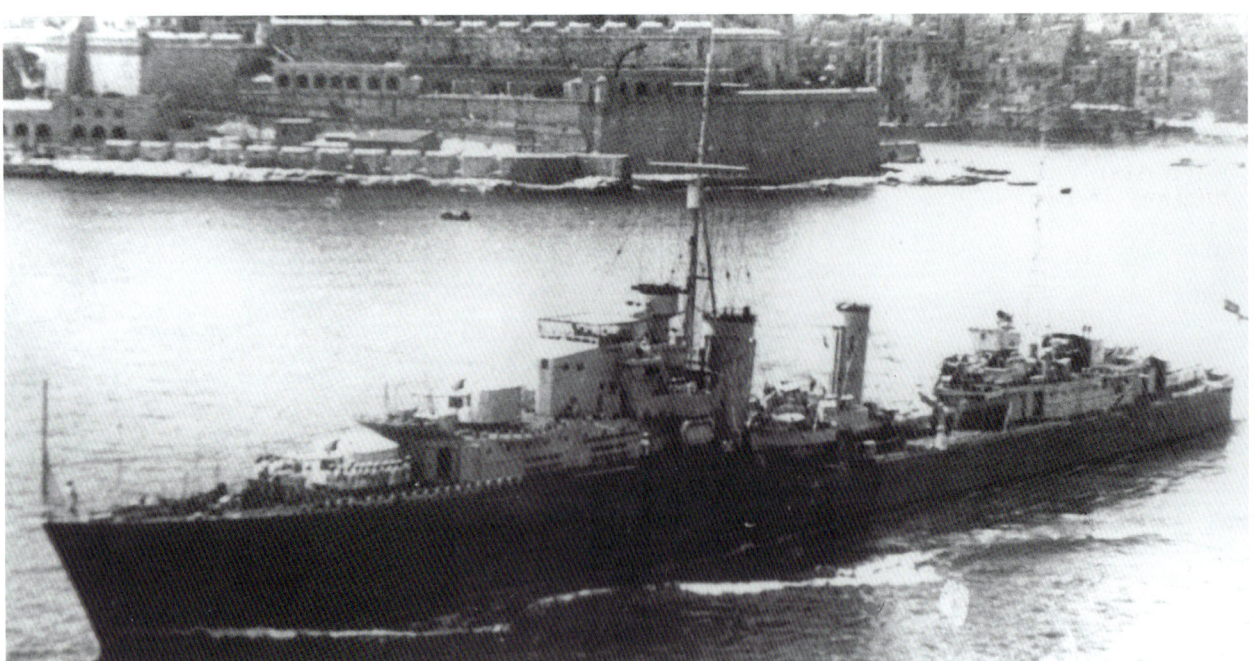

HMS Maori leaving Grand Harbour with Fort St Angelo in the background. Numerous attempts have been made to trace the owner of this photograph, which is displayed in many dive centres in Malta.

HMS *Maori* - St. Elmo Bay - Valletta

St Elmo Bay is situated on the south side of the entrance to Marsamxett harbour, on the lower-level road, below the city walls on the northern side of Valletta. Divers normally use this dive site when the weather conditions do not permit diving at the more popular dive sites, but in my opinion the *Maori* should be dived when the sea conditions elsewhere are good, your reward would be to find that you are the only divers here. The wreckage is beginning to deteriorate due to time and sea conditions but is still an interesting dive.

During weekdays parking can be a problem at this dive site, but you do have a choice of three entry points, all leading to HMS *Maori*, during these days maybe the best entry point is E3.

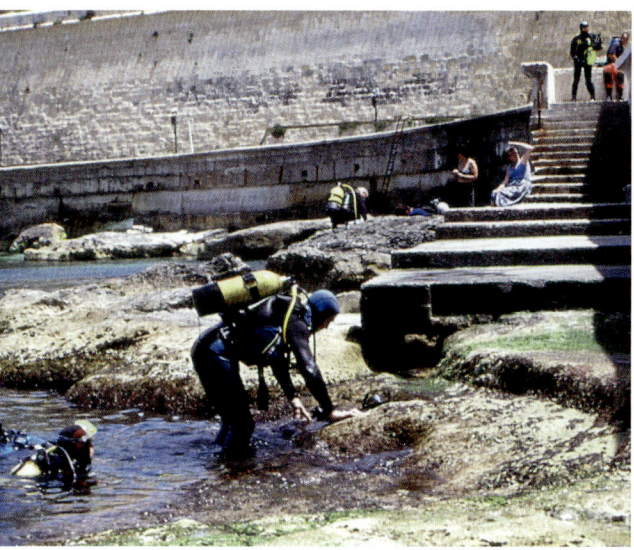

THE DIVES — Minimum time - 40 mins

Route 1 using entry point E1 at the bottom of the steps, which can be quite slippery; the depth here is less than 2m so care must be taken when entering the water. From this point take a compass bearing of 20°/30°. The distance is some 120 metres to the wreck and it will take you around 6 minutes at a slow fin to reach the top of the rocky slope, here the depth will be 8 or 9m. Continue over and down the rocky slope onto the sand or if your navigation has been 1st class, onto the wreck. If not, your direction now depends on the depth, if you find yourself at 13m or more, turn right or if less than 10m turn left. The Maori's bows are against the rocky slope, see plan.

Divers at entry exit point E1 for HMS Maori.

HMS *Maori* — Area 1

This 1870-ton Tribal Class British Destroyer built by Fairfield, Govan, Scotland was launched on 2nd September 1937. Other details, overall length 115m, breadth 11m, main armament 8 x 4.7 guns, 4 x 21 torpedo tubes, twin screws with a speed of 36 knots and a crew of 190 men. During World War Two HMS *Maori* was involved in the following campaigns, April/May 1940 Norway, Bismark May 1942. Malta Convoys during 1941 and 1942. She was one of the four destroyers, which sank two Italian cruisers near Cape Bon on the 13th December 1941.

During the early hours of February 12th 1942 the HMS *Maori* was moored in Grand Harbour Valletta, when a parachute flare dropped by enemy aircraft became trapped in her foremast. Soon after the illuminated destroyer received a direct hit by a bomb and caught fire. She was abandoned and shortly afterwards the aft magazine exploded. The destroyer sank stern first causing the bows to rise out of the sea, during that afternoon she slowly filled with water and sank. In 1945 she was cut in two and the forepart was re-floated, then towed to St. Elmo's Bay near the entrance to Marsamxett harbour and is still there today. The aft section was re-floated and sunk in deep water off the island.

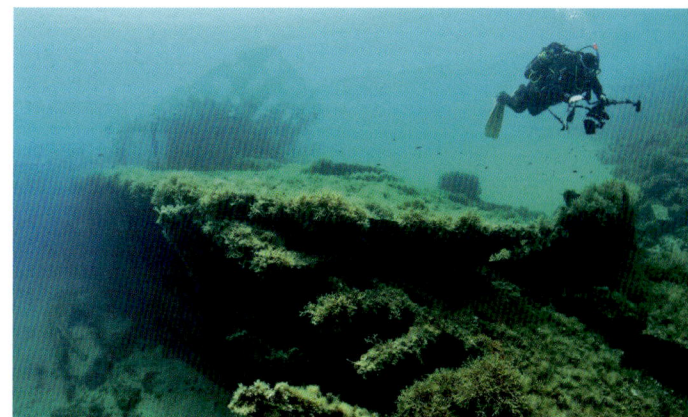

Diver over the bows and in the background the wall.

Below: The starboard side of HMS Maori.

PHOTO: ARKADIUSZ SREBNIK POLANDDIVINGPHOTO

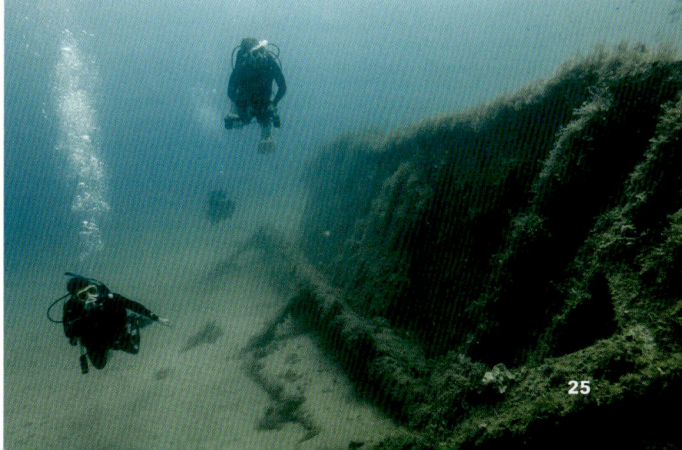

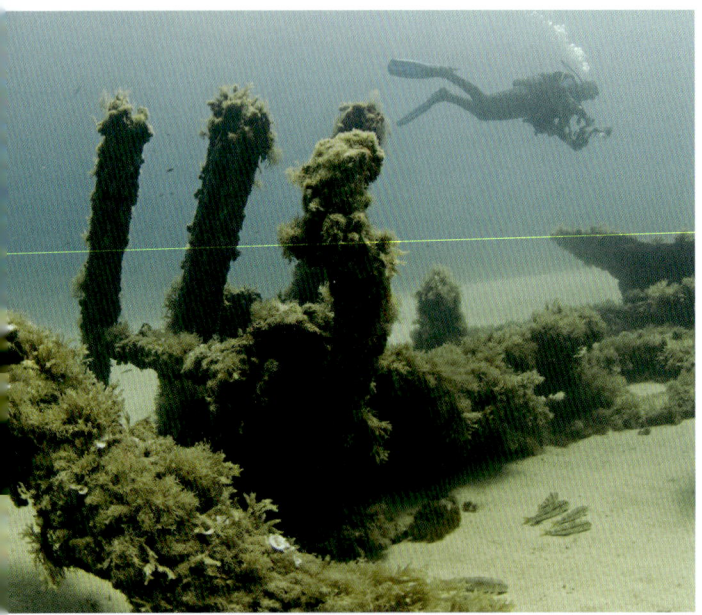

More wreckage of HMS Maori out on the sand.
PHOTO: SHARON FORDER

Route 2 to entry point E2 if this is your choice, I would suggest you check the route before kitting up and maybe consider E1 as your exit point. From the sea wall you will have to walk over the rocks to the most northerly point, where you will find a gentle slope giving easy access to the water, E2. When under the water take a north compass bearing and in less than 2 minutes you will reach the top of the rocky slope at 10m. Continue down and over the rocky slope to your chosen depth or to the sandy bottom at 30m. Now, keeping the rocky slope on your right, head in an easterly direction. It will take you approximately

A diver above the forward deck of HMS Maori.

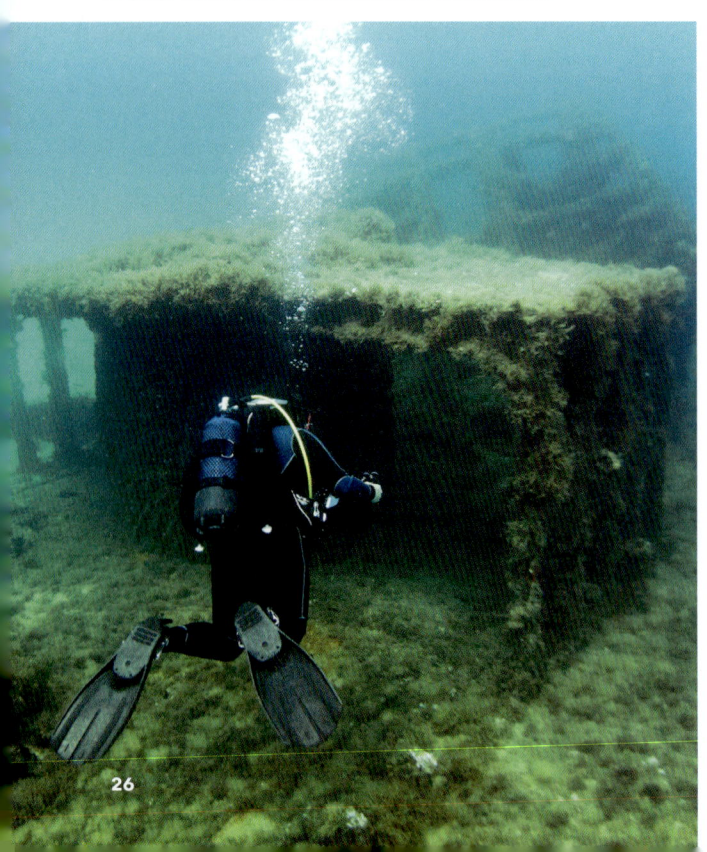

10 minutes at a slow swim to reach the Maori 14m. At a depth of 18m you will find a smooth step/slope in the sand, turn away from the rocky wall and head out over the sand for about 2 minutes, you will find a single rock called Photo Rock, a great place for macro photography.

Route 3 using entry point E3 in the little pool there will normally be a ladder, but this is removed during the winter, there are steps cut out in the rocks as an alternative. Once under the water and down to a depth of 7m, take a compass bearing of 240°/250°. Moving over the reef and down onto the sand at 14m, continue over the sand until you reach the wreck or the stony wall, if the latter and your depth is more than 14m turn left or right if its less than 10m. The distance and time are almost identical to route one, 120 metres approx. 6 mins.

HMS *Maori* & Return Routes

The deepest part of this dive is on the starboard side at 14m the bow of the wreck is resting on the rocky slope, two winches and bollards remain, the brass base of the forward gun is still in place. The upper structure for the second gun is collapsing, unfortunately both guns have been removed and were reused as shore battery guns in 1942. Move away from the main structure and explore the wreckage, which lies on the sand in an area at the rear of the *Maori*. The marine growth, the many small fish and occasionally seahorses are to be found here, with good visibility and sunlight it makes this an ideal spot for photography.

Return route to E1 leave the wreck by the bows and continue up the rocky slope, from here your exit point has a compass bearing of 200°. This shallow area allows you to spend time, if you have the air, to look around on your way back, if you are lucky, you may see large shoals of salema fish. Just to the right of entry point E1, there are two smooth flat steps in the rock below the water level, which I call the 'Throne', making an easy exit, even when there is a small swell.

Return route to E2 go to the top of the rocky slope and head in a westerly direction until you reach a marker which you hopefully placed at the start of your dive. Now head in a southerly direction to E2

Return route to E3 leave the wreck on the port side once away from the wreckage take a compass bearing of 80°/90°. Continue over the sand until you reach the reef, then follow it along where it meets the sand until reach a depth of 14m or if you have left one, your marker stone. Move up and over the reef on a compass bearing of 60°/70° towards your exit point E3. You can of course plan your own dive to the *Maori* using alternative routes.

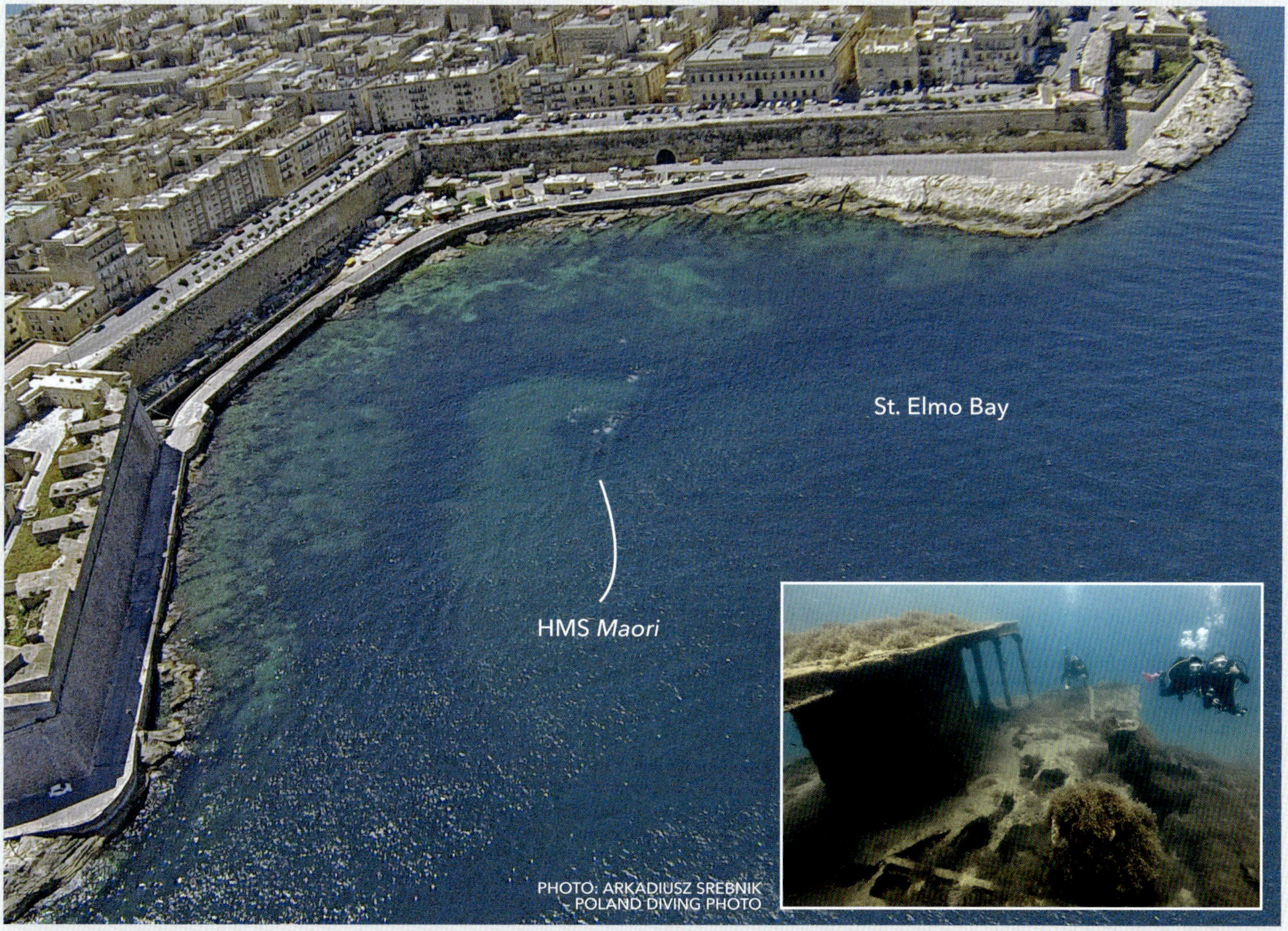

HMS *MAORI* - ST. ELMO BAY - VALLETTA

St. Elmo Bay

HMS *Maori*

PHOTO: ARKADIUSZ SREBNIK
POLAND DIVING PHOTO

PHOTO: JOE ABDILLA & PAUL GAUCI

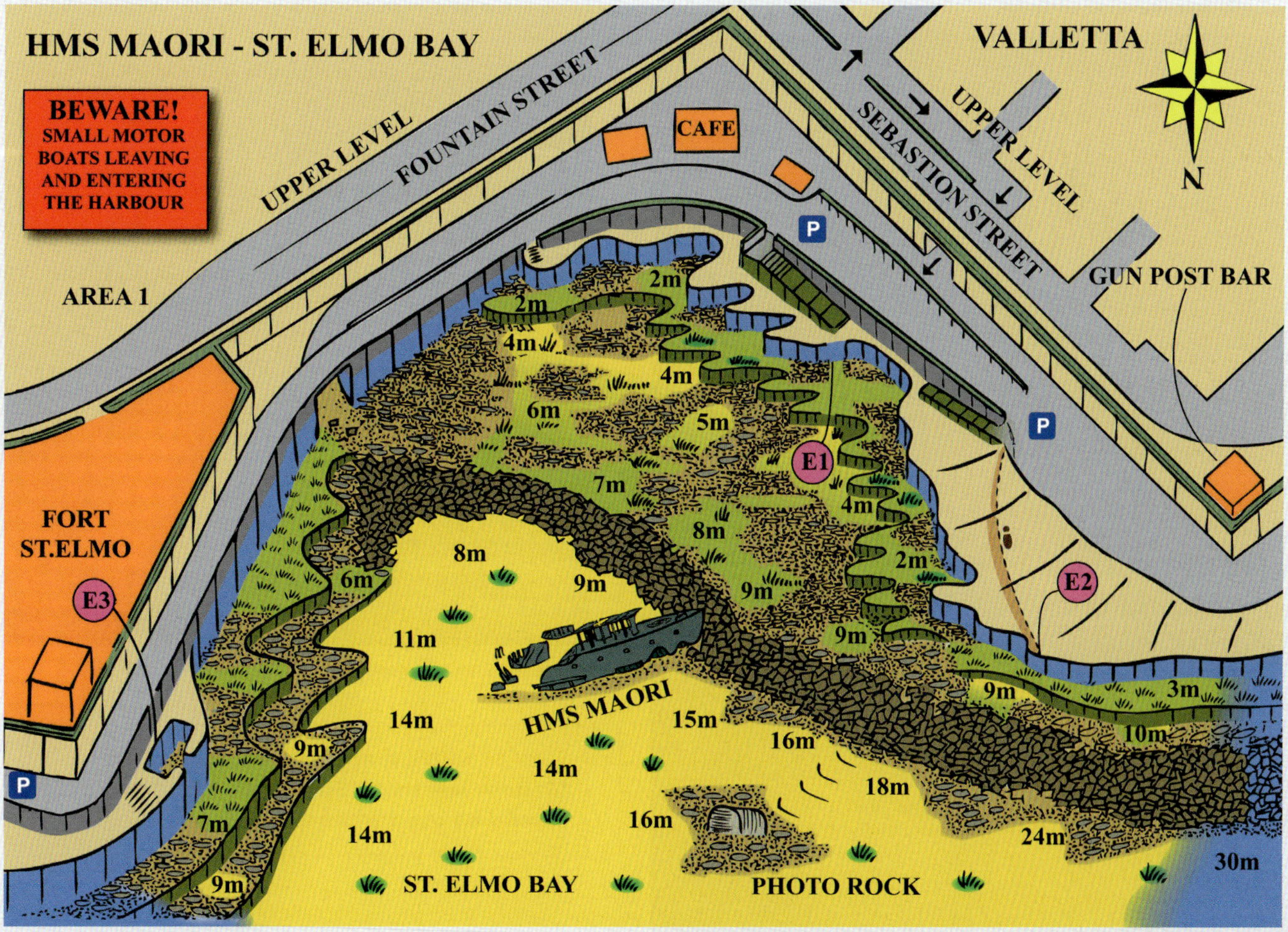

HMS MAORI - ST. ELMO BAY — VALLETTA

BEWARE! SMALL MOTOR BOATS LEAVING AND ENTERING THE HARBOUR

AREA 1

FORT ST. ELMO

UPPER LEVEL
FOUNTAIN STREET
CAFE
SEBASTION STREET
UPPER LEVEL
GUN POST BAR

E1, E2, E3

P (parking)

HMS MAORI
ST. ELMO BAY
PHOTO ROCK

Depths: 2m, 2m, 4m, 4m, 6m, 5m, 7m, 8m, 4m, 2m, 6m, 8m, 9m, 9m, 9m, 11m, 14m, 15m, 16m, 9m, 9m, 3m, 14m, 9m, 18m, 10m, 7m, 14m, 16m, 24m, 30m, 9m

Fort St. Elmo — Area 2

This dive site is situated between the entrance to Grand Harbour and Marsamxett Harbour. The entry point I would use would be E3, it is on the northeast corner right of the bay, by the car parking area. Here you will find a ladder during the summer period, if not there are steps cut into the rocks. Check your exit points E if no ladder, I would exit the water from one of the two little pools, one each side of entry point E3 this can be difficult and you may have to use a de-kit routine. This dive should not be attempted in rough sea conditions, as exit would be difficult.

THE DIVE — Minimum time - 40 mins

Using entry point E3 surface swim round in an easterly direction until in front of the black post, descend to the seabed, from here take a north to northeast compass bearing and within 3 minutes you should reach a depth of 12/13m with a drop off down to 20m, this is the start of the main reef. From here travel in an easterly direction follow the base of the drop off, after some 6 minutes you will reach a valley which runs up to the top of the reef. This of course can be your turning point or you can continue until reaching a depth of 35m then ascend to the top of the reef, now head in a westerly direction until reaching the top of the valley.

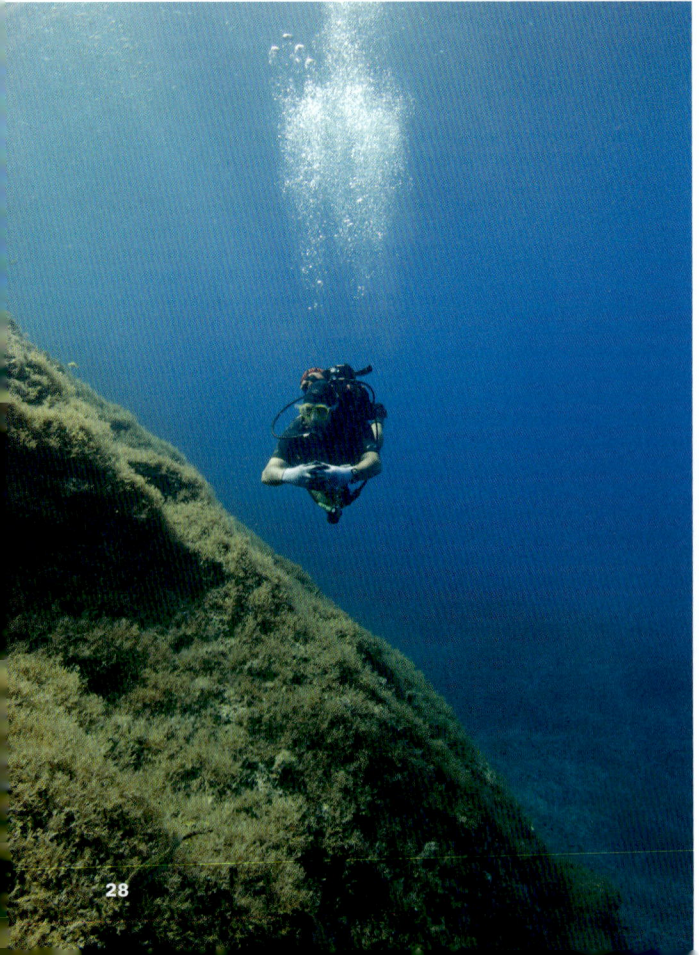

The reef with its drop off.

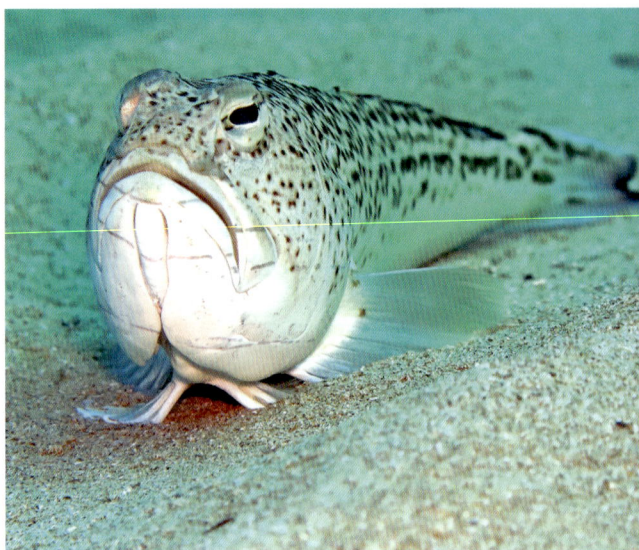

Stargazer normally covered in sand.   PHOTO: JOE FORMOSA

A compass bearing from here of 180° will take you to the coastline reef and a depth of 9m; from here to your exit point keep the reef on your left. Alternatively, you could plan your own dive using the same entry/exit points and the coastline reef for your navigation. I found this site to be a place to explore and rummage with a maximum depth of approximately 16m, within this large area there are many gullies, small rocks and boulders to explore. This dive would also be suitable for a second dive or training. A wide variety of marine life can be found here, such as moray octopus, groupers, damselfish, red mullet and shoals of salema fish.

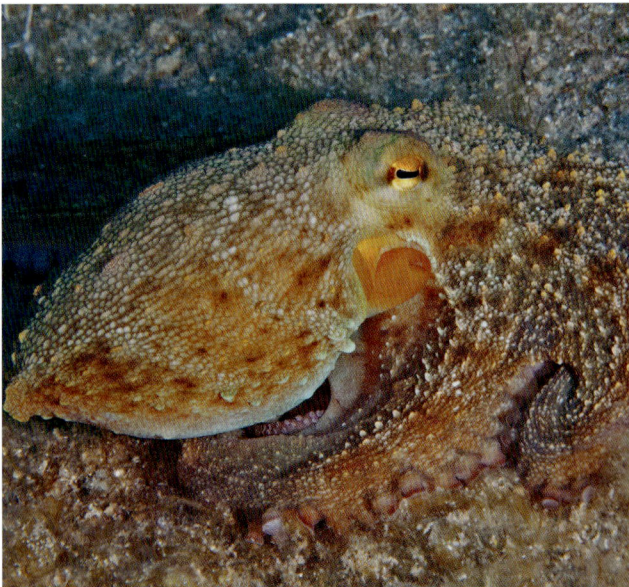

Octopus (Octopus vulgaris) out for a nights hunting.

PLEASE NOTE that it is a requirement of Maltese law that a Surface Marker Buoy should be used when diving in the harbour.

Grand Harbour
E
E
E

PHOTO: PGL AERIAL PHOTOS

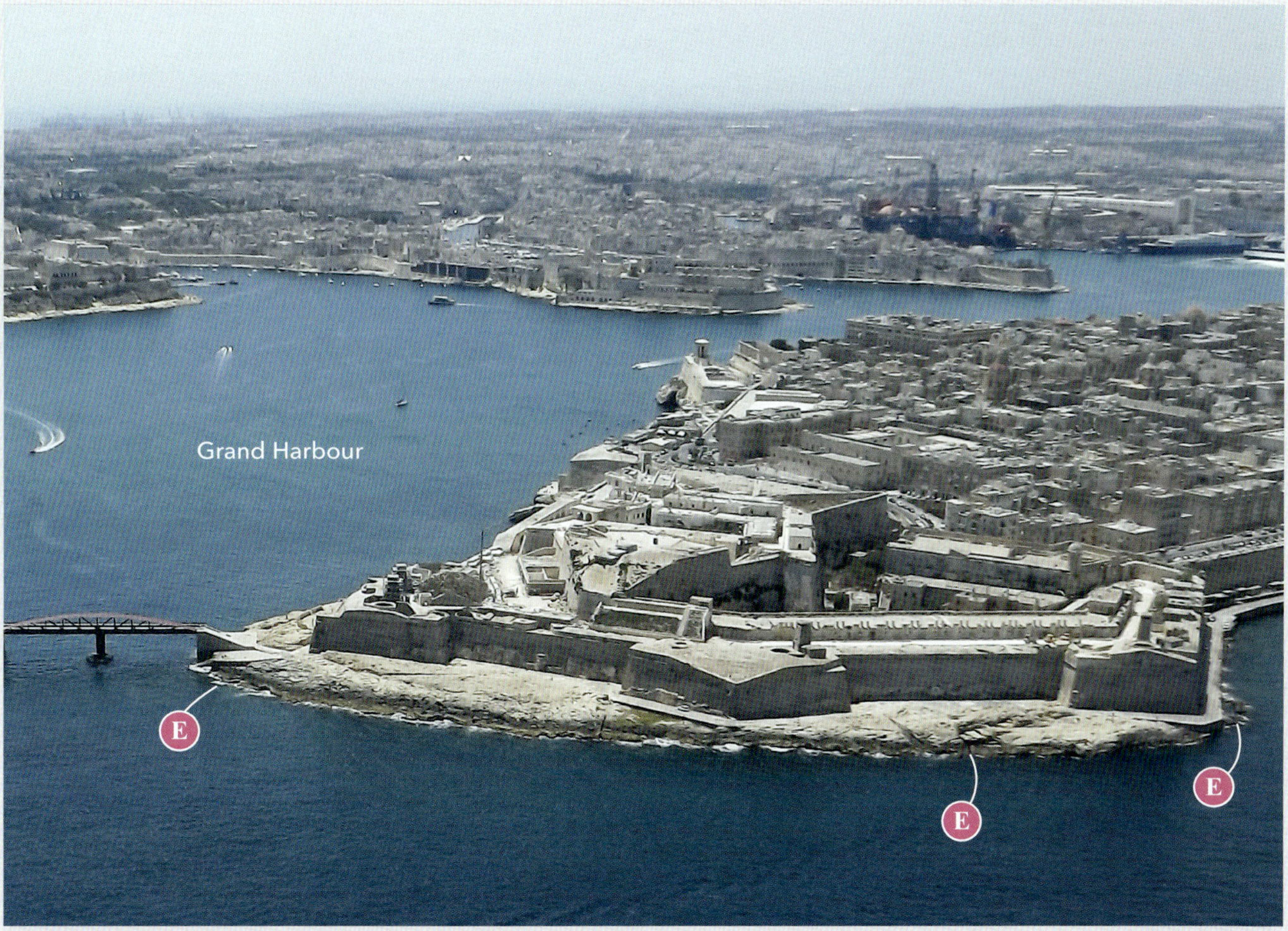

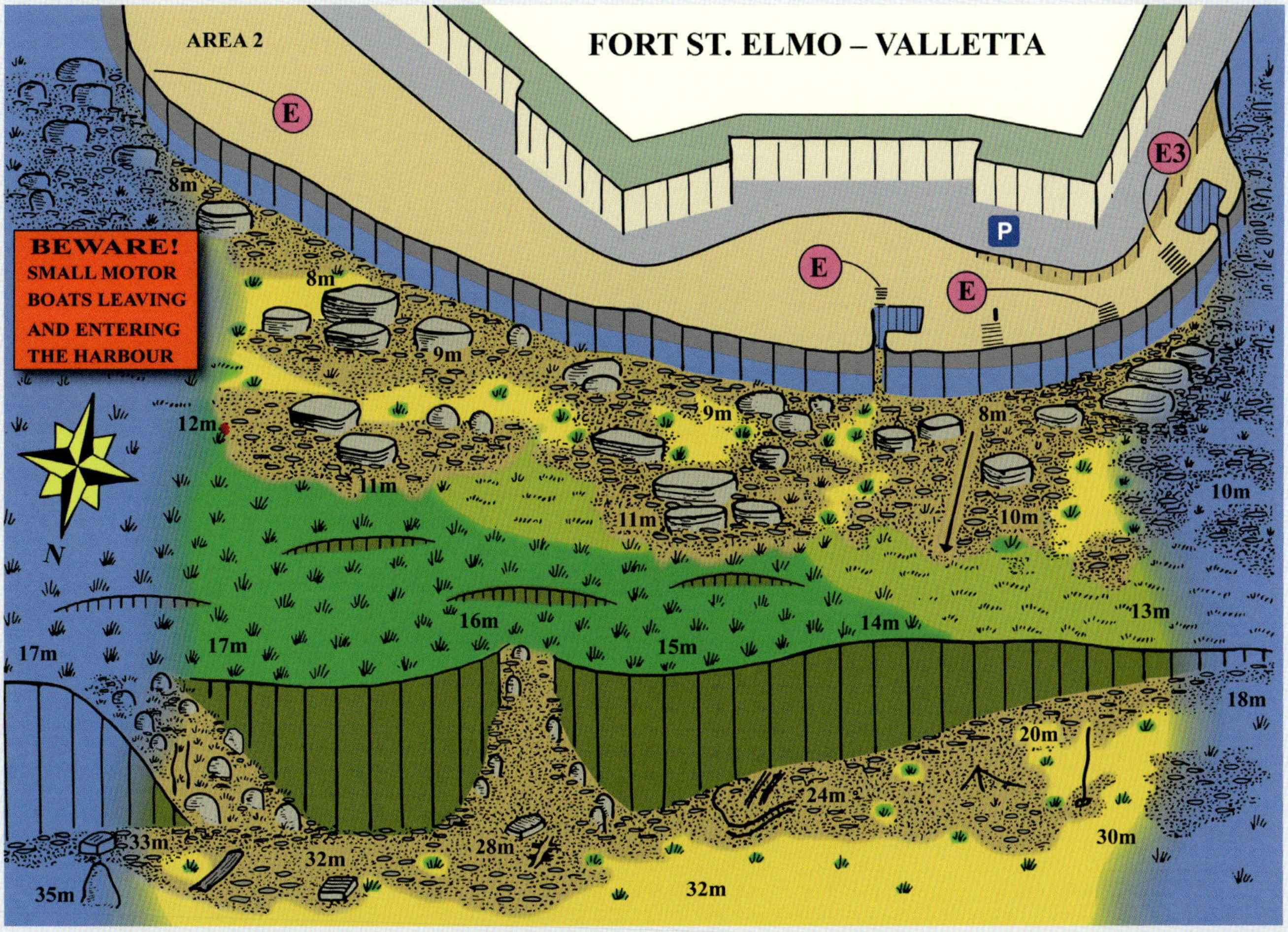

FORT ST. ELMO – VALLETTA
AREA 2
E
E3
P
E
E
BEWARE!
SMALL MOTOR
BOATS LEAVING
AND ENTERING
THE HARBOUR
N
8m
8m
9m
12m
9m
8m
11m
11m
10m
10m
13m
16m
14m
17m
15m
17m
18m
20m
24m
33m
28m
32m
30m
35m
32m

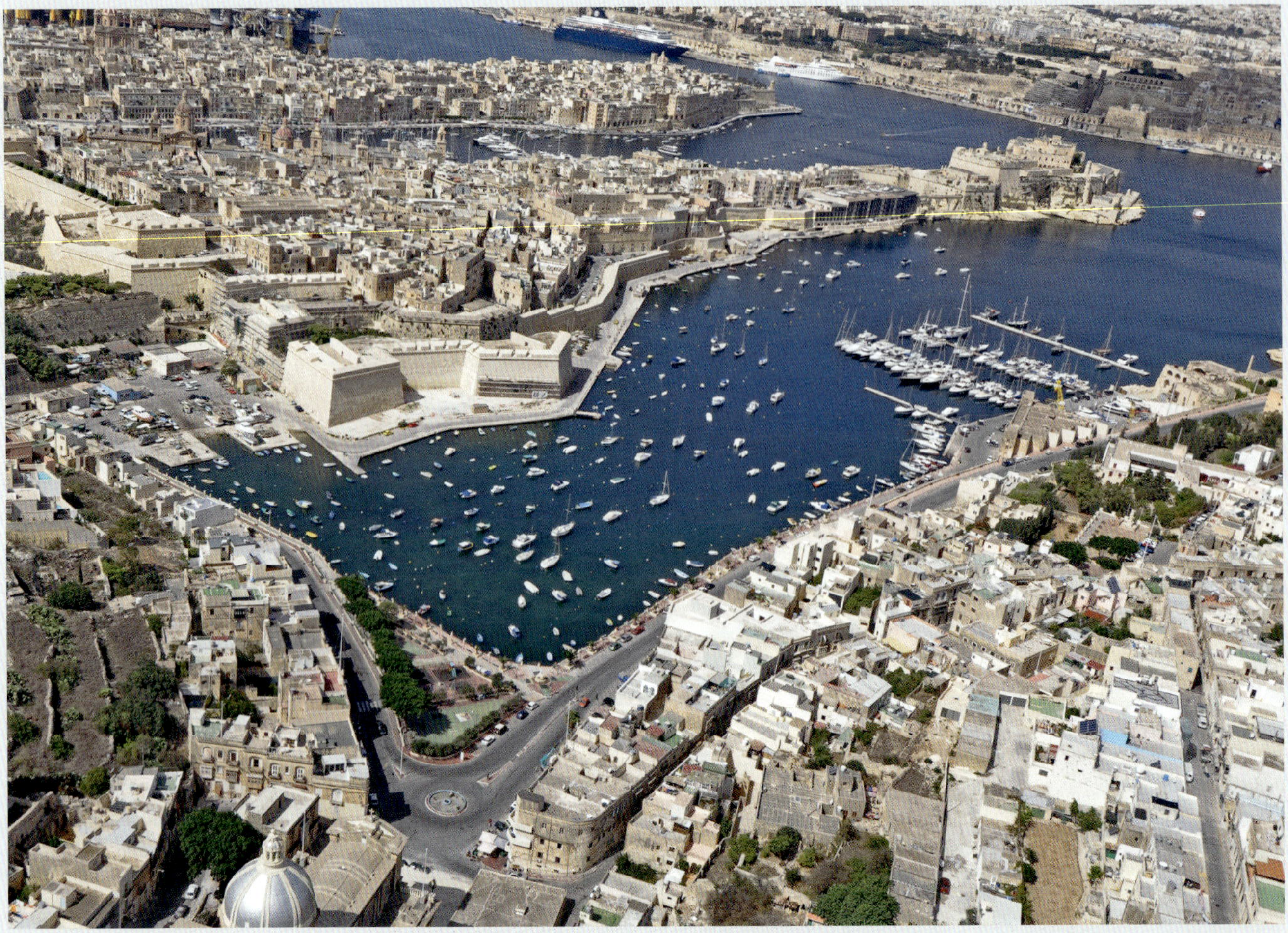

SS *MARGIT* - KALKARA CREEK

PHOTO: PGL AERIAL PHOTOS

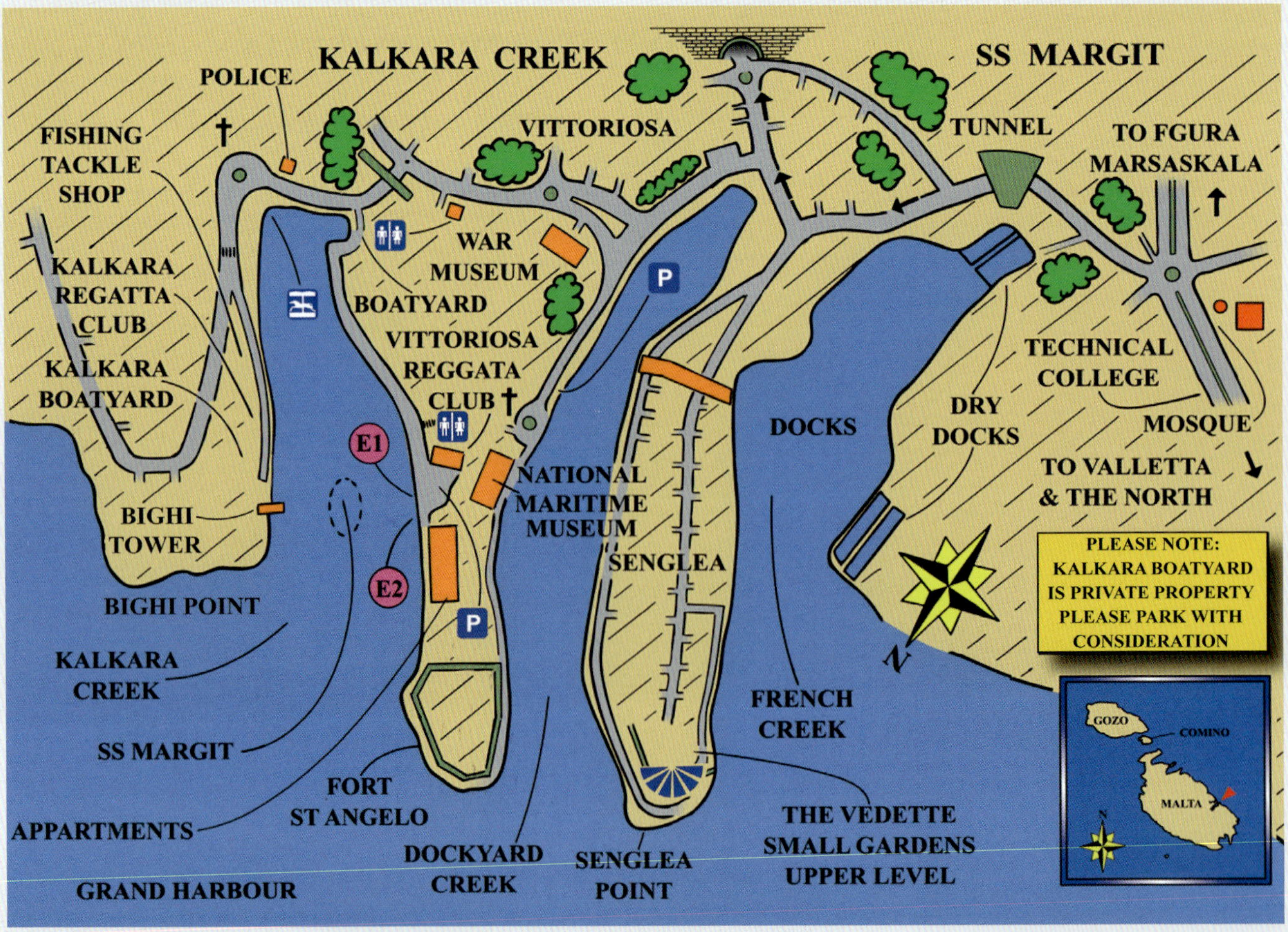

KALKARA CREEK — **SS MARGIT**

- POLICE
- FISHING TACKLE SHOP
- KALKARA REGATTA CLUB
- KALKARA BOATYARD
- BIGHI TOWER
- BIGHI POINT
- KALKARA CREEK
- SS MARGIT
- APPARTMENTS
- GRAND HARBOUR
- VITTORIOSA
- WAR MUSEUM
- BOATYARD
- VITTORIOSA REGGATA CLUB
- E1
- E2
- NATIONAL MARITIME MUSEUM
- SENGLEA
- FORT ST ANGELO
- DOCKYARD CREEK
- SENGLEA POINT
- DOCKS
- FRENCH CREEK
- THE VEDETTE SMALL GARDENS UPPER LEVEL
- TUNNEL
- TO FGURA MARSASKALA
- TECHNICAL COLLEGE
- MOSQUE
- DRY DOCKS
- TO VALLETTA & THE NORTH

PLEASE NOTE: KALKARA BOATYARD IS PRIVATE PROPERTY PLEASE PARK WITH CONSIDERATION

GOZO — COMINO — MALTA

SS *Margit* - Kalkara Creek

Kalkara Creek is situated on the eastern side of Grand Harbour on the opposite side of the water to Valletta. On one side of the creek is the city of Vittoriosa and on the lower-level road is their Regatta Club, here along the water's edge is your parking area right next to entry points E1 & E2. On the opposite side of the creek is the old Bighi Hospital, now after several years of development is the Esplora, Malta's Interactive Science Centre for all the family.

The SS *Margit* sits upright at a depth of 22m on a silty seabed and lies under the main channel so boat traffic is a problem if you need to surface above the wreck, a DSMB would be required.

The puzzle of its name - SS *Odile*

This 3496-ton passenger ship 105.5 metres in length with a 13.7 metre beam was built in 1912 by Forges & Chantiers de la Mediteranee at La Seyne (Yard No. 1055) and named 'Theodore Mante' over the next twenty-seven years her name was changed several times, in 1939 she was re-named Margit and arrived in Malta on April 17th the same year from Marseilles under a Panamanian flag. She stayed in Malta for the next two years, when war broke out. During the early hours of 19th April 1941 while moored to buoy No. 14 at the entrance to Kalkara Creek, during an air raid, she was hit, set on fire, listed to port and sank. Only her two masts remained sticking out of the water to mark her grave, in 1943 the two masts and her funnel were removed by explosives, this was to make anchorage available for use during the forthcoming invasion of Sicily. Wreck No 37448 Admiralty Chart HN/52.

Many Maltese in post-war years claimed that the ship sunk at No. 14 buoy on the 19th April 1941 was the ex-Italian ship Odile. In the mid-1980s the National War Museum Association of Malta made an investigation about this merchant ship, there was no Italian ship named Odile during the war – indeed there was no ship of that name in WW2. The only Odile that could be traced, was a 3206 GRT steamer built in 1907 which was re-named Katvaldis in 1929/1930; as Katvaldis, she was torpedoed and sunk in the Atlantic on 24th August 1942.

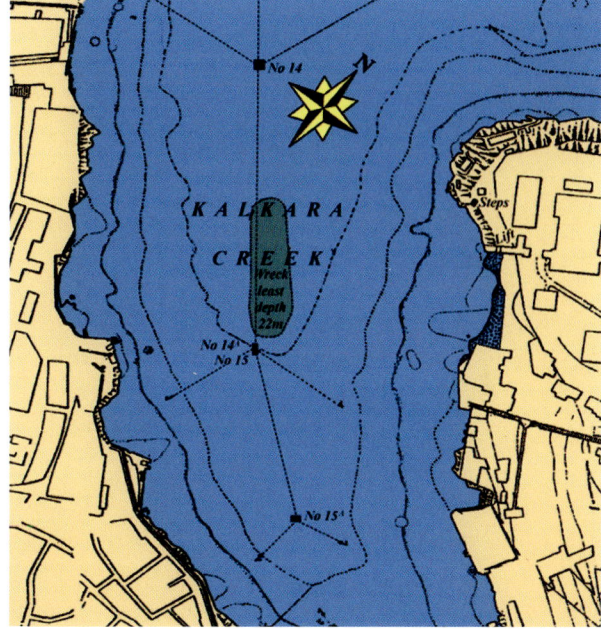

A chart of Kalkara Creek showing the wreck of the SS Margit and the network of mooring chains.

Below: The entry and exit points for the SS Margit on the west side of Kalkara Creek, in the background Malta's capital Valletta and the entrance to Grand Harbour.

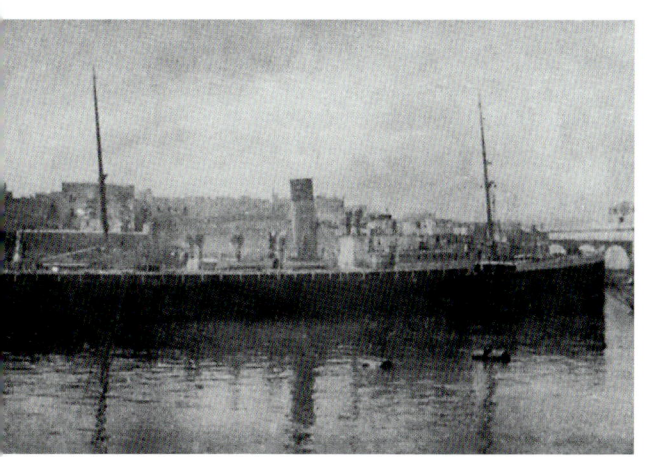

SS Margit in Kalkara Creek, with fort St Angelo in the background.

PHOTO: BY KIND PERISSION OF JOSEPH CARUANA
THE MALTA MARTIME MUSEUM

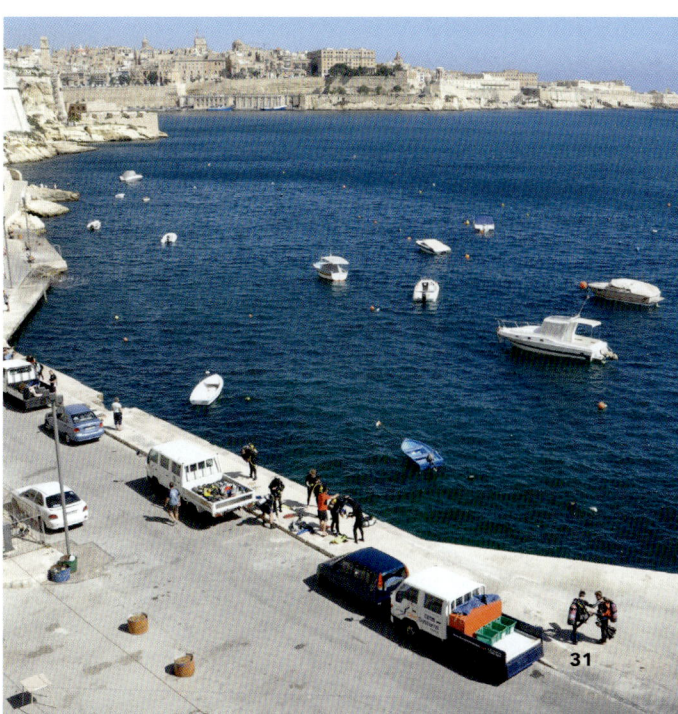

How did this name *Odile* come about?

On the 9th June 1940 the Italian steamer SS *Rodi* arrived in Malta, when Italy declared war on the 10th June, she was seized by the Contraband Control Service Malta. She was moored to No. 14 buoy, when on the 9th July 1940 the Royal Navy took her and other merchant ships to Alexandria so that they were not caught up in the war. The Rodi was taken away; she was renamed the Empire Patrol and was sunk in 1945. She was replaced at No. 14 buoy by the Margit.

Up to here is fact.

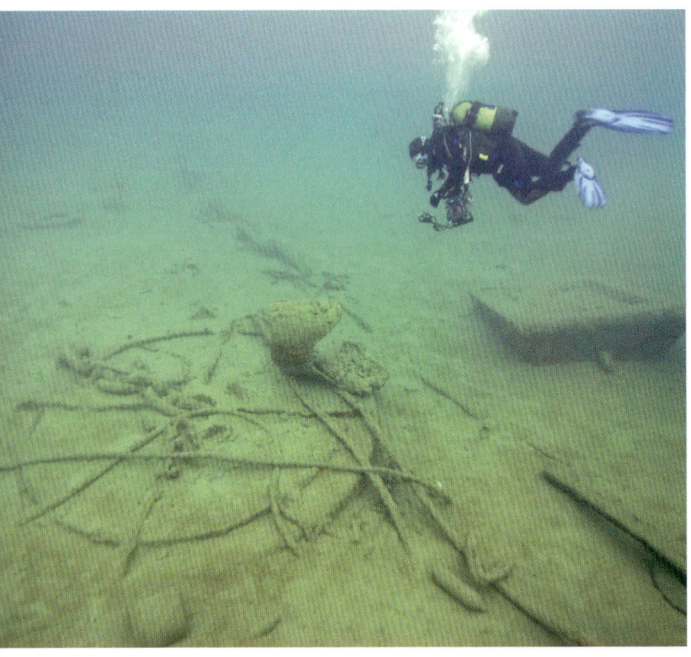

A diver hovers over a large sunken mooring buoy these can be seen on the surface with Battleship at the Malta Experience visual spectacular show, in Valletta.

Below: The engine room of the SS Margit and the top part of the pistons with the driving cogs below.

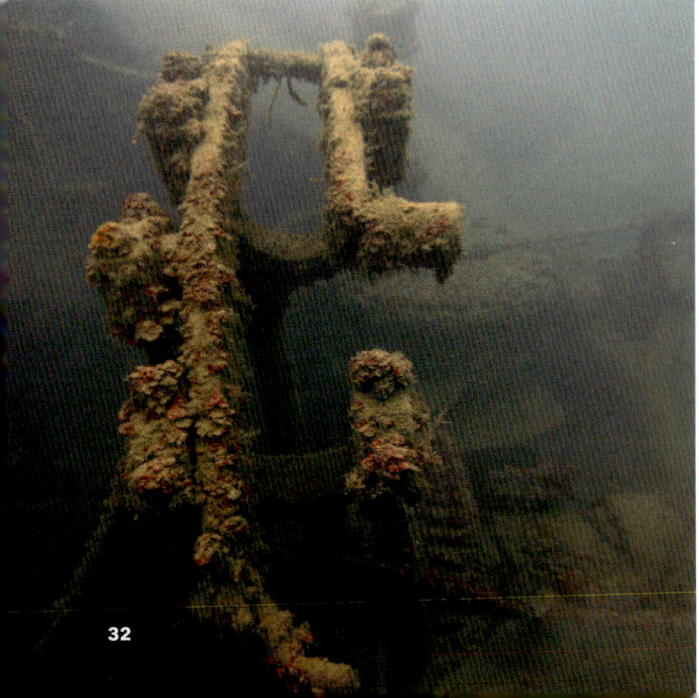

What follows is conjecture!

Note:

Rodi has 3 letters in sequence ODI - RODI
Odile has 3 letters in sequence ODI – ODILE

Now in June 1940 the British authorities suspected Malta was a hive of Italian spies. So, perhaps, to mislead these spies, they painted out the R of *RODI* and added LE, thus making the ship apparently to be named the *ODILE* and was so seen by the Maltese. Shortly after this time most of the inhabitants of Bighi and Kalkara were evacuated to the country, so that when they returned, they failed to realise that the ship which was moored at No. 14 buoy was not the same ex-Italian ship that was there before they were evacuated – one could well imagine that 2 years of rust had made the ships; name unreadable. So, they continued to think that the ship was the one they knew as the ex-Italian named *RODI*.

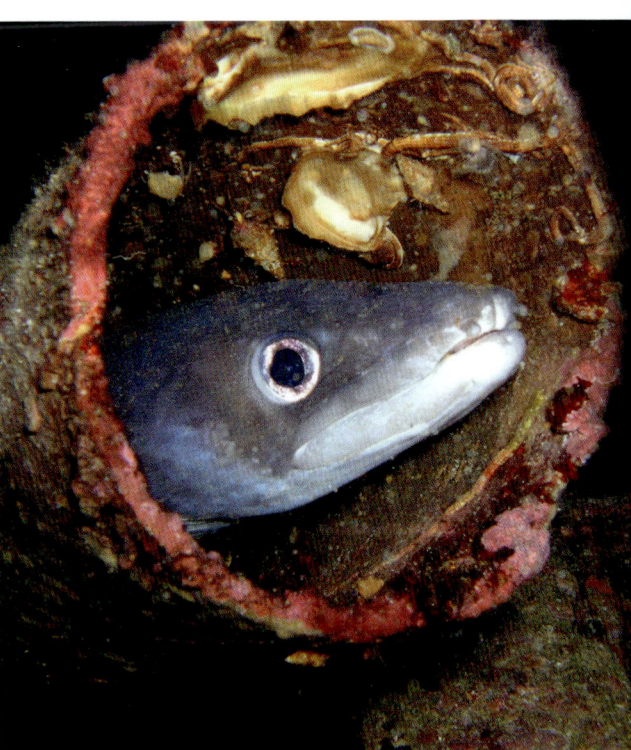

Conger eel (Conger conger, Linnaeus) are experts in finding good hiding places within wrecks.

THE DIVES — Minimum time - 50 mins

This is a great dive although within the harbour, it is still possible to get good visibility but not if there is a strong north easterly wind or you are following a large group of divers. The best time to dive this wreck is when sea conditions are good elsewhere. The normal rule is if you can see the seabed at your entry point then the visibility should be reasonable.

From E1 or E2 surface swim to the starboard buoy (green) or use the transits on the dive site plan, do not stray into the channel it can be busy.

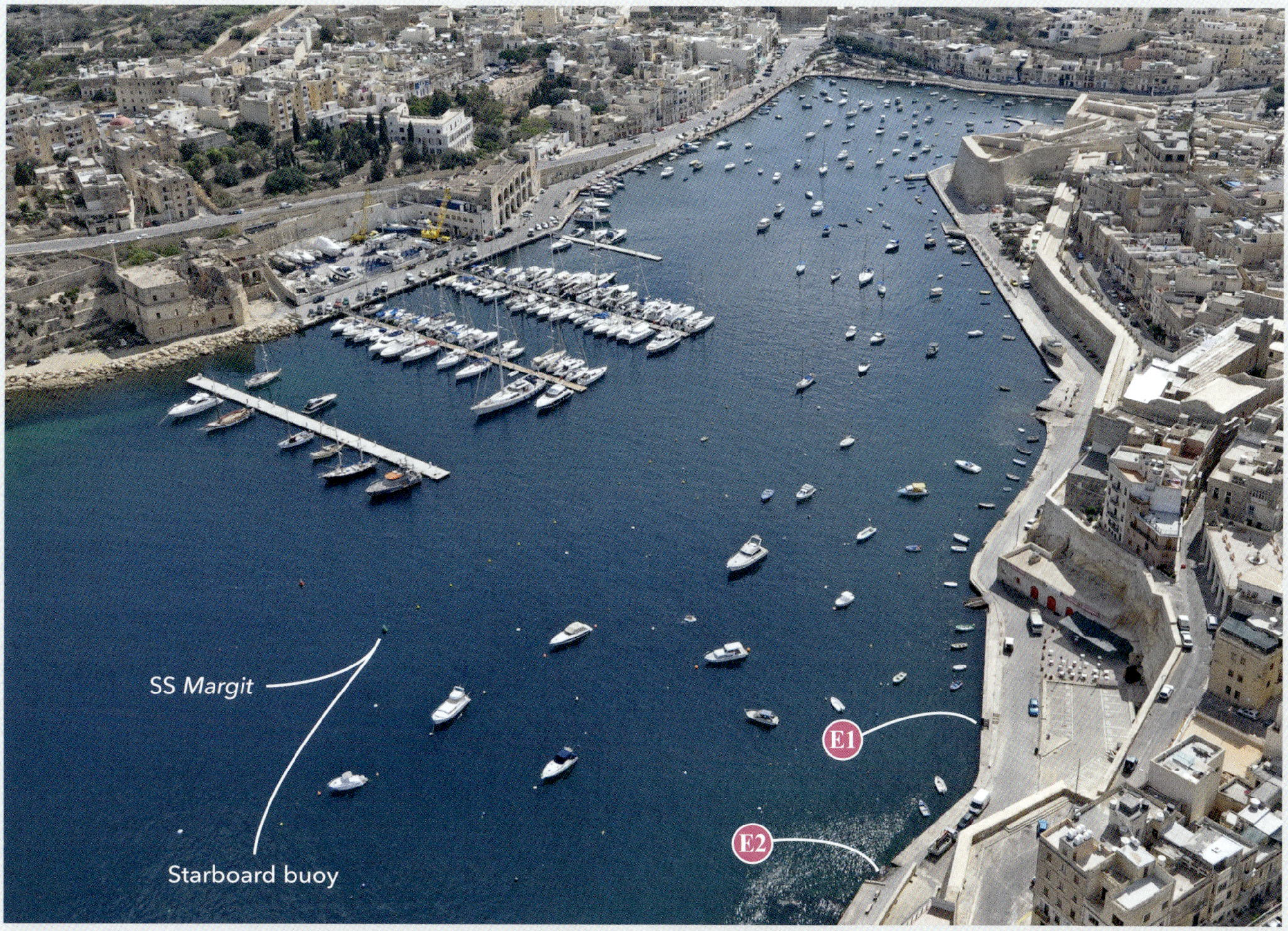

SS *MARGIT* - KALKARA CREEK

SS Margit

Starboard buoy

E1

E2

PHOTO: PGL AERIAL PHOTOS

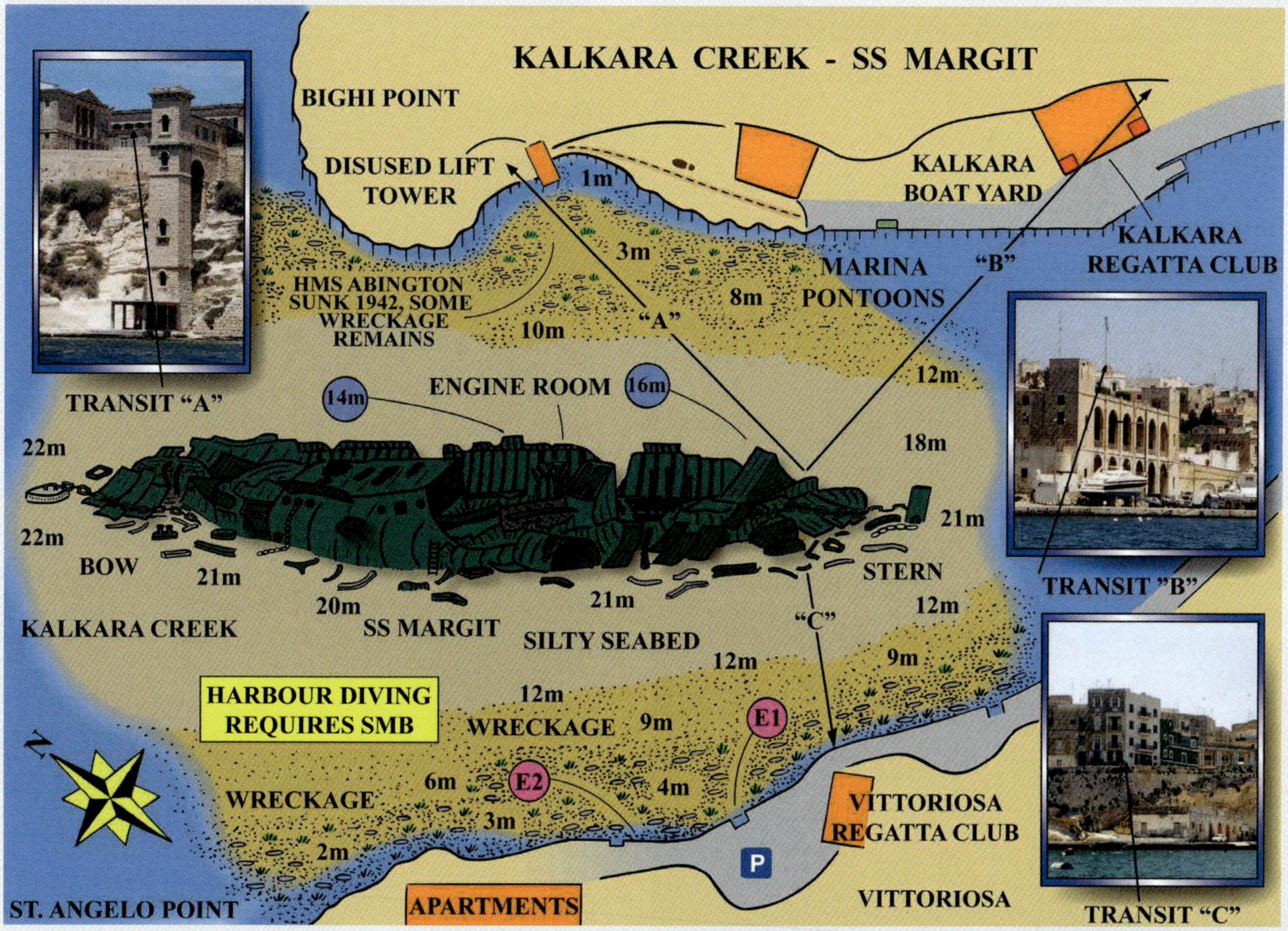

KALKARA CREEK - SS MARGIT

BIGHI POINT

DISUSED LIFT TOWER

1m

KALKARA BOAT YARD

TRANSIT "A"

3m

HMS ABINGTON SUNK 1942, SOME WRECKAGE REMAINS

"A"

8m

MARINA PONTOONS

"B"

KALKARA REGATTA CLUB

10m

14m ENGINE ROOM 16m

12m

18m

22m

21m

TRANSIT "B"

22m BOW 21m

20m

SS MARGIT

21m

STERN

21m

12m

KALKARA CREEK

SILTY SEABED

"C"

9m

HARBOUR DIVING REQUIRES SMB

12m

WRECKAGE

9m

E1

WRECKAGE

6m

E2

4m

VITTORIOSA REGATTA CLUB

3m

2m

ST. ANGELO POINT

APARTMENTS

VITTORIOSA

TRANSIT "C"

SS MARGIT - KALKARA CREEK

You can of course descend at your entry point and swim under the water to the wreck, to do this you will need the following compass bearings: from E1 30° from E2 60°.

If you get your transit right, you should land some 25m along the wreck from the stern, if the visibility is not too good, the starboard side of the wreck is the easiest to navigate along, as it is, in places 5m proud of the seabed.

Points to note or look for are: the stern mooring chain, prop shaft, gangway and supports, engine room with the piston rods, upper structure of the forward deck the bow mooring buoy and chain.

There are a variety of fish on the wreck including groupers, but look out for nudibranchs, to see these colourful little creatures on this silt covered wreck is quite remarkable.

Return route to the E1 and E2 once away from the wreck set your compass at 230° it will take you at least five minutes to clear the level silty seabed which will give way to a sandy bottom which gently slopes upwards, it will take you a about five minutes to reach a depth of 9m and less. Just off the harbour wall around this depth are small areas of wreckage, small rocks also a little reef, lots to explore and the wall itself is alive with marine life, soft corals, cuttlefish, small morays, sea hares and many other small fish, a really good area for macro photography.

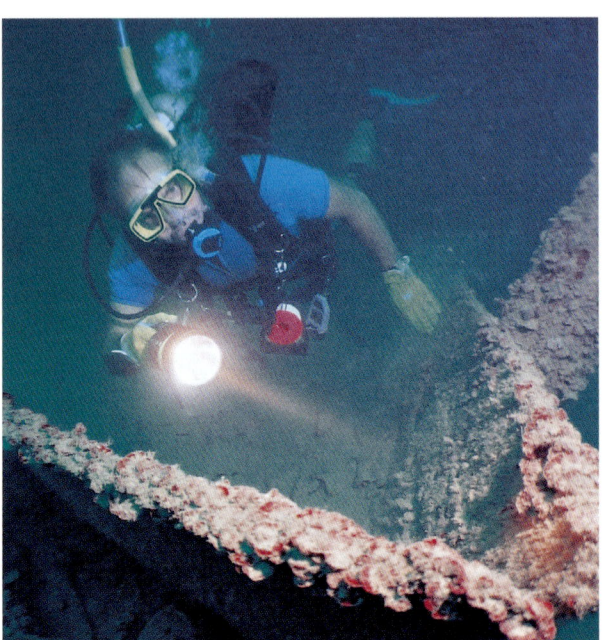

One of the ships lifeboats now covered in soft coral.

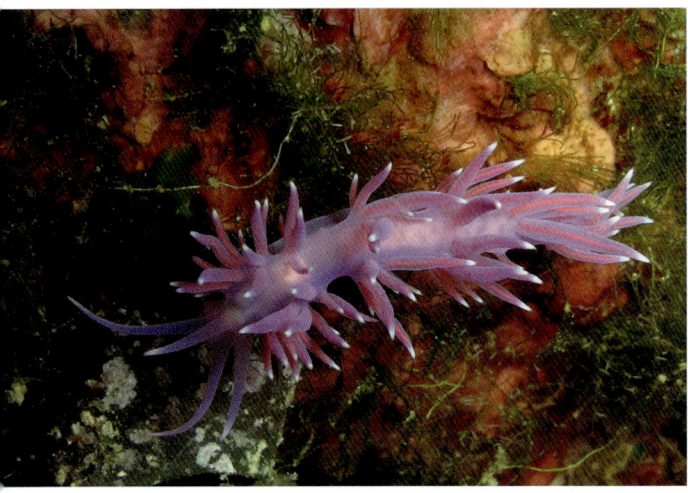

Colourful nudibranch (Flabellina affinis) can sometimes be found in very unusual places. PHOTO: JOE FORMOSA

Below: Just me taking photographs of the wreckage, fantastic visibility on this particular day. PHOTO: SHARON FORDER

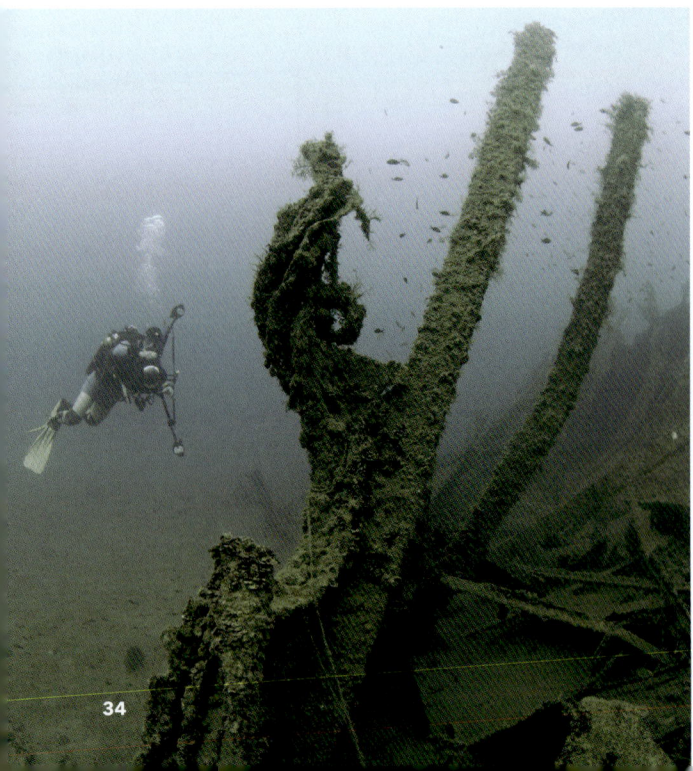

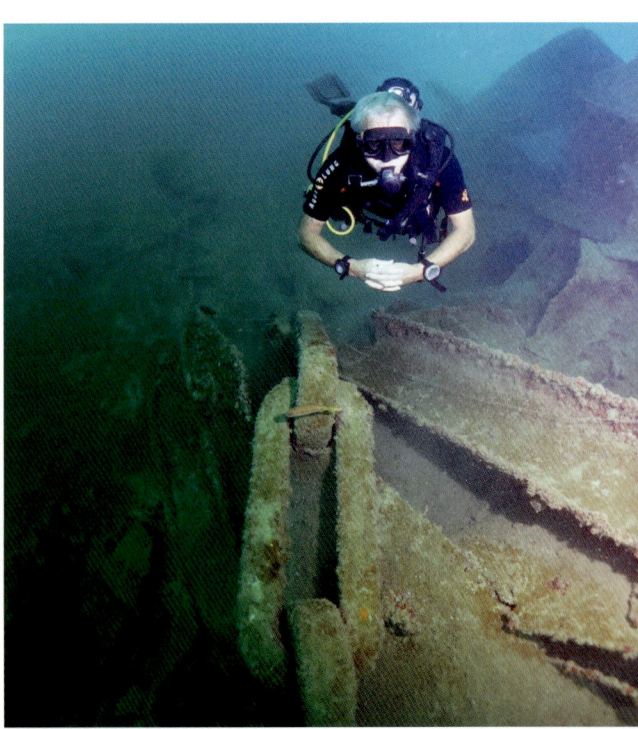

A diver following the route of this massive mooring chain, over the wreckage of SS Margit.

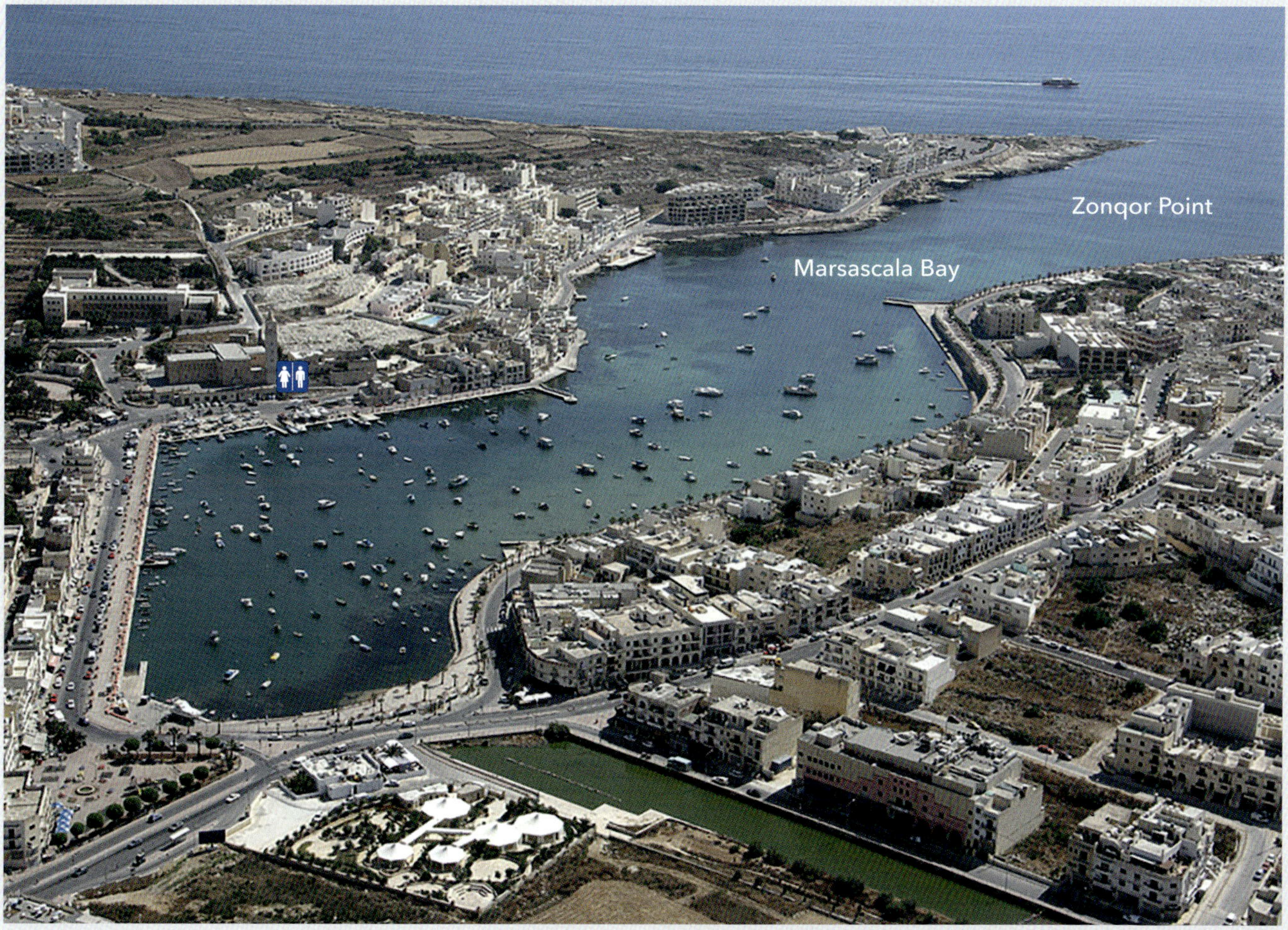

TUGBOATS - ZONQOR POINT - MARSASCALA

Zonqor Point
Marsascala Bay

PHOTO: PGL AERIAL PHOTOS

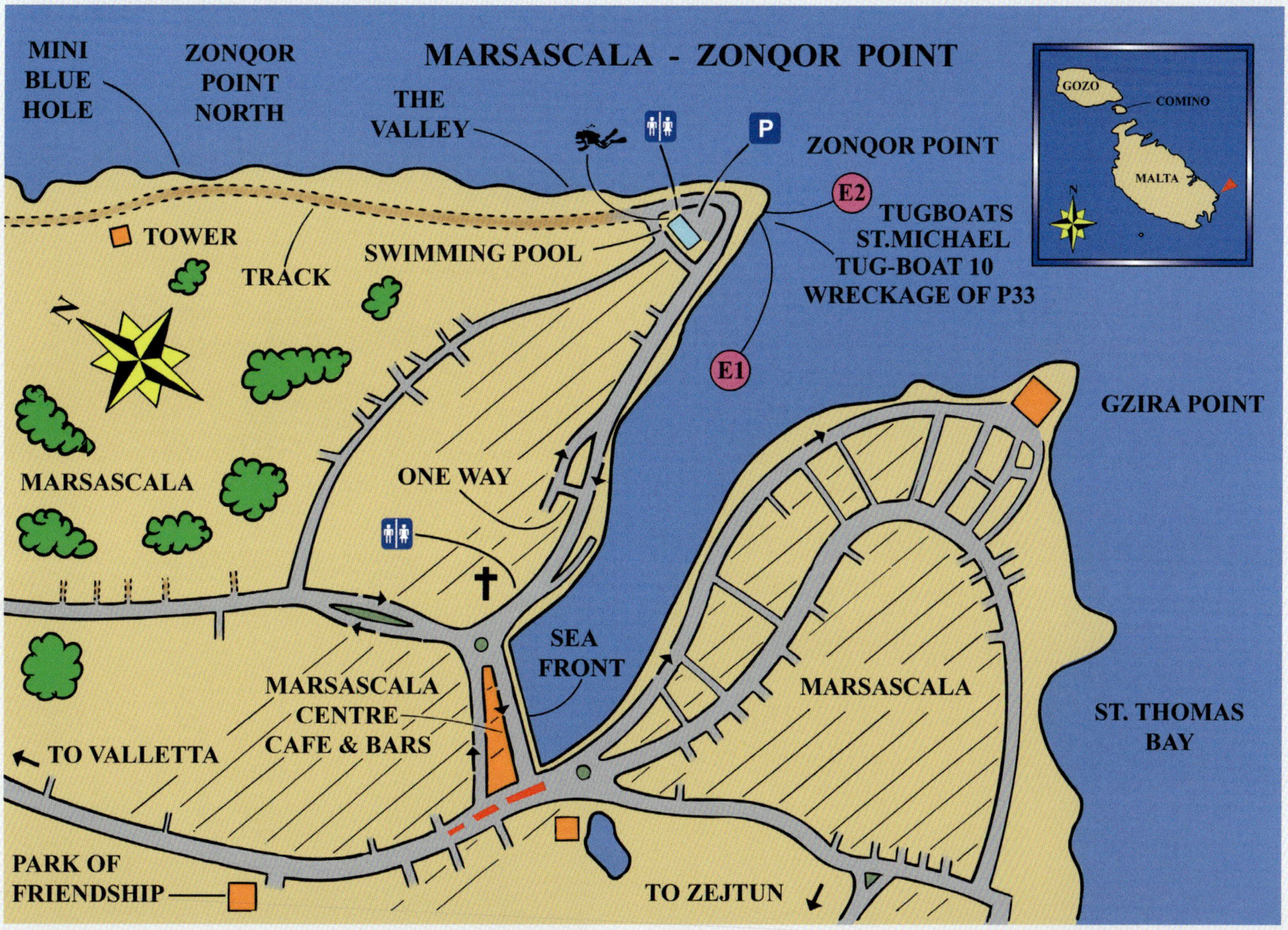

MARSASCALA - ZONQOR POINT

- MINI BLUE HOLE
- ZONQOR POINT NORTH
- THE VALLEY
- ZONQOR POINT
- E2
- TUGBOATS
- ST. MICHAEL
- TUG-BOAT 10
- WRECKAGE OF P33
- TOWER
- TRACK
- SWIMMING POOL
- E1
- GZIRA POINT
- MARSASCALA
- ONE WAY
- SEA FRONT
- MARSASCALA
- ST. THOMAS BAY
- MARSASCALA CENTRE CAFE & BARS
- TO VALLETTA
- PARK OF FRIENDSHIP
- TO ZEJTUN

GOZO — COMINO — MALTA

Tugboats - *P33* - Zonqor Point - Marsascala

Situated on the south east coast of Malta, on the north side of the entrance to Marsascala bay is an area of land jutting out into the sea, this is called Zonqor Point. When driving into Marsascala from Valletta watch out for the central reservation, for then you will need to turn left into a one-way system before you reach the harbour, this route will take you along the north side of Marsascala bay to Zonqor Point. On your return the one-way system takes you past the cafes and little bars on the water front. At Zonqor Point there is a large swimming pool, once Malta's National Pool, a new Olympic sized pool and complex is situated between Valletta and Sliema, near the University.

Within this area there are a number of dive sites, I have selected the tugboats *St Michael*, Tugboat *10* and the *P33* Patrol boat these can be completed in one dive, this is an excellent site to test your navigation skills. Other sites include the Mini Blue Hole and Zonqor North. These dives all add to the variety of diving on the island, away from the busy dive sites. Though it tends to be more crowded when sea conditions elsewhere are not good.

Tugboats: *St Michael* - Tugboat *10*

The two tug boats, *St Michael* and *10* were scuttled on the 16th May 1998 as part of a plan to create an artificial reef at Zonqor Point in Marsascala. At a depth of 21m and 22m they are upright on a flat sandy bottom and have created an oasis for marine life, transforming an ecologically barren area into a shore dive location which is accessible to divers of all levels. The site is particularly well chosen because it is protected from the prevailing northwesterly winds and can therefore be dived when other areas are unreachable due to bad weather conditions. The two tug boats, 20 and 16 meters in length, saw many years of service, working in and around Grand Harbour. They underwent a clean-up operation, made environmentally and diver friendly all glass, doors and hatches were removed. The preparation, towing and scuttling operations were undertaken by Charles and Anthony Cassar Boat and Ship Repair Ltd of Marsa. They both are now covered with sponges and corals, creating a lovely artificial reef and an oasis for a variety of marine life.

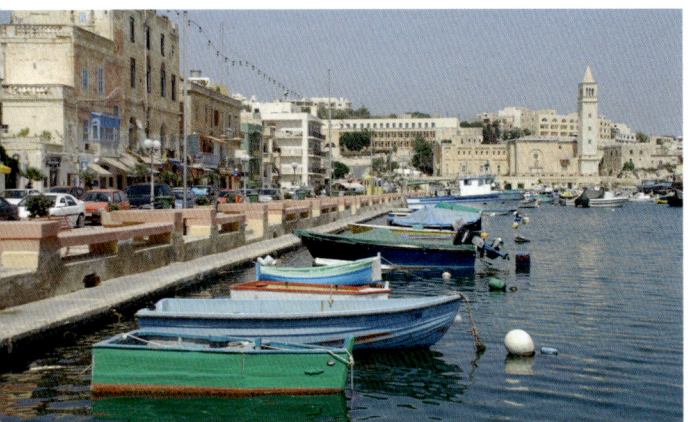

A short drive from the dive site is Marsascala promenade with its many cafes and bars to visit and chill out, after your dive.

Below: A diver above the Tugboat St Michael laying on the sand. PHOTO: ARKADIUZ SREBNIK POLANDDIVINGPHOTO

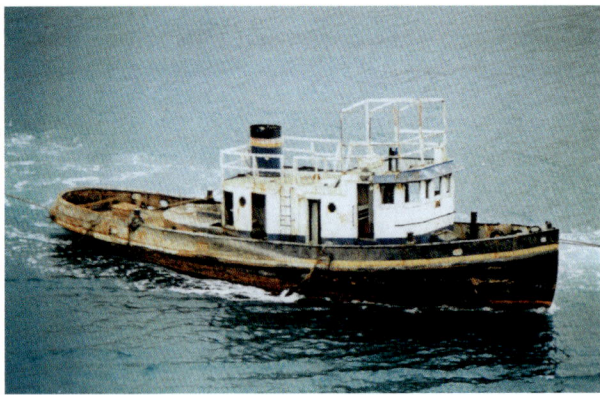

Tugboat St Michael being towed to Marsascala Bay to be Scuttled.
PHOTOS: MARK BALUCI

Below: Tugboat 10 being scuttled in Marsascala Bay Zonqor Point

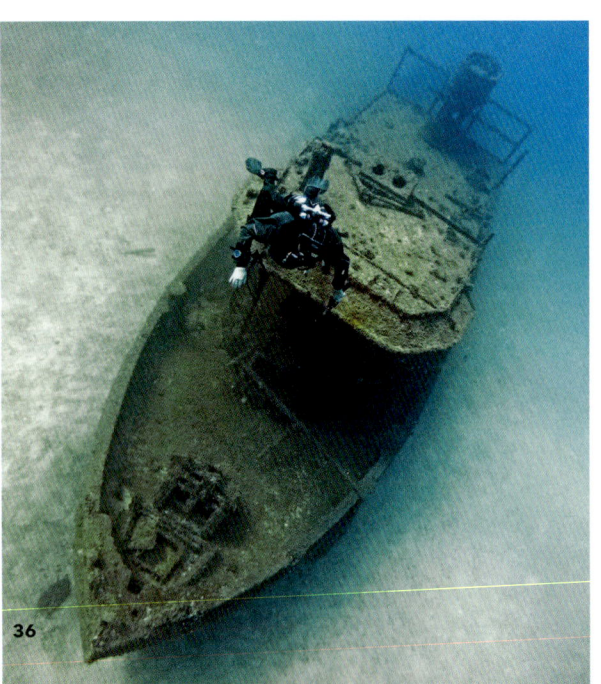

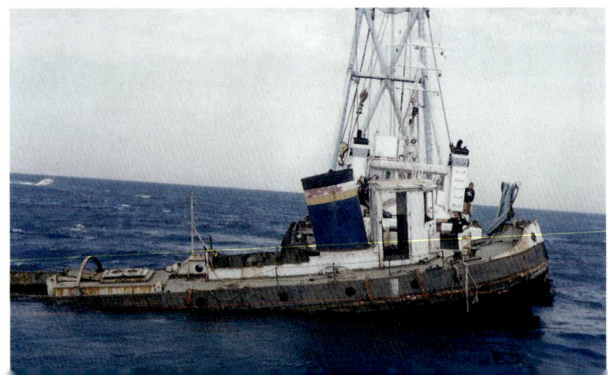

TUGBOATS - ZONQOR POINT - MARSASCALA

P33 Patrol Boat - wreckage

The *P33* was a Bremse class vessel built in 1972 in East Germany 23 metres in length with a beam of 5 metres arrived in Malta in 1972 and served as a patrol boat in the Maritime Squadron of the Armed Forces of Malta until she was decommissioned in 2005. Scuttled between the two tug boats on the 31st July 2021 at a depth of 22m. Unfortunately, due to her lightweight construction the wreck did not stand natures forces for long and has been well broken up by movement of the sea. Now the wreckage lies around the sandy seabed between the two tug boats.

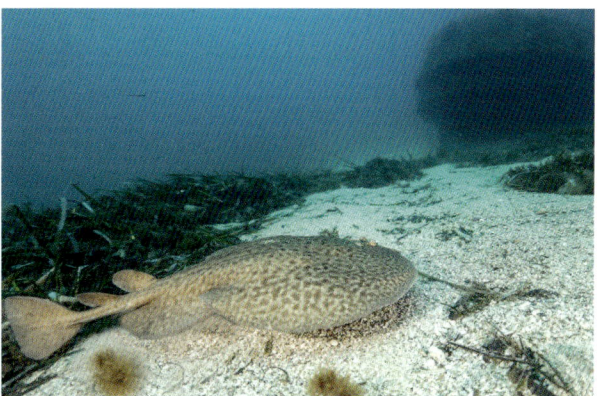

Common torpedo (Torpedo torpedo) near the stern of Tugboat 10. PHOTOS: JURIJS BICKINS DIVE MED

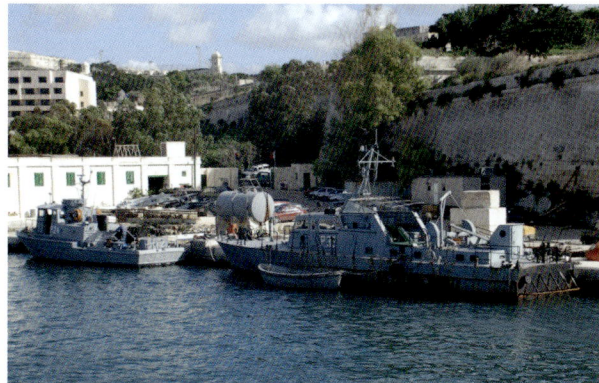

P33 Patrol Boat in Marsamxett harbour at the AFM base.

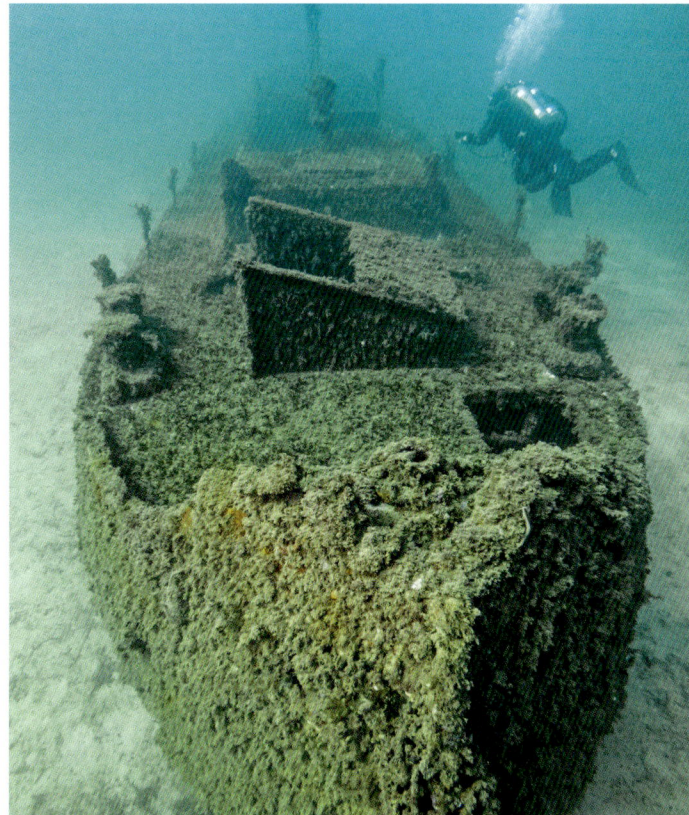

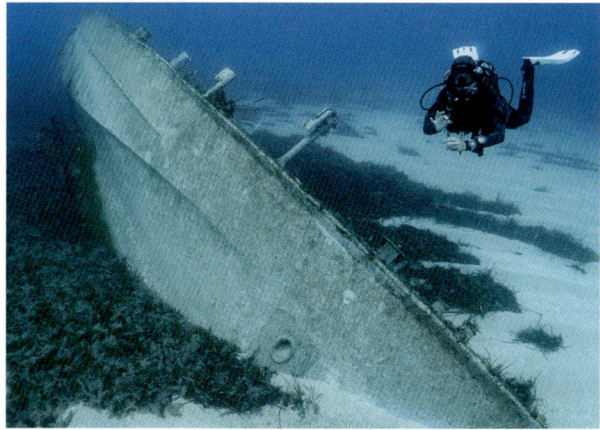

The damaged hull of the P33 after being broken up by a winter storm. PHOTOS: JURIJS BICKINS DIVE MED

Exploring Tugboat 10 now covered in marine growth where many fish and a variety of small living creatures have made their home here. PHOTOS: ARKADIUZ SREBNIK POLANDDIVINGPHOTO

Below: This panorama unusual photo of the P33, shows all the damage.

Below: Tugboat 10 on the sand just off the edge reef at a depth of 21m.

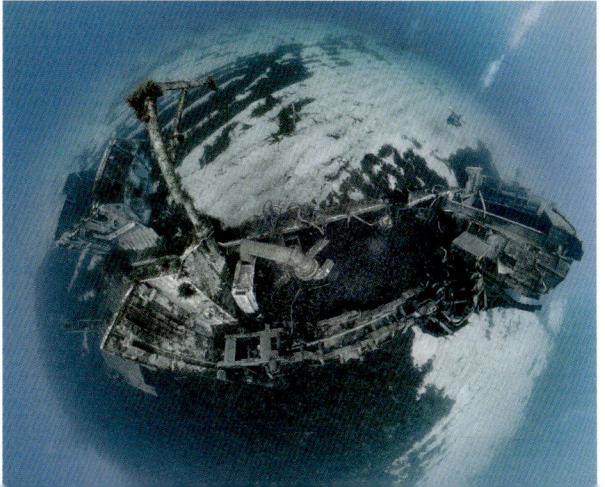

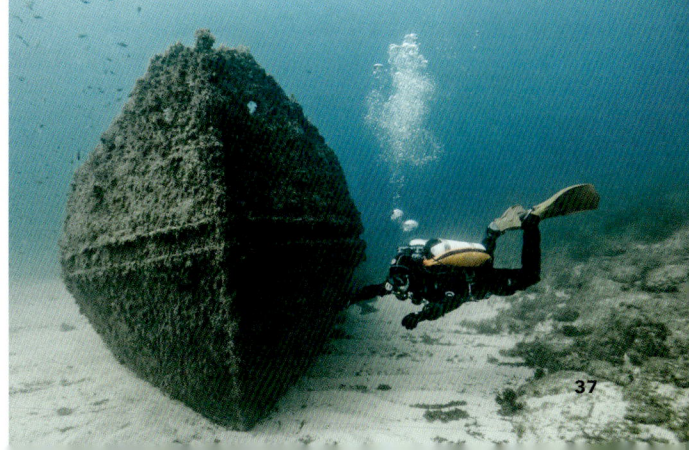

TUGBOATS - ZONQOR POINT - MARSASCALA

THE DIVES — Minimum time 40 mins

Here you have a choice of entry points. The most popular is **entry point E1**, turn right after walking through the gap in the wall, and continue until you are on the lower level just past a ridge which appears on your left, it is now possible to reach the water's edge E1. From here with a compass bearing of 140° and a gentle swim, it will take you some 6/8 minutes, to reach the bottom of the reef where it meets the sand. Your depth could be 18/22m depending on your navigation skills. **Your second choice E2**, is to walk towards the salt pans at the far end, passing between the two little buildings, you will find a distinct cut-out in the shoreline from here your compass bearing is 180°.

Possibly the best way to start this dive is to use the nearest entry point E1, surface swim out until you can just see the reef below you, descend, with a compass bearing of 140° follow the gently sloping reef down to the sand. Once you reach the sand your depth will determine your route 21m you will be close to the Tugboat *10*, 18m or less turn left, 22m or more turn right.

The bows of Tugboat *10* lie on the sand almost against the base of the reef, with its stern some 3 metres away from it.

Beware; the first area of sand may be covered by dead sea-grass making it difficult to determine where the reef ends and the sand starts especially in areas where the depth is 18m or less.

The tugboat *St. Michael* lies 15 metres off the reef and 60 metres off the bow of Tugboat *10*, taking a compass bearing of 90°, once moving off the wreck. Sometimes there is a line attached between the two tugs.

When it is time to head for shallower waters, especially from the *St. Michael*, take a compass bearing of 330° / 300° and follow the reef up to your required depth. At 9m and 6m and possibly below the furthest entry point, E2, the rocks and seabed are covered with marine growth of many colours and this makes an excellent area for photography. This is also an ideal place to test your skills in finding octopus and other marine life. To the west of the nearest entry point, E1, the reef becomes more rugged, but beware of the local fishermen if you travel too far along the reef in this direction before you exit the water.

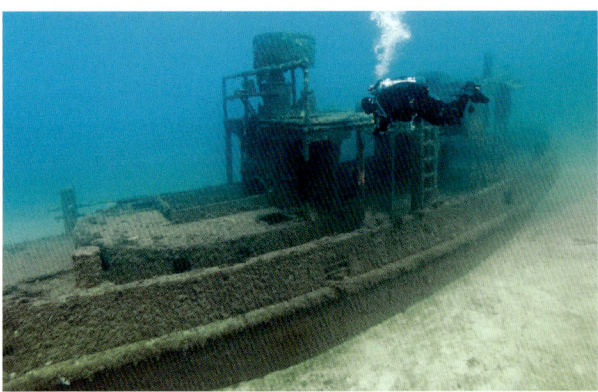

The starboard side of the Tugboat St Michael on the sand at 22m.   PHOTO: ARKADIUZ SREBNIK POLANDDIVINGPHOTO

Below: A view from the stern of the Tugboat St Michael.

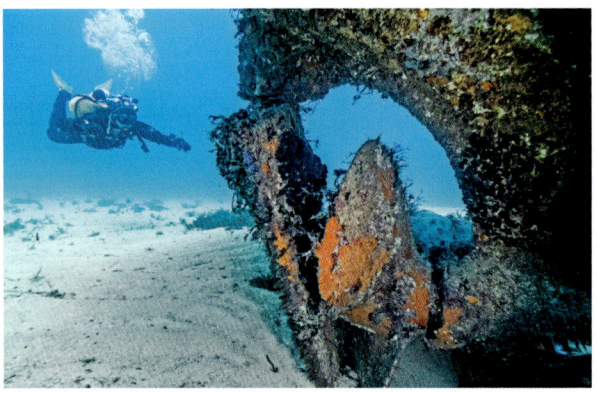

The propeller and rudder of the largest Tugboat St Michael.
PHOTO: ARKADIUZ SREBNIK POLANDDIVINGPHOTO

Below: Two-banded sea bream (Diplodus vulgaris) these shoals of fish and other marine life have made their home on the St Michael.

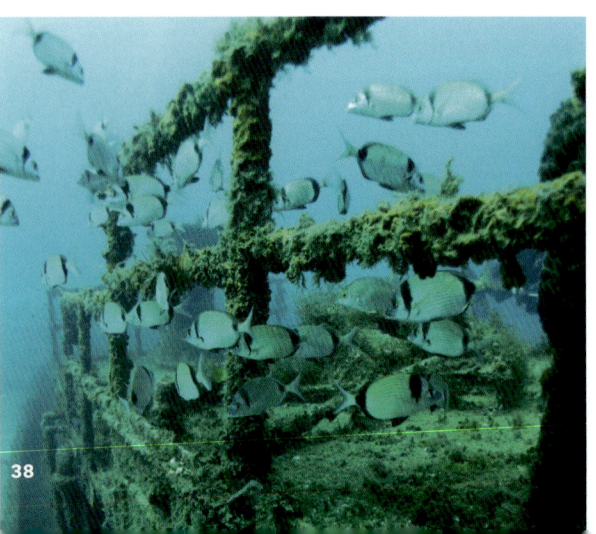

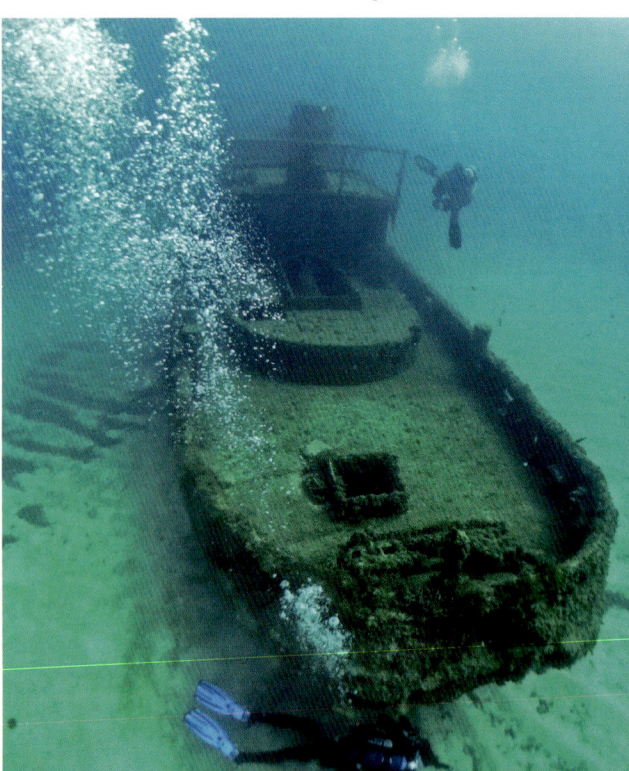

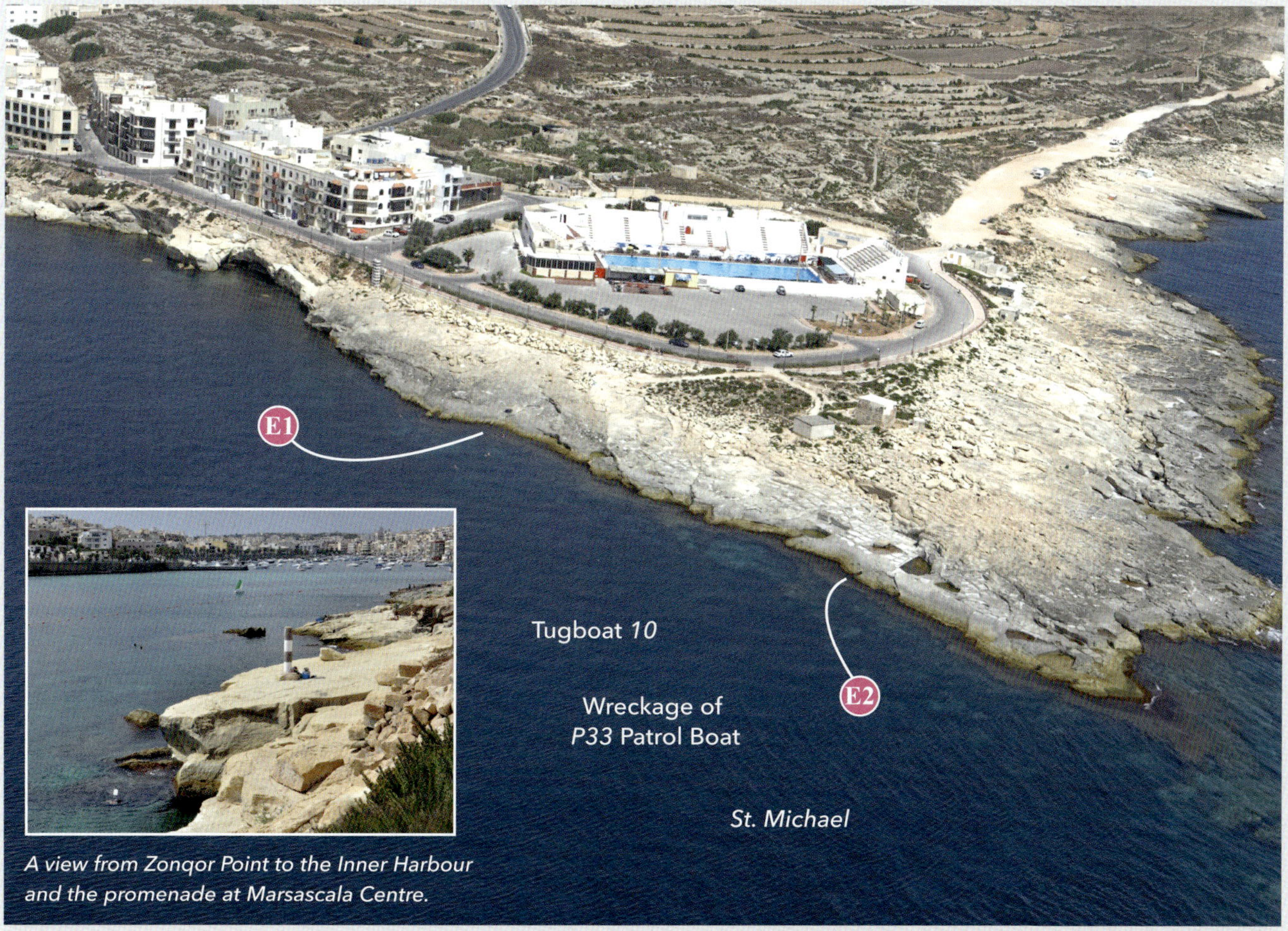

MARSASCALA - ZONQOR POINT

E1

Tugboat 10

Wreckage of P33 Patrol Boat

E2

St. Michael

A view from Zonqor Point to the Inner Harbour and the promenade at Marsascala Centre.

PHOTO: PGL AERIAL PHOTOS

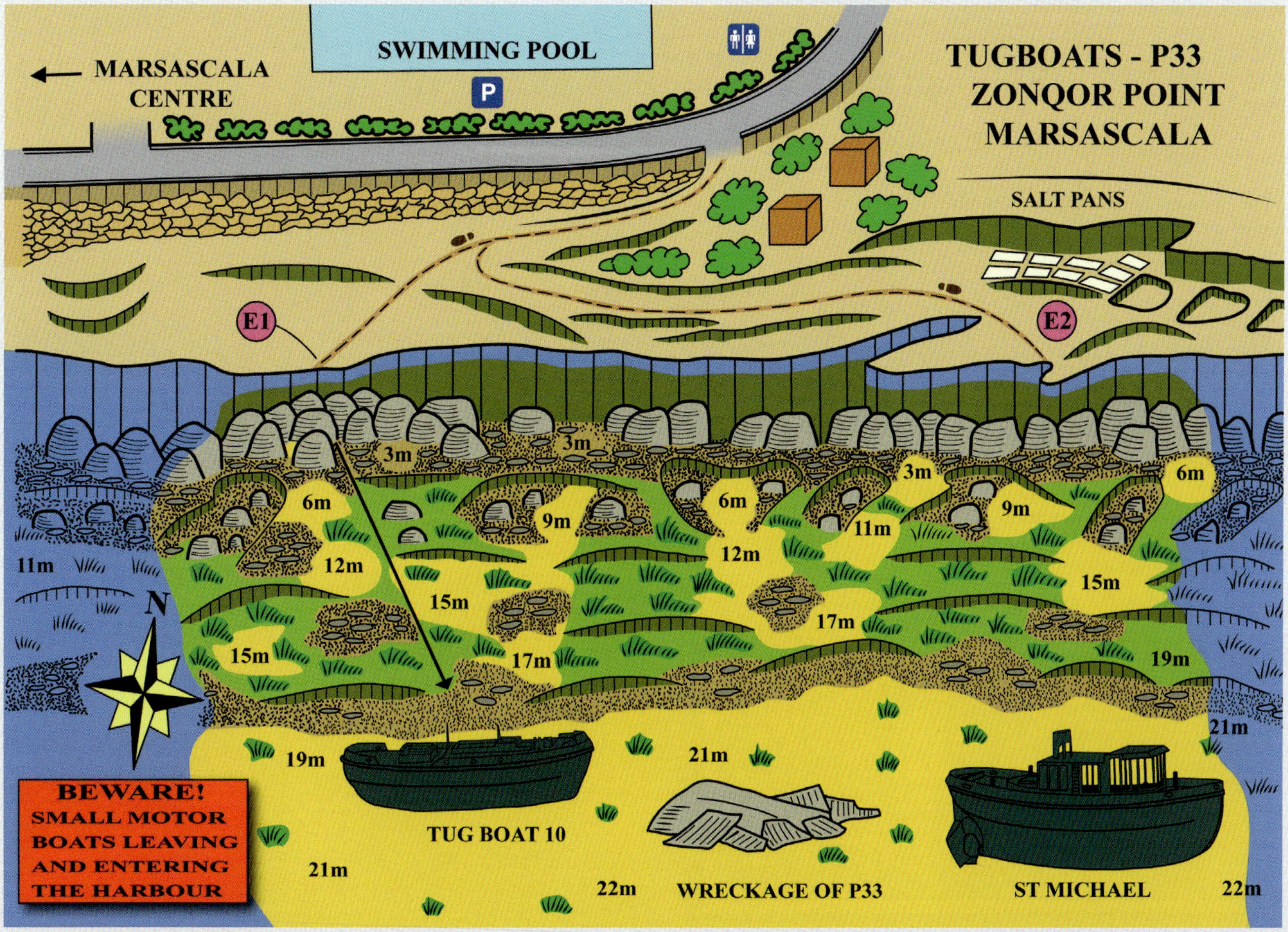

← MARSASCALA CENTRE

SWIMMING POOL

TUGBOATS - P33 ZONQOR POINT MARSASCALA

SALT PANS

E1

E2

3m, 3m, 6m, 9m, 6m, 3m, 9m, 6m
11m, 12m, 12m, 11m, 15m
15m, 15m, 17m, 17m, 19m
19m, 21m, 21m
21m

BEWARE! SMALL MOTOR BOATS LEAVING AND ENTERING THE HARBOUR

TUG BOAT 10 — 21m
WRECKAGE OF P33 — 22m
ST MICHAEL — 22m

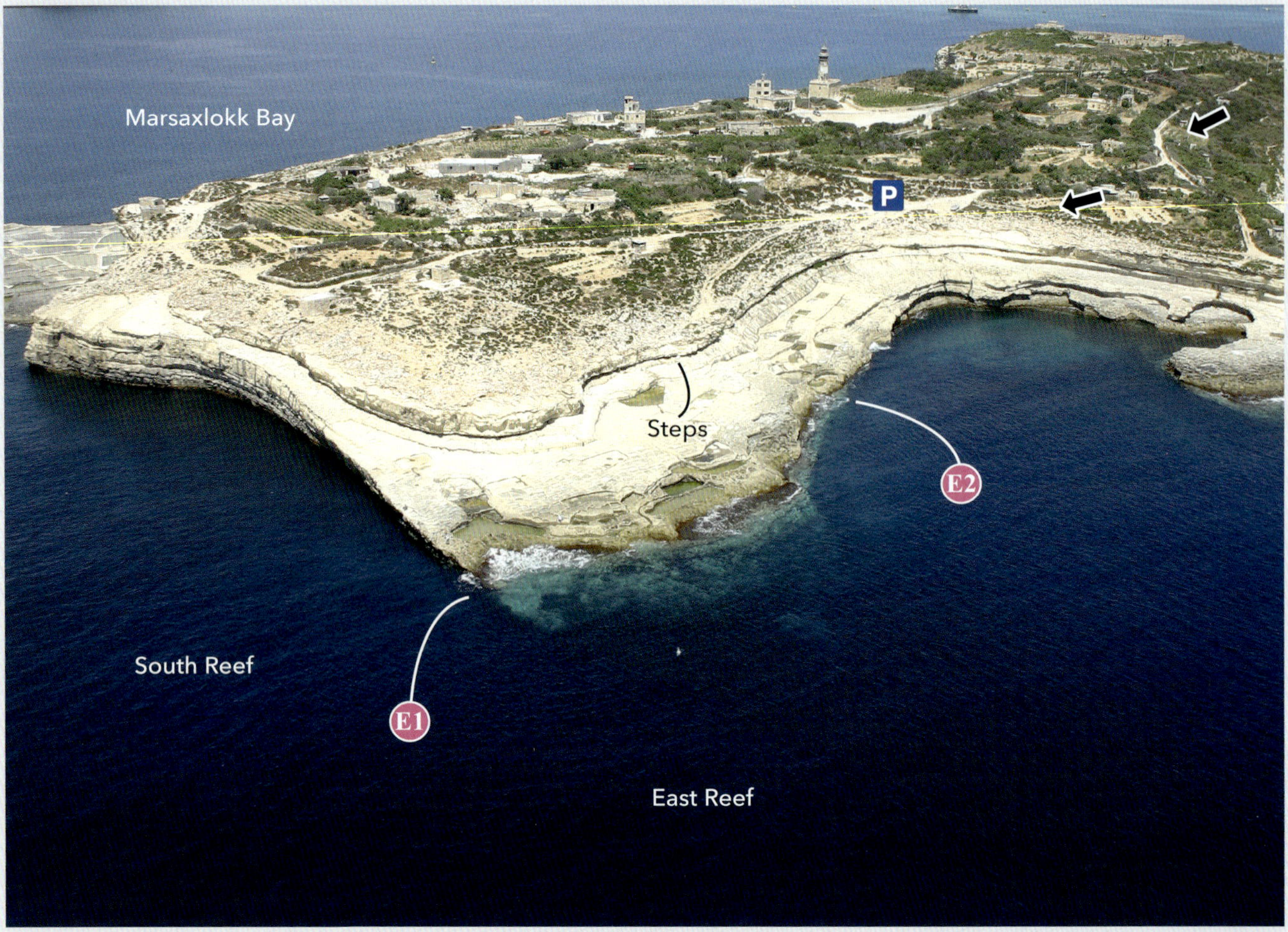

MARSAXLOKK - DELIMARA POINT

Marsaxlokk Bay
Steps
E2
South Reef
E1
East Reef

PHOTO: PGL AERIAL PHOTOS

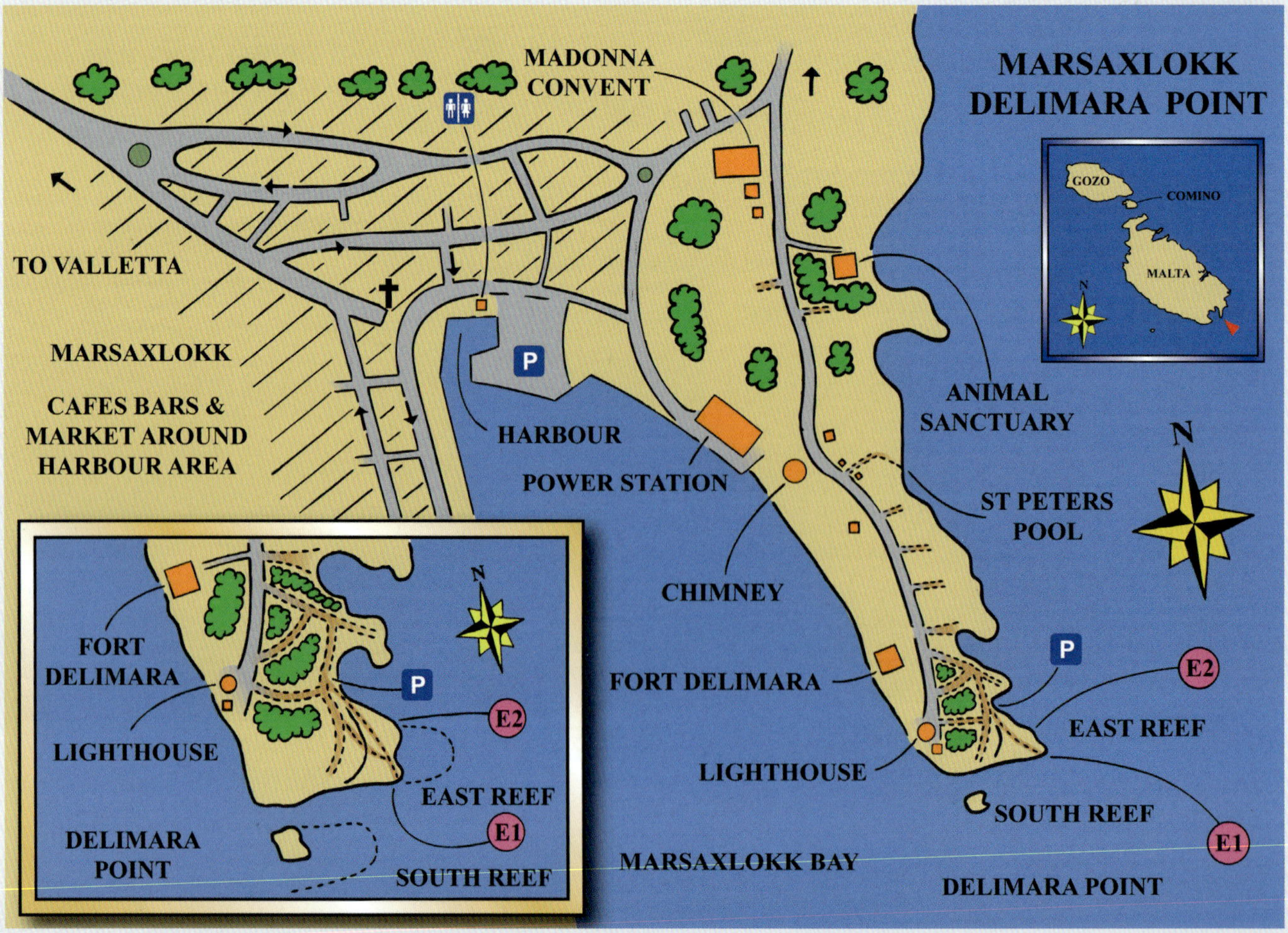

MARSAXLOKK DELIMARA POINT

GOZO
COMINO
MALTA

MADONNA CONVENT
TO VALLETTA
MARSAXLOKK CAFES BARS & MARKET AROUND HARBOUR AREA
HARBOUR
POWER STATION
ANIMAL SANCTUARY
ST PETERS POOL
CHIMNEY
FORT DELIMARA
LIGHTHOUSE
E2
EAST REEF
SOUTH REEF
E1
MARSAXLOKK BAY
DELIMARA POINT

FORT DELIMARA
LIGHTHOUSE
DELIMARA POINT
E2
EAST REEF
E1
SOUTH REEF

MARSAXLOKK - DELIMARA POINT

Delimara Point - East Reef - South Reef

This dive site is situated on the south of the island, about 4.2km or a 15-minute drive from the town of Marsaxlokk, which is popular with visitors for its fish market, colourful boats and harbour.

Leave the village heading east, at the roundabout head up the hill to the Madonna Convent, here, turn right to Delimara point, this narrow road passes the rear of the Power Station, continue on to Fort Delimara on your left. after another 50 metres, fork left down a track, for a distance of approximately 500 metres. On your left you will pass two small brick-built viewing platforms, take the second track to your right. Follow this track into the open area. with the sea on your left, this is your parking area. See aerial photograph.

There are a number of ways which you can plan and dive this under rated dive site with excellent reefs with depths of 30m plus. There are two main reefs in this area, for easy reference I will refer to them as East or South reef. For the East reef I have three dive plans and one for the South reef.

Depending on your required dive time it may be worth considering using a 15-litre cylinder for this dive site.

All dives will start at entry point E1 which is some 220 metres from the parking area, but in my opinion, it is well worth the effort, it was here that my buddy found the largest octopus that I have ever seen in Maltese waters, also a good area to locate the locust lobster.

Your route from the parking area to E1, follow the track which leads towards Delimara Point, keeping the cliff edge on your left after about 170 metres, now look for the steps down to the lower level, they are slightly hidden by an overhanging rock, see aerial photo above East Reef dive site plan.

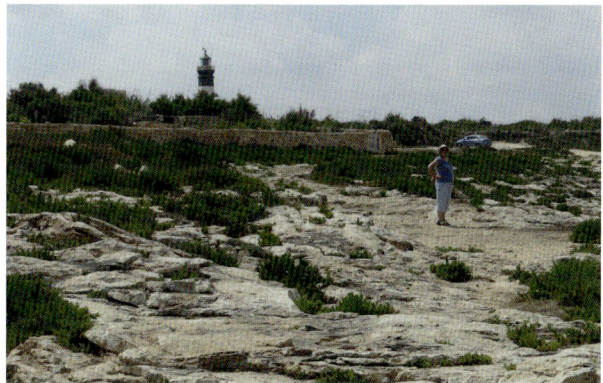

The track leading to the steps, that enable you to reach the lower level, these steps have been cut out by the kind fishermen.

Below: To the right of the lighthouse, parking to the left the steps leading down to the lower level and your entry exit points.

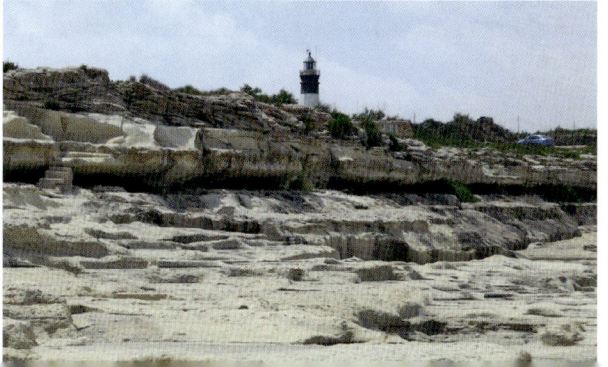

Delimara Point — East Reef

THE DIVES — Minimum time - 50 mins

This reef is U shaped and runs out from the furthest point of land in an easterly direction from entry point E1.

Dive plan 1. Once in and under the water follow the top of the reef in an easterly direction all the way along to the corner, where your depth will be 14m, this will take approximately 6 minutes. Here there are normally large shoals of fish to see and photograph. Now descend to the bottom at 23m passing an interesting ledge at 16m, continue your dive in an easterly direction, down this gently sloping area of grass, rugged boulders and sand. At a depth of 30m and some 12 minutes into your dive you will find another small reef, turn left follow this reef in a northerly direction for some 50 meters or 4/5 minutes. At this point take a westerly compass bearing this will take you back to the East Reef, any further and you will require a more south-westerly bearing.

Two divers just below the entry exit point E2 of this unusual underwater stepped wall which can be used for navigation.

PHOTO: JURIJS BICKINS DIVE MED

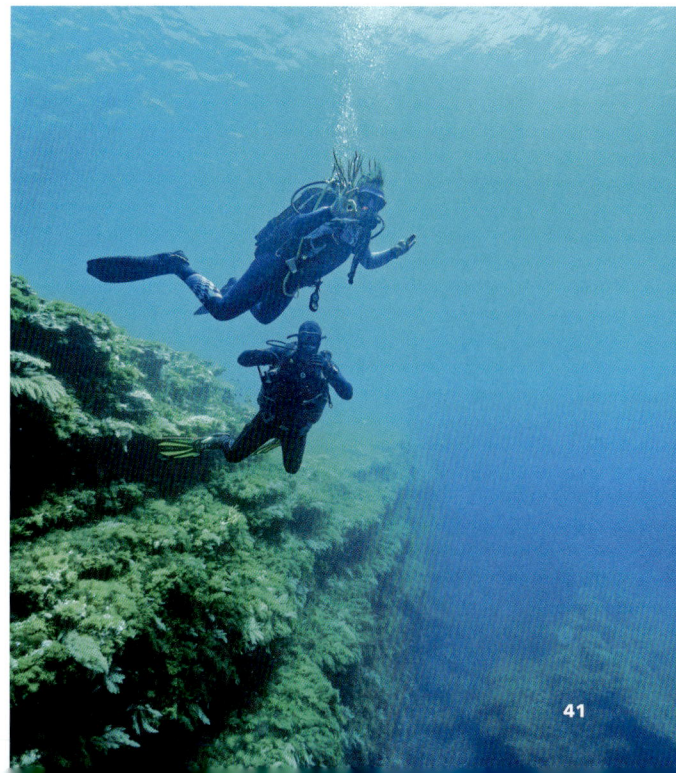

EAST REEF - DELIMARA POINT

Once you reach the reef, head north keeping the reef on your left, the reef will now change direction to westerly, until it reaches the coastline where you will have to bear right and head north. After a short time, the seabed below you will open up to a flat area of sand and small rocks with a depth of 9m, here you will be very close to E2 entry/exit point.

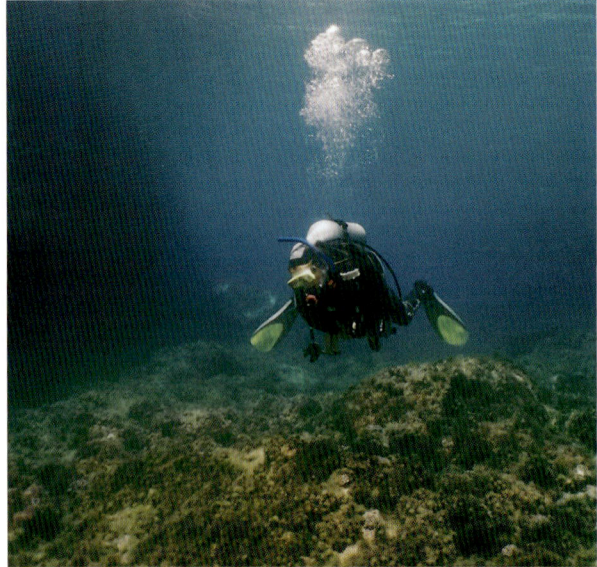

Exploring the shallows of East Reef on the return route to E2.

Dive plan 2. Using entry point E1 descend to the seabed at 13m, the choice is now yours, either follow the reef keeping it on your left to The Corner where your depth will be 23m: or move away from the reef for some 2 to 3 minutes and then head east. Take your time to explore this area with its large boulders, overhangs, grass and small sandy patches; this is a good area for locating the locust lobster. Once you reach a depth of about 20/22m, or the Lone Boulder at 25m, now head north to The Corner at 23m This is an excellent area where you normally find large shoals of fish, bring your camera.

A free-swimming octopus (Octopus vulgaris) seems to have found a friend and attached itself to the diver's arm.

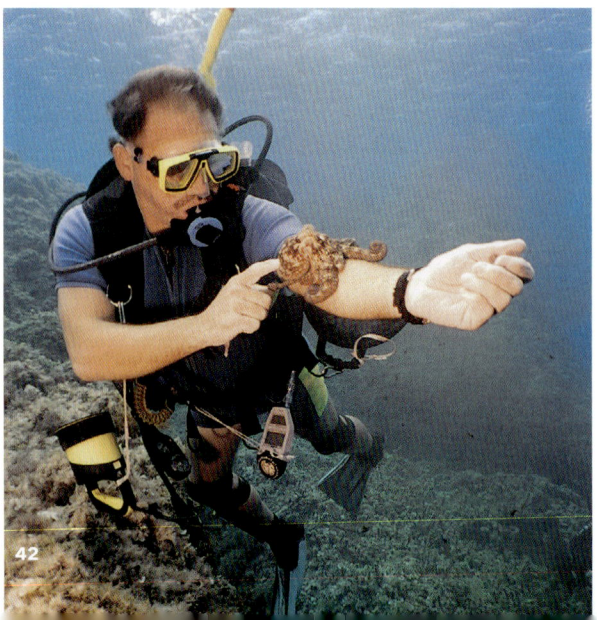

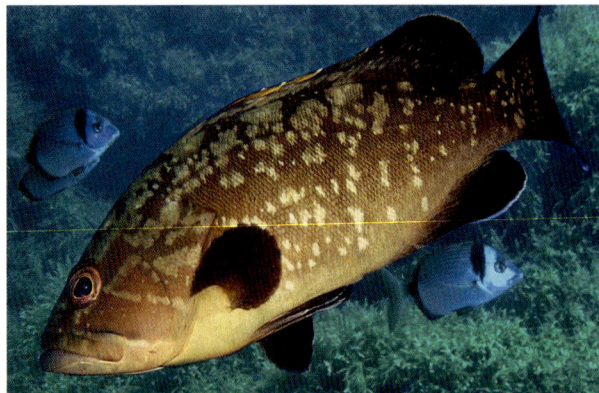

Here is a friendly grouper (Epinephelus guaza) normally very shy.
PHOTO: VICTOR FABRI

Now follow the reef keeping it on your left, head in a northerly direction, either at its base or on the top, after a short time the bearing of the reef will change to northwesterly then westerly towards the coastline, where the reef bears to the right towards entry /exit point E2.

Dive plan 3. Using the same entry point E1, descend to the seabed at 13m, leaving the main reef behind you, swim in a southerly direction and within 5 minutes another reef will appear in front of you, here your depth will be 16m. Now take an easterly direction until you reach the end of the reef, where the depth is 21m; to reach this point will take approximately 10/12 minutes. Continue in the same direction down over the grass and small rocks to an area of sand and a number of small boulders at 34m. Here keep the reef on your left it is quite steep and rises up to 25m and to assist you with your bearings keep it in view. When it is time to return, ascend the reef to the top, follow it in a westerly direction along its ridge, until you reach the single boulder at 25m. When the visibility is good, from this point you will be able to see the corner on the East Reef, if not, take a northerly bearing and within 3 minutes you will reach the corner of the reef. At this point I would ascend to 13m at the top of the reef, then follow the ridge, on the south side of the East reef, in a westerly direction to my entry /exit point E1.

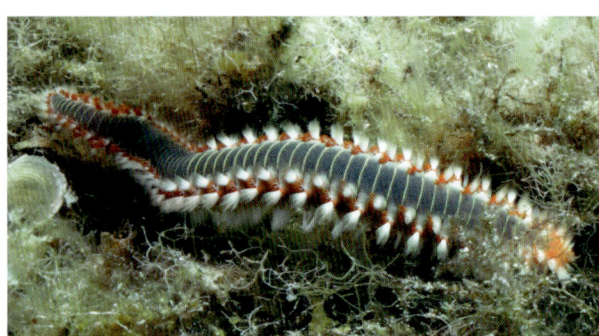

Fireworm (Hermodice carunculate) do not handle these creatures.

It must be noted that there is a possibility of strong currents in this area or swell following a storm, which also may affect the visibility, making navigation more difficult. A good guide for visibility is that you should be able to see the seabed from your entry point.

Delimara Point
Steps
E2
E1
East Reef
P

PHOTO: PGL AERIAL PHOTOS

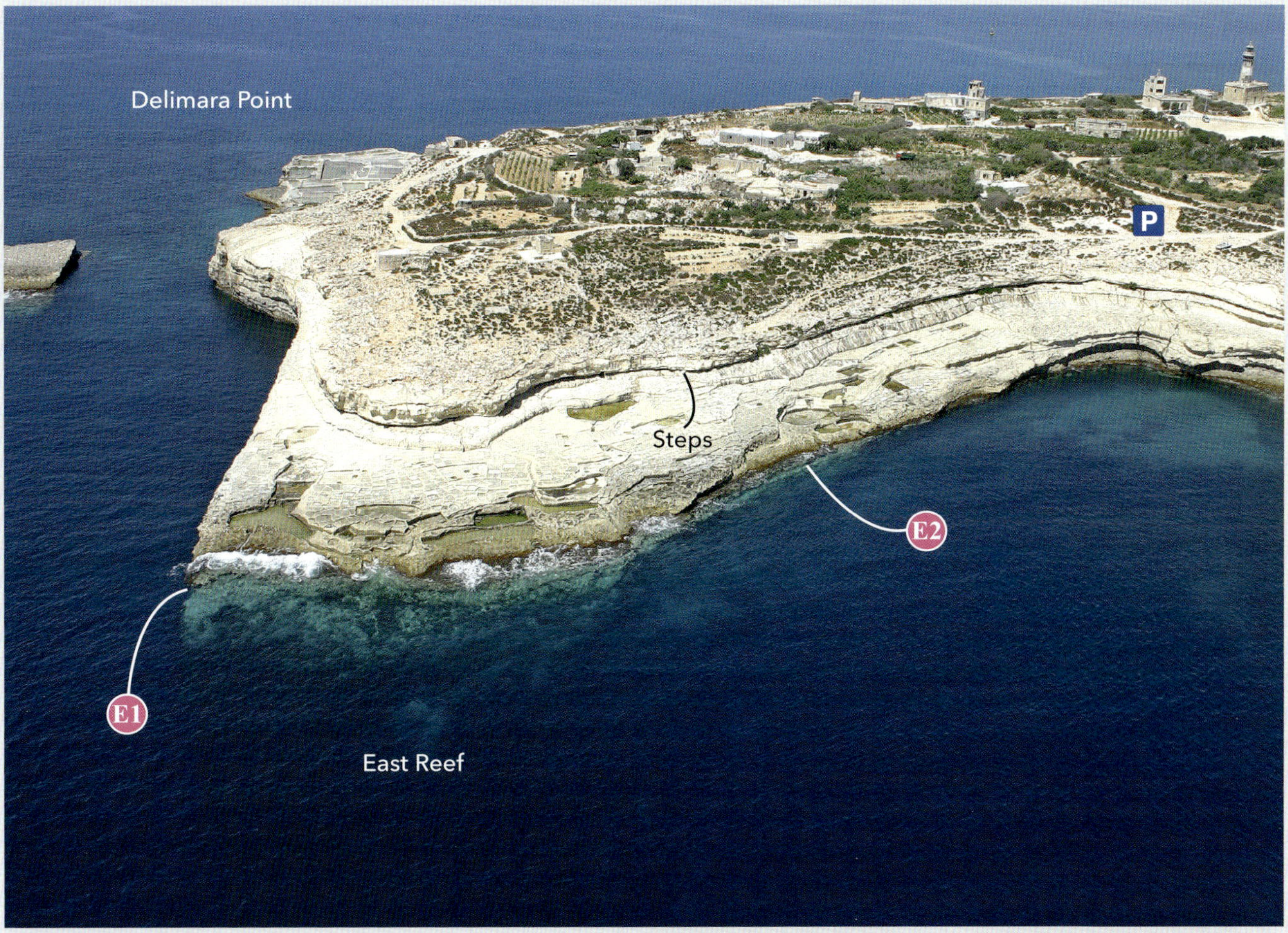

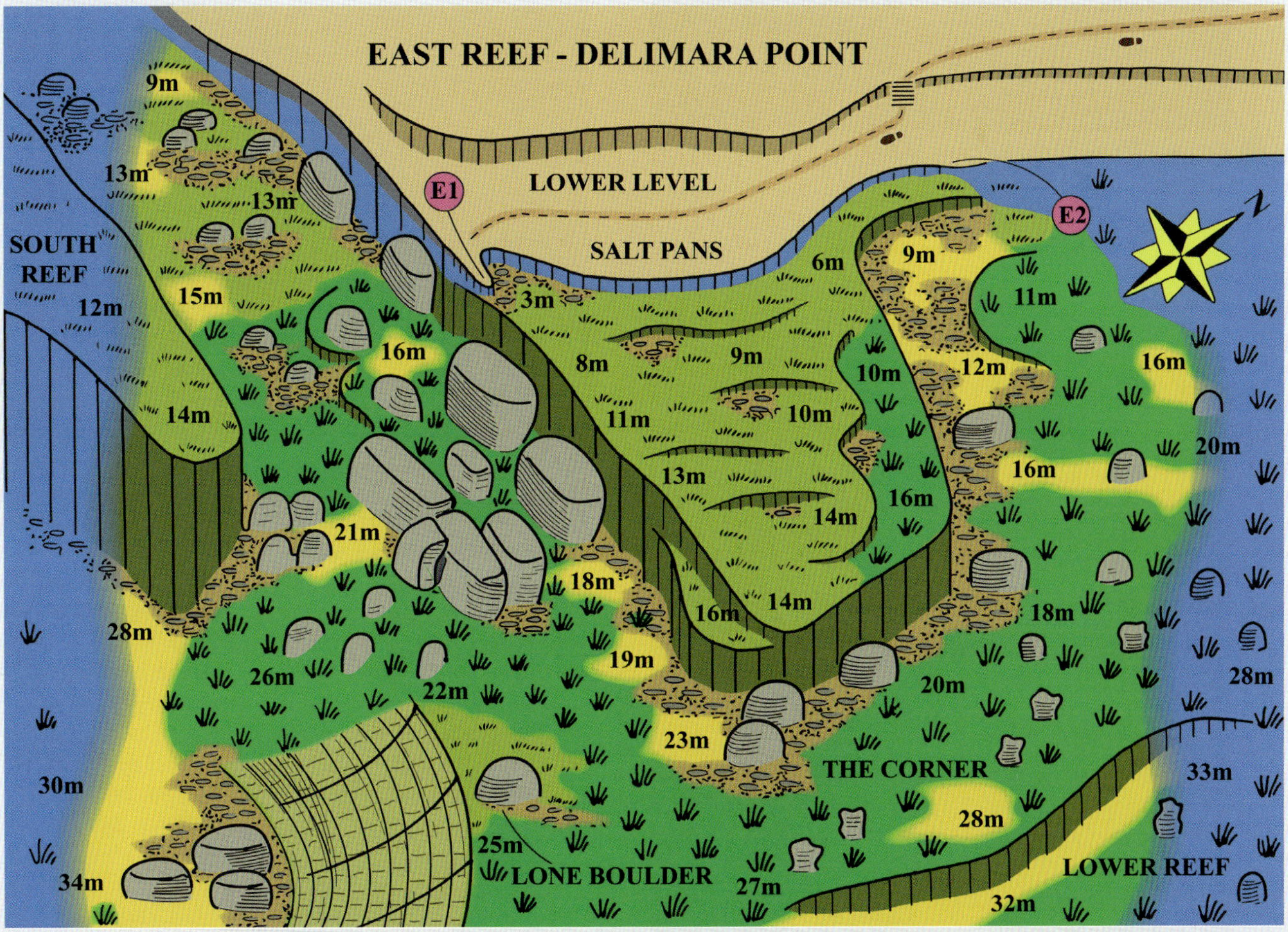
EAST REEF - DELIMARA POINT
LOWER LEVEL
SALT PANS
E1
E2
SOUTH REEF
9m
13m
13m
12m
15m
16m
14m
3m
6m
8m
9m
11m
10m
13m
14m
16m
14m
9m
11m
10m
12m
16m
16m
20m
21m
18m
19m
18m
28m
26m
22m
23m
20m
THE CORNER
28m
28m
30m
33m
25m
LONE BOULDER
27m
34m
LOWER REEF
32m

Delimara Point — South Reef

THE DIVES — Minimum time - 55 mins

This reef is U shaped and runs out from the furthest point of land in an easterly direction from entry point E1.

Dive plan 1. Once in and under the water follow the top of the reef in an easterly direction all the way along to the corner, where your depth will be 14m, this will take approximately 6 minutes. Here there are normally large shoals of fish to see and photograph. Now descend to the bottom at 23m passing an interesting ledge at 16m, continue your dive in an easterly direction, down this gently sloping area of grass, rugged boulders and sand. At a depth of 30m and some 12 minutes into your dive you will find another small reef, turn left follow this reef in a northerly direction for some 50 meters or 4/5 minutes. At this point take a westerly compass bearing this will take you back to the East Reef, any further and you will require a more south-westerly bearing.

Continue over the top of the reef in the same direction until you can see the drop-off, which goes down to 25m. Descend from the top of the reef and head in a westerly direction, slowly descending the reef and in this area, you will find three large boulders which I have called the Three Peaks. Now continue along the base of the reef to the end, depth 22m: from here when the visibility is good you will be able to see Arrow Head Rock, otherwise a southerly compass bearing will take you across the valley to its base at 24m. The next reef is shaped like a U, follow it all the way round until the reef turns to a southerly direction, keeping it on your right-hand side, your average depth here will be 22m, within in a short distance you will see two large boulders on your right, they will be slightly obscuring the entrance to Abigail's Cave at 18m, your dive time could be 35 minutes.

Once inside the cave it is quite light due to two openings in the roof, of which you will be able to exit easily onto the top of the reef at 16m. Your choice of return route depends on the time and air you have remaining, you can either reef hop from one to the other taking a north to north-easterly bearing which would be the most direct route to your exit point or you can navigate the tops of the reefs, only crossing at their narrowest parts back to your exit point. Of course, at any time during your dive, if you wish, you could ascend to the top of the reef and return to your exit point E1.

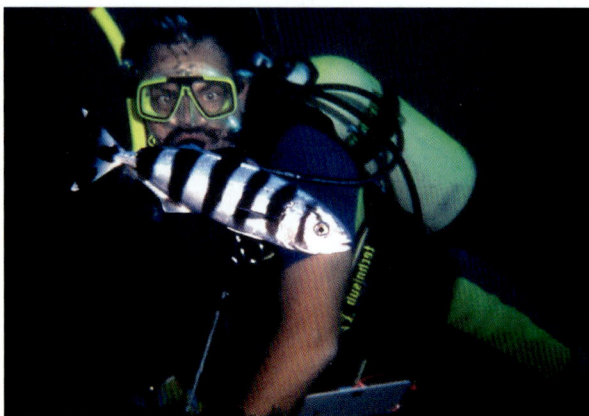

Pilot fish (Naucrates doctor) a diver makes eye to eye contact with this energetic, inquisitive fish, during a dive on this reef.

Below: At the end of the third reef from your entry point at the top is Arrowhead Rock this rock is a distinct navigational point.

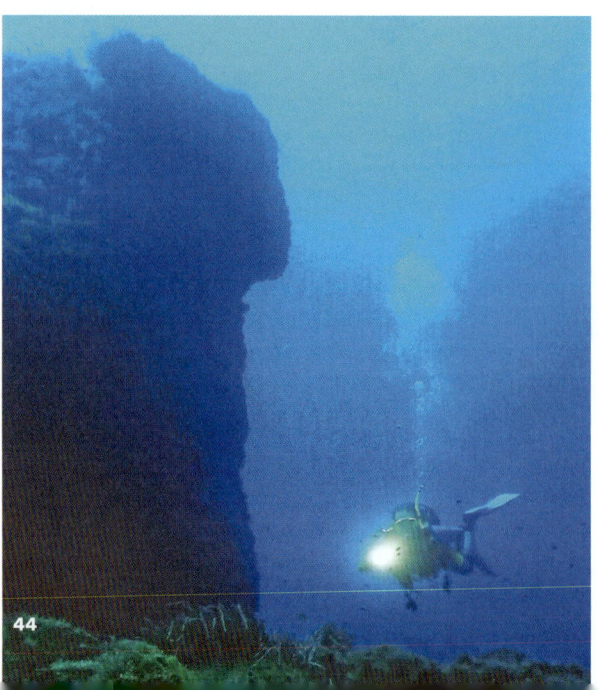

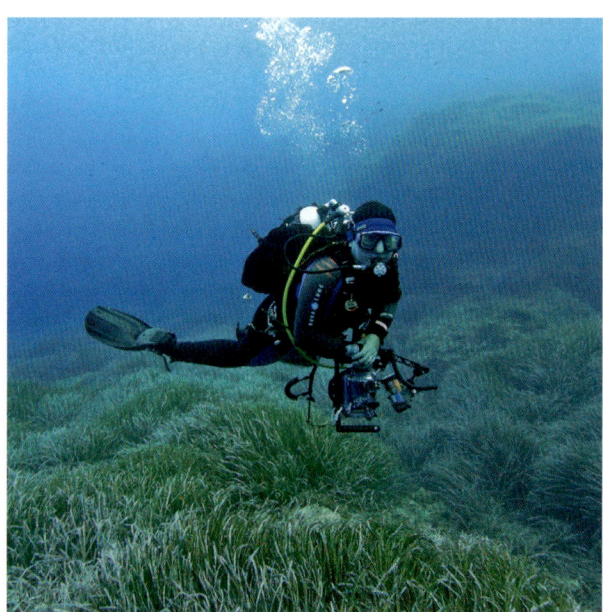

The areas of posidonia sea grass between the South Reefs.

Remember that this site is well away from any amenities in the village of Marsaxlokk, if you require refreshments, it is advisable to take them with you. If you do not have any non-divers with you do not leave any valuables in the car. The market is a daily event, but the Sunday fish market is very popular, with not only the local people but also tourists, so you can expect heavy traffic and crowds of people in Marsaxlokk.

Marsaxlokk Bay
P
South Reef
E1
Delimara Point

PHOTO: PGL AERIAL PHOTOS

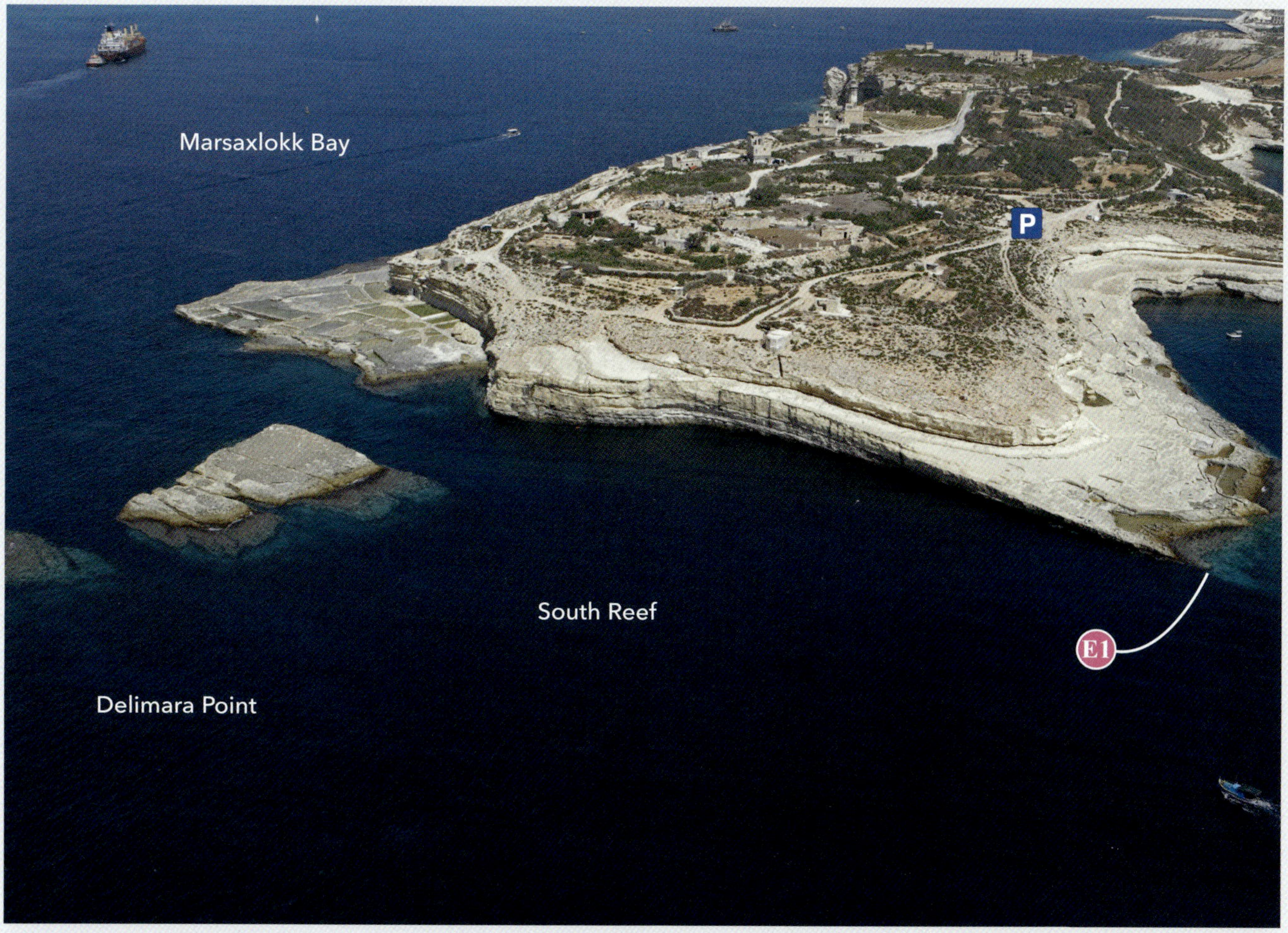

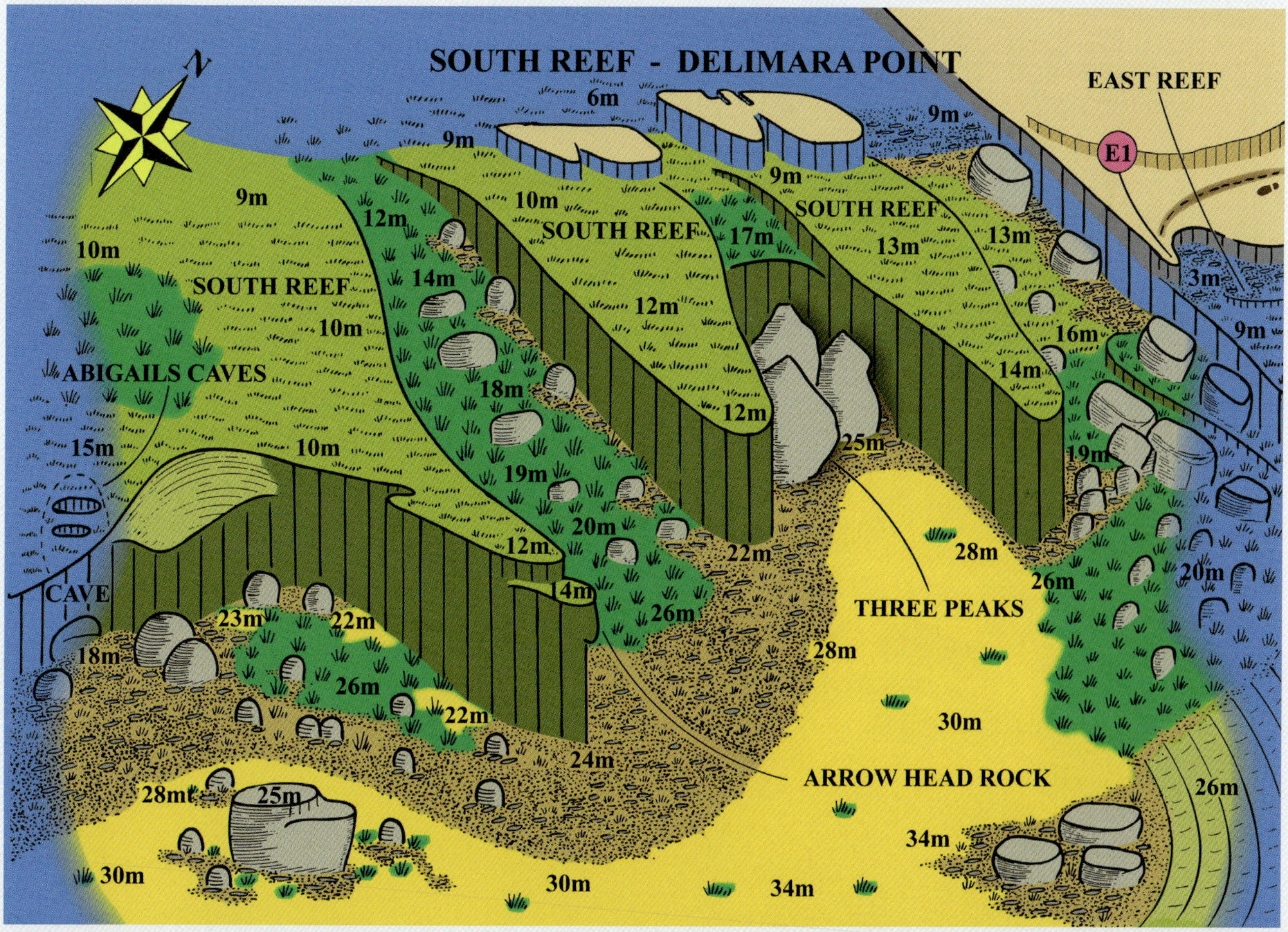
SOUTH REEF - DELIMARA POINT
N
EAST REEF
E1
6m
9m
9m
9m
9m
10m
12m
10m
SOUTH REEF
17m
SOUTH REEF
13m
13m
10m
SOUTH REEF
14m
12m
3m
9m
10m
16m
ABIGAILS CAVES
18m
14m
12m
15m
10m
25m
19m
19m
20m
12m
28m
22m
20m
14m
26m
CAVE
26m
THREE PEAKS
23m
22m
18m
28m
26m
30m
22m
24m
ARROW HEAD ROCK
26m
28m
25m
34m
30m
30m
34m

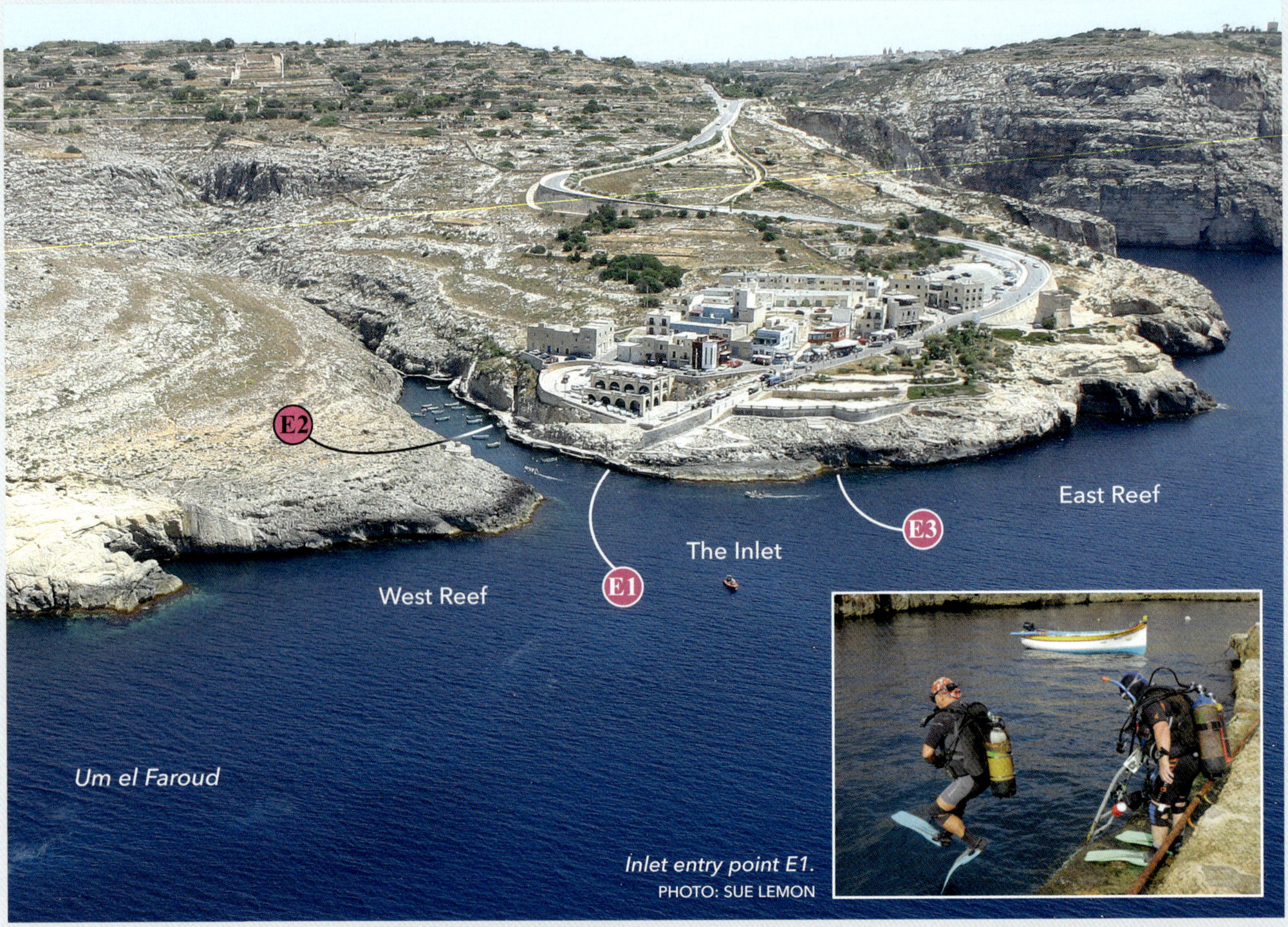

WIED IZ-ZURRIEQ (BLUE GROTTO) - UM EL FAROUD

East Reef
The Inlet
West Reef
Um el Faroud

Inlet entry point E1.
PHOTO: SUE LEMON

PHOTO: PGL AERIAL PHOTOS

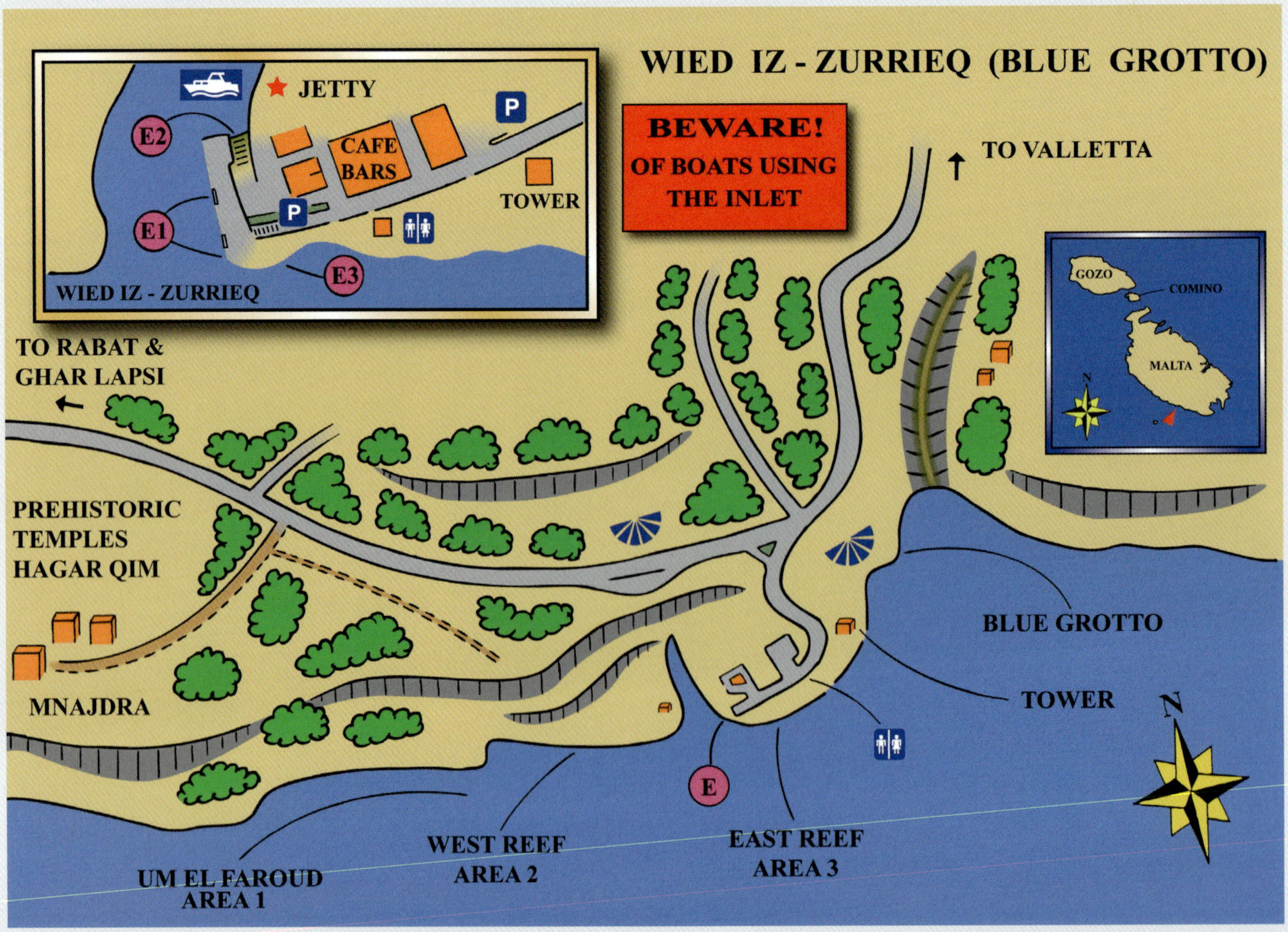

WIED IZ - ZURRIEQ (BLUE GROTTO)

JETTY
CAFE BARS
TOWER
WIED IZ - ZURRIEQ

BEWARE! OF BOATS USING THE INLET

↑ TO VALLETTA

GOZO
COMINO
MALTA

TO RABAT & GHAR LAPSI

PREHISTORIC TEMPLES HAGAR QIM

MNAJDRA

BLUE GROTTO
TOWER

N

UM EL FAROUD AREA 1
WEST REEF AREA 2
EAST REEF AREA 3

Wied iz-Zurrieq (Blue Grotto) - *Um el Faroud*

Wied iz Zurrieq is a small village situated on the south coast, there are two main routes to this site, one from Rabat 10km along a country road, or from Luqa 7km taking the road which passes under the airport runway. The dive site is very popular, with divers for the *Um El Faroud*, possibly the best wreck dive in the Mediterranean, also tourists visiting this village and inlet for a boat trip to the Blue Grotto.

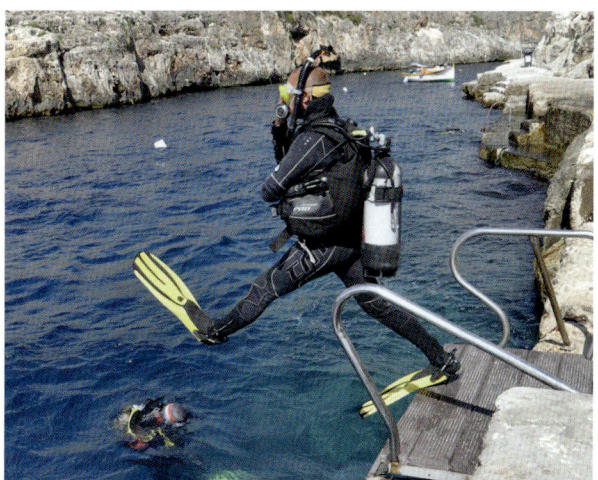

The main entry point at this dive site E1 in the inlet at Wied iz-Zurrieq.   PHOTO: SUE LEMON

The Blue Grotto

This dive site is normally referred to as the Blue Grotto, but is approximately half a mile to the west of the inlet and can only be reached by boat, there is a viewing area up on the main road above the Grotto, see plan.

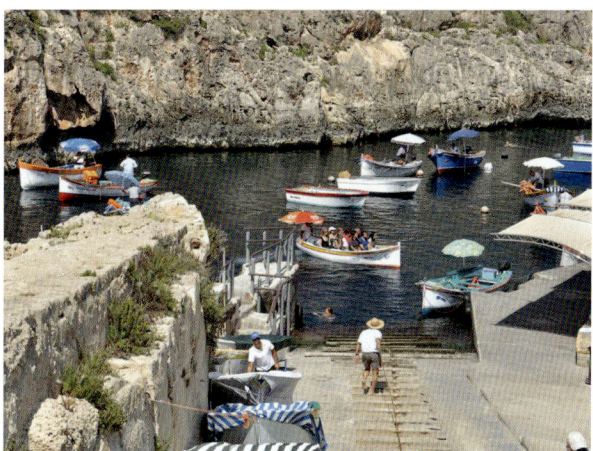

The exit point E2 normally used when there are no ladders at E1.

Parking for divers is at the bottom of the hill where the road ends, this is close to your entry / exit points. Sea conditions must be checked here, for although there is virtually no tide, sometimes there are currents even when sea conditions are calm. If there are divers leaving the water you could ask them if they have experienced any during their dive.

Remember the small inlet is your only exit area, and depending on the sea conditions you might have to consider use of the slipway, E2, which is sheltered from the open sea. Beware of the boats taking tourists to the Blue Grotto, they travel quite fast so if you intend to surface swim across the inlet, stay together and keep a look out.

There are three diving areas here, but the dive plan can be varied depending on experience and depth required. Please note the ladder at E1 may be removed during the winter period. If using E2 be careful, this area is very slippery and the boats may be running.

Um el Faroud — Area 1

The 3,147 gross ton vessel is a Single Screw Motor Tanker, built by Smith Dock Co. Ltd., Middlesborough England in 1969. The port of registry was Tripoli and owned by General National Maritime Transport. The engine room, bridge and accommodation are arranged aft. The overall length is 110 metres and the breadth is 16m metres, still in place are the propeller and rudder at 36m.

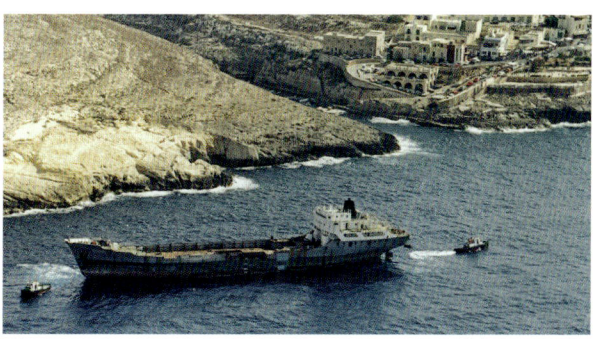

Sinking of the Um el Faroud on the 2nd September 1998 just off the village of Wied iz-Zurrieq.

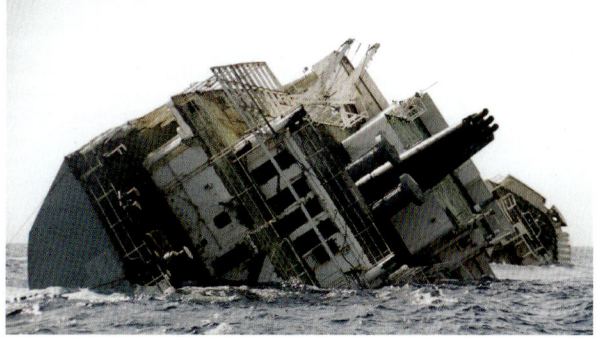

WIED IZ-ZURRIEQ (BLUE GROTTO) - UM EL FAROUD

Um el Faroud the ill-fated tanker

The ill-fated tanker *Um el Faroud* was scuttled on Wednesday 2nd September 1998. three and a half years after the explosion that killed nine dockyard workers in Grand Harbour Valletta, this tragic event shocked the people of Malta. Her final voyage started in the early hours of the morning, arriving off Wied iz Zurrieq around 9.30am. It then took over three hours to get her into position, due to a moderate south-easterly swell. Finally, around 3.30pm she sank quietly beneath the surface, down onto the sand at 35m. At this moment in time, she is upright on the seabed in two sections with the bow separated just in front of the bridge.

In the centre of the bridge at the front, below the remaining top floor, is a brass plaque in memory of the workers killed in the explosion.

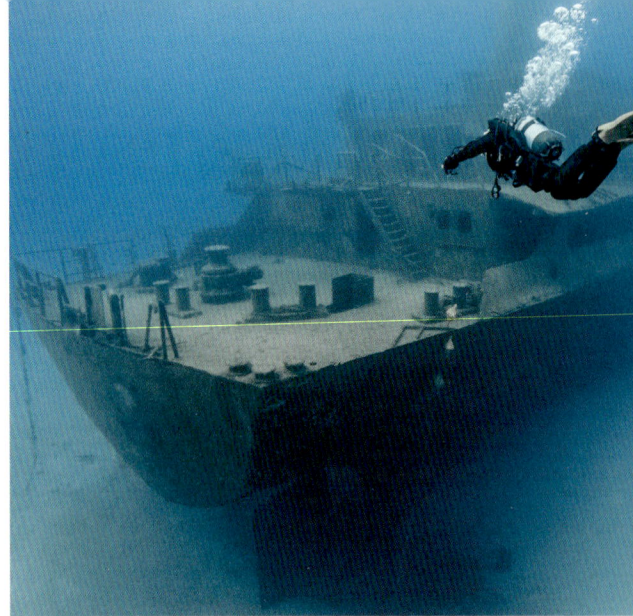

The stern section of this massive wreck at a depth of 22m plus.
PHOTO: ARKADIUSZ SREBNIK POLANDDIVINGPHOTOS

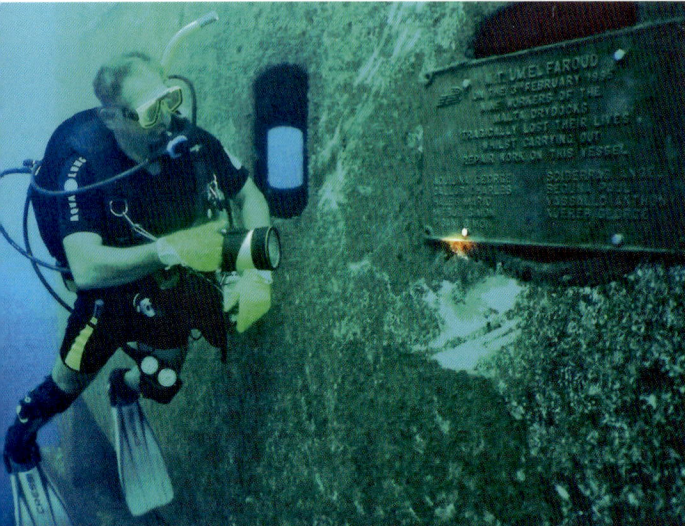

A plaque in the centre of the bridge in memory of nine dock workers who sadly lost their lives in the explosion.

Below: The bow of the Um el Faroud and the anchor chain.

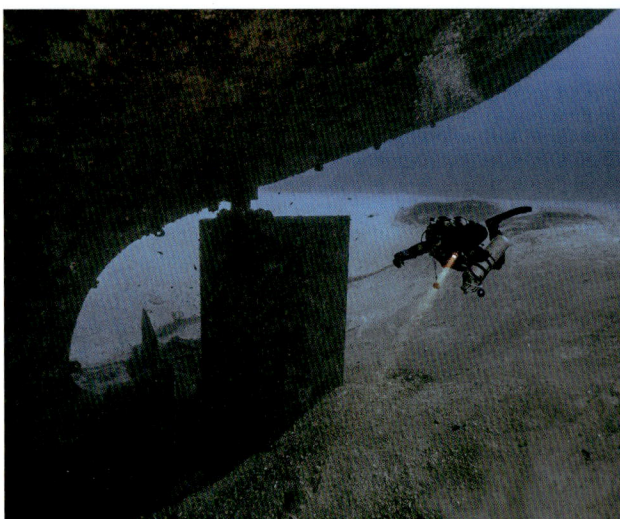

A diver explores the area below the stern where the propeller and rudder can be found.
PHOTO: JON BORG - www.jonborg.com

Below: The huge propeller and rudder of the Um el Faroud.

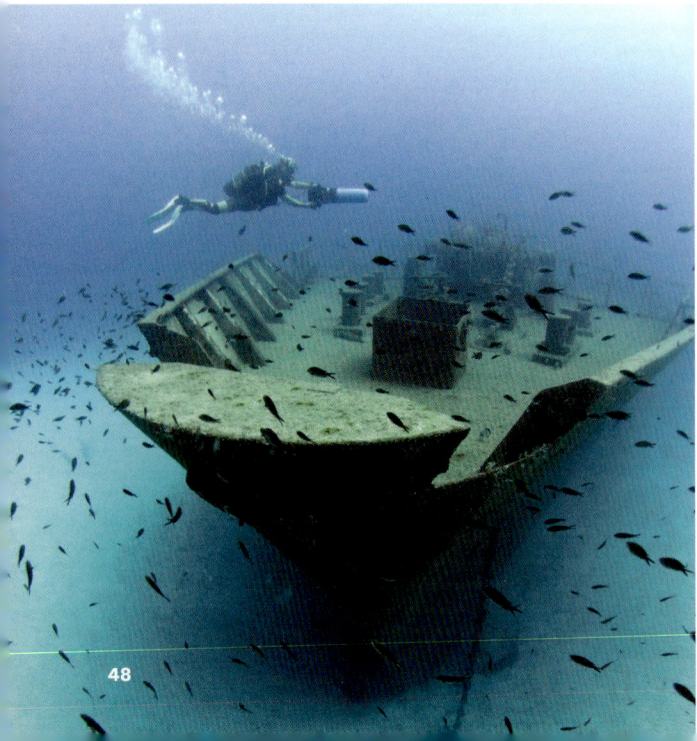

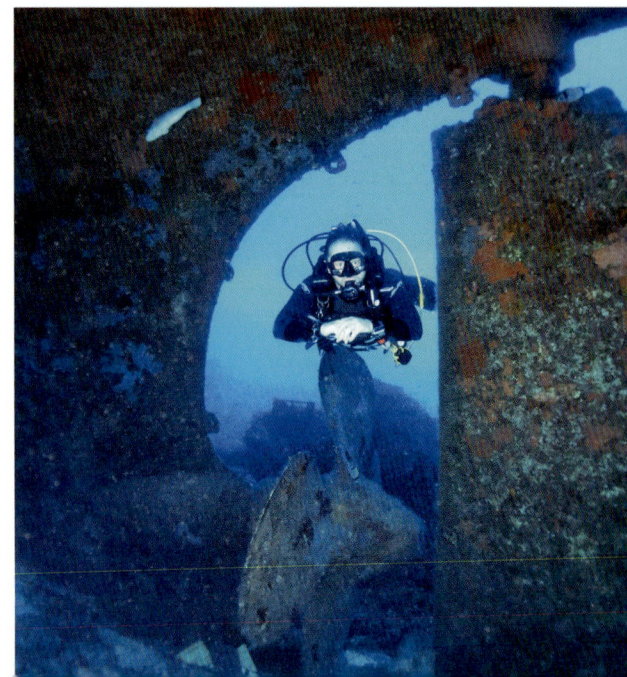

WIED IZ-ZURRIEQ (BLUE GROTTO) - UM EL FAROUD

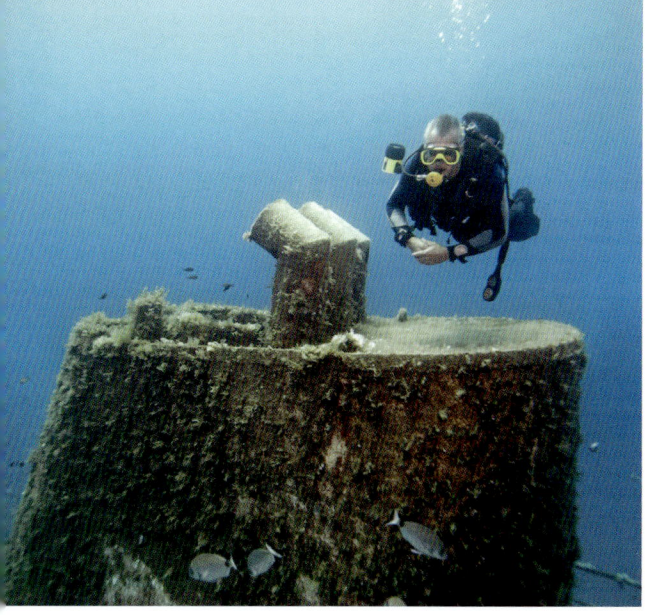

The ship's chimney is a good place to take a souvenir photo.

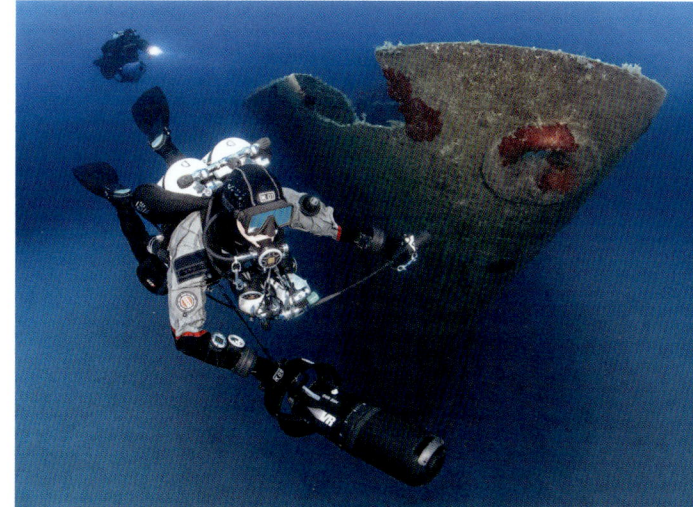

Exploring this wreck with a DPV at the bow of the Um el Faroud.
PHOTO: DAN - MARCELLO Di FRANCESCO - ORANGE SHARK

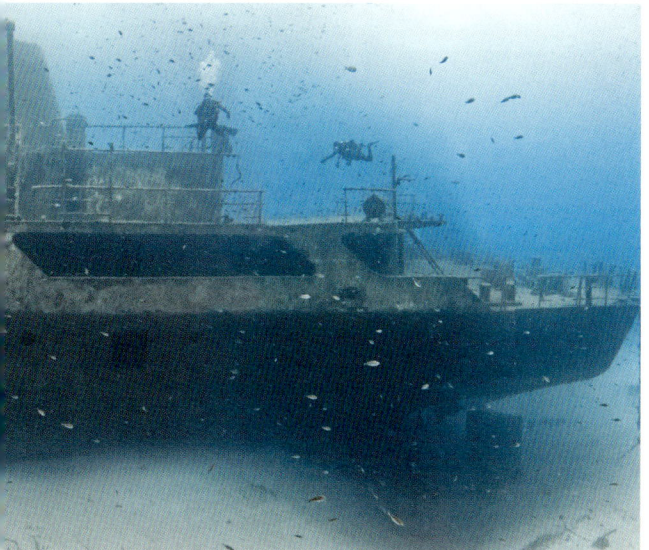

A view of the bow section of the Um el Faroud from the portside. PHOTOS: ARKADIUSZ SREBNIK POLANDDIVINGPHOTOS

Below: A diver explores the engine room, the power house of this ship.

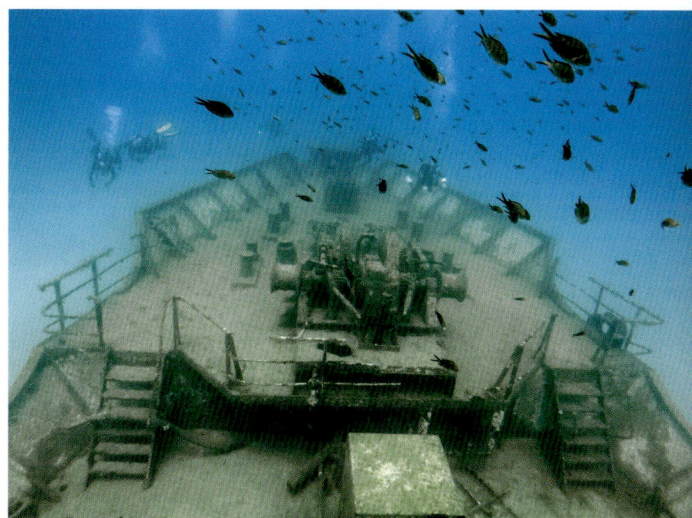

Small fish above the bow, which attract the larger fish at feeding times. PHOTOS: ARKADIUSZ SREBNIK POLANDDIVINGPHOTOS

Below: Divers leaving the bridge area, heading back to the inlet.

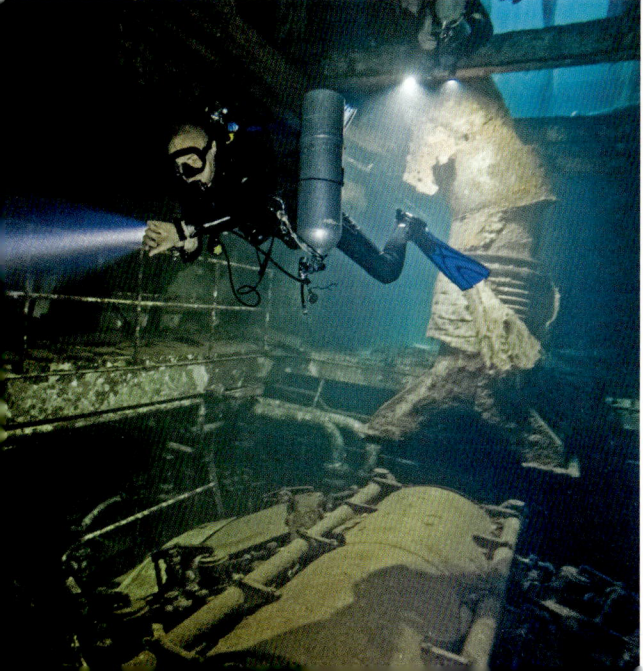

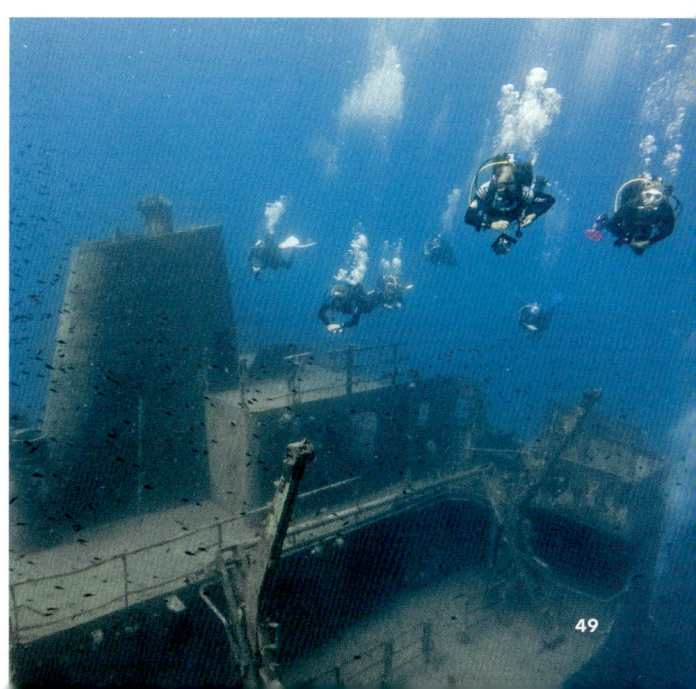

WIED IZ-ZURRIEQ (BLUE GROTTO) - UM EL FAROUD

THE DIVE — Minimum time - 50 mins

There are number of ways to reach the wreck of the Um el Faroud, above or below the surface. If they are available, by boat this does not happen very often. I personally have two different routes for reaching the Um el Faroud, and for both, my entry point is E1 just at the bottom of the steps.

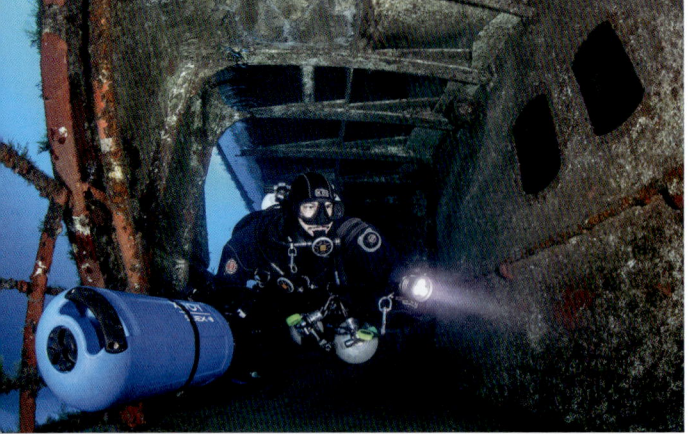

DPV diver in the starboard gangway heading towards the bridge. PHOTO: DAN - MARCELLO Di FRANCESCO ORANGE SHARK

Route 1 If Sea conditions are perfect, surface swim taking a compass bearing of 240° until you have a 20° compass bearing on the flat faced sandy coloured rock, which can clearly be seen in the aerial photograph. The surface swim is some 200 metres from your entry point, E1 and will take some 8/15 minutes. This route should not be attempted if there are any off shore currents.

Route 2 In my opinion the best way to dive this wreck is to surface swim across the inlet entrance, west along coast for approximately 100 meters until you reach a little cove, even at a slow swim, this will take no more than 8/10 minutes.

Below: A shoal of amberjacks (Serola dumerili) on a feeding frenzy. PHOTO: VERONICA BUSUTTIL

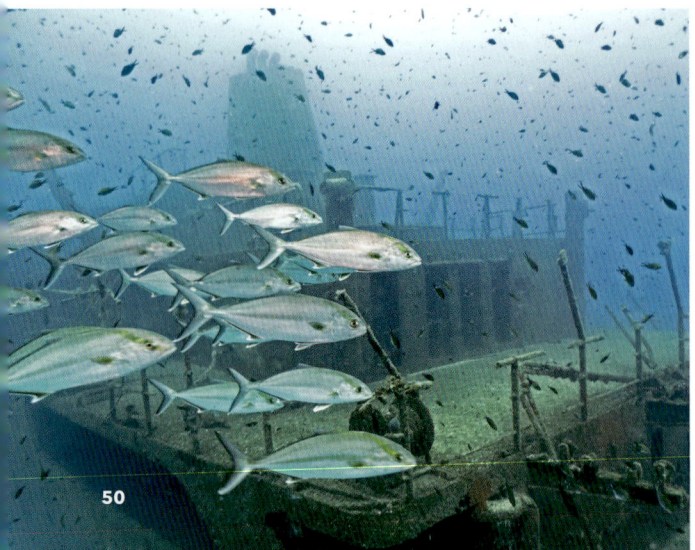

If you are facing out to sea, behind you will be a large sandy coloured flat faced rock and below you a 10m ledge. From this ledge, take a compass bearing of 200°. Your distance from here to the wreck is about 70 metres and takes about 3/4 minutes.

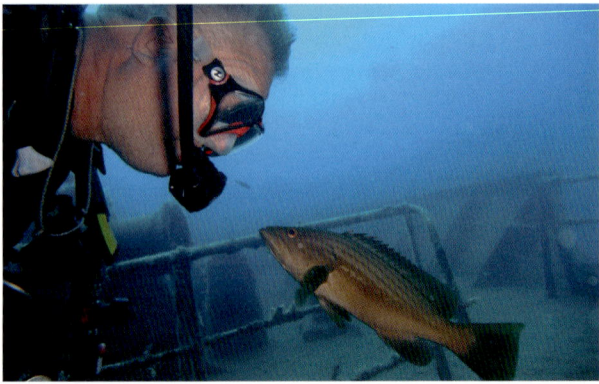

A friendly brown wrasse (Labrus marla) has eye to eye contact with diver Paul. PHOTO: DEBBIE ADAMS

For the depths on this ship, see plan. If penetration is in your dive plan ensure that all diving safety procedures are carried out. For your safety all doors and windows have been removed also holes have been cut in the hull for entry and exit. Do not be tempted to stay too long, I recommend that you leave the wreck with a minimum of 100 bar which will give you time to explore the reef on your return journey, leaving from the bridge and once away from the wreck, take a compass bearing of 330°. This compass bearing will not lead you directly back towards the inlet, but to the closest reef to the wreck, which is approximately 50 metres, here the depth will be 18m.

To ascend this reef to a depth of 6m will take approximately 5/6 minutes from the bridge of the wreck. Once you have reached your required depth, bear right heading in an easterly direction; follow the reef all the way round back to the inlet and your planned exit point. You should allow for this return journey, some 20/25 minutes, but can be done quicker if you do not explore the reef on the way. If you do not have sufficient air when leaving the wreck, take a compass bearing of 60° this will lead you directly back to your exit point, do not miss the inlet entrance. In my opinion unless you have boat cover, this dive is for experienced divers only and a 15-litre cylinder should be used.

Below: Passing by the Um el Faroud's chimney with a torpedo DPV.

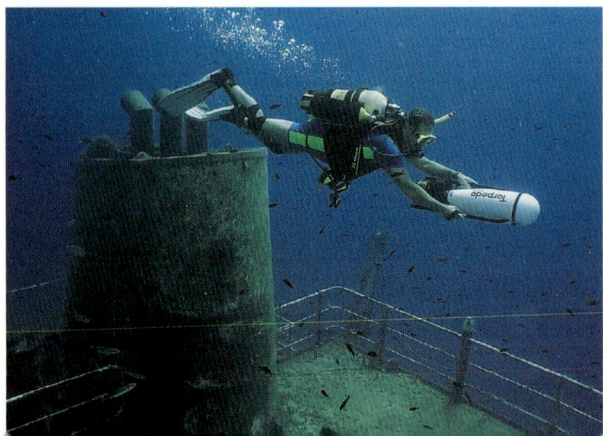

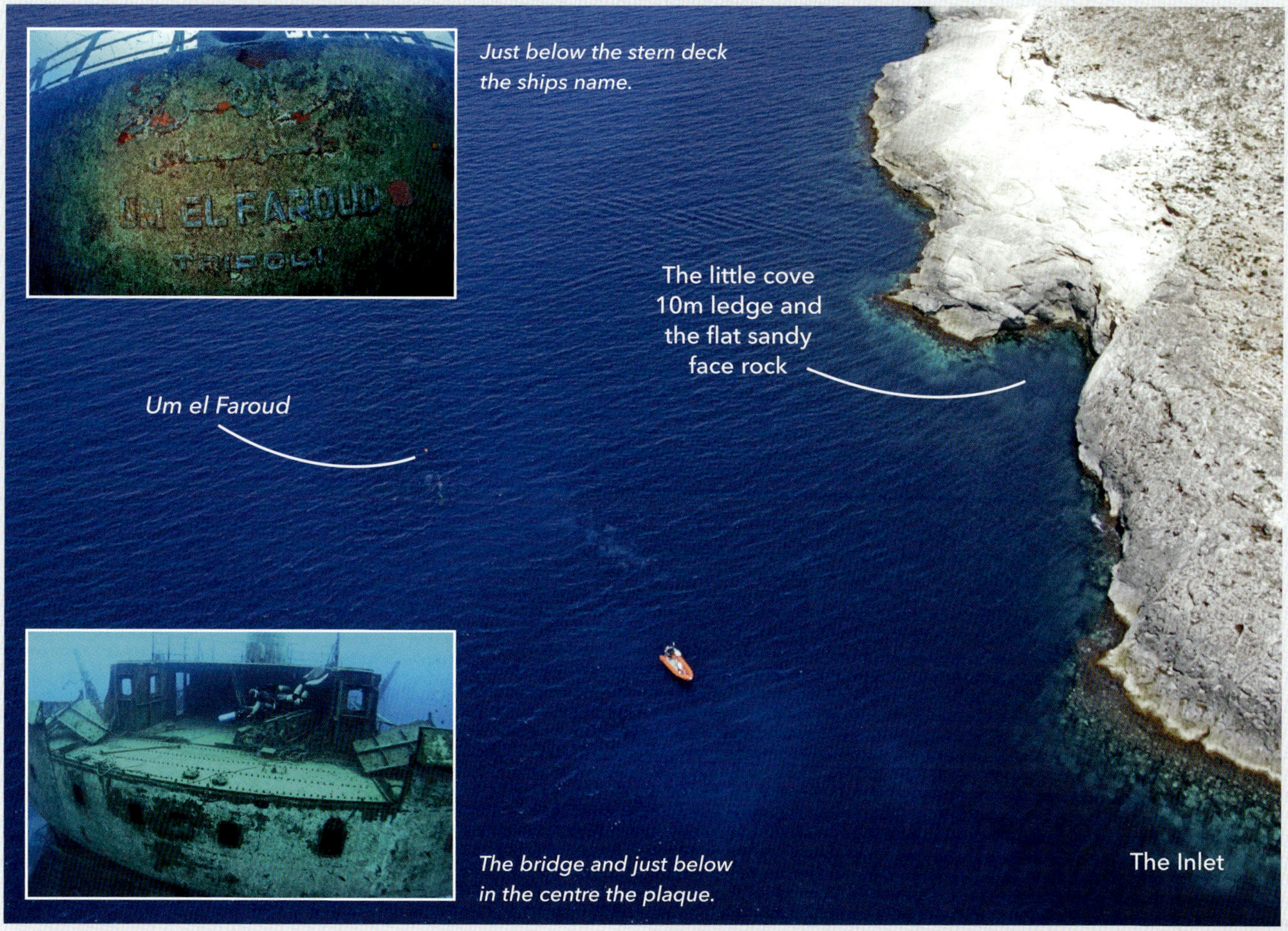

The little cove
10m ledge and
the flat sandy
face rock
Um el Faroud
The Inlet

Just below the stern deck the ships name.

The bridge and just below in the centre the plaque.

PHOTO: PGL AERIAL PHOTOS

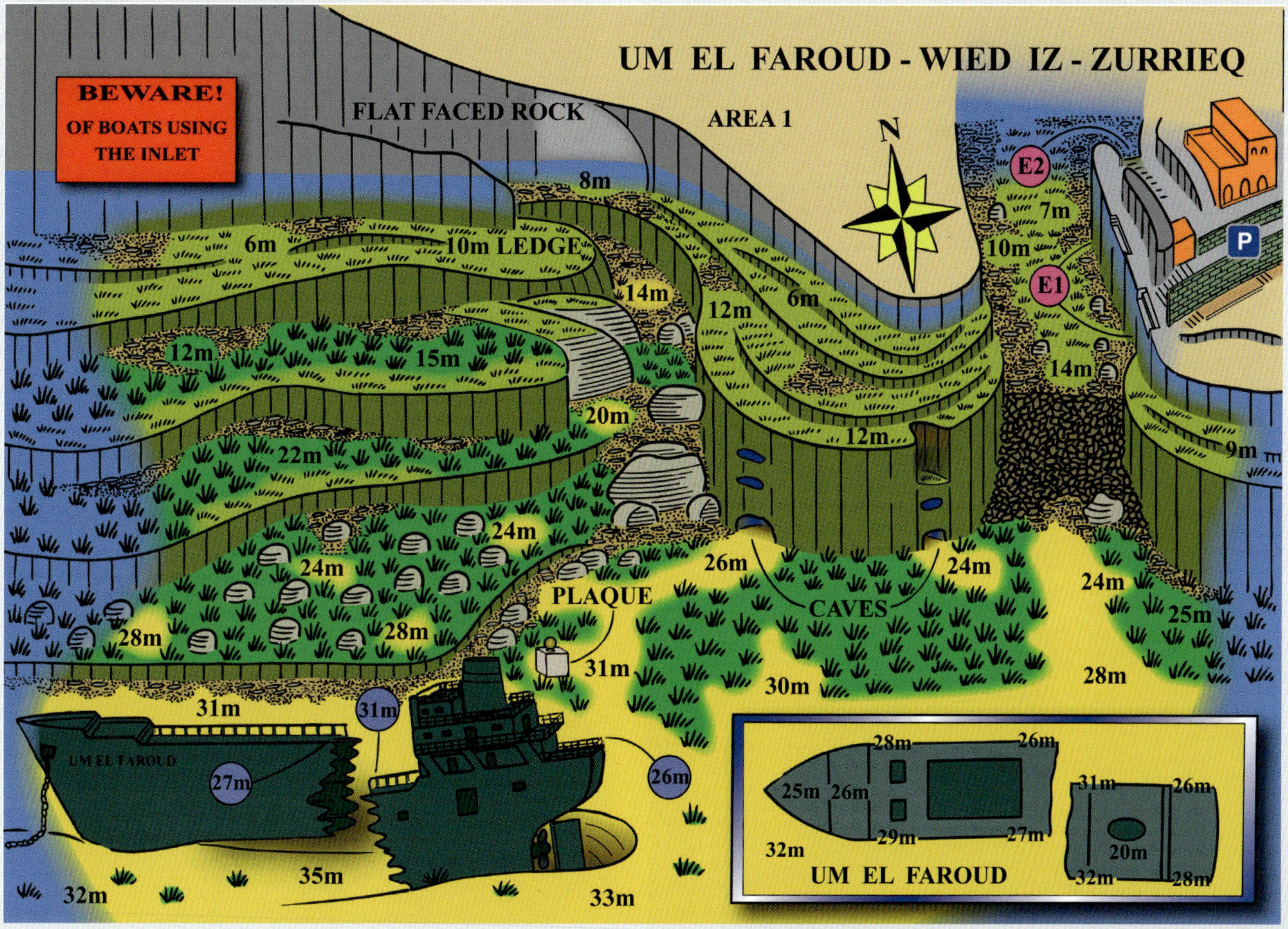

UM EL FAROUD - WIED IZ - ZURRIEQ
BEWARE!
OF BOATS USING
THE INLET
FLAT FACED ROCK
AREA 1
N
E2
E1
P
8m
6m
10m LEDGE
7m
10m
14m
12m
6m
12m
15m
14m
20m
12m
9m
22m
24m
24m
26m
24m
24m
25m
PLAQUE
CAVES
28m
28m
31m
30m
28m
31m
31m
UM EL FAROUD
27m
26m
32m
35m
33m
28m
26m
25m
26m
31m
26m
32m
29m
27m
20m
32m
28m
UM EL FAROUD

West Reef & Inlet — Area 2

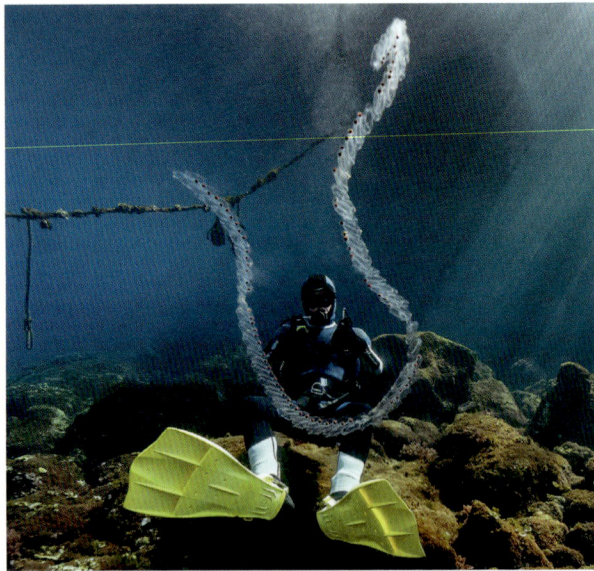

Spectacular show of salps (Jellyfish eggs) and only just below your entry point E1.   PHOTO: JON BORG www.jonborg.com

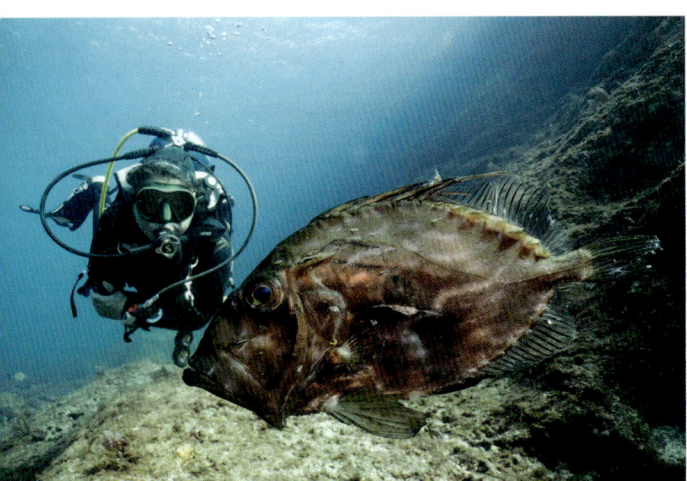

In the Inlet a John Dory (Zeus faber) and a diver enjoys it's company.   PHOTO: VERONICA BUSUTTIL

Below: A shoal of small fish in the shallows on West reef.
PHOTOS: JON BORG www.jonborg.com

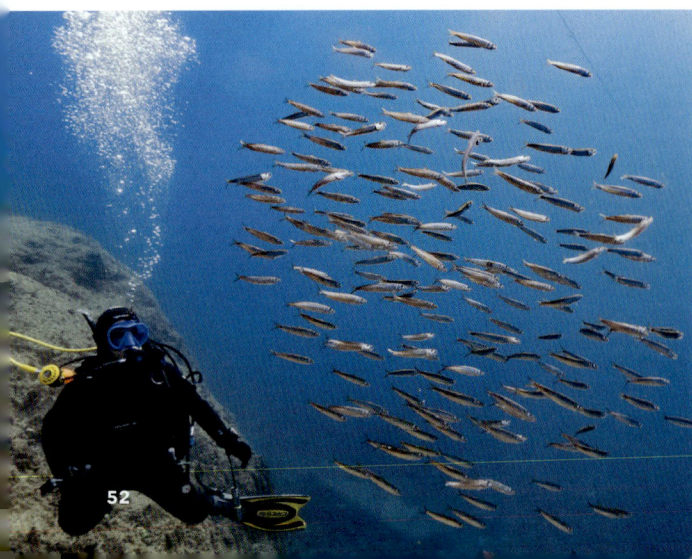

THE DIVE — Minimum time - 40 mins

This dive site is situated on the western side of the inlet and there are a number of different areas to explore. There are drop offs, ledges, gullies and boulders surrounded by sea grass and sandy areas. There are also two caves, the walls of which are covered in a wide variety of brightly coloured corals and inside many cardinal fish using them as their home.

Enter the water at E1 and down to 10m cross the inlet to the western side, down over the rocky slope onto the small area of sand at 24m. Follow the reef around to the right heading west; over the sea grass, the first of the two caves are at 24m, further round you will find a small area of sand where you will find the entrance to Bell Tower cave at 26m, when entering the cave be careful not to kick up the sand. You can exit the cave at 21m. On the left-hand side of the cave exit is a large rock, from this point follow a line where the grass, rocks and boulders meet the sand with a compass bearing of 240° this will lead you to the divers helmet plaque at 31m, placed there by BS-AC Atlam Dive Club to commemorate fifty years of their club.

When it is time to return ascend the reef to your required depth. Follow it along and on the ridge, just before the inlet you will find a fissure, which runs from 16m to the top of the reef, another good place to explore. If you intend to cross the inlet underwater, remember the pleasure boats using the inlet, so leave enough depth to be safe.

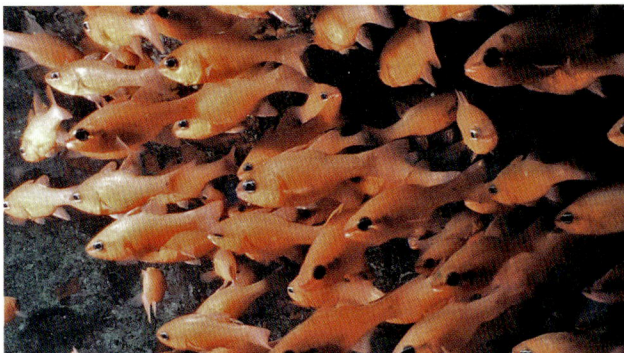

Cardinal fish (Apogon imberbis) can be found below 10m in overhangs where they can retreat to if necessary.

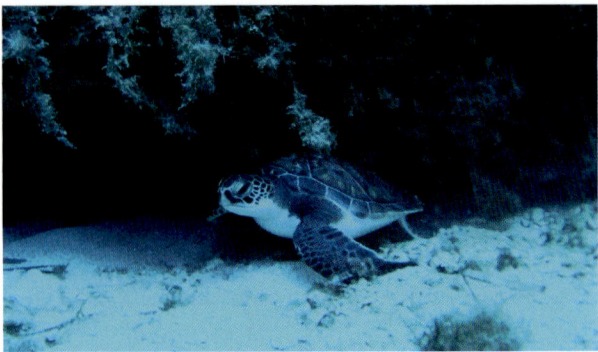

A visit to Zurrieq by a turtle (Eretmochelis imbricata) fantastic.
PHOTO: SERGEY MARKOV DIVE SYSTEMS DIVE CENTRE

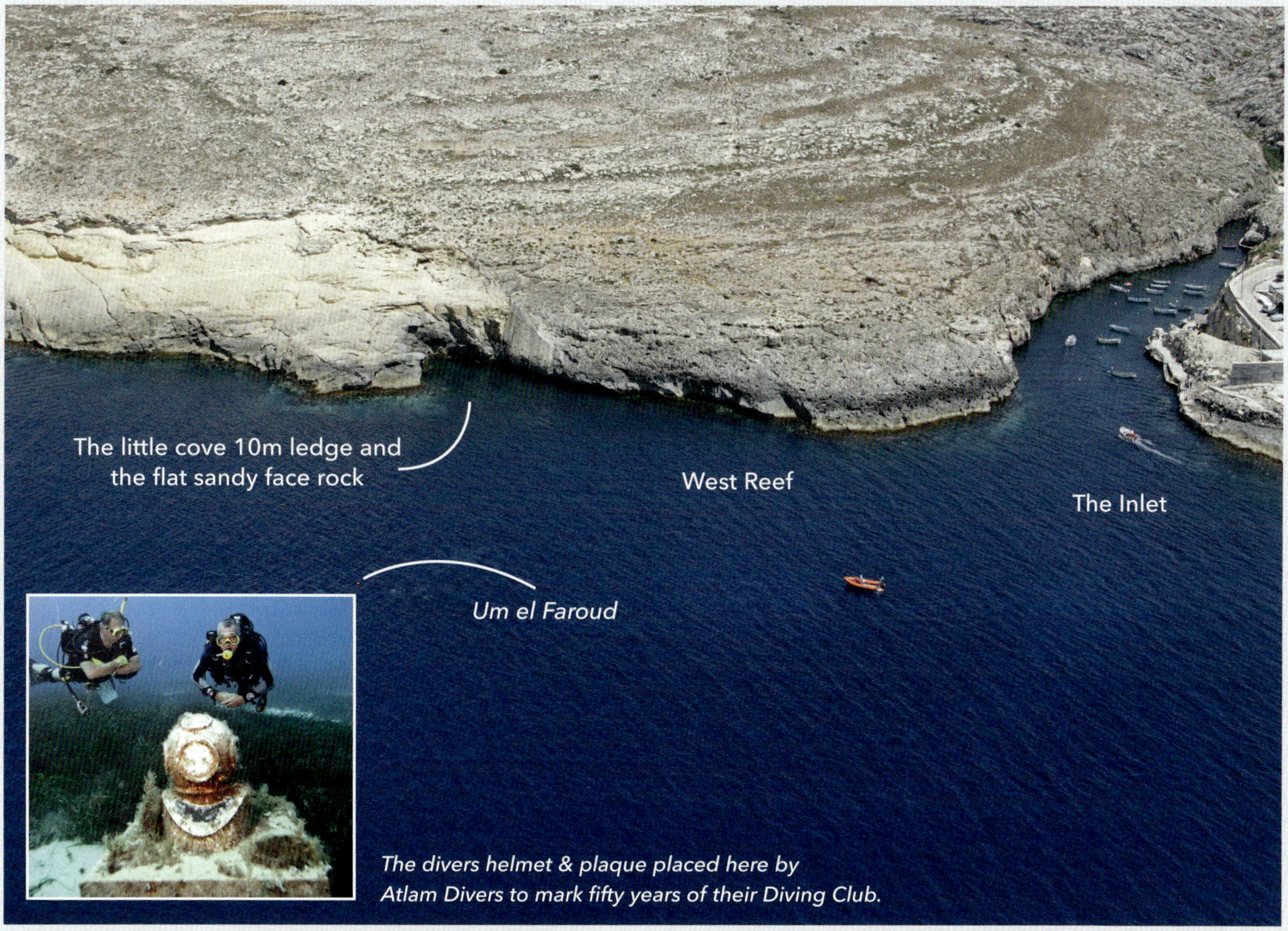

WIED IZ-ZURRIEQ (BLUE GROTTO) - WEST REEF & INLET

- The little cove 10m ledge and the flat sandy face rock
- West Reef
- The Inlet
- Um el Faroud

The divers helmet & plaque placed here by Atlam Divers to mark fifty years of their Diving Club.

PHOTO: PGL AERIAL PHOTOS

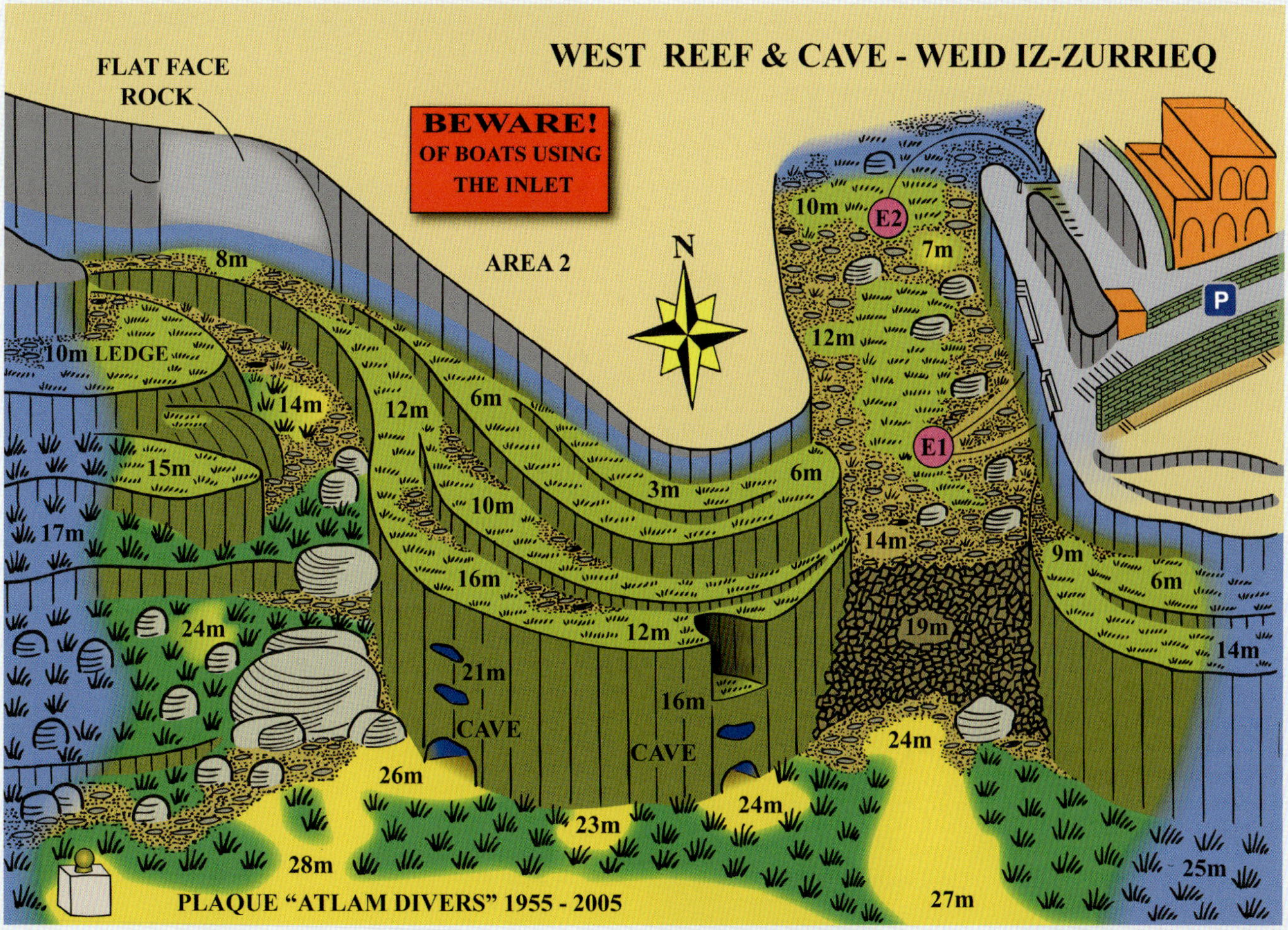

WEST REEF & CAVE - WEID IZ-ZURRIEQ

FLAT FACE ROCK

BEWARE! OF BOATS USING THE INLET

AREA 2

N

8m
10m LEDGE
14m
15m
17m
24m
12m
6m
10m
16m
12m
3m
6m
21m
CAVE
16m
CAVE
26m
23m
24m
28m
27m
10m
E2
7m
12m
E1
14m
19m
9m
6m
14m
24m
25m

P

PLAQUE "ATLAM DIVERS" 1955 - 2005

East Reef & Inlet — Area 2

This straight line reef continues in an easterly direction for 300/400 metres. At the start of this reef is a large ledge with depths from 9m to 16m, the maximum depth to the seabed is 36m. Of course, moving away from the reef the depth will increase, but this area is mostly sand and sea grass.

Here the visibility here can be excellent, with clear water up to 40 metres plus. Usually, large shoals of small fish can be seen on the reef, also keep an eye out into the blue for those larger fish that may be coming in to feed.

THE DIVE — Minimum time - 45 mins

Entry for this dive can be made directly below the steps E1, or further round to the east there is another entry point, E3, bearing in mind that exit is not possible from the latter. Once under the water you can follow the ledge along for some 60 meters and at varying depths of 9m to 16m. at the end of the ledge descend the drop-off down to 28m plus, if you have decided to use entry point E1 descend to 9m then down over the rocky slope to 24m. and out of the inlet bearing left and heading east, follow the bottom of the reef at 28m.

This is where both routes meet

Continue to follow the line where the bottom of the reef meets the sand past the small overhang, staying close to the base of the drop off the seabed in front of you will begin to rise, passing a number of large boulders on the seaward side until you reach a depth of 9m. You are now immediately beneath the overhang on the surface, this could be your turning point from here return to the ledge at your required depth. Follow the reef all the way along heading west, round into the inlet and your planned exit point.

This moray out in the open over the sand makes a great photo shoot.   PHOTO: LELI SCEBRIS CALYPSO SUB AQUA CLUB

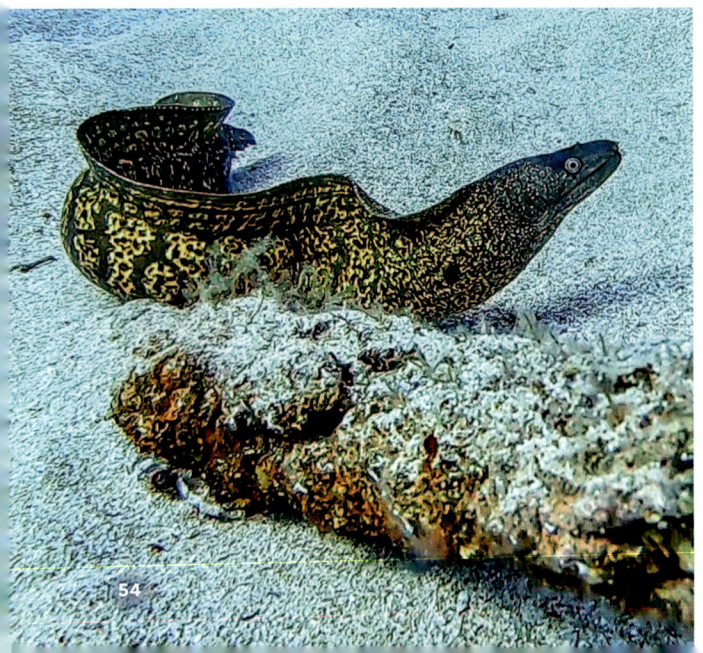

Alternatively, if you wish to be a little more adventurous, the best way to dive the reef is to surface swim to the overhang (see aerial photograph) be sure to check for currents and keep to the shoreline, as the pleasure boats also use this route to the Blue Grotto. Once you have reached the surface overhang, which should take you 6 to 8 minutes from E3, descend to 8m on the eastern side of the reef, from here you will be able to descend a drop off to 35m. Follow the line of the reef staying at a depth of 30m keeping the reef on your right and heading in a westerly direction, once you meet the main reef ascend to your required depth until you return to the inlet and your exit point.

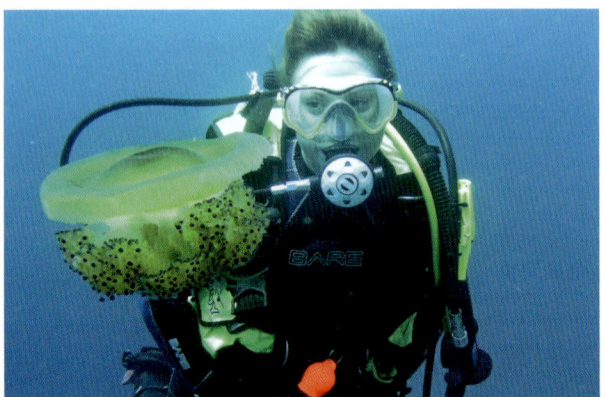

A diver, admires a fried egg jelly fish (Cotylorhiza tuberculata).   PHOTO: PAUL ADAMS

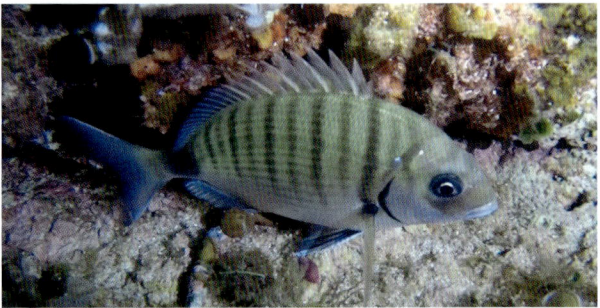

Sharpsnout sea bream (Diplodus puntazzo) normally solitary, but the young swim in shoals near the shore.   PHOTO: LELI SCEBRIS CALYPSO SUB AQUA CLUB

Night diving at Weid iz-Zurrieq

Wied iz-Zurrieq is an excellent venue for a night dive, for there is an abundance of marine life to see around the small overhangs and rocks within the inlet. There are reef walls to navigate by, safe exits, lighting and footpaths, and if you are very lucky a full moon will shine down and glisten over the sea while you sit and enjoy a drink of your choice after the dive.

There are many fish to see here during the day or night, just to name a few, damselfish, red mullet, cardinalfish within the caves, painted combers, scorpionfish, moray-eels, cuttlefish, wrasse, john dory and it was here at 6m in the inlet, I saw my first seahorse in Malta.

Restaurants, cafés and gift shops are open during the day and evening over the summer period but close earlier in winter.

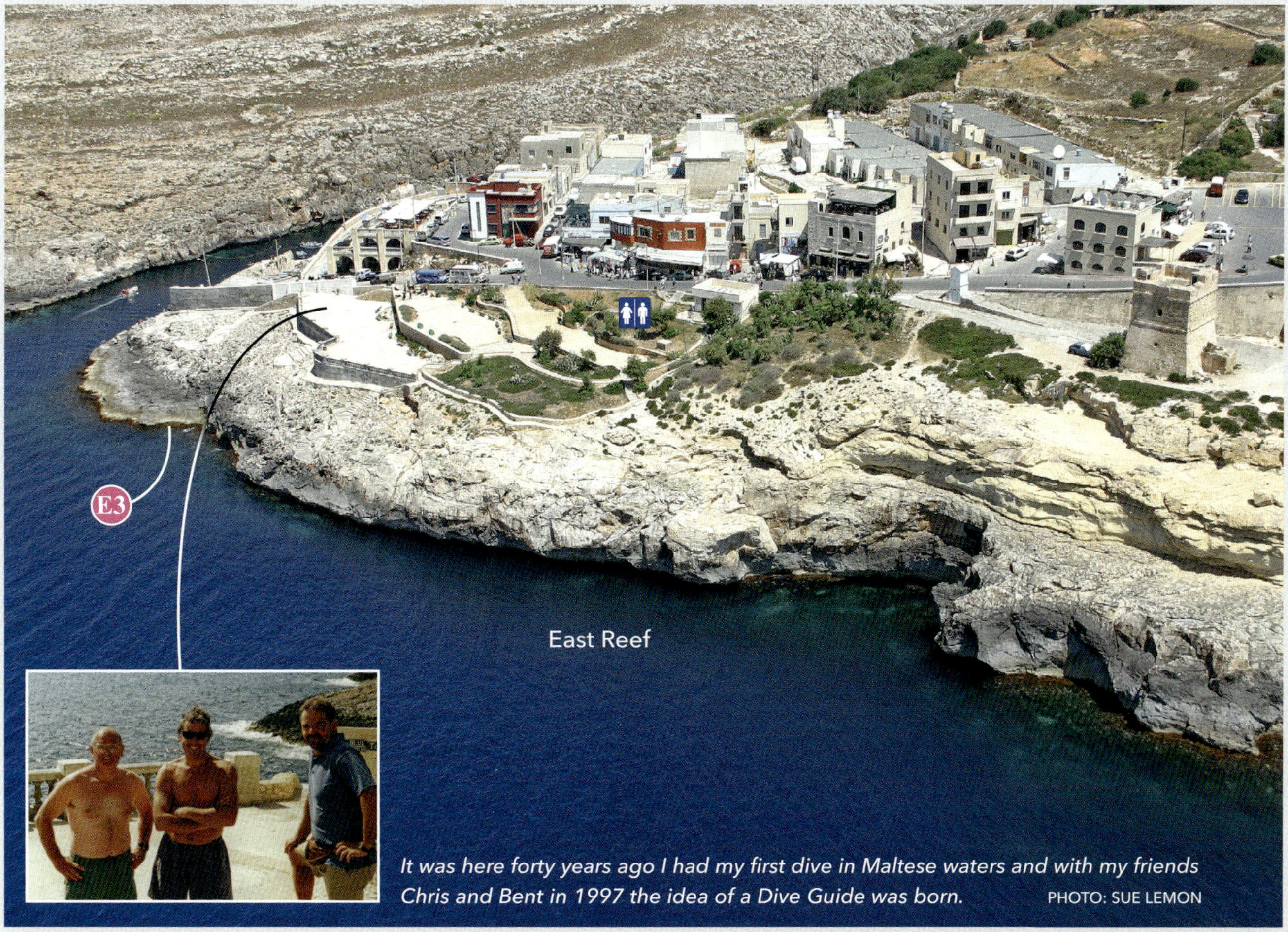

E3
East Reef

It was here forty years ago I had my first dive in Maltese waters and with my friends Chris and Bent in 1997 the idea of a Dive Guide was born. PHOTO: SUE LEMON

PHOTO: PGL AERIAL PHOTOS

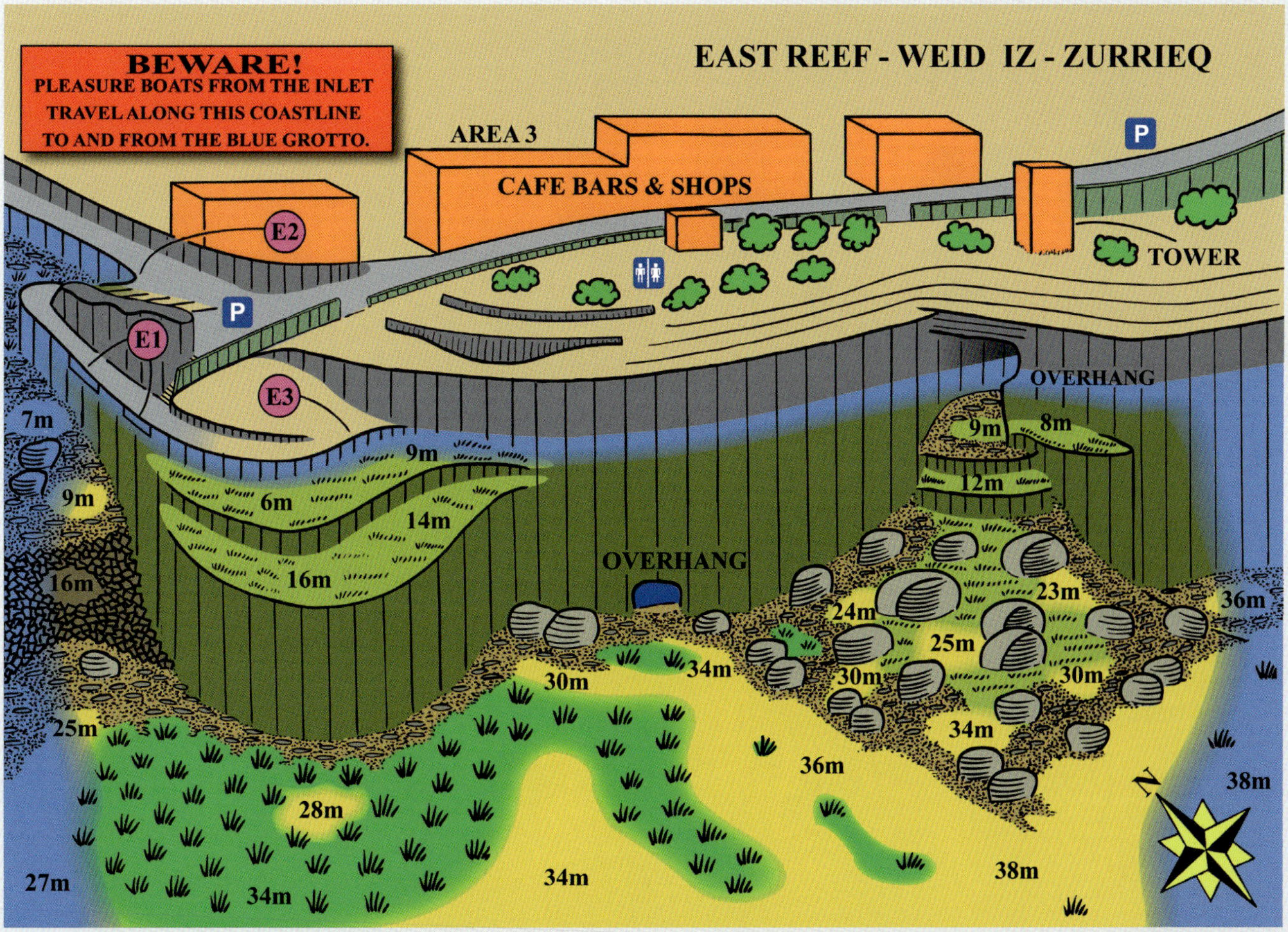
EAST REEF - WEID IZ - ZURRIEQ
BEWARE!
PLEASURE BOATS FROM THE INLET TRAVEL ALONG THIS COASTLINE TO AND FROM THE BLUE GROTTO.
AREA 3
CAFE BARS & SHOPS
P
P
TOWER
E2
E1
E3
OVERHANG
OVERHANG
7m
9m
16m
25m
27m
9m
6m
14m
16m
9m
8m
12m
23m
24m
25m
30m
30m
34m
34m
30m
36m
36m
38m
38m
34m
28m
34m
N

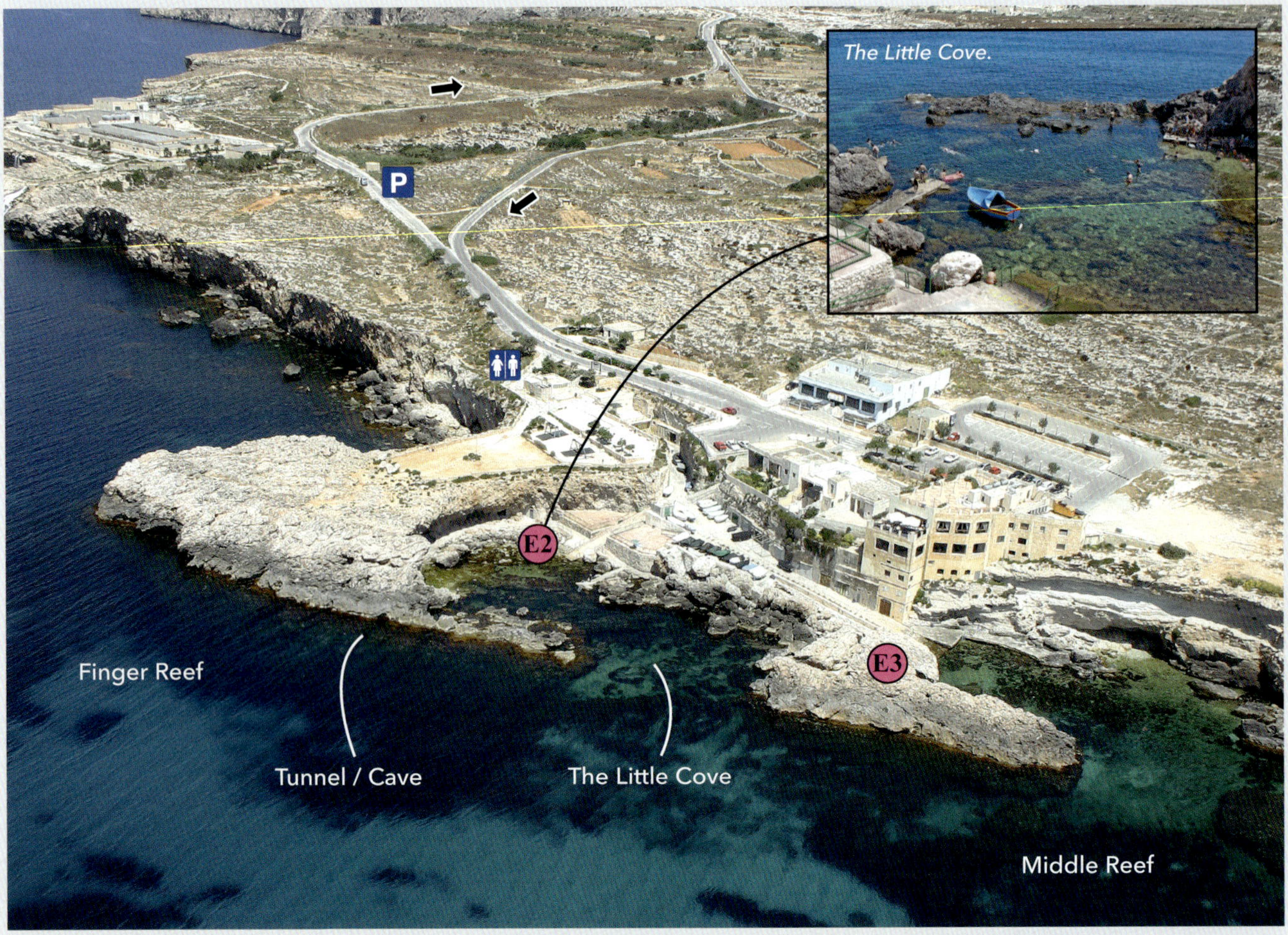

GHAR LAPSI - BLACK JOHN

The Little Cove.

Finger Reef
Tunnel / Cave
The Little Cove
Middle Reef

PHOTO: PGL AERIAL PHOTOS

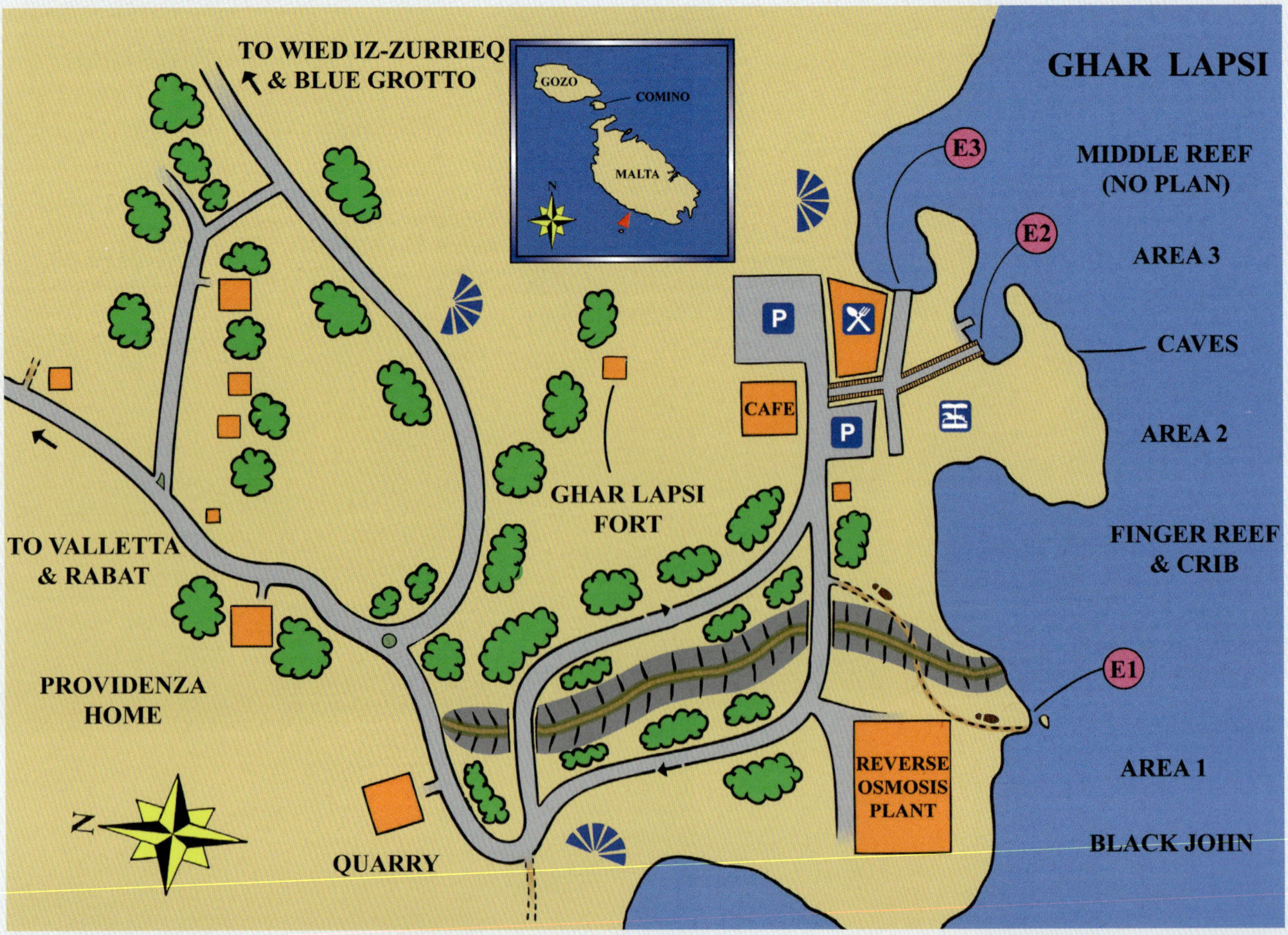

GHAR LAPSI

TO WIED IZ-ZURRIEQ & BLUE GROTTO

GOZO COMINO MALTA

TO VALLETTA & RABAT

PROVIDENZA HOME

CAFE

GHAR LAPSI FORT

QUARRY

REVERSE OSMOSIS PLANT

MIDDLE REEF (NO PLAN)
AREA 3
CAVES
AREA 2
FINGER REEF & CRIB
AREA 1
BLACK JOHN

Ghar Lapsi - Black John - Finger Reef

Ghar Lapsi is a very small hamlet which has a pretty little cove and is situated in the south of the island and is one of the few places where the sea can be entered along this coastline. To reach Ghar Lapsi from the north you will probably travel from Rabat/Mdina 9km in distance along single lane country roads. From Wiedi z-Zurrieq and the south continue along the coast road to Ghar Lapsi, 5km. passing the Prehistoric Temples (Haga Qinn) At the roundabout turn down the hill and past the quarry to where the road splits in two and a one-way system is operated. Here you will find two car parks, next to the small car park is a steep road with steps leading down to the cove where your entry/exit points E2, E3 are, parking to dive Black John is near the Osmosis Plant, see plan.

Black John — Area 1

The dive at Black John takes you away from the popular dive sites and it is almost a certainty that you will be the only divers here. The dive site is situated at the rear of the Osmosis Plant; this involves a 200 metre walk over uneven ground.

Follow the rough track down to a small concrete hut then follow the pathway into a little valley, a short climb up the other side, turn left, follow the fence around the Osmosis Plant going under the water outlet. Keep following the fence until you find steps cut into the rock. This leads down to a small concrete platform, which is your entry point and to the right is your exit point E1. Check this route before you rig.

Remember it is not possible, with safety in mind, to dive this site during rough sea conditions for there is only one entry/exit point. The next nearest exit point is the cove at Ghar Lapsi, which is some 400 metres away.

I have two dive plans for this off shore reef but of course you can plan your own dive.

THE DIVE — Minimum time - 45 mins

Dive Plan 1 entry is a 2m drop to the water and below you a depth of 10m, once on the seabed move away from this area.

With the reef on your left heading east past a large rock and under an arch/overhang. Coming through the other side do a part U-turn and take a compass bearing of 200° to the main reef. On reaching the reef keep it on your left; follow it all the way round until it is heading east.

If you stay reasonably close to the reef your maximum depth will not exceed 25m, but further away from the reef, depths of 30m or more are possible around the large rocks, grass and sandy areas. After some 25 minutes into your dive, depending on the time you have taken to explore and you are close to the base of the reef you will find what appears to be a large crack which leads diagonally upwards to the top of the reef.

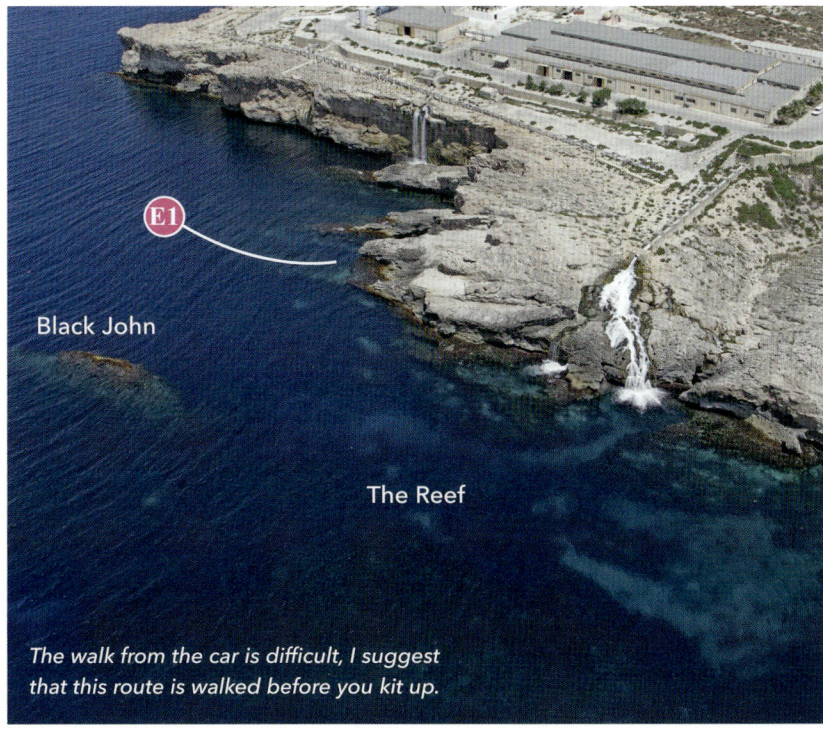

The walk from the car is difficult, I suggest that this route is walked before you kit up.

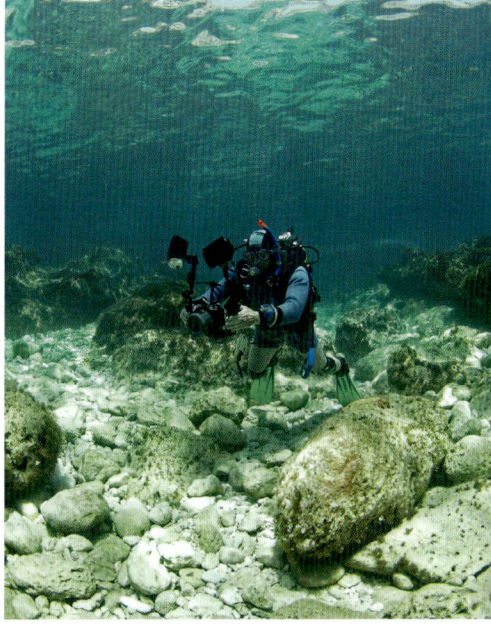

Above: Below the surface at the exit, entrance to the little cove, Ghar Lapsi.

PHOTO: SHARON FORDER

GHAR LAPSI - BLACK JOHN

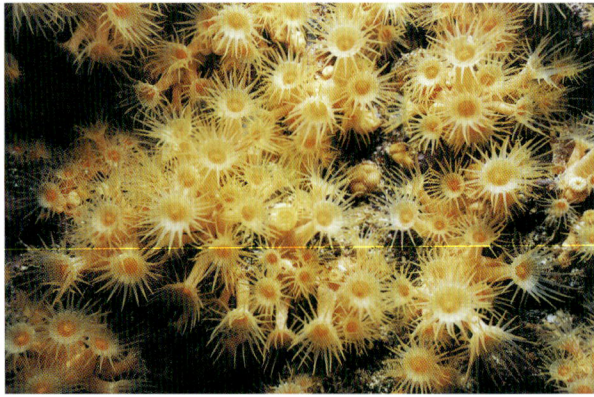
Golden zoanthid (Parazoanthus axinellae) lives on rocky slopes.

Once at the top of the reef head in a westerly direction along the ridge, it will take you no more than 6 minutes to reach the base of the reef at 10m that leads up to Black John itself.

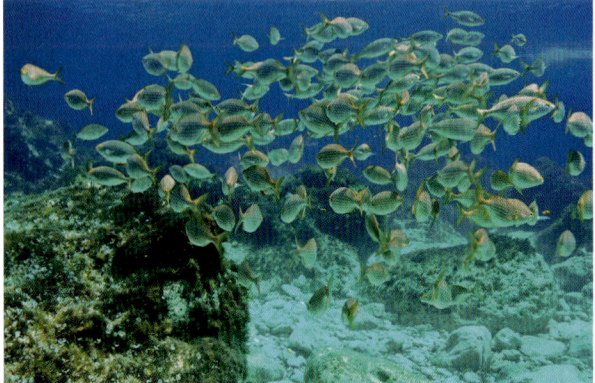
A shoal of salema fish (Sarpa sarpa) below the plant outfall.

Below: Practising the use of a Delayed Surface Marker Buoy.

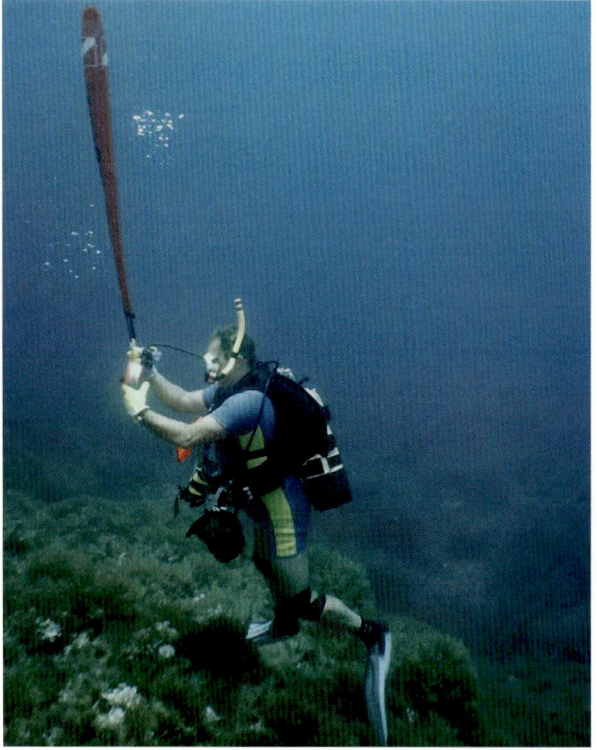

Now a northerly compass bearing will take you towards the coastline, first over the reef to Propeller rock and then over the sand where the water from the Osmosis Plant falls into the sea, here there is normally an abundance of marine life.

To find your exit point head west and you will pass over the large rock and overhang where your dive began, then ascend to the 6m ledge where you can do your safety stops and explore at the same time, bear round to the right for your exit point.

Dive Plan 2 the alternative way to do this dive with a depth of 38m is to surface swim to the far side of Black John continue on until you are clear of the shallow reef. Now descend keeping clear of the boulders, once on the seabed head in an easterly direction with the large boulders and grass on your left and the sandy area on your right, depth 38m. Keeping to this route and in approximately 9 minutes you should reach a depth of 32m.

Turn to your left and head in a northerly direction you should be able to see in front of you, a very large boulder, which has its base at 30m. Ascend to the top of this boulder and then on to the main reef, now follow the ridge in a westerly direction, it should take you no more than 10 minutes to reach the base of Black John itself. **From this point of your dive the route to your exit is the same as Dive Plan 1.**

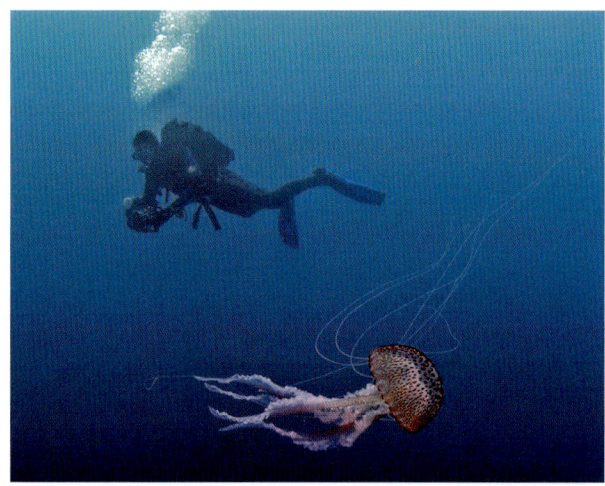
Jellyfish (Peleegi noctiluca) artistic photography underwater.
PHOTO: SHAROM FORDER.

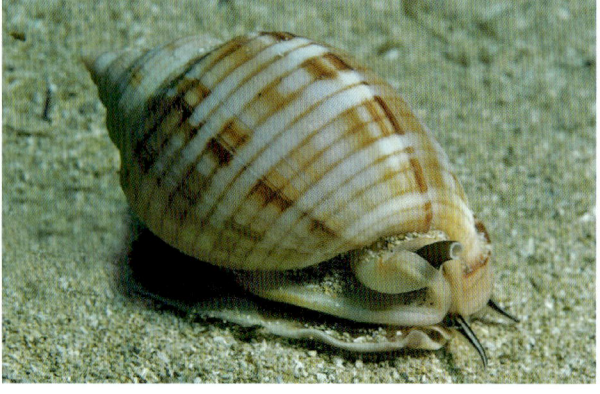
Very pretty ribbed helmet shell (Phalium granulatum).

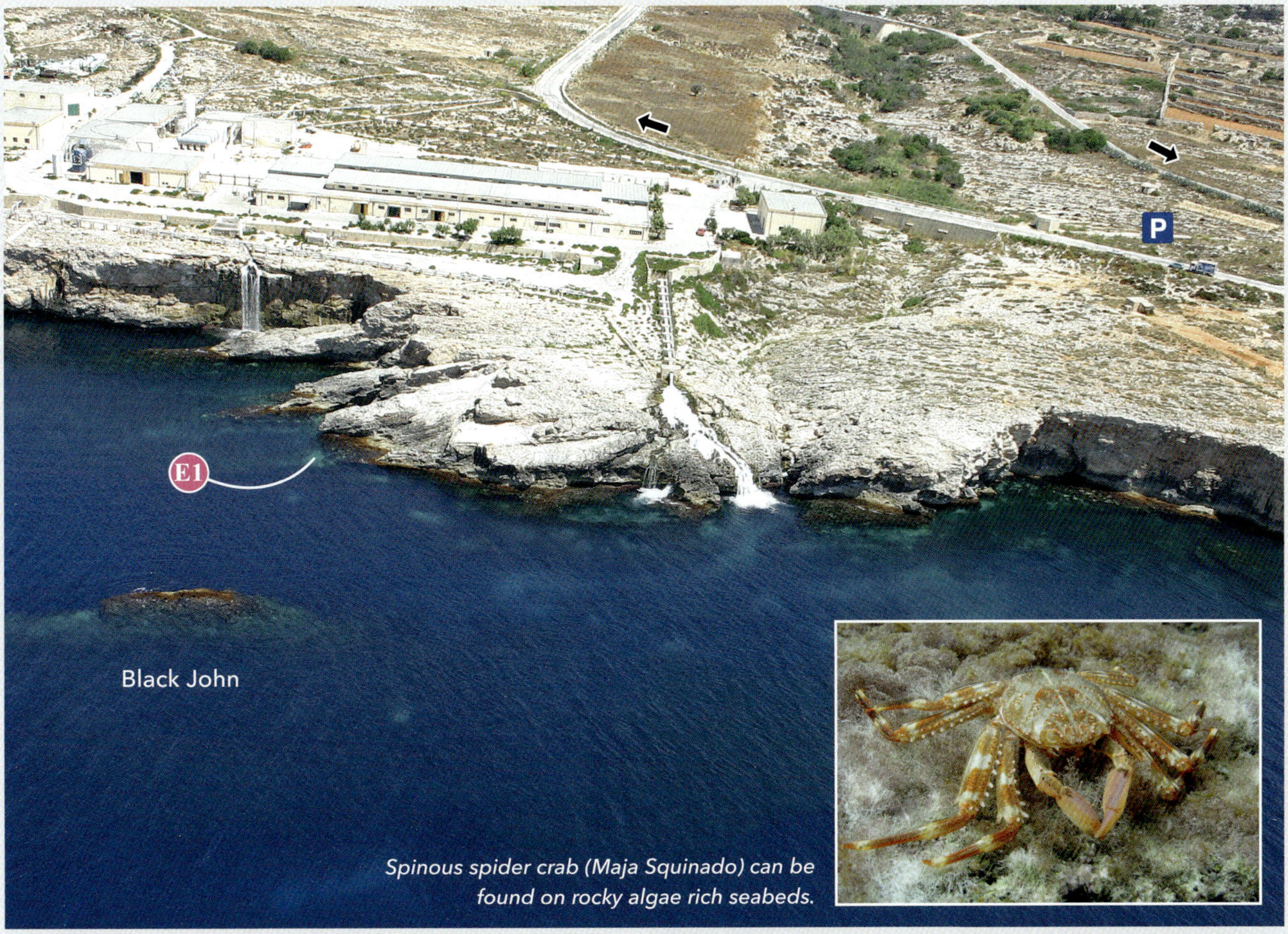

GHAR LAPSI - BLACK JOHN

Black John

Spinous spider crab (Maja Squinado) can be found on rocky algae rich seabeds.

PHOTO: PGL AERIAL PHOTOS

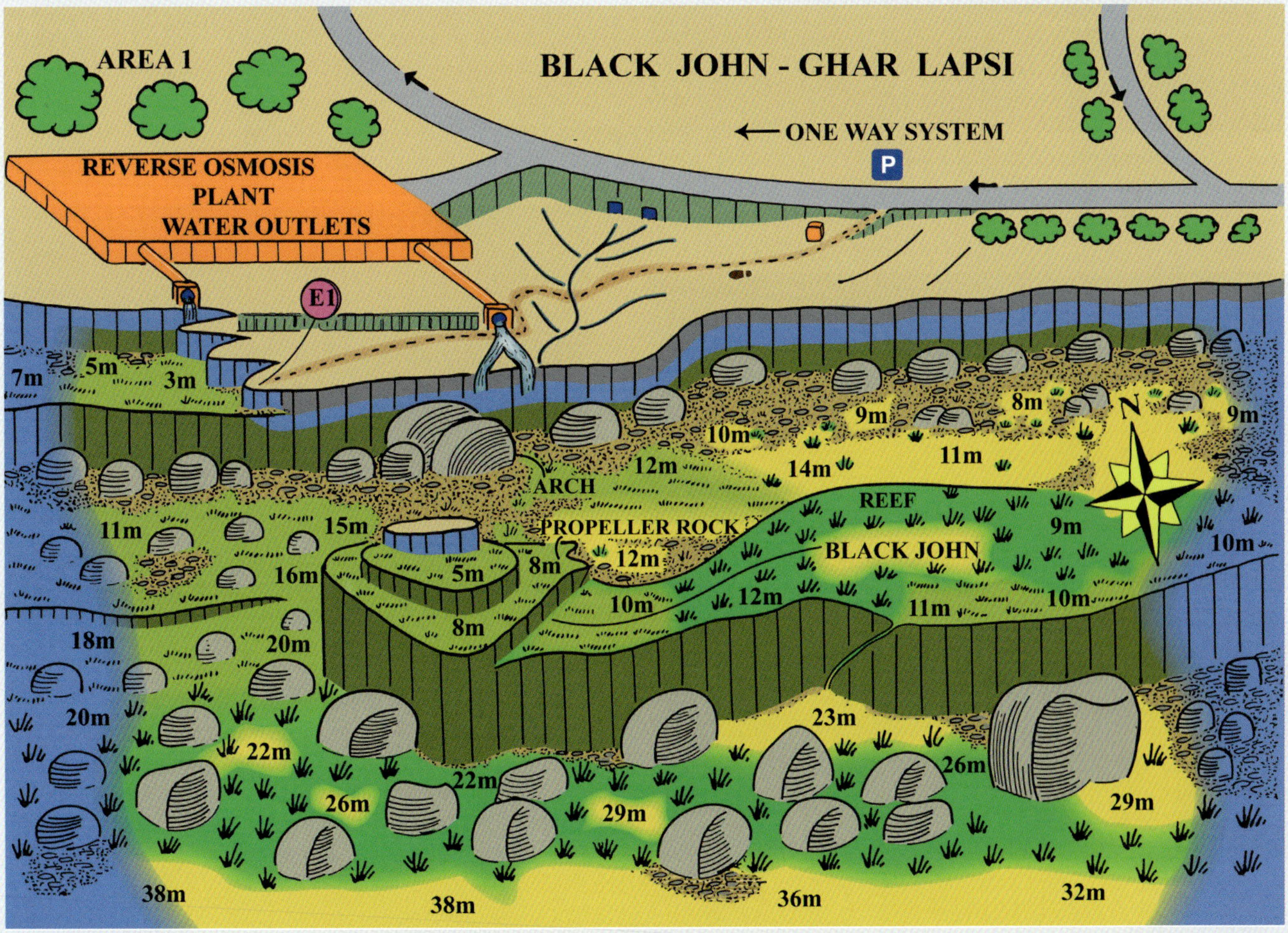

BLACK JOHN - GHAR LAPSI

AREA 1

REVERSE OSMOSIS PLANT WATER OUTLETS

← ONE WAY SYSTEM

ARCH
PROPELLER ROCK
REEF
BLACK JOHN

GHAR LAPSI - FINGER REEF & CRIB

Finger Reef & Crib — Area 2

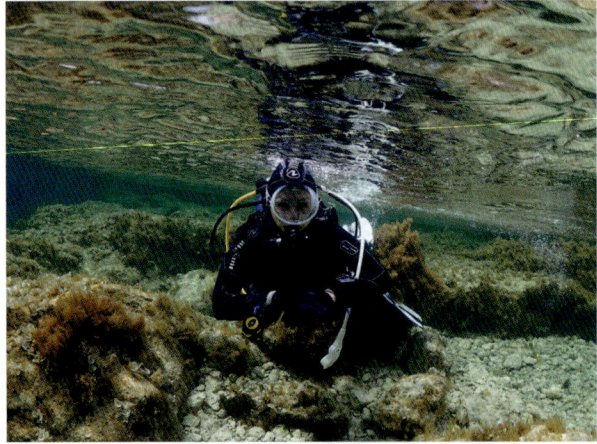

The crystal-clear waters in the little cove at entry E1 below the steps. PHOTO: SERGEY MARKOV DIVE SYSTEMS DIVE CENTRE

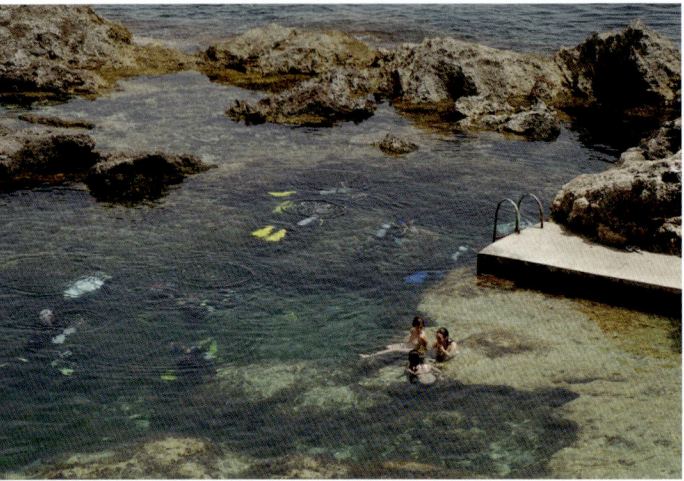

Calm waters today so it's safe for diver head for the tunnel, caves.

Below: the outer area of the cove before you reach the open sea. PHOTO: ARKADIUSZ SREBNIK POLANDDIVINGPHOTO

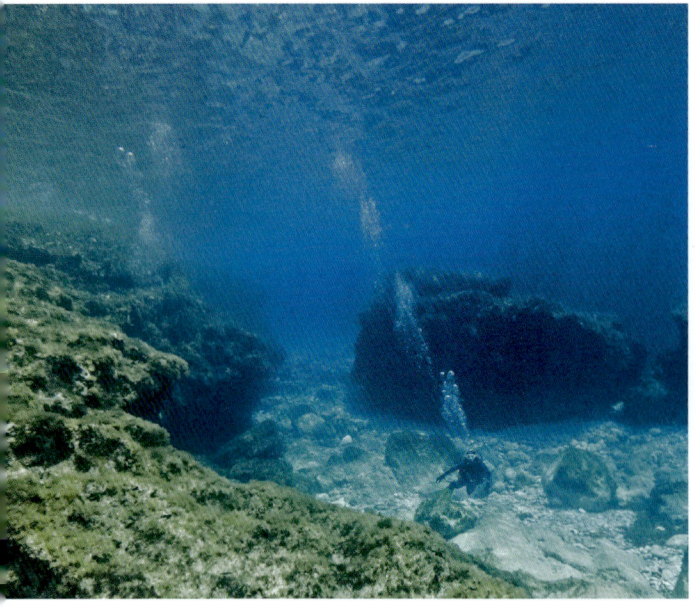

Before diving this area, you will have to decide which route you are going to follow.

Route 1 via Finger Reef, its western side is shaped like a finger hence its name, then to the cave at 19m with the hole in the roof, this dive is the shorter distance of the two dives.

Route 2 via the Crib at 22m, this will be your maximum depth. This reef twists and turns until it reaches the cave at 19m. The Crib, a nativity scene, is of almost life size figures cut from plate metal, welded to a tubular frame, placed under the water within an overhang, by the Calypso Diving Team.

Around both these reefs are areas of boulders, rocks and Posidonia grass. Of course, within this area there are many permutations of dives giving you the opportunity to create your own dive plan.

Your entry point, E2, is immediately below the small car park at the bottom of the steep track and steps.

THE DIVE — Minimum time - 55 mins

Route 1 from entry point E2 to the open sea from the centre of the cove near the end of the little jetty, descend, then swim out of the cove underwater with the reef wall on your right, once out of the cove, continue down over the seabed in a westerly direction, until you reach the sand at 11m.

Alternatively, if the weather conditions permit and there is no surge in the cave it could be used for the start of the dive, or if you prefer at the end. Surface swim directly across the cove, descend, swim under a small arch depth 1m, into a little pool. The entrance to the cave is on your right, which is small, but once inside there are many small openings in the cave which allows rays of light to shine in. When you reach a depth of 8m your exit will be on the left, leave the cave here swim out through a gully, down onto the sand at 11m.

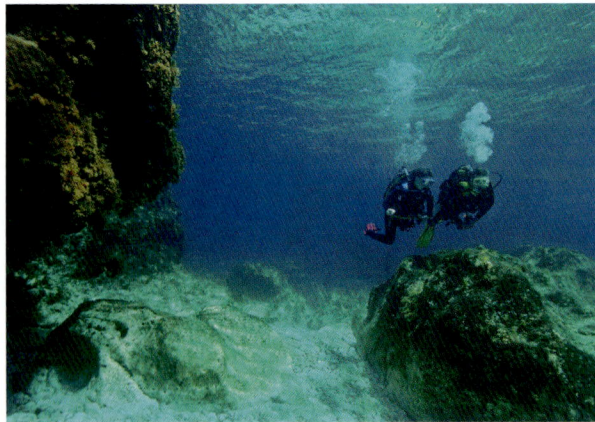

The alternative way for divers leaves the little cove for the open seas.

Here the two dives meet. Now follow the line where the sand meets the reef in a westerly direction for approximately 2 minutes where you will see a mound covered in sea grass on your left, this is the point where the two dives separate at a depth of 12m. **See route 1 or route 2.**

GHAR LAPSI - FINGER REEF & CRIB

Route 1 to go to the cave with the hole in the roof via Finger reef, continue in a westerly direction over the sand into an area where there are many small boulders, the depth here is 12m. Now bear slightly to your left and the reef will start to rise beside you, here your depth will decrease to around 9m and you will be about 10 minutes into your dive. Dropping over a small ridge to a depth of approximately 11m, on your left you will see the start of what I call Finger Reef. Here it is easy to follow this reef all the way to the end, but take your time to explore the many little over-hangs filled with colourful marine life. When you reach the end of the reef you will possibly be 20/25 minutes into your dive, here the depth will be 20m. From the end of the reef take a compass bearing of 60°, this will lead you in an easterly direction over the sea grass to a ridge at 16m.

Drop over this ridge down to 18m, turn left and the cave entrance at 19m; will be just in front of you. When entering take great care, for you may be lucky to see the groupers that are sometimes here. After you have explored the cave, leave through the hole in the roof emerging on the top of the reef 12m. At this point you will be some 30/35 minutes into your dive and from here to your exit point, E2, is a minimum time of 15 minutes. **See return route.**

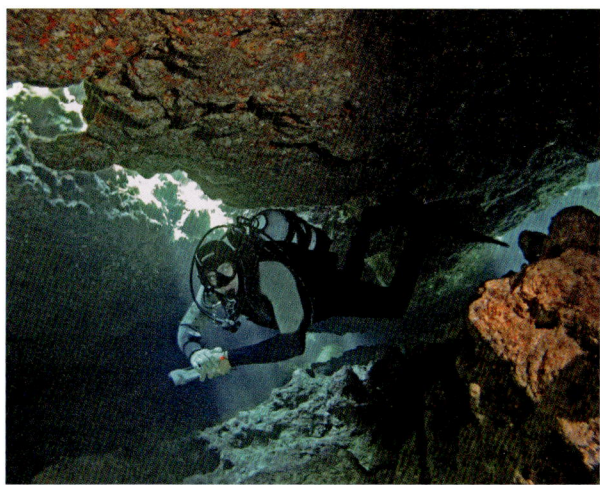
Inside the cave system near the exit to the open sea at 8m.
PHOTO: SERGEY MARKOV DIVE SYSTEMS DIVE CENTRE

Route 2 to go to the cave with the hole in the roof via the Crib take a compass bearing of 210° this will lead you in a southerly direction, for the next 7/8 minutes this area on your left will be mostly sand and, on your right, will be mostly posidonia grass with small patches of sand.

On reaching a depth of 14m on the sand in front of you will be an area of sea grass, continue straight on up and over the sea grass and within 2 minutes, at a depth of 12m you will be on top of the reef. Descend to the bottom at 16m and turn right, follow the base of the reef along for approximately 5 minutes when you should reach a depth of 22m, this is the deepest part of your dive and the Crib is in an overhang on your right-hand side. Make sure that you stay close to the reef at this point or you may miss it altogether.

When it is time to move on, almost immediately the reef starts to head in a northerly direction and from here it will take you around 5 minutes to reach the Double Hooks.

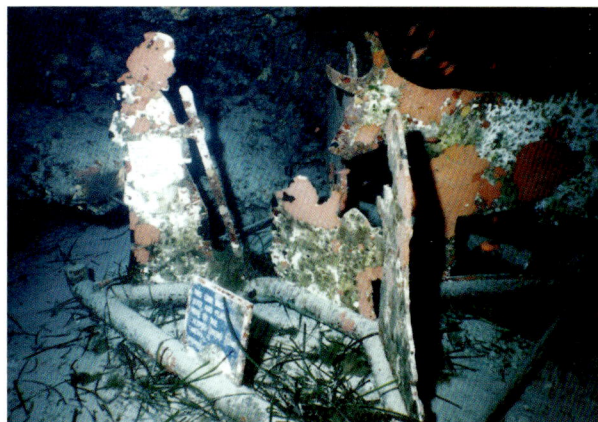
The Crib, placed here by Calypso Sub Aqua Club, December 1992.

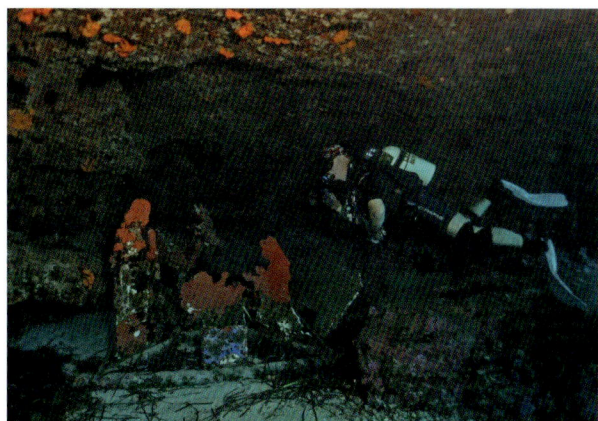
The Crib with almost life-size figures cut from plate metal at 22m.

Below: Two divers heading towards the end of Finger Reef at 18m.   PHOTO: ARKADIUSZ SREBNIK POLANDDIVINGPHOTO

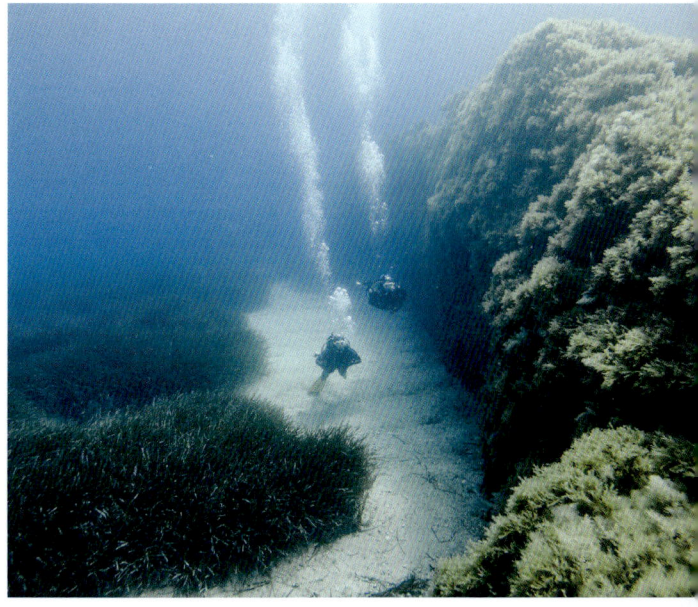

GHAR LAPSI - FINGER REEF & CRIB

Cross over to the opposite reef, and from here it will take you some 5 minutes to reach the Elephant Rock, be careful for his trunk almost reaches the seabed. Once more cross to the opposite reef, from here to the cave will take you no more than 4 minutes. When you have explored the cave ascend through the hole in the roof to the top of the reef at 12m. At this point you will possibly be 40/45 minutes into your dive. Of course, you can at any time go up on top of the reef take a northerly compass bearing and return to the main coastline.

Normally the entrance to the cave is marked with a small heap of stones; at this point your maximum depth should be 6m this will enable you find the reef and follow it into the cove and your exit point. If you wish you can use the route through the cave, into the cove and your exit point, E2.

Return Route. From the hole in the roof of the cave follow a compass bearing of 70° until you reach a 9m drop-off to an area of small boulders at 12m. **Alternatively** once out of the hole head north to the ridge of Finger Reef, then in a north easterly direction follow it all the way along, then down to the area of small boulders at 12m. Now head in an easterly direction and in a very short time the main coastline will be on your left. Continue along this reef at your required depth.

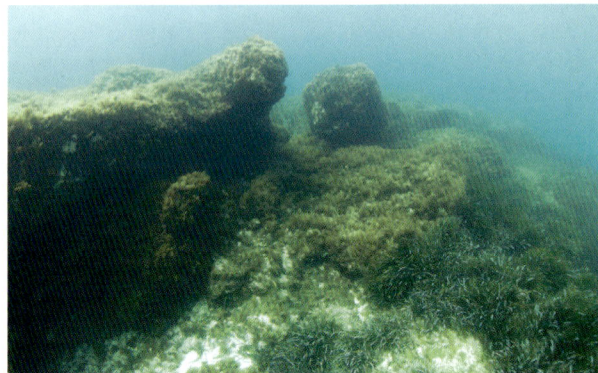

These two boulders mark the north-easterly end of Finger Reef.

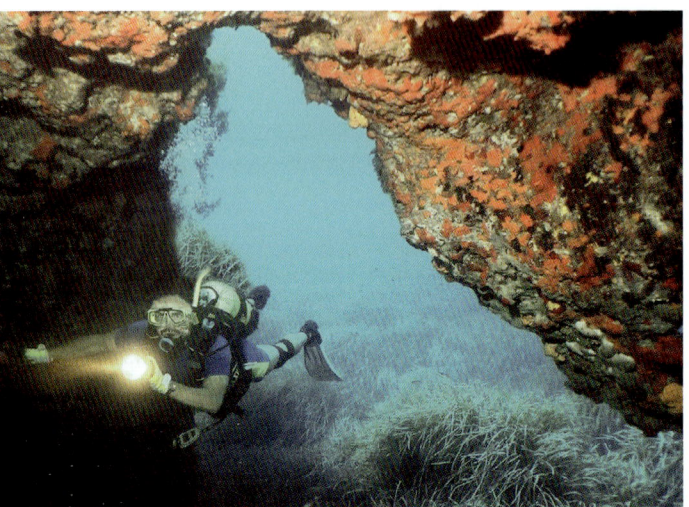

The entrance to the cave with the hole in the roof, which leads you out onto the top of Finger reef, enter slowly look out for the Grouper.

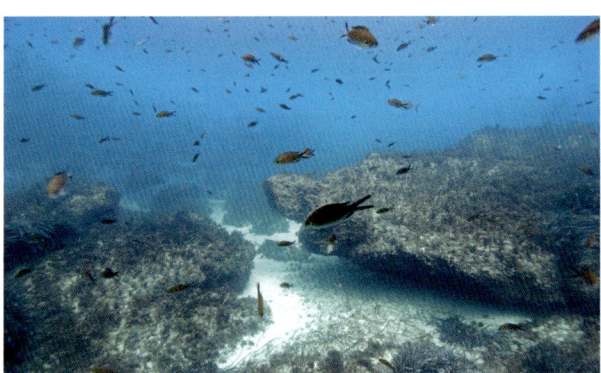

Above: The Lizards Head an area to the east of the little cove, Middle Reef.

Situated next to the car parks are two nice restaurants, which are very popular with the Maltese and at weekends can be quite busy. In the late autumn and winter, they are not always open. Ghar Lapsi is ideal for snorkelling, swimming or sunbathing within the cove, there is a children's playground, also public toilets. A whole day could be spent in this area maybe diving at Wied iz Zurrieq as a first dive and then on to Ghar Lapsi for a second dive, but remember that you will need to take two cylinders with you.

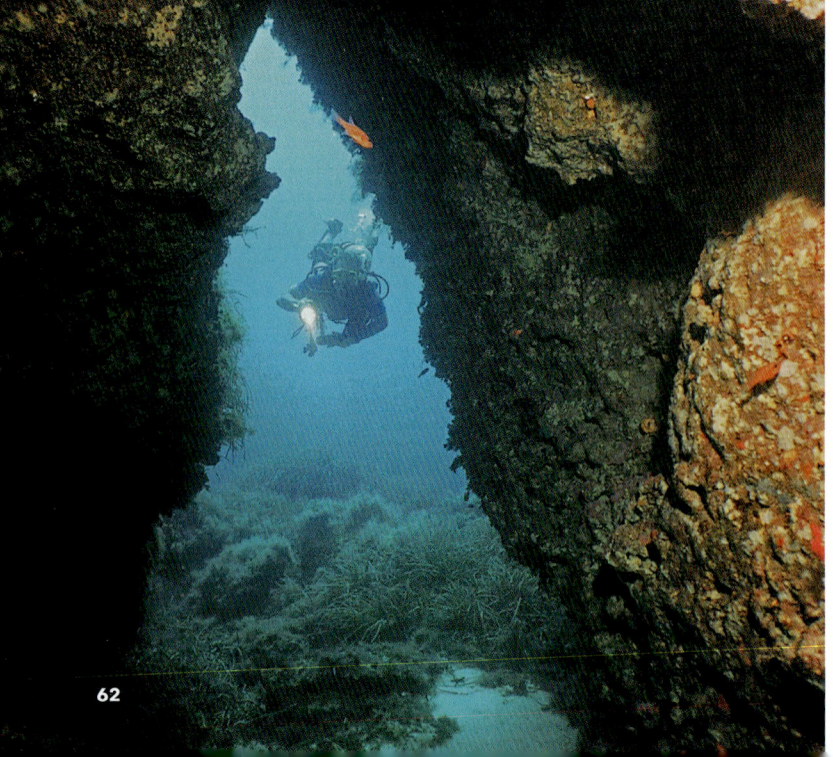

Left: A diver enters the area where to his right is a rock which resembles an elephant's head and trunk.

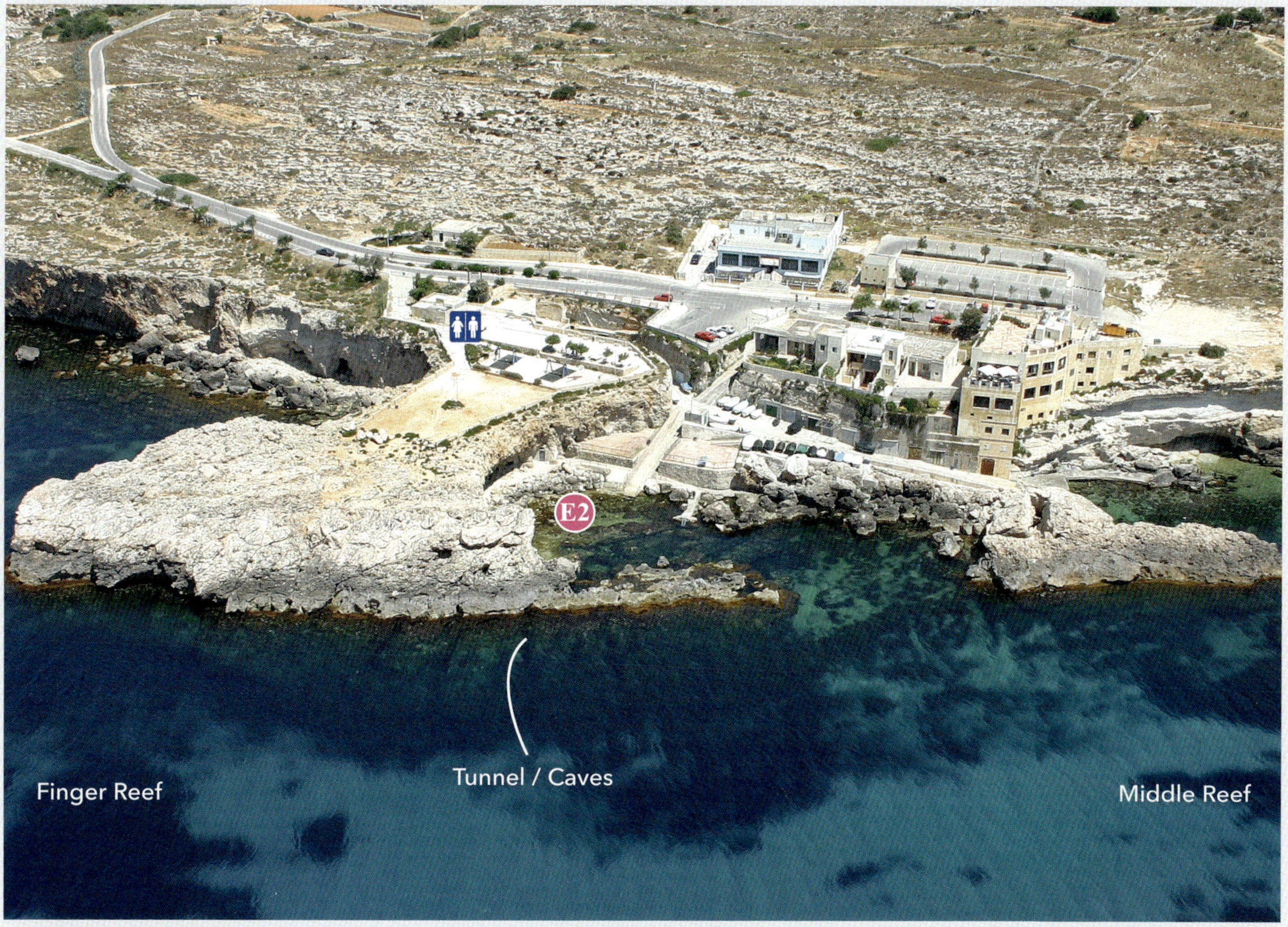

E2
Tunnel / Caves
Finger Reef
Middle Reef

PHOTO: PGL AERIAL PHOTOS

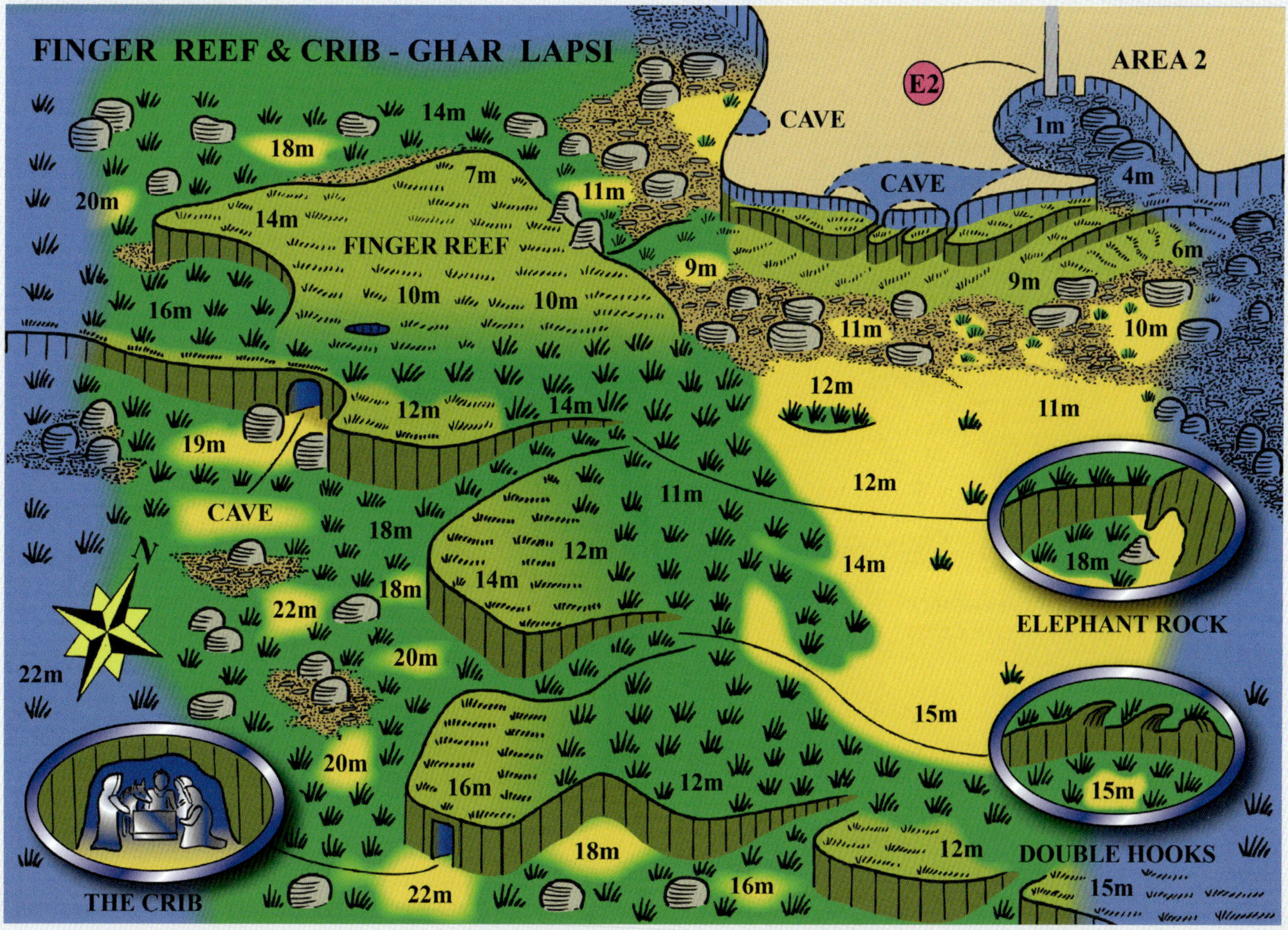
FINGER REEF & CRIB - GHAR LAPSI
AREA 2
E2
CAVE
CAVE
1m
4m
6m
14m
18m
7m
11m
20m
14m
FINGER REEF
9m
9m
16m
10m
10m
11m
10m
12m
12m
14m
11m
19m
CAVE
11m
12m
18m
12m
N
18m
14m
14m
18m
ELEPHANT ROCK
22m
20m
22m
15m
20m
15m
16m
12m
12m
DOUBLE HOOKS
18m
THE CRIB
22m
16m
15m

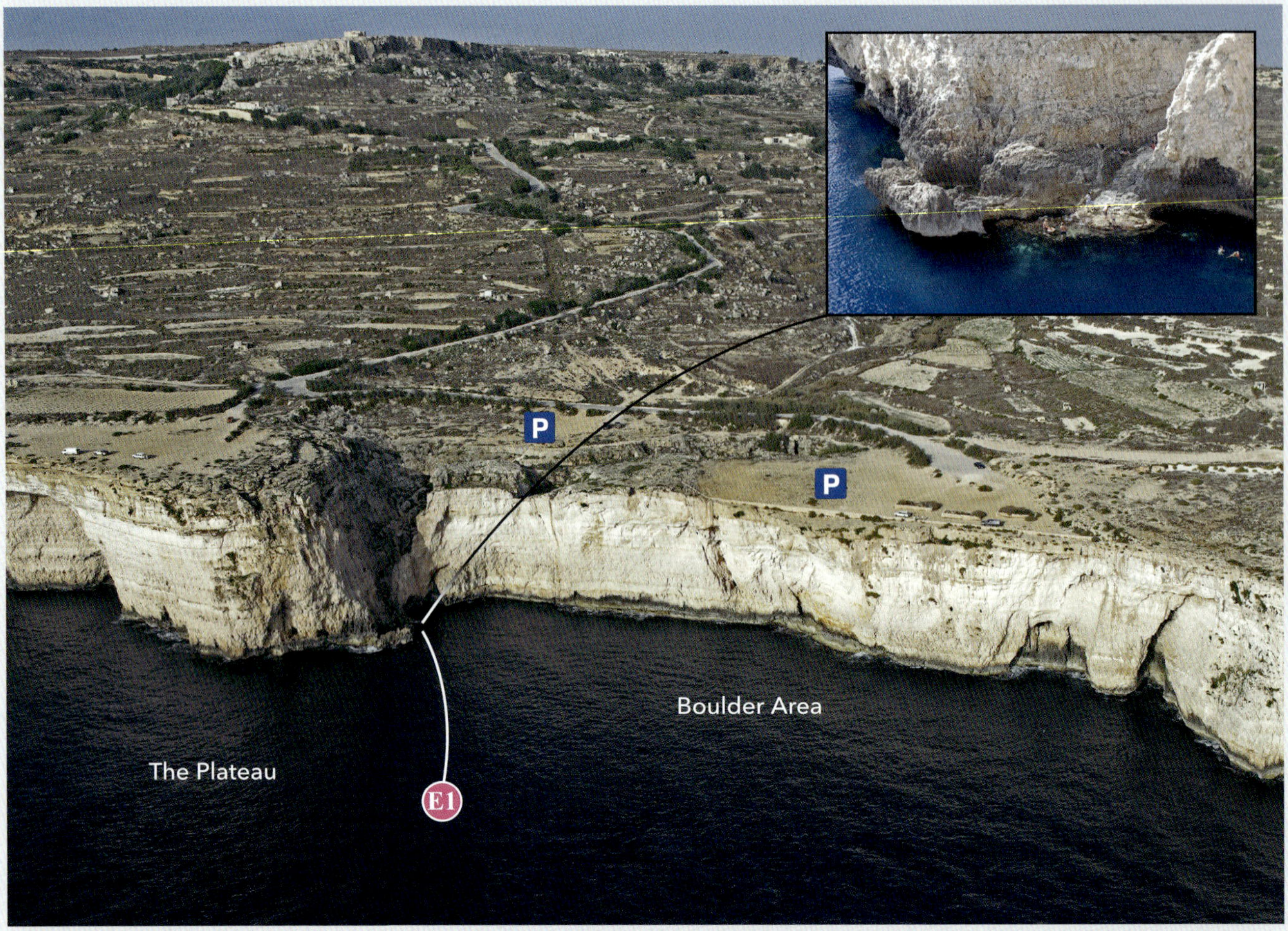

MIGHRA FERHA

Boulder Area

The Plateau

E1

PHOTO: PGL AERIAL PHOTOS

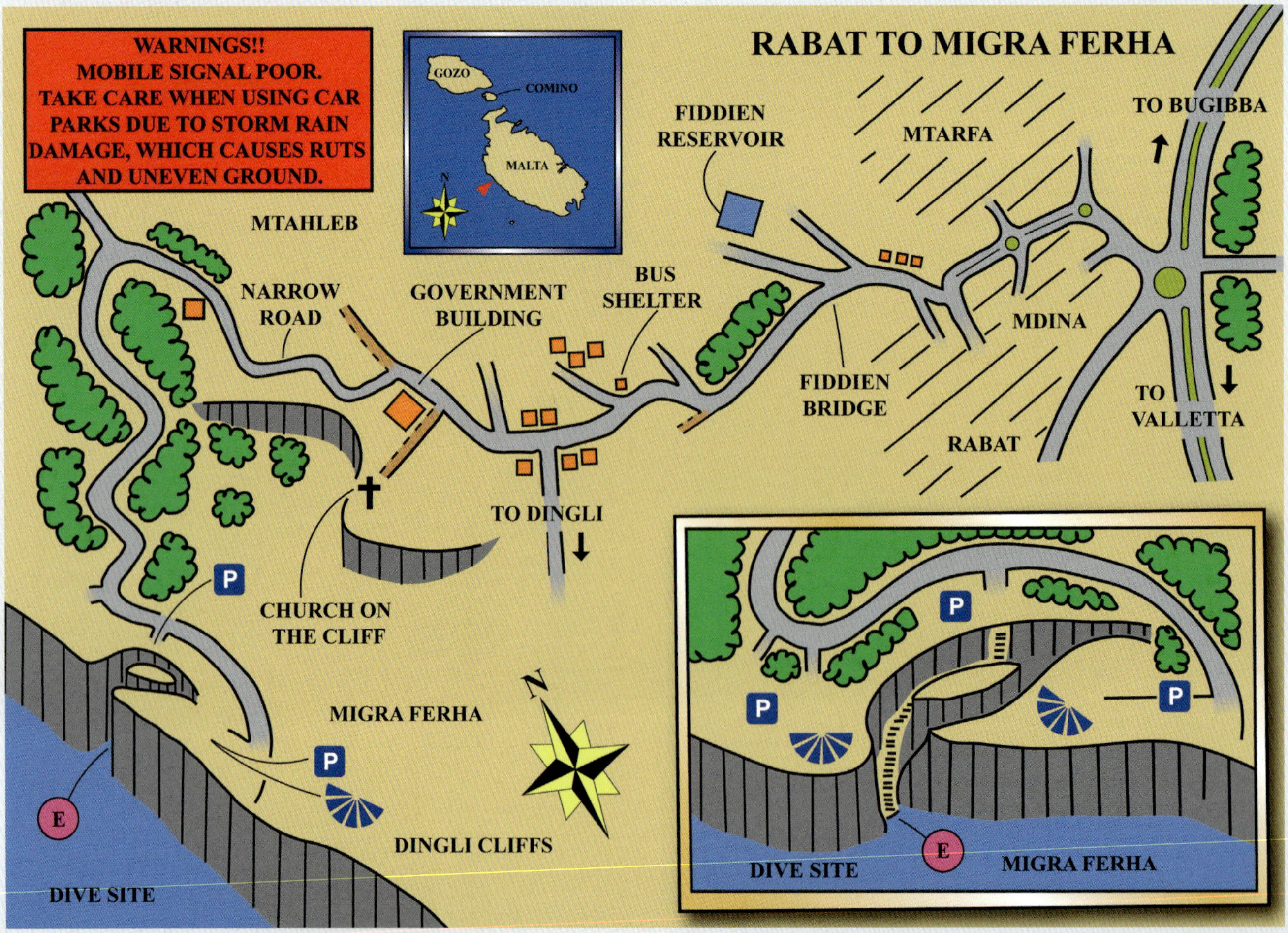

RABAT TO MIGRA FERHA

WARNINGS!! MOBILE SIGNAL POOR. TAKE CARE WHEN USING CAR PARKS DUE TO STORM RAIN DAMAGE, WHICH CAUSES RUTS AND UNEVEN GROUND.

GOZO COMINO MALTA

FIDDIEN RESERVOIR
MTARFA
TO BUGIBBA
MTAHLEB
NARROW ROAD
GOVERNMENT BUILDING
BUS SHELTER
MDINA
FIDDIEN BRIDGE
RABAT
TO VALLETTA
TO DINGLI
CHURCH ON THE CLIFF
MIGRA FERHA
DINGLI CLIFFS
DIVE SITE
E

DIVE SITE   E   MIGRA FERHA

Mighra Ferha

The route to this dive site will take you some twenty minutes from the main road that runs up the valley between Mdina, known as the Silent City, this was once the ancient capital of Malta, on the other side, the village of Mtarfa, famous for its clock tower. Leaving Mdina/Rabat heading northwest, you will pass Fiddien Bridge, a bus shelter and a government premises. Now bear left on to a very narrow road/track, looking to your left over the valley you will see a Church which is built in the cliff face. After a short distance the road gets much better and this will lead you down to Migra Ferha. There are two car parks here, **beware of the surface conditions at the entrance to the first car park.** Once parked check out your route to the dive site before kitting up.

It's important to remember that you are some distance from any amenities, the nearest are in Rabat. Reception for mobile phones is very poor and do not leave valuables on display in your vehicle.

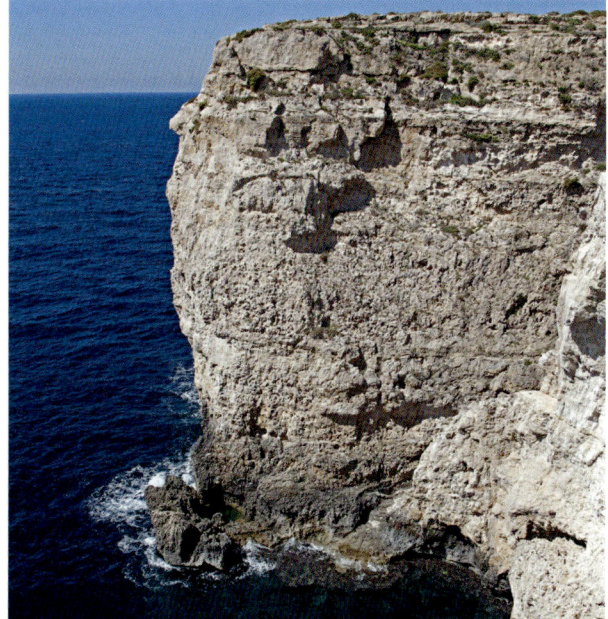

Your only entry exit point along this coastline, below the magnificent cliff and down the 150 steps, visit just once it's well worth it!

This unique and unspoilt dive site should only be attempted by experienced and very fit divers, due to the fact that there are approximately 150 steps to be negotiated to reach the entry/exit point below the Dingli Cliffs, which run along this westerly coastline in each direction. Please do not upset the fishermen for they made the steps that enable us to reach sea level and they also have to replace them after heavy rain, as the gully becomes a river. Before you dive this site, you must check the sea conditions, as this is your **only** exit for a number of kilometres. Once in the water be aware that there can be offshore currents.

There are two dive area's here.

Dive Area 1 to the north a large reef with depths of 16m to 9m and over the drop-off 30/50m plus.
Dive Area 2 to the south a large area of boulders to explore, depths to 25m, once you move away from the reef or the boulders, within 30 metres distance your depth will be at least 36m, from this point the bottom drops away very quickly. If you decide to dive this site, take a 15-litre cylinder and make the most of one good dive.

It is always a good idea, even for the very fit diver, to rest for 20/30 minutes after your dive before attempting the climb back up the 150 steps! unless you came by boat.

The Plateau Reef — Area 1

THE DIVE — Minimum time - 50 mins

Once on the ledge that you will be using for your entry/exit turn to your left and you will find some little steps to assist you especially with your exit. Into the water, depth below you is 15m, when on the bottom head in a westerly direction keeping the reef on your right-hand side, within 8 minutes you will reach the corner of the reef, depth 27m.

Now, keeping the reef on your right-hand side, head in a northerly direction. Within 10 minutes, you will come to an area where you will see cars littered around the boulders at 36m and more on the sand at 50m. From this point ascend the cliff face to the plateau at 15m, here you will also find more cars, they have all been pushed over the cliff top. This should be your turning point; from here you will be able to see the shoreline cliffs, that rise out of the sea, now ascend to your required depth.

Below: A diver explores the small caves along the back of the plateau, home for many cardinal fish (Apogon imberbis).

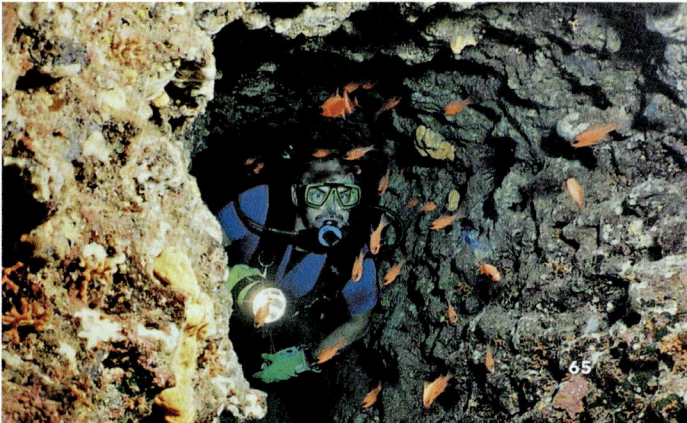

MIGHRA FERHA

Keeping the reef on your left, head in a southerly direction and you will find two small caves and a large over-hang, almost immediately you will have to bear round to your left, you should now be above your outward route and almost at your exit point. The return journey should not have taken more than 10/15 minutes, plus exploring time.

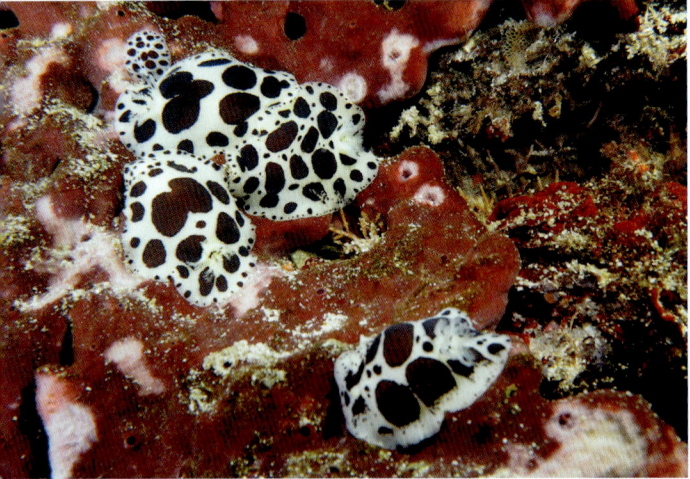

Nudibranch (Peltodoris atromaculata) with its distinctive colours.   PHOTO: DAVID AGUIS CALYPSO SUB AQUA CLUB

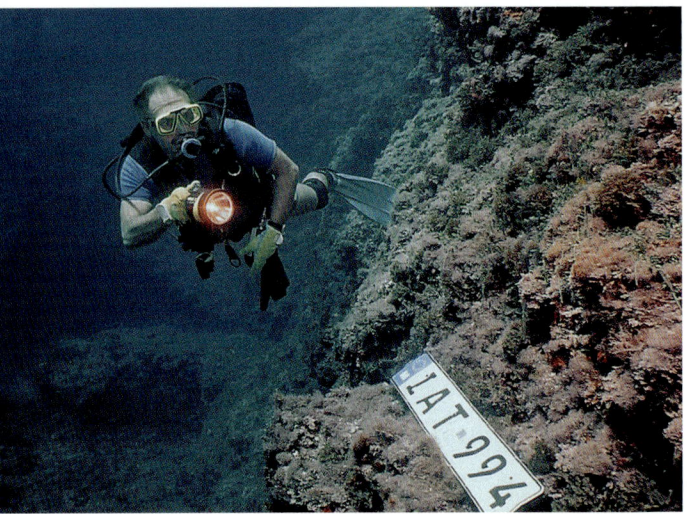

Just below the entry point a diver finds a car's number plate.

Below: Laying on the sand at 50m vehicles that have been pushed over the cliff into the sea below, this practise has now been stopped.

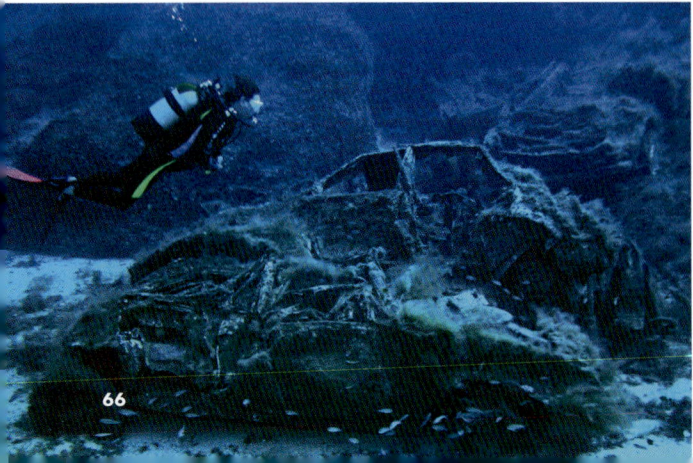

The Boulder Site — Area 2

THE DIVE   Minimum time - 50 mins

Once on the bottom follow the cliff wall in a southerly direction, almost immediately you will come to a large over-hang, this is worth a look inside, continue on the same course keeping the reef on your left. This area is littered with large boulders and between them small rocks, a haven for marine life with many places to explore. Within 15 minutes, depending on the time spent exploring, on your left you will see a very large rock that seems to be leaning up against the cliff wall, it is also a corner where the reef changes direction, depth 25m. At this point you should turn and swim in a northerly direction, keeping the boulders on your right and the flatish area on your left staying at a depth of around 25m, remember this is a good area for finding octopus and moray. In approximately 15/20 minutes you should reach the reef wall, depth 27m, if you turn to your right follow it in an easterly direction, this will lead you into a corner below the ledge at your exit point. Alternatively, you can explore the area on top of the reef before returning to your exit point. Of course, you can plan your own dive, but to fully complete both areas in one dive is really just too much and will give you no time to explore. In my opinion, the plateau is the best dive.

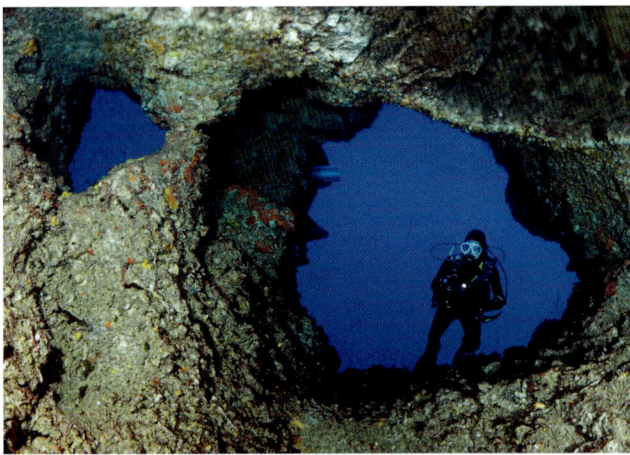

One of the many caves and overhangs to explore.
                    PHOTOS: DAVID AGUIS CALYPSO SUB AQUA CLUB
Below: Divers on the underwater drop-off below the plateau.

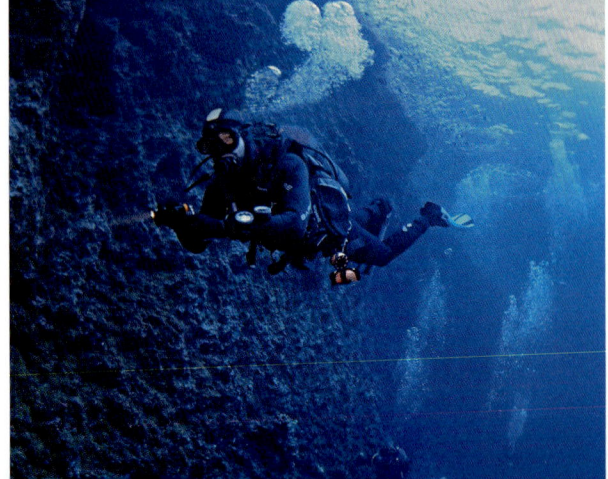

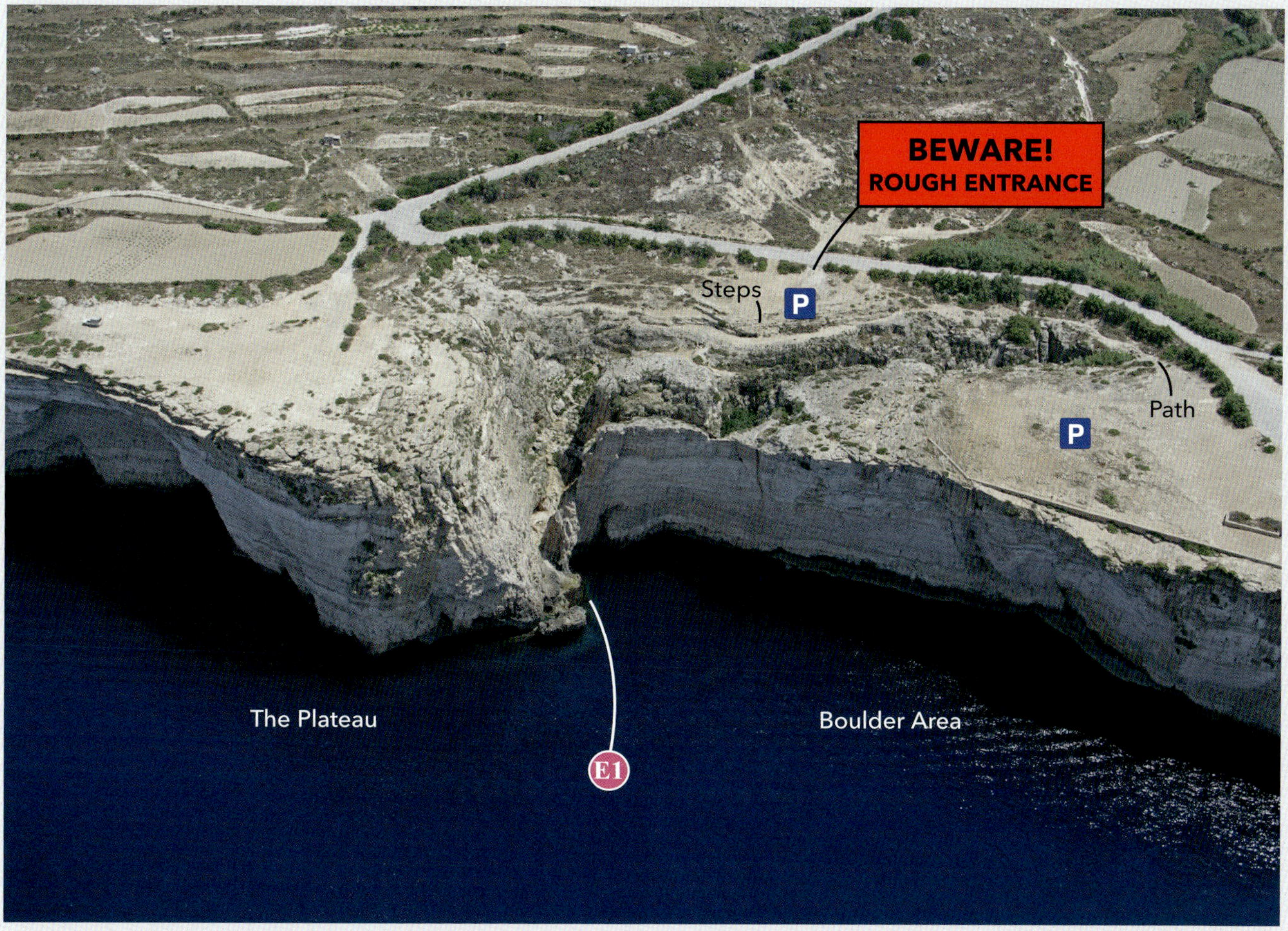

MIGHRA FERHA

BEWARE! ROUGH ENTRANCE

Steps P

Path

P

The Plateau

Boulder Area

E1

PHOTO: PGL AERIAL PHOTOS

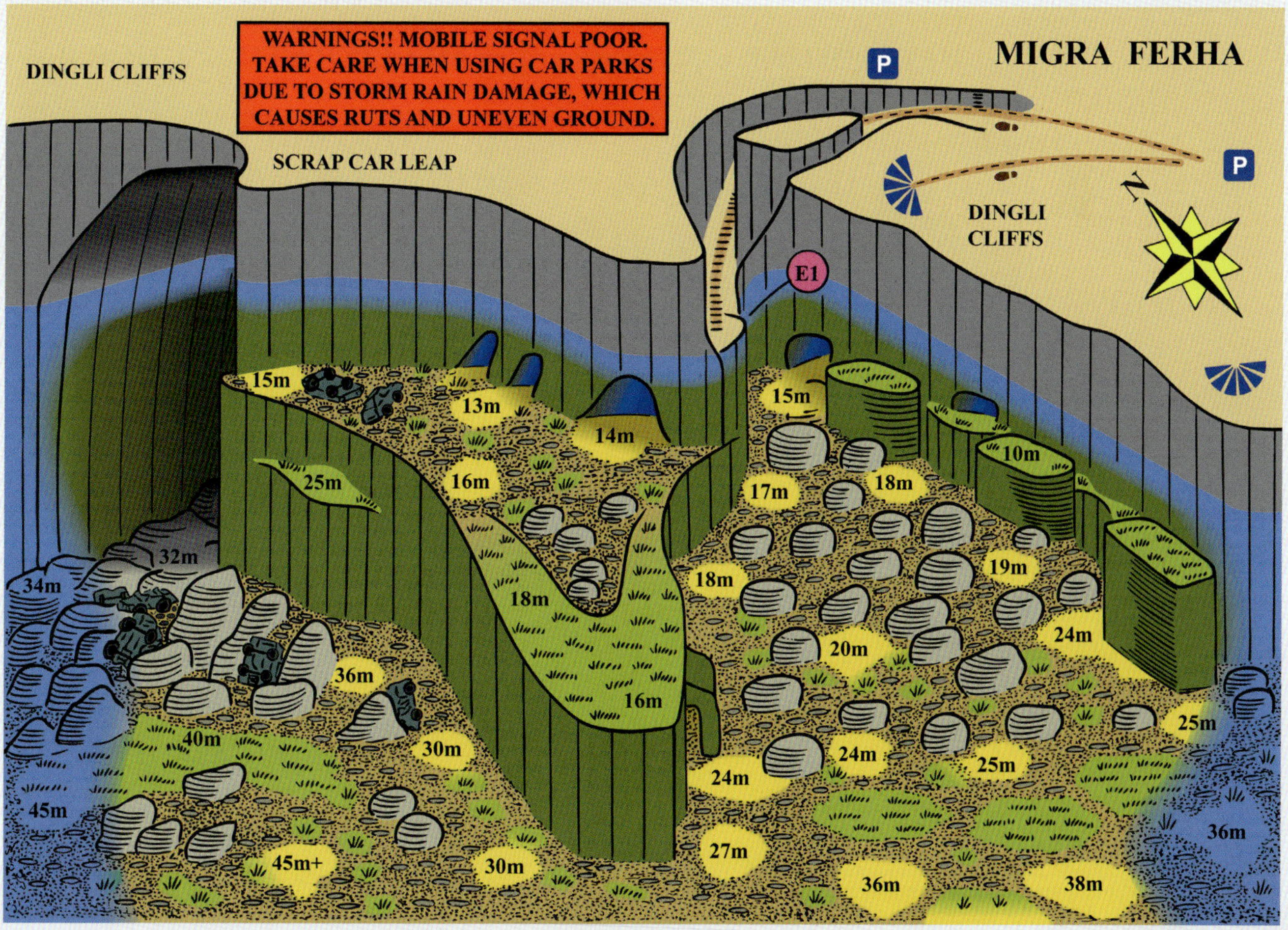

DINGLI CLIFFS

WARNINGS!! MOBILE SIGNAL POOR. TAKE CARE WHEN USING CAR PARKS DUE TO STORM RAIN DAMAGE, WHICH CAUSES RUTS AND UNEVEN GROUND.

SCRAP CAR LEAP

MIGRA FERHA

P P

DINGLI CLIFFS

E1

15m, 13m, 14m, 15m, 10m, 25m, 16m, 17m, 18m, 32m, 18m, 19m, 34m, 16m, 20m, 24m, 36m, 24m, 24m, 25m, 25m, 40m, 30m, 45m, 45m+, 30m, 27m, 36m, 38m, 36m

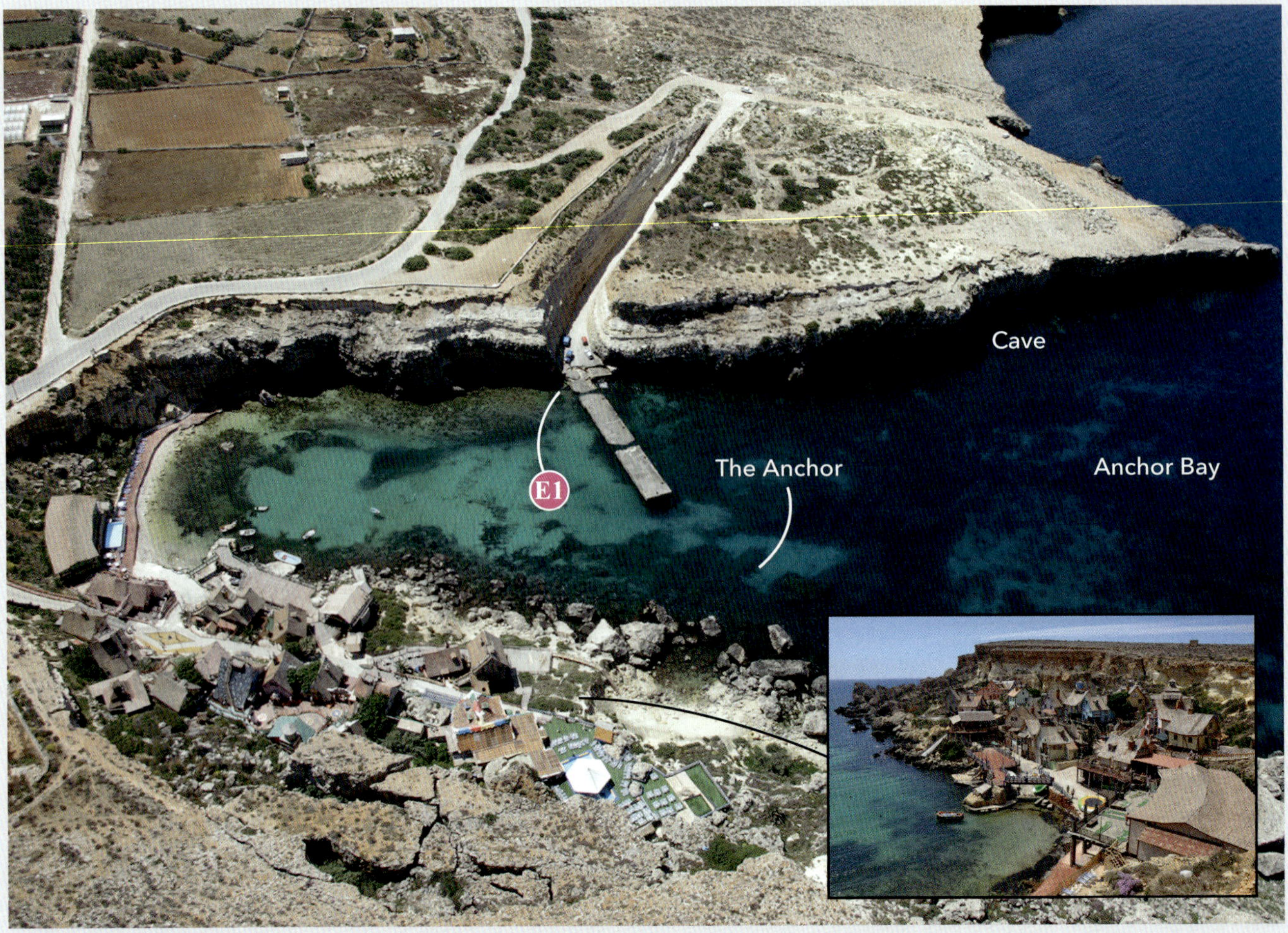

ANCHOR BAY

Cave
The Anchor
Anchor Bay
E1

PHOTO: PGL AERIAL PHOTOS

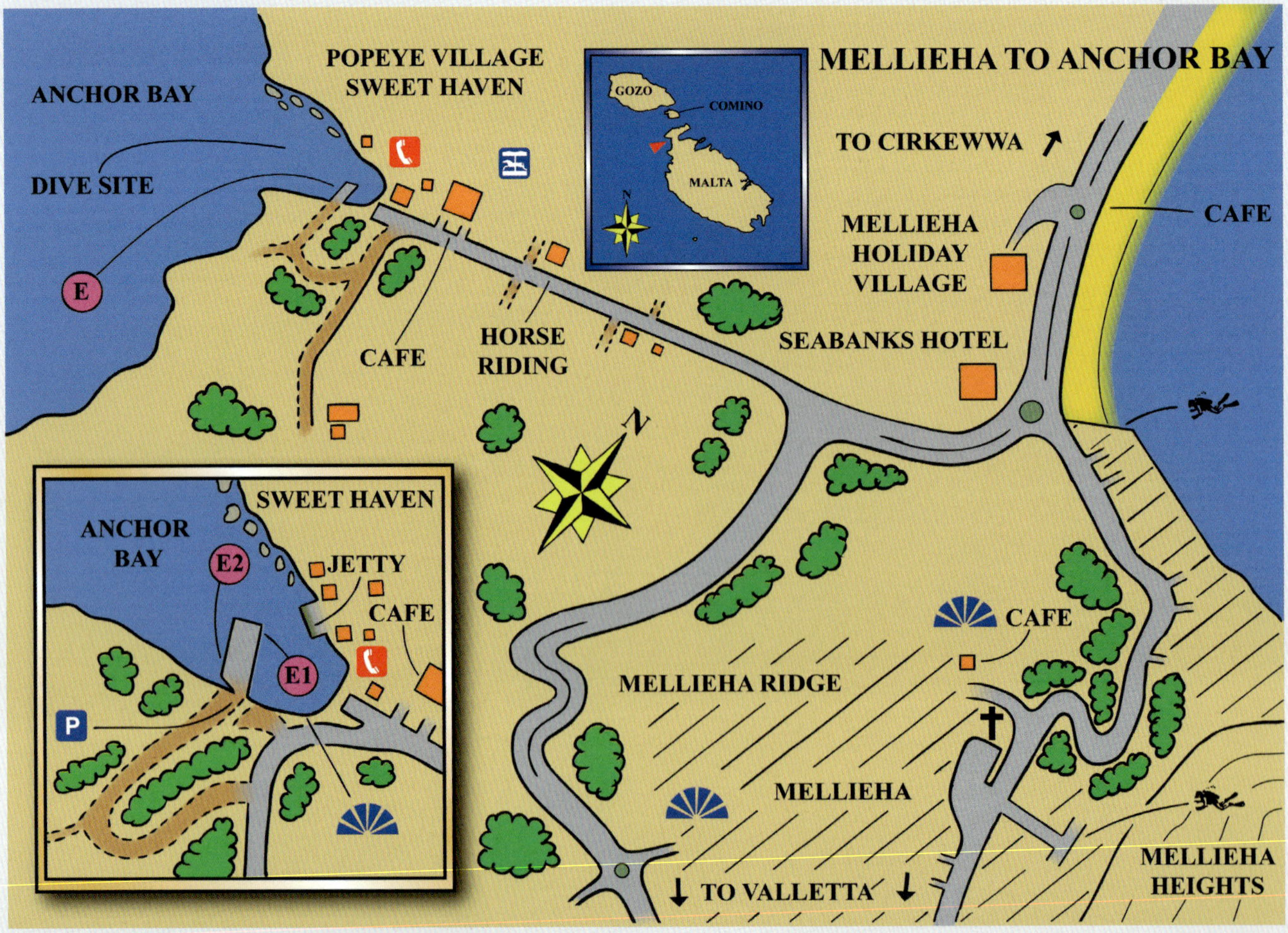

MELLIEHA TO ANCHOR BAY

ANCHOR BAY
DIVE SITE
E

POPEYE VILLAGE
SWEET HAVEN

GOZO   COMINO
MALTA

TO CIRKEWWA
CAFE
MELLIEHA HOLIDAY VILLAGE
SEABANKS HOTEL

CAFE
HORSE RIDING

N

CAFE
MELLIEHA RIDGE
MELLIEHA
MELLIEHA HEIGHTS

TO VALLETTA

Inset:
ANCHOR BAY
SWEET HAVEN
E2
JETTY
CAFE
E1
P

Anchor Bay and Cave

Anchor bay is a small inlet situated on the north west coast of Malta, only a short drive from Mellieha. The views from Mellieha ridge are quite breath taking of the bay and 'Popeye' village. Here is one of the only places on Malta where you can see both coastlines. This site is usually used as a second dive or when there are strong north to north east winds. Depth ranges are from 2m to 18m within the bay. The Anchor at 8m, on the south side of the bay and on the north side there is a small cave at 9m at the entrance.

Please note the jetty has been severely damaged by storms and is no longer nicely attached to the shore line. Check your entry/exit point before kitting up, a de-kit exit may be required. Please do not leave anything of value in your vehicle, unless you have shore cover. In a emergency there is a telephone in the entrance kiosk to Popeye Village, the owners will allow you to use, when it is closed it is manned by security personnel.

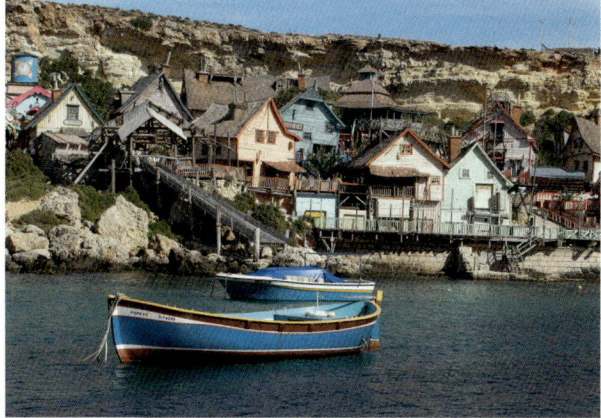

The village of Sweethaven, originally built for the film Popeye; it is now a very popular tourist attraction.

On to the approach road to the Anchor Bay there are some riding stables for visitors. As you leave the road and turn right onto the track, stop at the top of the cliffs, this viewpoint is a good position to take photographs of the village and bay. There is a restaurant and gift shop next to the car park, the 'Popeye' village itself is worth a visit.

This bay was made famous by the building of the timber village called Sweethaven, which was the film set

Below: The damaged jetty with the exit ladder. First check it out!

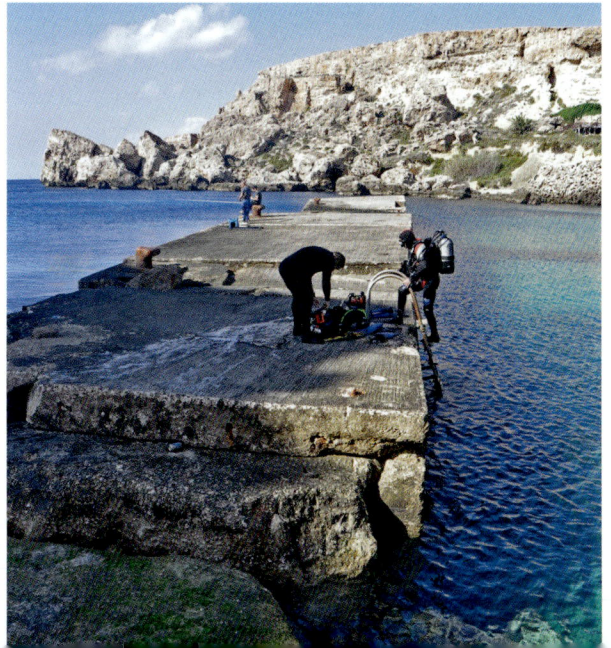

for the production of the film Popeye with Robin Williams. A jetty was constructed to enable boats to unload materials at this isolated bay when they constructed the village, one of these boats being the Scotscraig which is now a popular boat dive and lies just around the headland. The name Anchor Bay came from the anchor which was used as a mooring, it is still here with its long heavy chain, **see plan.**

THE DIVE — Minimum time - 50 mins

From the entry point E1 proceed to the end of the jetty continue over the sand you will reach a bank with sea grass on the top of it. Now head about 320° but do not miss the very large anchor chain, for in places it is covered in marine growth. Once you have found it turn left and follow it, at the end you will find a very large anchor, 8m. From here head 210° to start off with, there is a small reef on your left, it helps with navigation.

Eventually you will pass an area of small rocks on your left, here leave this small reef but remain on your present compass bearing until you reach the base of the shoreline cliff face on the south side of the bay, if your depth is less than 8m turn right, if more than 11m turn left. The entrance to the cave is on the open seaward side of a very large boulder, which is hiding the cave entrance. From your entry point to the cave, allowing for time to look around, will take you some 24 minutes. The depth at the entrance of the cave is 10m, inside the cave the depth ranges from 8m to 2m. There is a large cavern above water level in which you may surface and admire this impressive dome shaped ceiling.

Below: Tompot blenny PHOTO: JOE FORMOSA

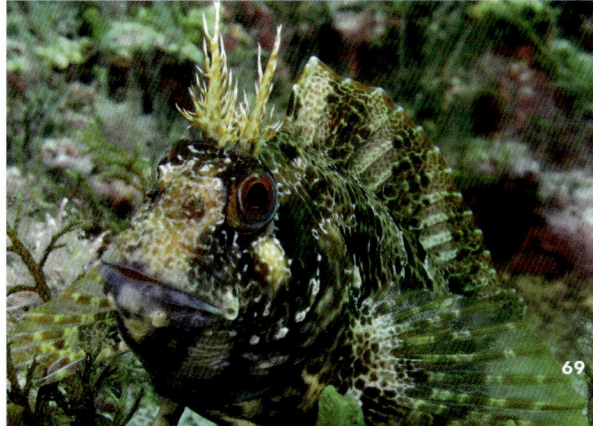

ANCHOR BAY

> **BEWARE,** for there are boats leaving and arriving with parties of tourists from the little jetty in front of the Popeye village.

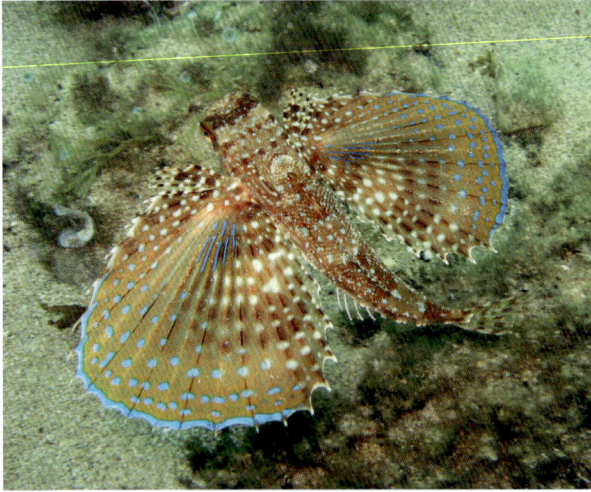

Flying gurnard (Dactylpterus volitans) hovers over the sand.

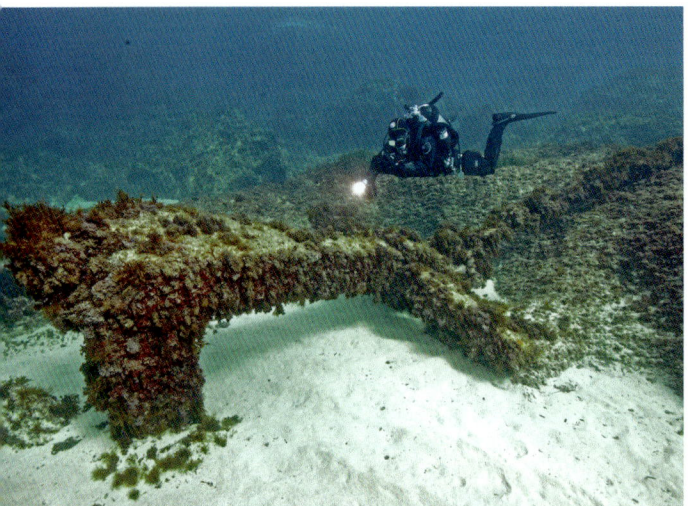

The anchor and large chain, which gave its name to the bay,
PHOTOS: MAX VALLI - ORANGE SHARK DIVE CENTRE
Below: Divers enter the cave along the south side of the bay.

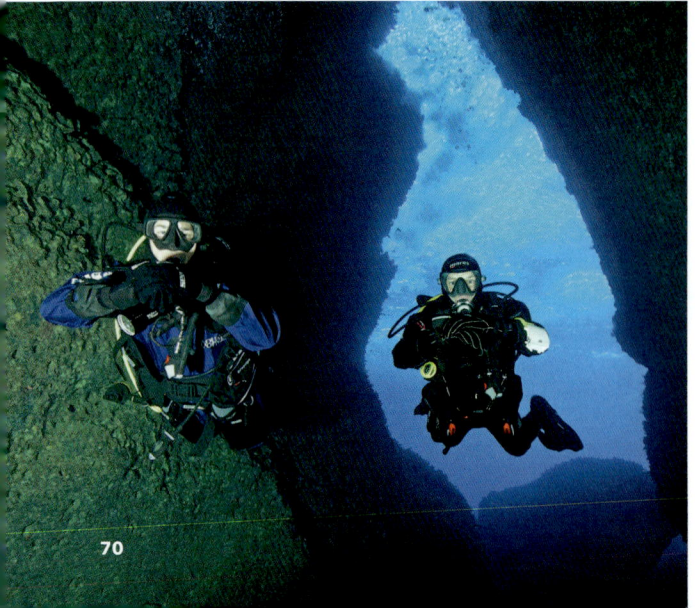

The area on the westerly side of the cave entrance is quite rugged and if you have the time and air, is worth exploring. When it is time to return, head 60° east keeping the cliff face on your right, from the cave to your exit point it will take you approximately 15 minutes, longer if you wish to explore. You can of course complete this dive in reverse, by going directly to the cave from your entry point.

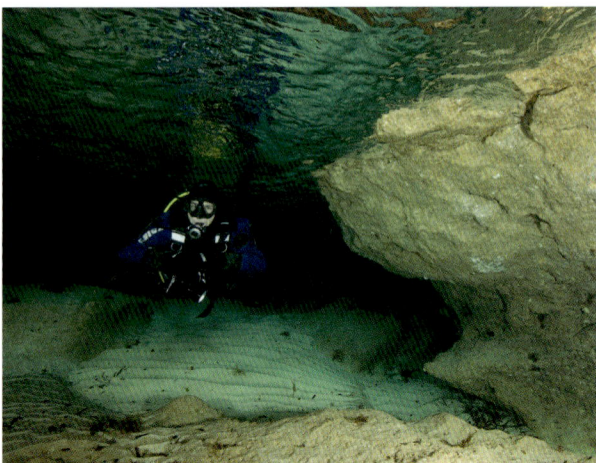

At the end of the cave at depth of 2m where you can surface. Check the air before removing your regulator.
PHOTO: MAX VALLI - ORANGE SHARK DIVE CENTRE

Another area to dive, on the north shore of Anchor Bay, not far from the anchor is an area of large boulders surrounded by a sandy seabed, often to be found here is the Tun Shell. You can of course plan your own dive but remember, the swim from the cave to your exit point will take you approximately 15 minutes, with no time spent exploring.

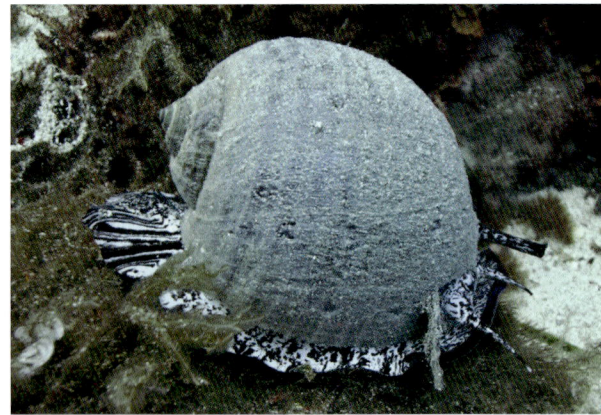

The giant tun shell (Tonna galea) lives on sandy seabeds.

Mellieha has a busy shopping centre and the steep main street is lined with a variety of shops, small bars and restaurants. Perched on the hill side in front of the church with fantastic views over the north coast of Malta with Gozo in the distance is a small family run café / bar and a children's playground, a great place to relax after a dive. In an effort to preserve both local and migratory birds, the wetland inland from Mellieha Bay has been turned into a bird sanctuary.

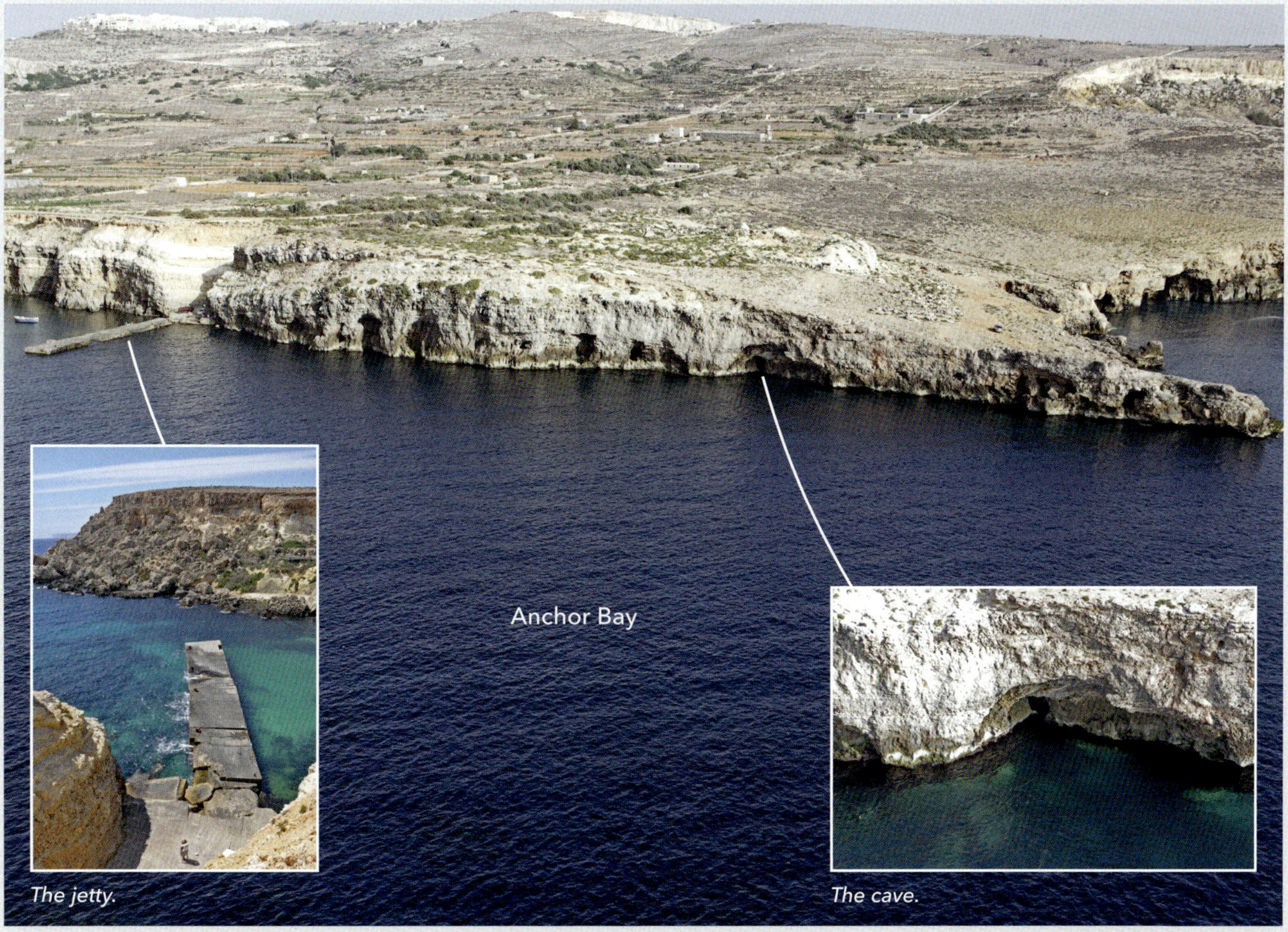

ANCHOR BAY

The jetty.

Anchor Bay

The cave.

PHOTO: PGL AERIAL PHOTOS

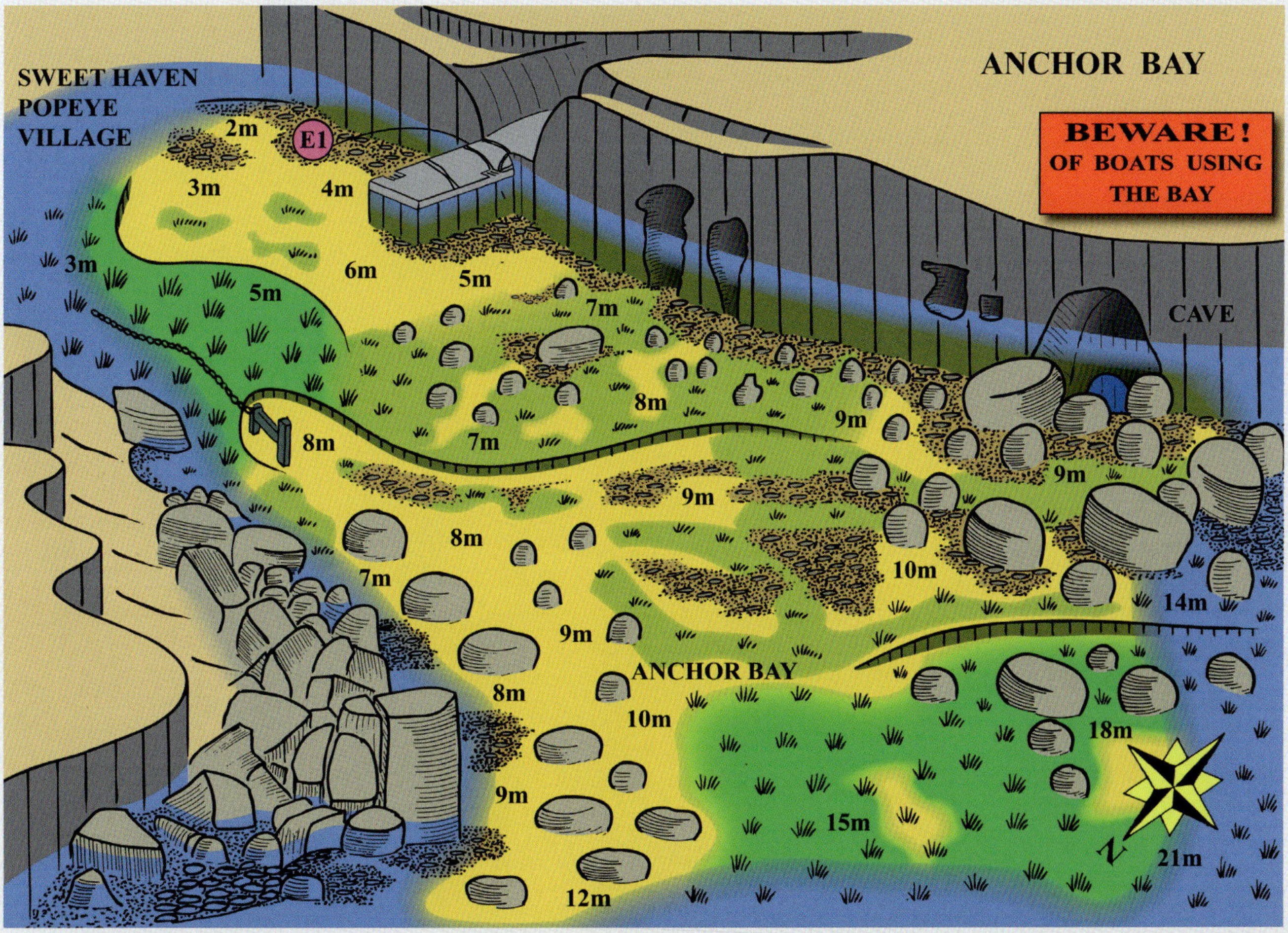

SWEET HAVEN POPEYE VILLAGE

ANCHOR BAY

BEWARE! OF BOATS USING THE BAY

CAVE

ANCHOR BAY

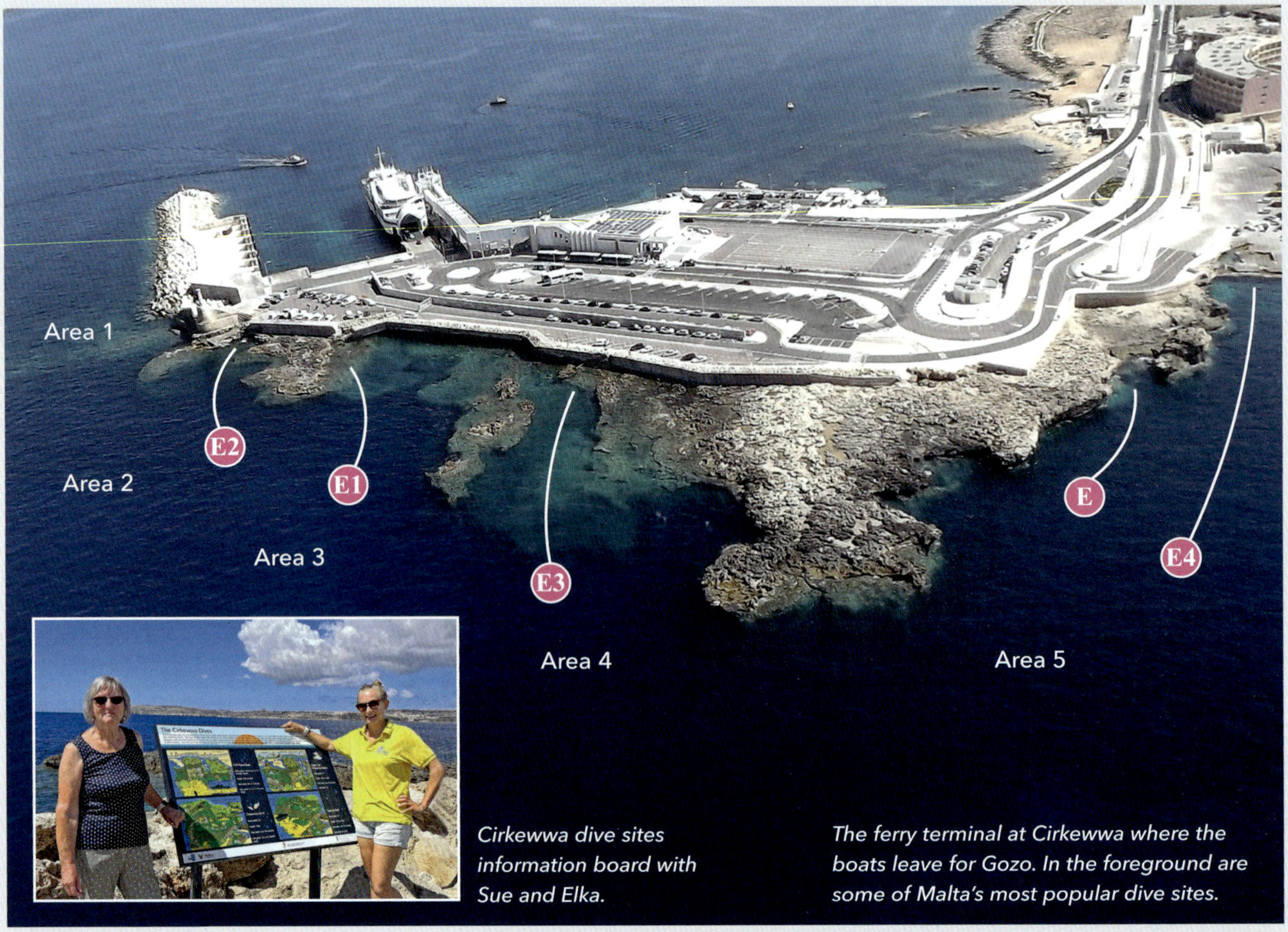

CIRKEWWA MARINE PARK

Area 1
Area 2
Area 3
Area 4
Area 5

E2
E1
E3
E
E4

Cirkewwa dive sites information board with Sue and Elka.

The ferry terminal at Cirkewwa where the boats leave for Gozo. In the foreground are some of Malta's most popular dive sites.

PHOTO: PGL AERIAL PHOTOS

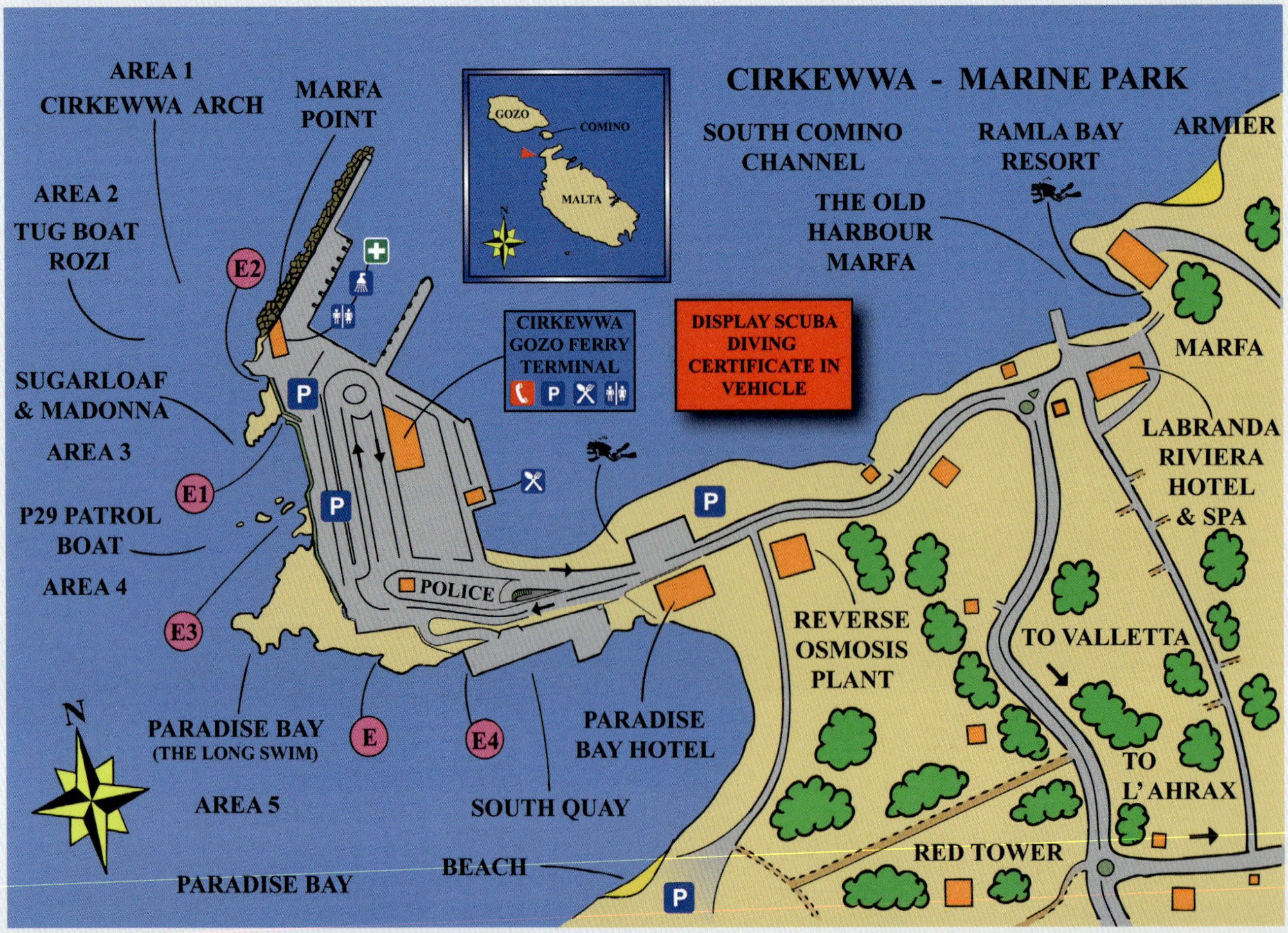

CIRKEWWA - MARINE PARK

AREA 1
CIRKEWWA ARCH

AREA 2
TUG BOAT ROZI

SUGARLOAF & MADONNA
AREA 3

P29 PATROL BOAT
AREA 4

PARADISE BAY
(THE LONG SWIM)
AREA 5

PARADISE BAY

MARFA POINT

GOZO — COMINO
MALTA

SOUTH COMINO CHANNEL

THE OLD HARBOUR MARFA

RAMLA BAY RESORT

ARMIER

MARFA

LABRANDA RIVIERA HOTEL & SPA

CIRKEWWA GOZO FERRY TERMINAL

DISPLAY SCUBA DIVING CERTIFICATE IN VEHICLE

E2
E1
E3
E
E4

POLICE

REVERSE OSMOSIS PLANT

TO VALLETTA

TO L'AHRAX

PARADISE BAY HOTEL

SOUTH QUAY

BEACH

RED TOWER

Cirkewwa Marine Park - Marfa Point

Cirkewwa is situated on the north west coast of the island and is the main terminal for the car and passenger ferries to Gozo. Most divers refer to this area as Marfa and is the most popular dive location on the island of Malta. **To park here you will be required to display your diving qualification card on the dashboard of your vehicle.**

Many years ago, before the terminal was built, the rocks below the lighthouse were not part of the mainland, these outcrops of rocks were known as Marfa Point. The actual hamlet of Marfa itself is approximately 1 km along the coast where there is a small harbour.

There are two quays at the Cirkewwa terminal, the north quay, which is the normal one used; the south quay is used when weather conditions dictate otherwise. The car ferries are not a problem for divers unless you leave the main dive areas and surface well out to sea. It is the small craft, fishing and pleasure boats that can be a problem; a few tend to cut the corner when rounding the headland, even though both wrecks are buoyed. Dive boats visit this area, so beware of anchors and shot lines. Due to the fact that it is so popular it can become really busy at times. There are five dives here which of course can be interchanged to suit your qualifications and dive plan requirements, with depths down to 36m.

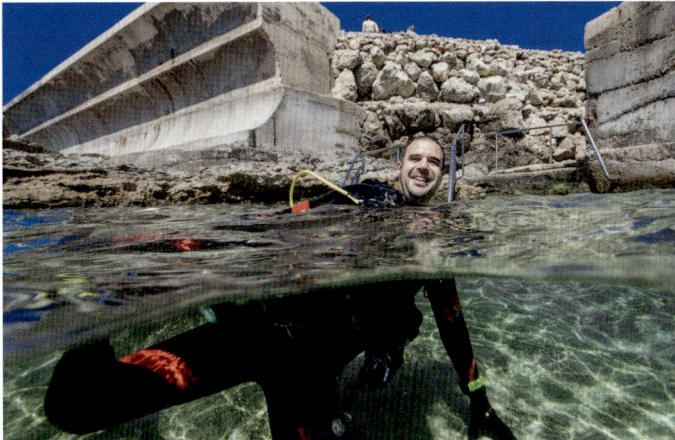
A happy diver in Susie's Pool after a great dive.
PHOTO: JON BORG www.jonborg.com

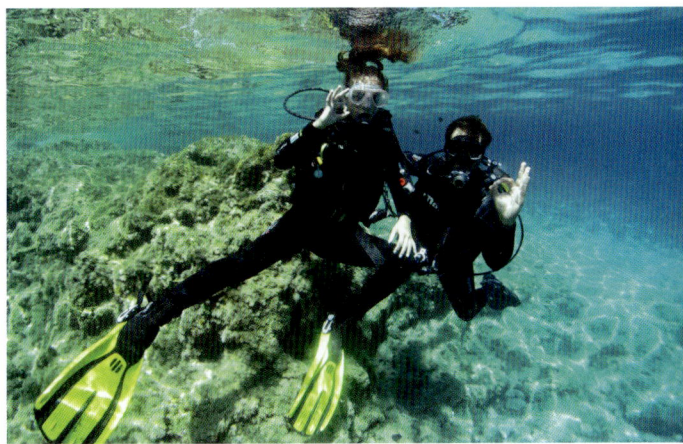
Cirkewwa is a fantastic place for that first dive.

Below: A variety of fish to be found in this Marine Park.
PHOTO: VERONICA BUSUTTIL

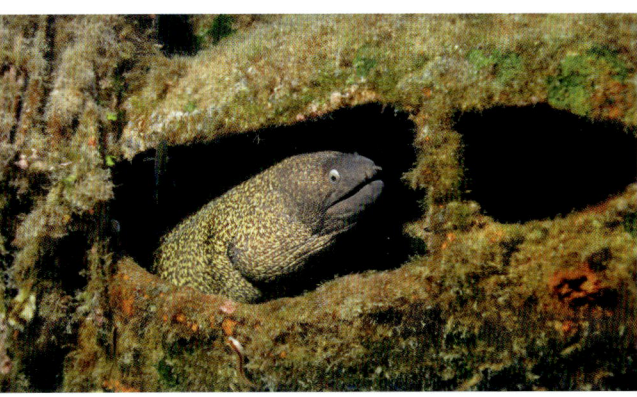
Moray (Muraena Helena) a home found on the Rozi.

Below: Divers heading towards the Swimthrough.

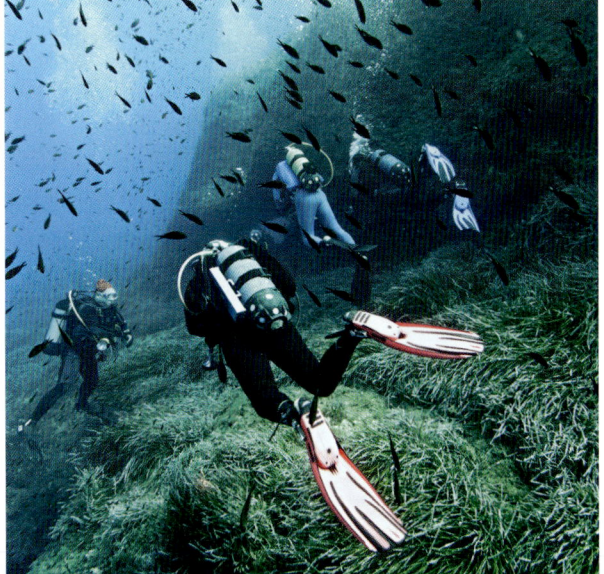

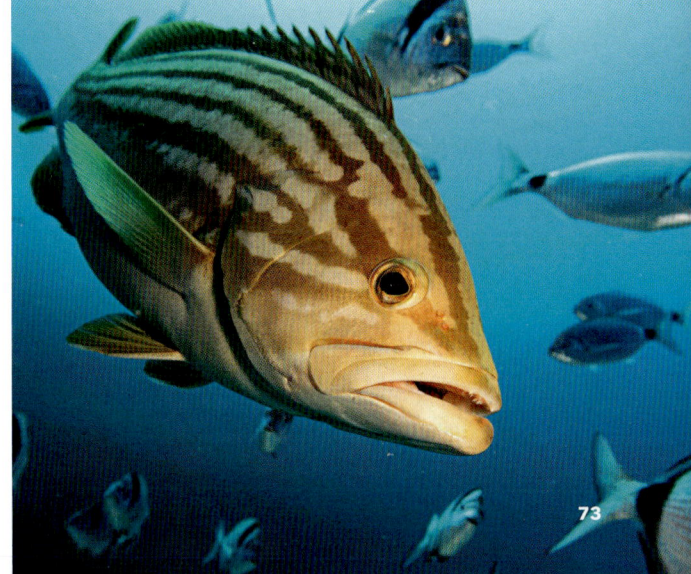

Cirkewwa Arch — Area 1

This unusual arch some 12m below the surface and 8m above the sea bed has a compass bearing from the lighthouse directly over the reef of 320°. Your route is not direct but will take you along the side of the reef, which can be used for navigation, the approximate distance for this route is 180 metres. Most of the sea bed area of this dive site is covered in sea grass with large boulders and small areas of sand. On your outward journey you will find a small cave, which can be explored, while returning along the shallow depths of the reef, where the marine growth is short, there are many nooks and crannies which make good hiding places for marine life.

THE DIVE — Minimum time - 40 mins

Entry point E2 is just below the lighthouse. From the entry point surface swim around to the end of the reef, once on the north west side of the lighthouse descend to 6/7m, now swim in an easterly direction past a large reef/boulder when the next reef appears in front of you, descend bearing to your left continue down to a depth of 14m, here the bottom is covered in sea grass and the main reef will be on your right-hand side.

Continue along the reef until you come to an area of sand, be sure not to miss the little cut out in the reef, for on the left-hand side of this cut out is the entrance to the cave. Once you have entered the cave leave by the first exit on your left, as the other exit is too small for divers, continue to follow the reef on your right. Within a short distance the reef bears sharply to the right, at this point you can either follow the reef to the Arch or take a compass bearing of 350°

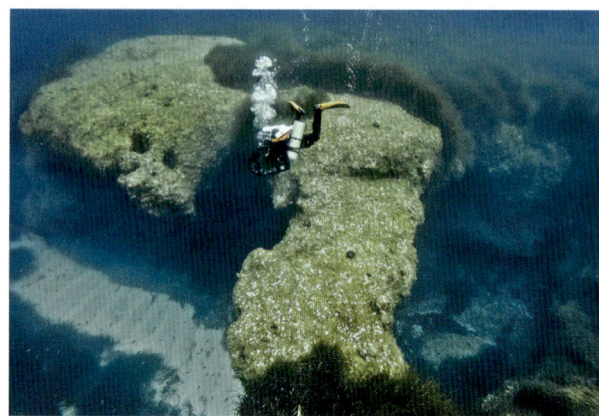

A divers view from above of this attractive arch
PHOTO: ARKADIUSZ SREBNIK POLANDDIVING PHOTOS

Below: The tunnel on the way to the Cirkewwa arch.

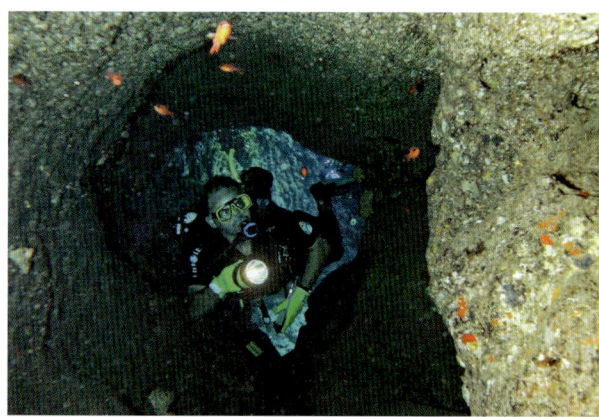

Take your time and explore this area while admiring the breath-taking view of the reef formation. If you are lucky, under the Arch there are sometimes large shoals of amberjacks, especially if there is a slight current, if you are really careful you can get very close to them, which makes a great photographic opportunity. When on the seabed below the Arch take care not to stir up the sand, moving under the Arch towards the reef wall at the far end, where there are a number of hiding places for groupers and moray eels. On your return route follow the reef until you are above the cave; if there are divers inside the bubbles form a curtain, again another chance for an unusual photograph. After you have passed the cave, bear right past the first boulder / reef then cross over to the main reef, you will now be below the lighthouse where you can exit at E2 or if the sea is choppy and you have the air then continue to Susie's pool E1, at your chosen depth.

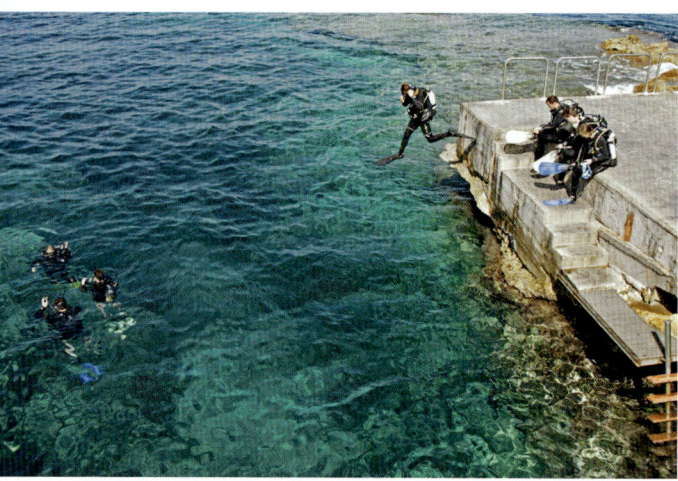

Entry point E1 normally used for Cirkewwa Arch and Rozi.

Below: Divers on the West side of the Cirkewwa Arch

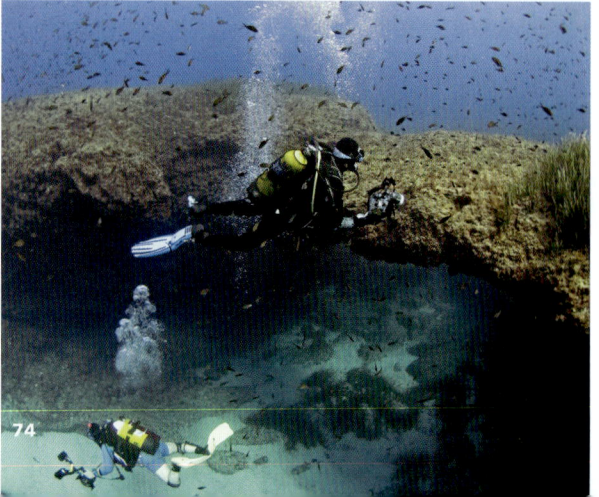

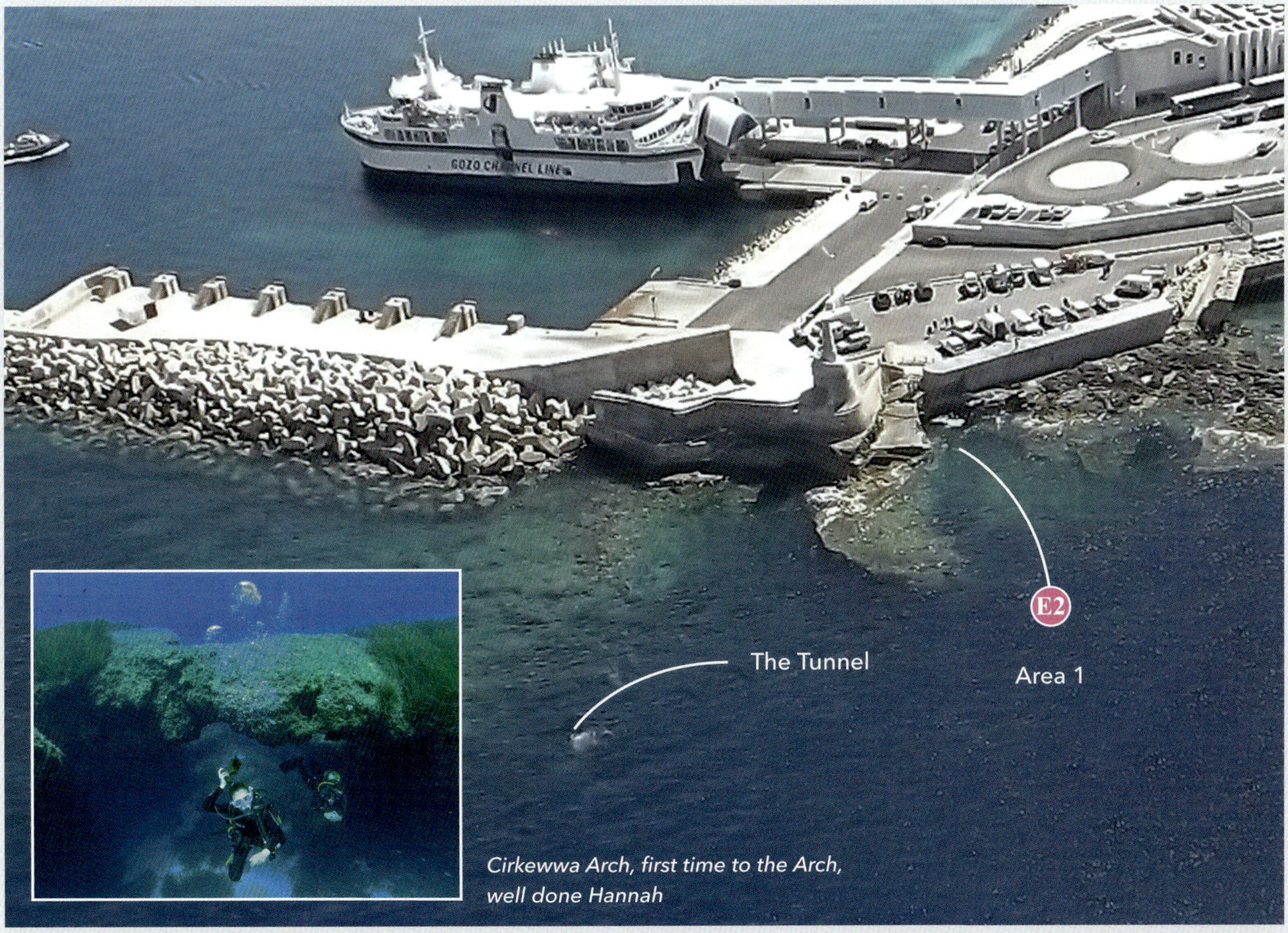

CIRKEWWA ARCH - CIRKEWWA MARINE PARK

The Tunnel

Area 1

Cirkewwa Arch, first time to the Arch, well done Hannah

PHOTO: PGL AERIAL PHOTOS

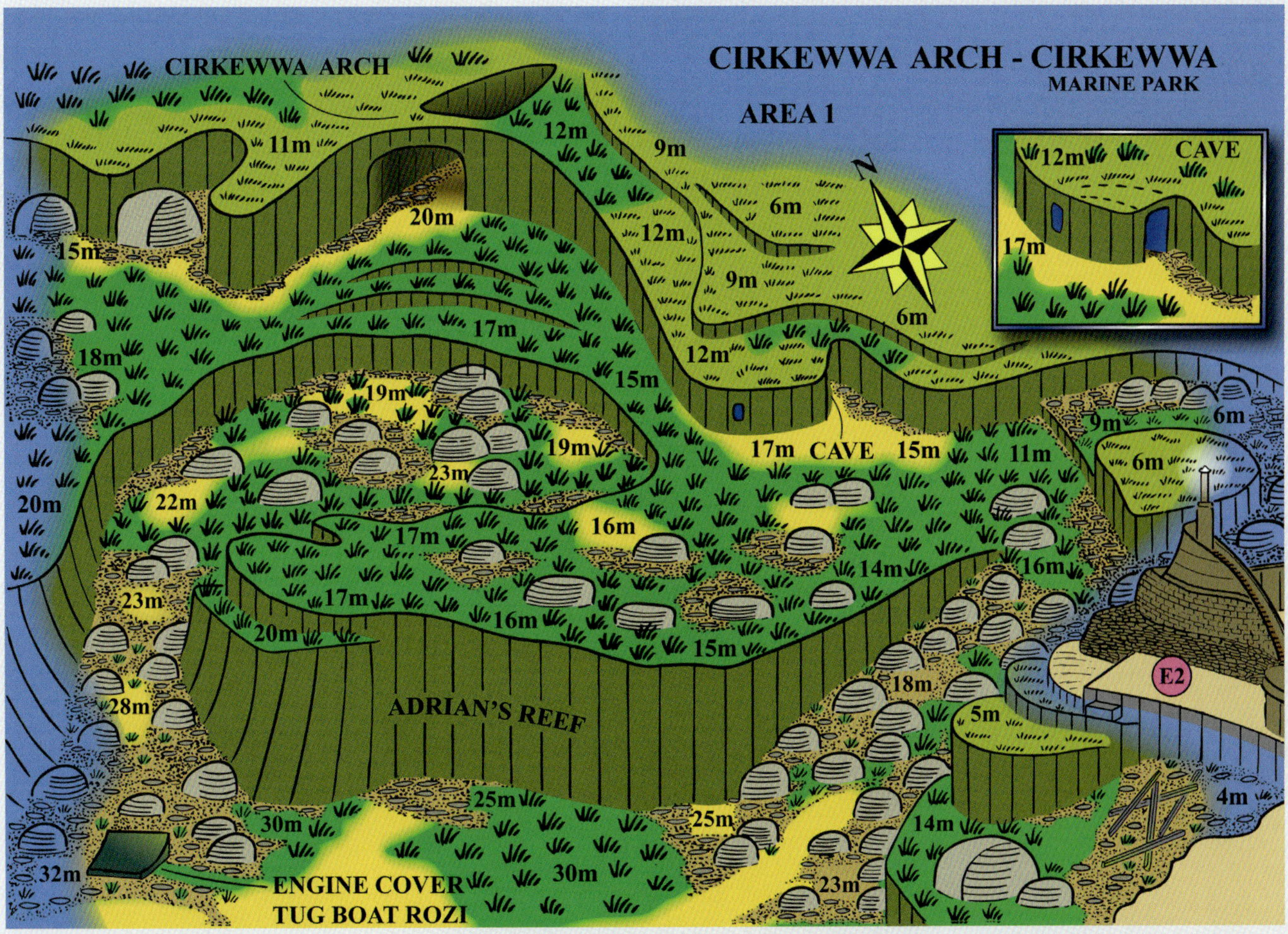

CIRKEWWA ARCH - CIRKEWWA MARINE PARK
AREA 1

CIRKEWWA ARCH

CAVE

ADRIAN'S REEF

ENGINE COVER TUG BOAT ROZI

A look around Cirkewwa Marine Park

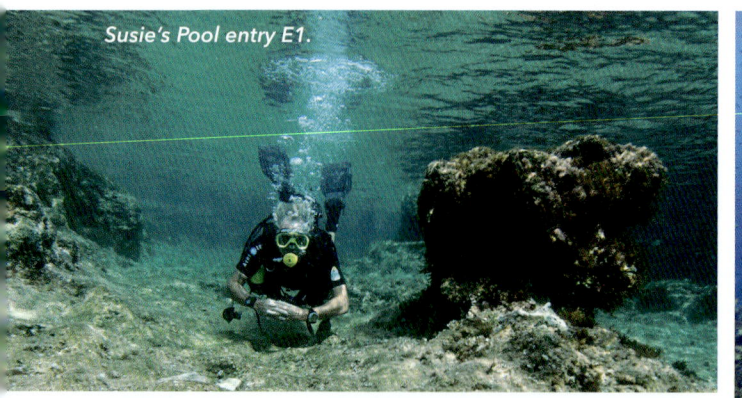
Susie's Pool entry E1.

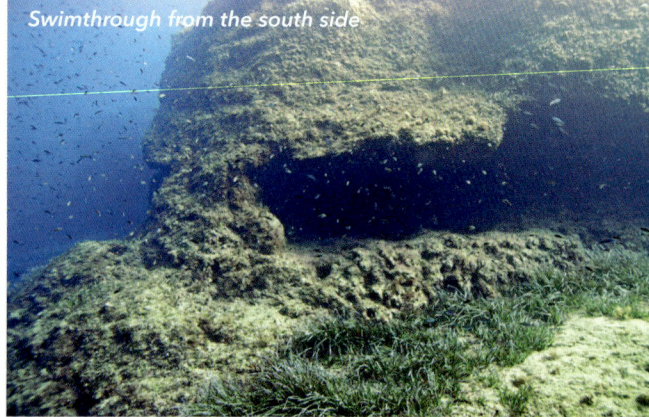
Swimthrough from the south side.

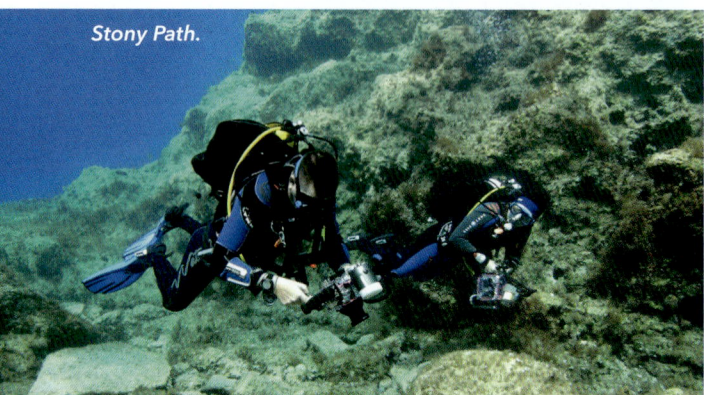
Stony Path.

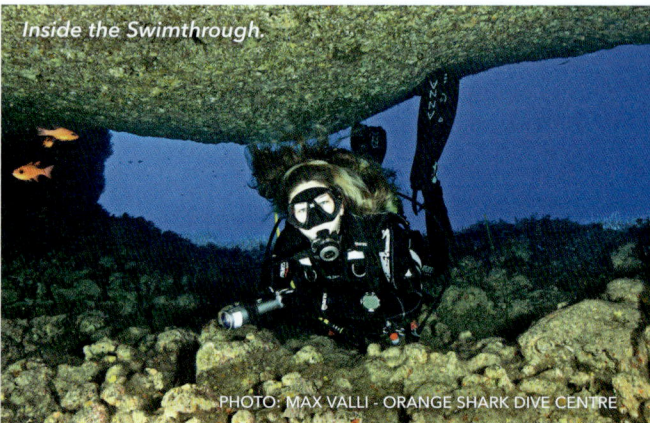
Inside the Swimthrough.

PHOTO: MAX VALLI - ORANGE SHARK DIVE CENTRE

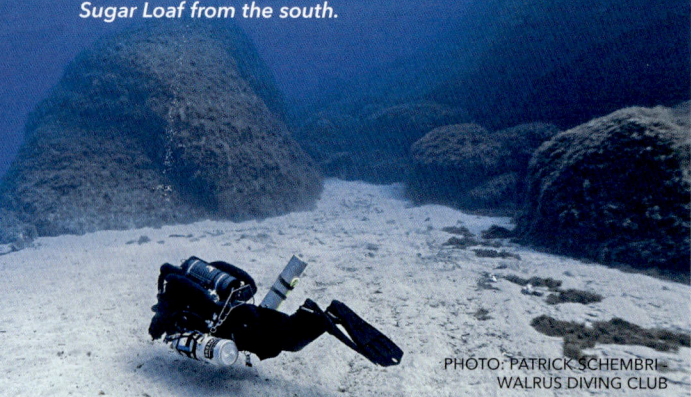
Sugar Loaf from the south.

PHOTO: PATRICK SCHEMBRI WALRUS DIVING CLUB

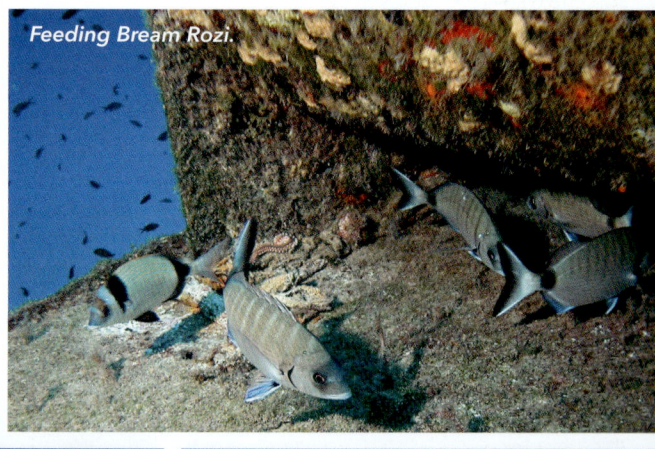
Feeding Bream Rozi.

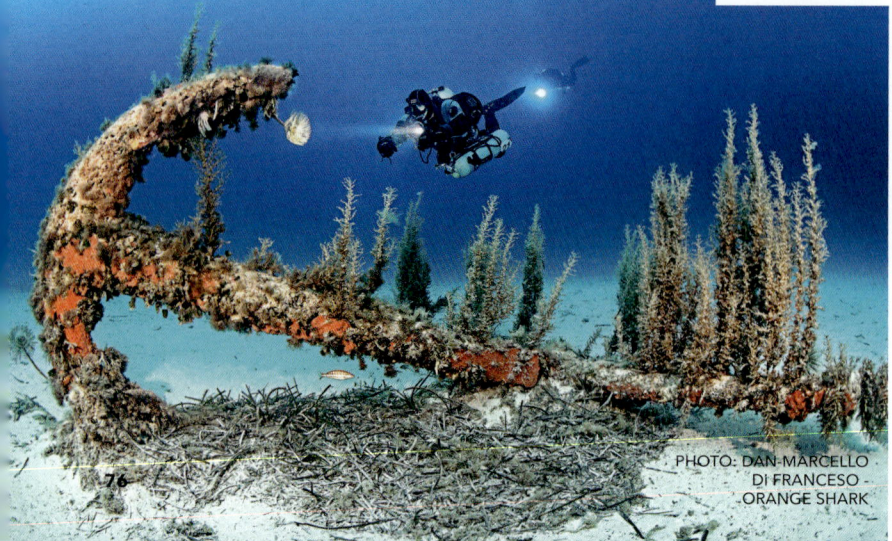
Cirkewwa Anchor.

PHOTO: DAN-MARCELLO DI FRANCESO - ORANGE SHARK

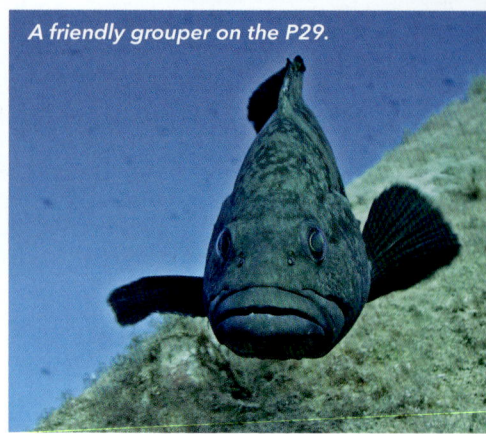
A friendly grouper on the P29.

The Tugboat *Rozi*

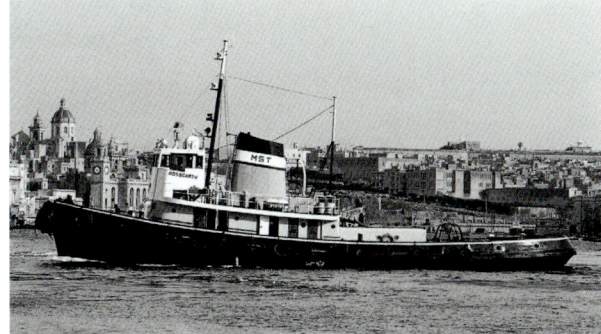

Tugboat Rossgarth (Rozi) working in Grand Harbour.
PHOTO: COURTESY OF BETTINA ROHBRECHT - HAMBURG

This 30m tug boat named *Rozi*, built in Bristol, England in 1958 by Charles Hill & Sons Ltd, for Johnston Warren Lines Ltd, of Liverpool and launched as *Rossmore*. She was renamed *Rossgarth* in 1969 and in 1972 was sold to Mifsud Brothers (Malta Ship Towage) Ltd, Malta, retaining her name. In the same year she sailed from Liverpool for Malta where in 1973 she was registered. She was sold to Tug Malta in 1981 and renamed *Rozi* and was sold to Captain Morgan Cruises, Malta who scuttled her as an artificial reef off Cirkewwa in 1992 as an attraction for a tourist submarine. Buoyed some 130 metres west of the lighthouse at a depth of 36m she sits upright on a sandy seabed. There was a time when tourists enjoyed seeing divers on the *Rozi*, but the submarine has long since gone. During the intervening years thousands of divers from all over the world have enjoyed diving on her, and seeing the marine life that have made the *Rozi* their home.

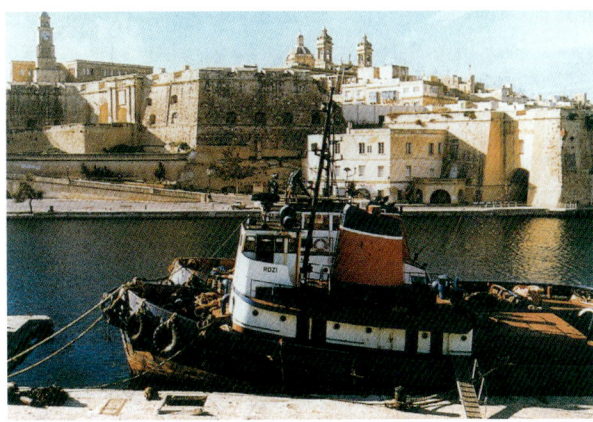

The Rozi in Grand Harbour with her new name on the bridge.
PHOTO: BY PERMISSION OF TUG MALTA

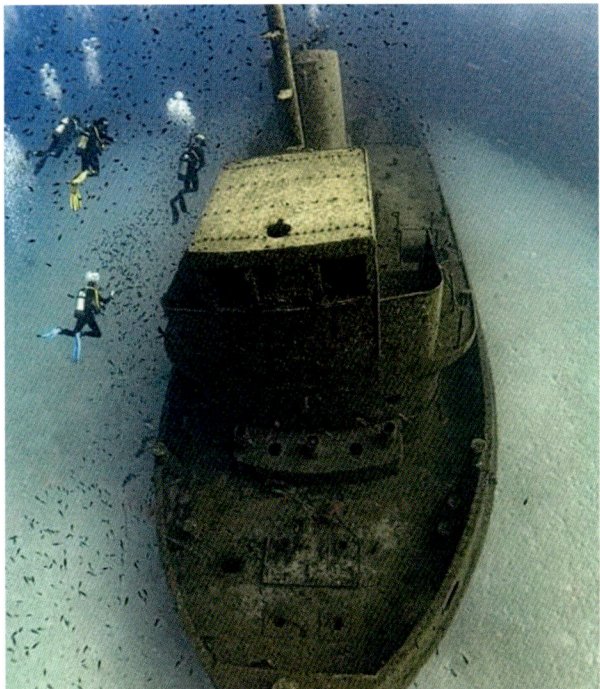

A excellent view of the Tugboat Rozi from above.
PHOTO: VERONICA BUSUTTIL

Below: Pointing away from the reef a diver above the stern.
PHOTO: JON BORG www.jonborg.com

Below: Ian, myself and the marine life, on the sand in front of the Rozi's bows.
PHOTO: SHARON FORDER

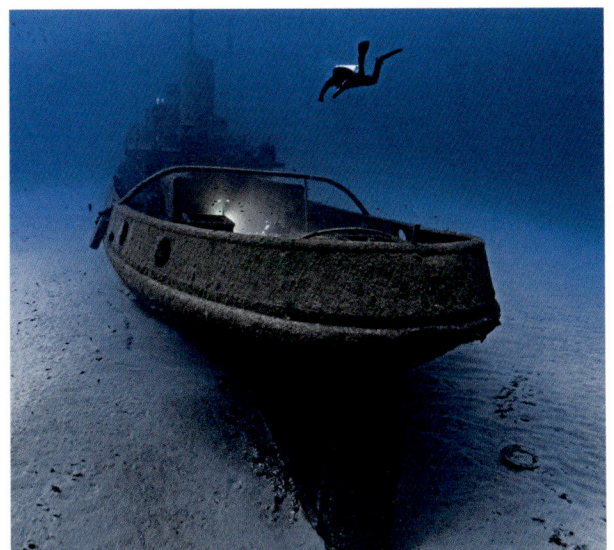

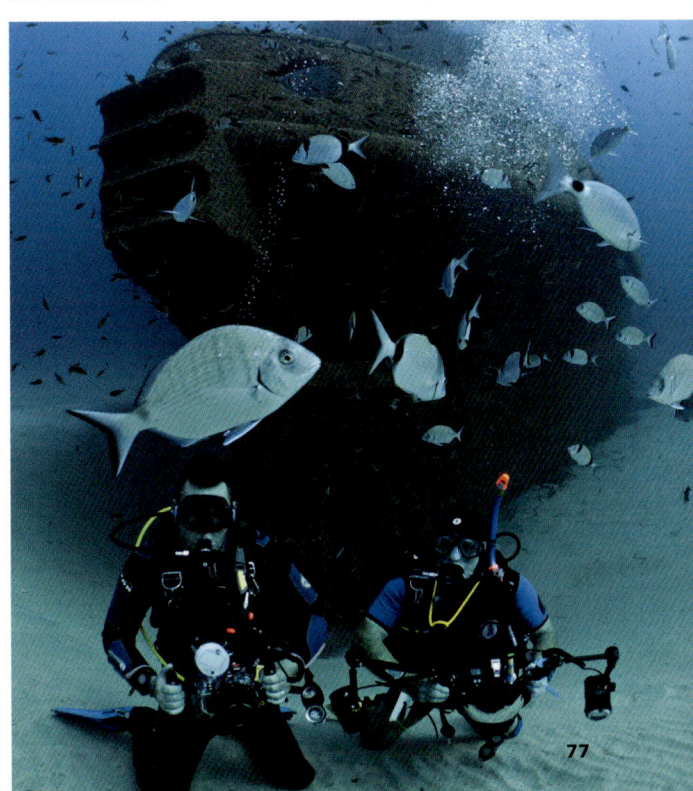

The Tugboat *Rozi* — Area 2

THE DIVE Minimum time - 50 mins

For this dive use entry point E2 at the south side of the lighthouse. Your dive plan will either be to surface swim to the end of the reef, then down to your chosen depth, maybe 6m, so you can see the reef below. Pass directly over the rocky valley to the reef on the other side, depth 15m. Follow the edge of the reef for about 70 metres, down on the seabed you will see an area of sand shaped like a banana which separates the sea grass. The Rozi's bows lie just to the right of this path; dive time to the wreck is approximately 6 minutes.

The alternative, is a surface swim, with a compass bearing of 300° from entry point E2, not required if she is buoyed. You will have to take great care and keep an eye out for small boats cutting the corner. Also, the currents that occur here from time to time will push you off course without you realising it. For your return journey you have three choices, most divers plan to return to Susie's Pool E1, but of course you can exit at E2.

Return route 1, mid-way port side of the wreck follow a compass bearing of 150°, to the anchor, which is 50 metres away at a depth of 32m. From this point continue on a compass bearing of 120°, this will lead you back on to the reef, when you have reached it, ascend to your required depth then head in a southerly direction keeping the main reef on your left. Once you have reached the swim-through at 11m and either passed through it or taken the short trip round, then continue to follow the reef wall. Within approximately 2 minutes at a depth of 11m you will find a ledge that will lead you up into the training area and Susie's Pool and E1.

Return route 2, leave the stern of the *Rozi* behind you and following a compass bearing of approximately 60° until you reach the top of the reef, at approximately 17m. At this point turn right; continue along the edge of the reef until you reach the rocky valley cross over to the other side. Here the reef rises to the surface, near E2, bearing in mind to reach this point from the wreck, will take you some 5/6 minutes. Once you have reached your required depth bear to the right, keeping the main reef on your left, you will pass the two small arches in the reef, continue on to the swim-through. Now follow the reef at 5/6m to Stony Path or the 11m Ledge and overhang both will lead you into the training area and exit point at Susie's Pool E1.

Return route 3, this I consider to be my favourite return route. Leave the stern of the *Rozi* passing over the engine cover, which lies on the sand, and follow a compass bearing of 30°. Continue in this direction following the gently sloping reef to higher ground.

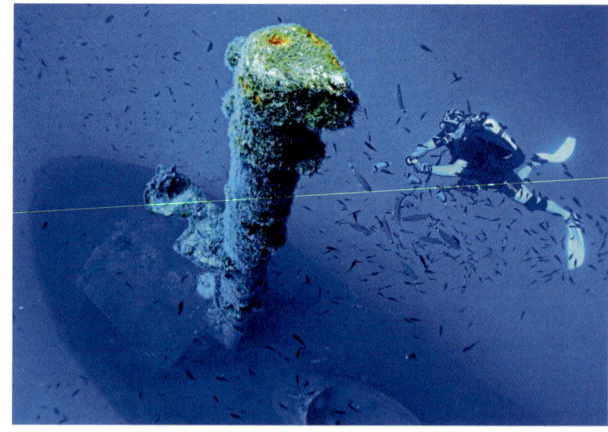

Above the mast looking down onto the Rozi.

The small damsel fish often found in shoals around wrecks and reefs. PHOTO: VICTOR FABRI

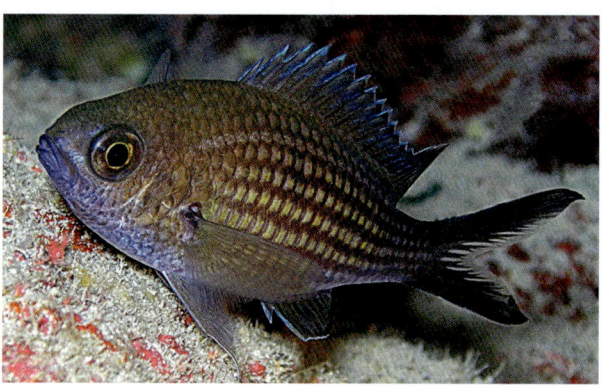

At a depth of around 20m you will find a small drop-off on your right, follow its edge until you have a reef in front of you, continue to the top of this reef, depth 11m. Taking a southerly compass bearing will lead you directly over the Arch and on to a reef where you can select your own depth; the minimum time from the wreck to this point will take you 6 minutes. Follow the reef all the way to your exit point E2, on the south side of the lighthouse.

Below: A diver in front of the bridge of the Rozi.

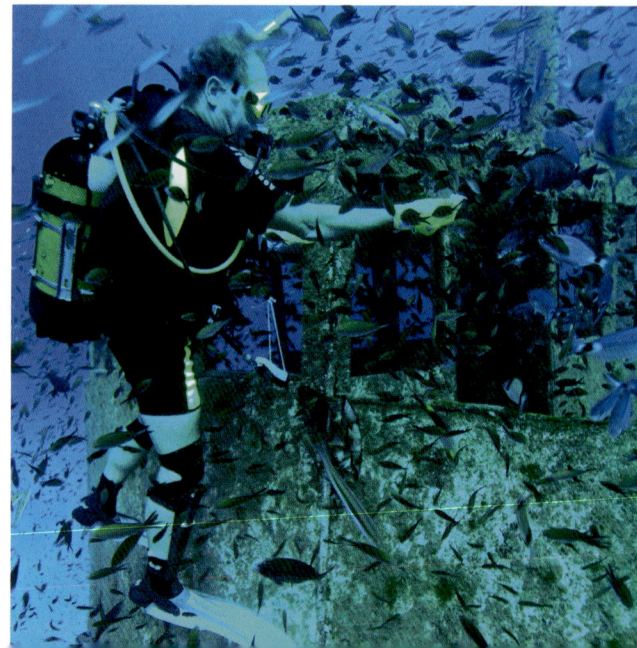

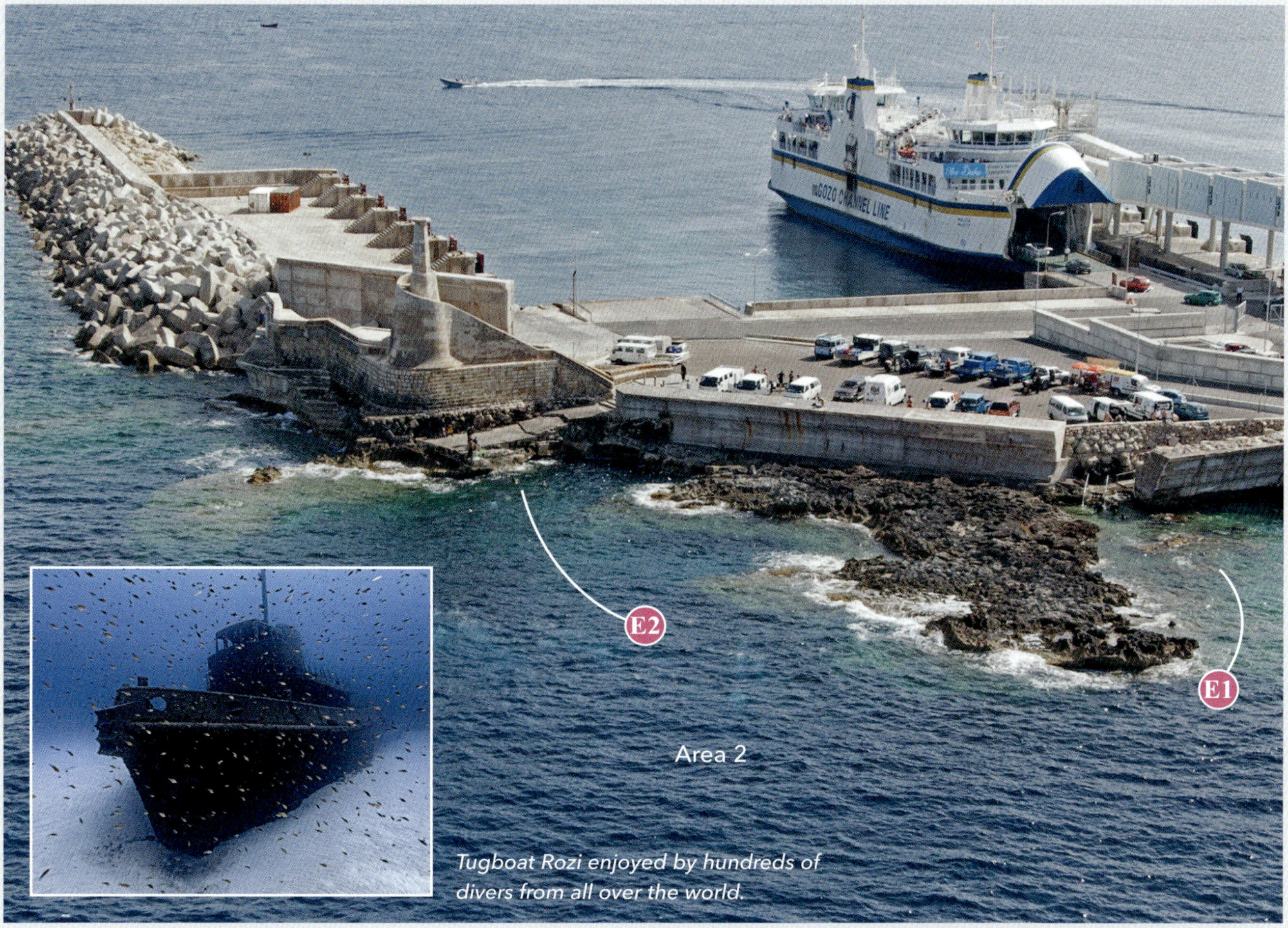

TUGBOAT ROZI - CIRKEWWA MARINE PARK

Area 2

Tugboat Rozi enjoyed by hundreds of divers from all over the world.

PHOTO: JON BORG www.jonborg.com

PHOTO: PGL AERIAL PHOTOS

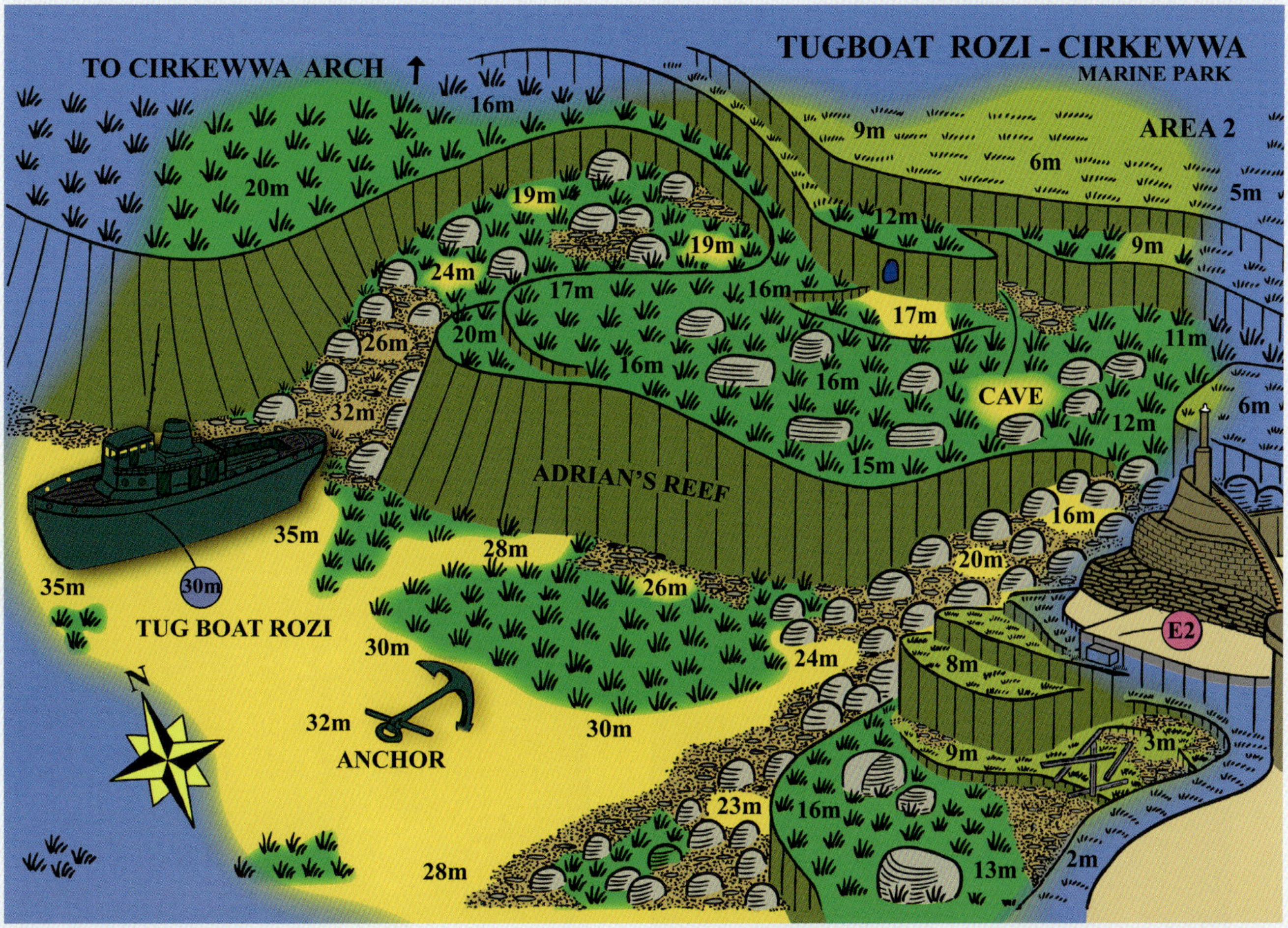

TUGBOAT ROZI - CIRKEWWA MARINE PARK

TO CIRKEWWA ARCH ↑

AREA 2

TUG BOAT ROZI

ADRIAN'S REEF

CAVE

ANCHOR

E2

Sugar Loaf, Madonna — Area 3

There are many ways you can dive this site, by using the reef to navigate your way around, generally, it runs south to north. Most divers who come to Cirkewwa (Marfa Point) normally dive this site first. A visit to the Madonna Statue, then on to Sugar Loaf, which is a huge rock detached from the main reef and rising some 8m from the seabed. Once out of the training area and over the drop off you will find the seabed sandy, flat, with boulders near the reef. Also there are overhangs within the reef to explore, which makes this an interesting dive site.

THE DIVE — Minimum time - 40 mins

Entry for this area would normally be made at Susie's Pool E1, once under water head in a westerly direction along the stony path to the drop-off, over and down on to the bottom. Now turn right in a northerly direction and in a very short distance, in a corner you will find a small fissure at a depth of 18m. Here you will find the Madonna statue, which is also the home for many cardinal fish.

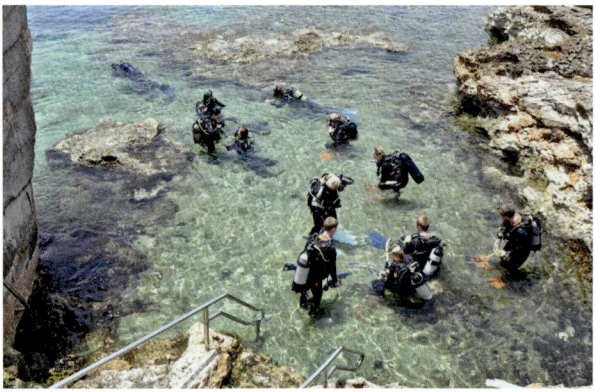

Susies Pool, your entry point E1 for Area 3.

Below: The Madonna in her little cave with her flowers and fish.

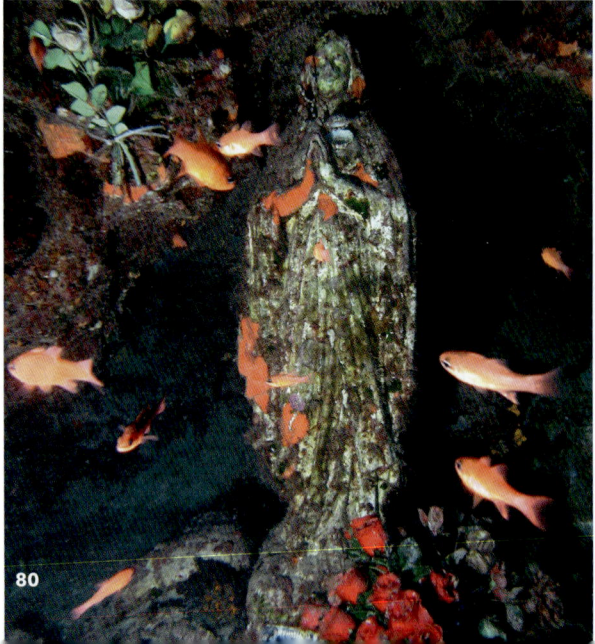

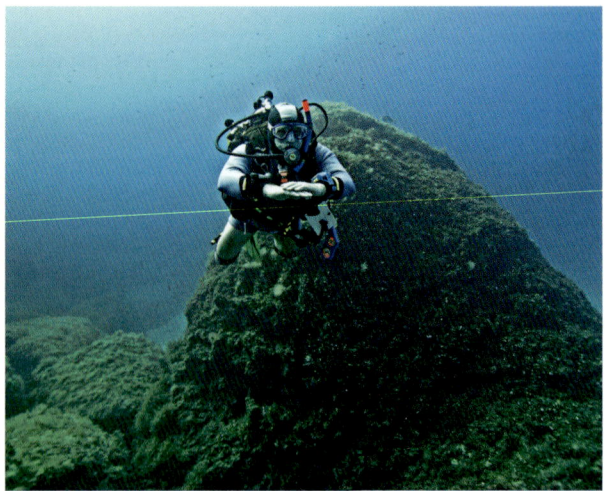

Behind me Sugar Loaf and to my left the main reef.

Now follow the reef down over the large boulders, round the corner, the large rock on your left is called Sugar loaf.

Watch out for groupers lying on the smaller round boulders, between the main reef and Sugar Loaf, but remember they are very shy, so you have to move slowly.

When it is time to return, ascend the reef to your required depth and head south, keeping the coastline reef on your left, you will come to the swim-through at 11m, once you have gone through or round to the other side, continue along the reef, over the Madonna cave. Within this area there are many small crevices and little overhangs to explore. Once at the ledge at 11m, move to your right and you will find a very large overhang, sometimes hiding right at the back on a small ledge you may see a grouper. The roof of this overhang is covered with brightly coloured small soft coral, this may be a good opportunity for photographs. Moving from the ledge there are depths of 6m and shallower areas for safety stops, through the training area and your exit point at Susie's pool E1.

The main training area mostly used for first time divers.

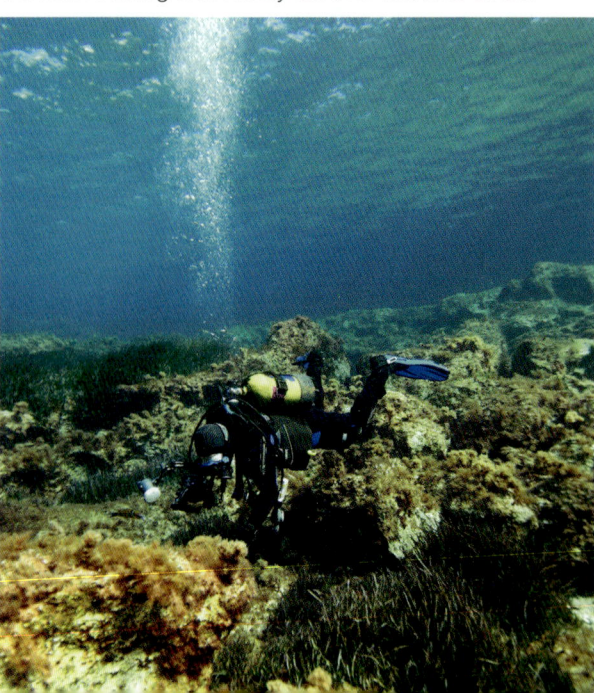

E2
Area 2
E1
Susies Pool
Training Area
Sugar Loaf
Madonna

PHOTO: PGL AERIAL PHOTOS

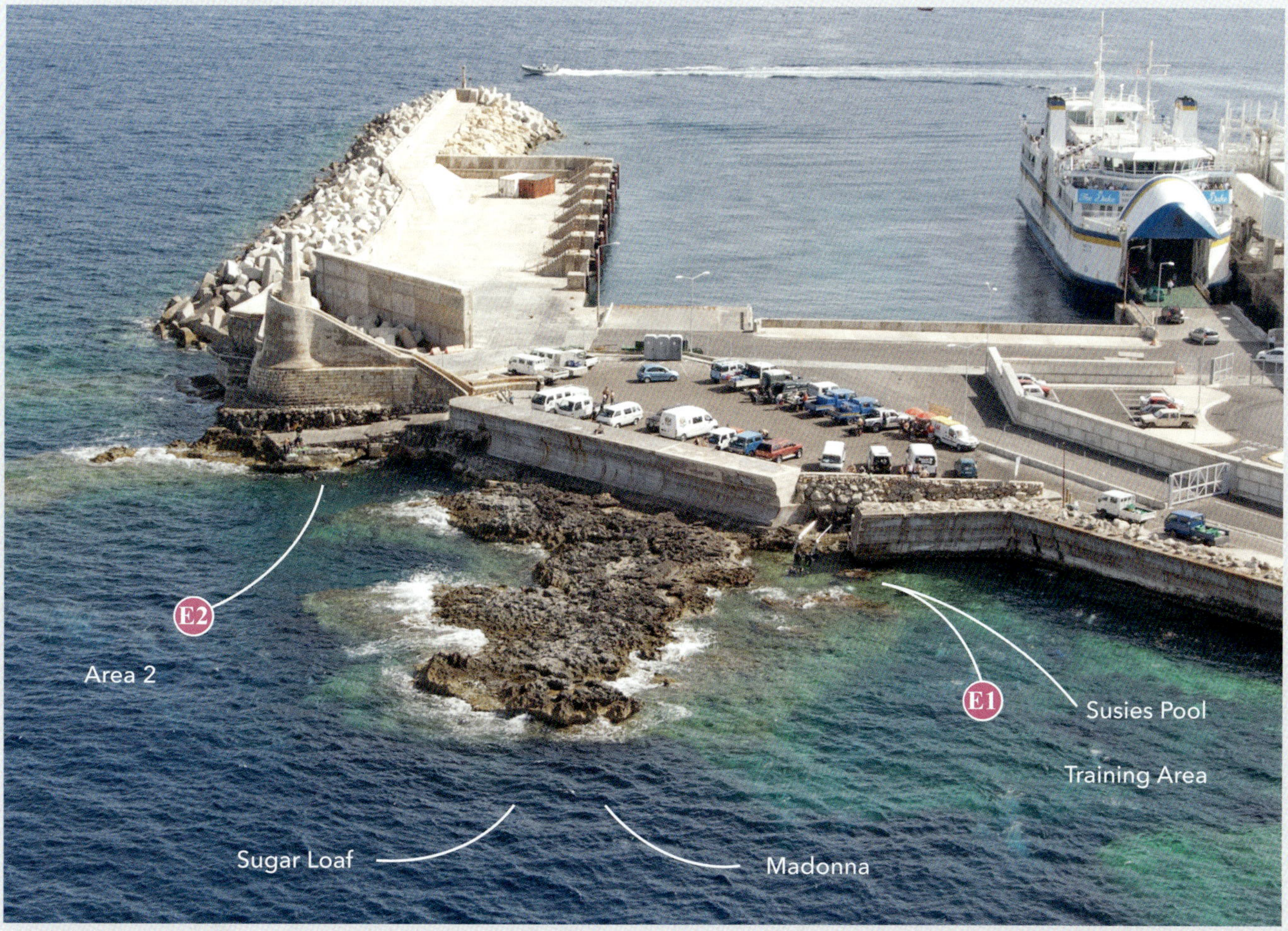

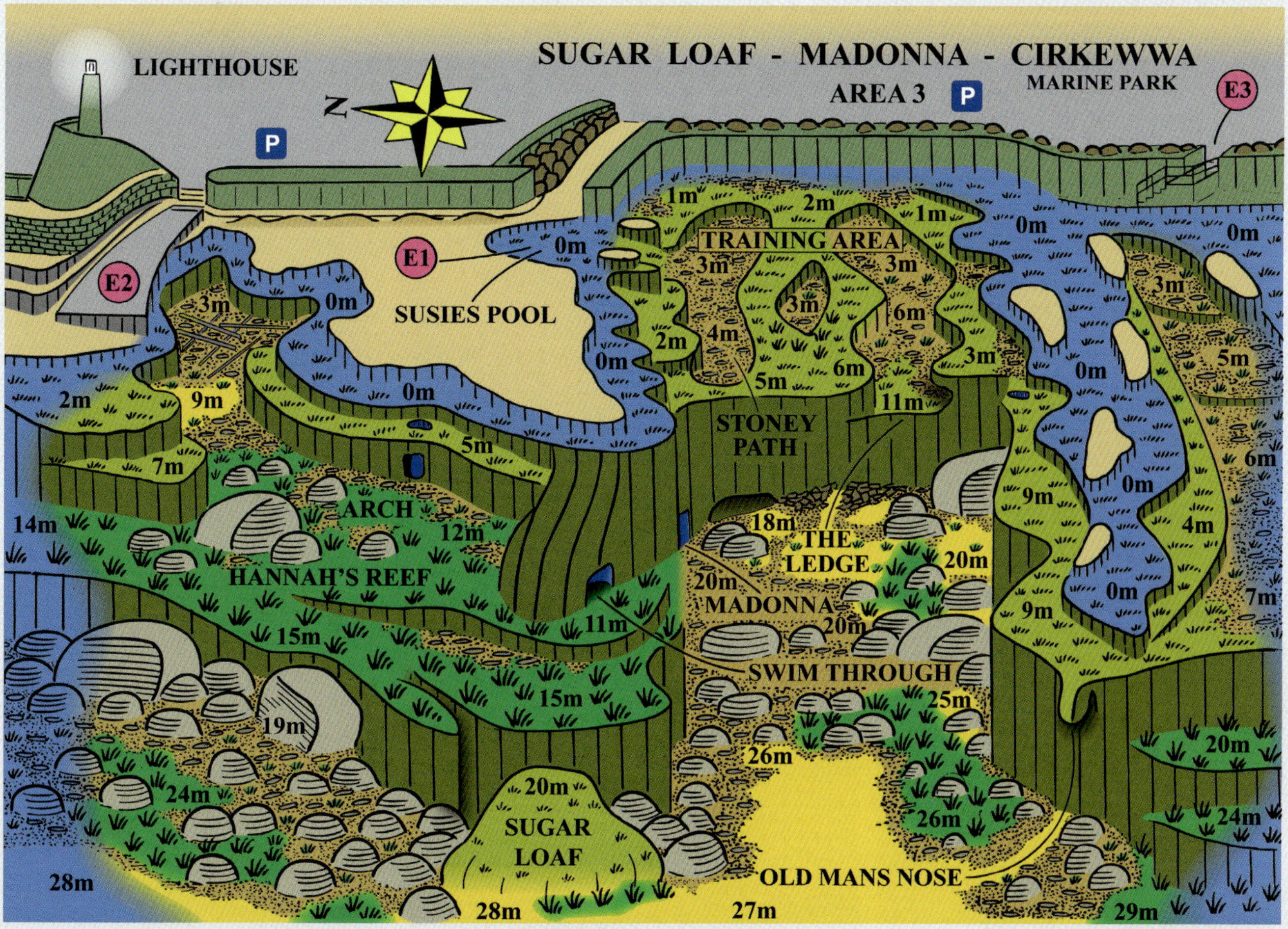
SUGAR LOAF - MADONNA - CIRKEWWA
MARINE PARK
AREA 3
E3
LIGHTHOUSE
N
P
E1
E2
SUSIES POOL
TRAINING AREA
STONEY PATH
ARCH
HANNAH'S REEF
THE LEDGE
MADONNA
SWIM THROUGH
SUGAR LOAF
OLD MANS NOSE
0m
1m
2m
3m
4m
5m
6m
7m
9m
11m
12m
14m
15m
18m
19m
20m
24m
25m
26m
27m
28m
29m

CIRKEWWA MARINE PARK

A look around Cirkewwa Marine Park

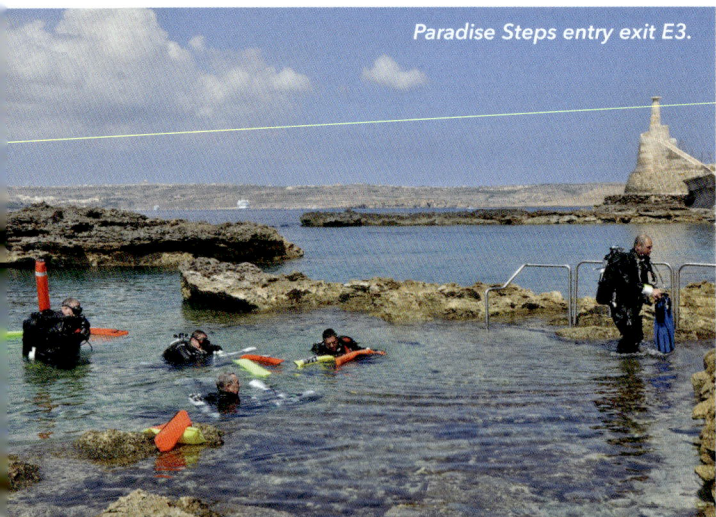
Paradise Steps entry exit E3.

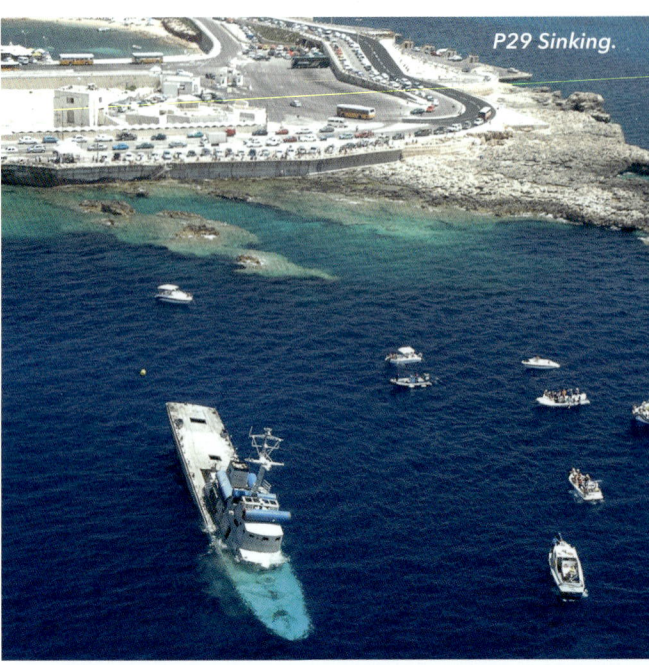
P29 Sinking.

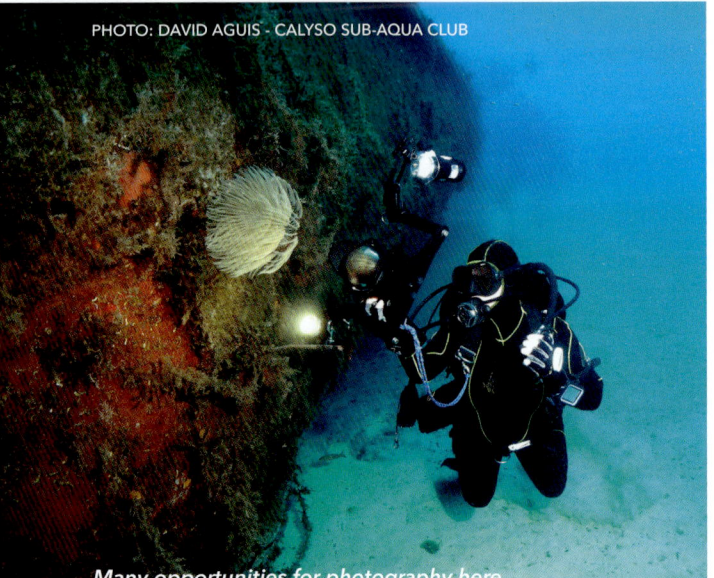
PHOTO: DAVID AGUIS - CALYSO SUB-AQUA CLUB
Many opportunities for photography here.

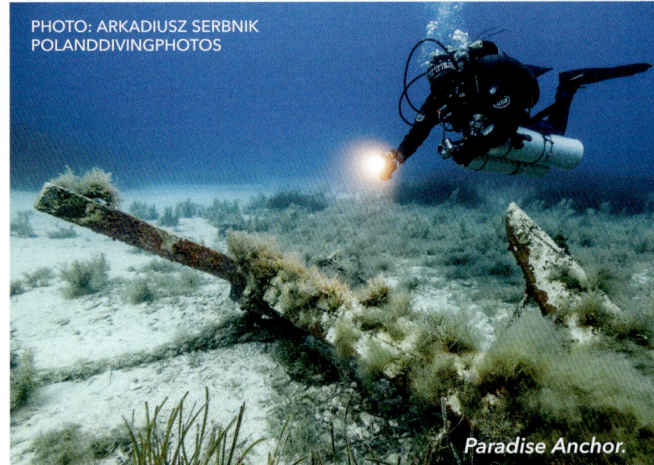
PHOTO: ARKADIUSZ SERBNIK
POLANDDIVINGPHOTOS
Paradise Anchor.

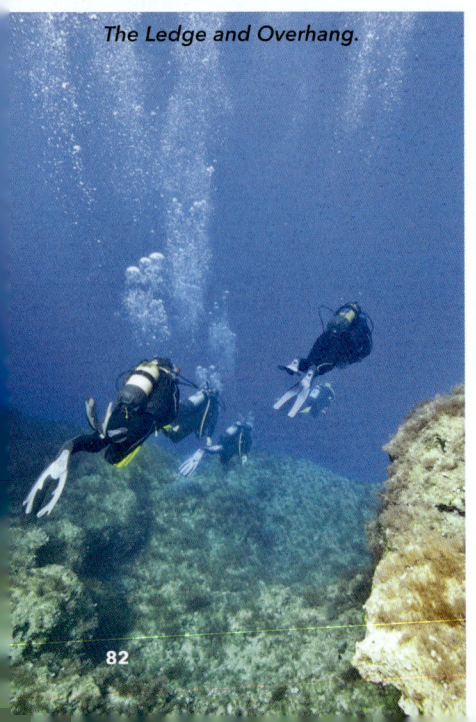
The Ledge and Overhang.

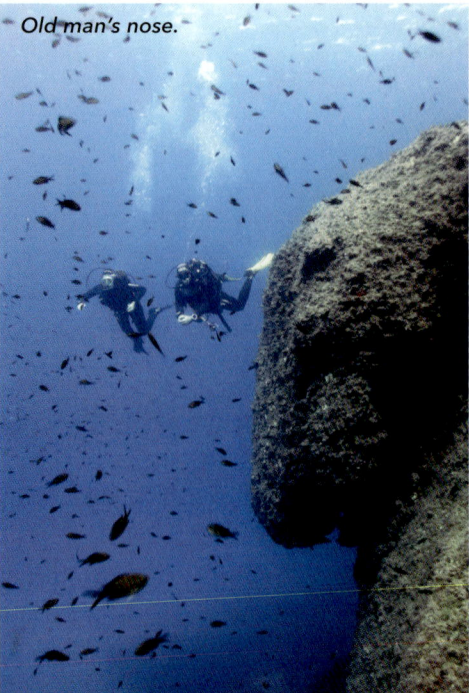
Old man's nose.

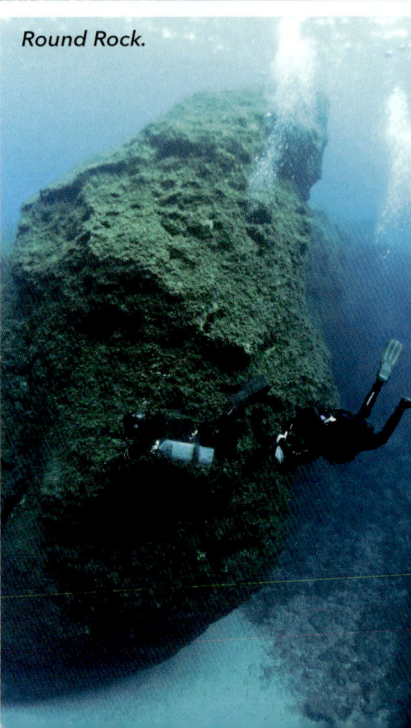
Round Rock.

P29 Patrol Boat

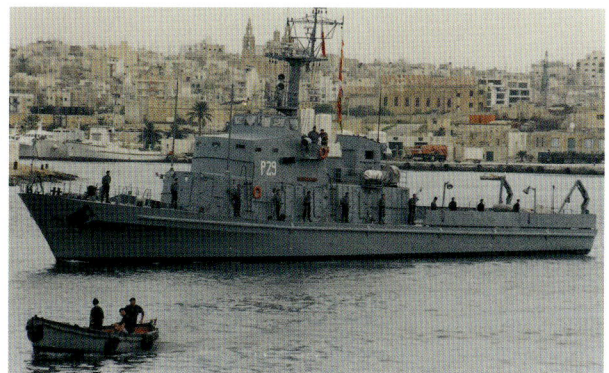

The arrival of the P29 in Grand Harbour in August 1997.

The *P29*, formerly *Boltenhagen* started life in former East Germany. She is a Kondor class boat designed and built on the Peenewerft, Wolgast in East Germany in the 1960's 52 metres in length weighing 360 tons. Originally designed as a minesweeper, other duties were, border control and fishery protection. She was also part of the German Democratic Republic logistical fleet.

In August 1997, after a three-week voyage from Germany, the Armed Forces of Malta's Maritime Squadron took delivery of their third Kondor vessel, the *P29*. When the ship arrived in Malta it was greeted by the family and friends of the crew.

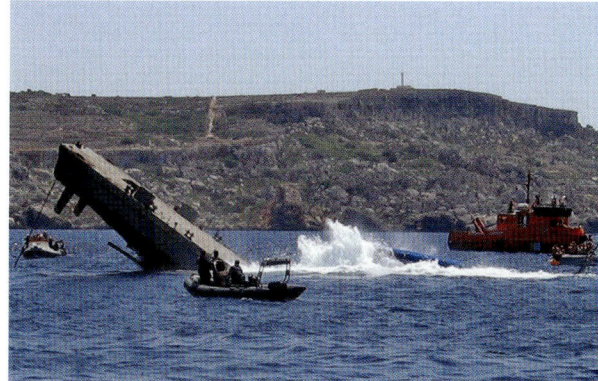

The sinking of the P29 off Cirkewwa August 2007.

Below: Grey triggerfish.   PHOTO: VERONICA BUSUTTIL

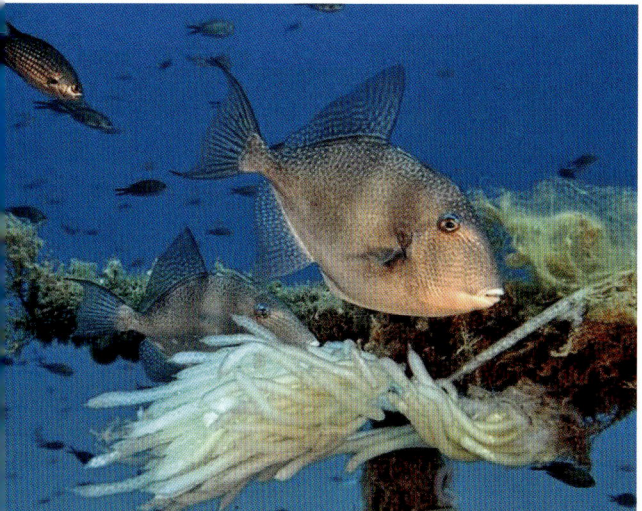

P29 PATROL BOAT - CIRKEWWA MARINE PARK

The Kondor vessels were the first war ships the AFM ever commissioned, and it was thanks to them that the Maritime Squadron was able to participate in naval exercises with other European fleets. From 1997 until 2004, when she was decommissioned, the *P29* patrolled the coastal waters of the Maltese Islands, fulfilling her duties with search and rescue operations, fisheries protection duties and exercises: of course, the naval exercises took her further afield into international waters of the Mediterranean. In 2000 and 2001 the Kondor's supported the prestigious Royal Malta Yacht Club's Middle Sea Race off Lampedusa.

In September 2005 the *P29* was sold to the Malta Tourism Authority to be scuttled as an attraction for divers. She was cleaned and made environmentally safe and was scuttled on the 14th August 2007 off Cirkewwa, buoyed and at a depth of 38m.

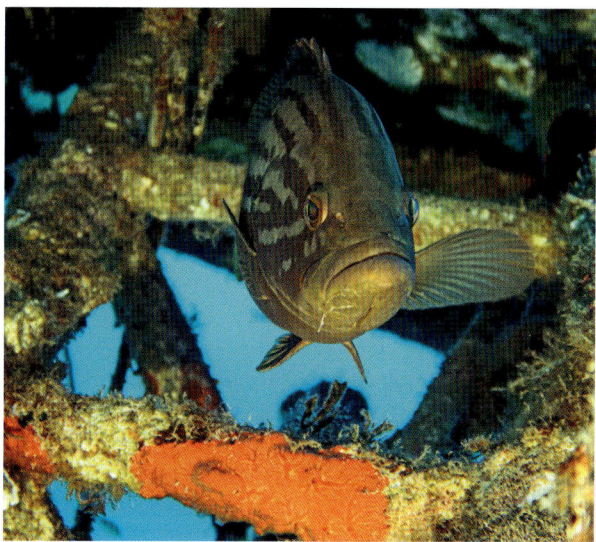

Hiding under the mast platform a large grouper.
PHOTO: VERONICA BUSUTTIL

Below: Above the bridge area next to the mast.

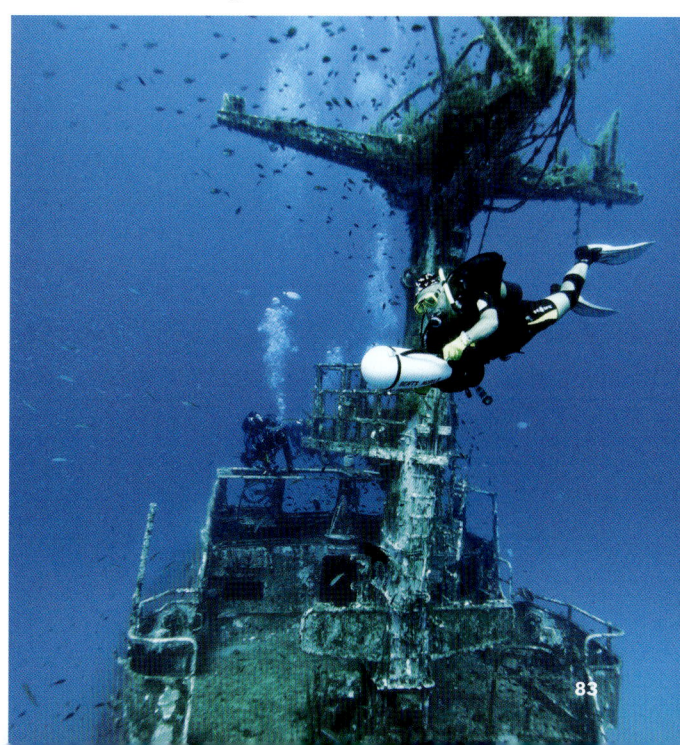

P29 Patrol Boat — Area 4

THE DIVE — Minimum time - 45 mins

Route 1 enter the water at Susie's Pool E1, surface swim out between the two rocks, now head in a westerly direction above stony path to the drop off and descend. From here the distance is 100 metres to the stern of the *P29*.

Take a compass bearing of 270° and if the visibility is good, you will be able to see the reef on your right-hand side until Sugar Loaf comes into view. In front of you and to the south of Sugar Loaf, on a sandy seabed will be a concrete block almost buried, at this moment in time there is a plaque on the far side. You are now half way there, if the visibility is not so good leave the drop off and drop down over the boulders, rocks and sea grass until you reach the sand; if you are taking a bearing of 270° you should find the concrete block and plaque. Continue with the same compass bearing. From the drop off to the *P29* should take you no more than 4 - 5 minutes.

Route 2 entry point E3 Paradise steps. I suggest that you surface swim to the 9m ledge above the Old Mans Nose, the best way is to go around the last rock of the reef on your right to reach the ledge, which is on the north side of the rock. From here the *P29* is 100 metres with a compass bearing of 310° the same distance as Route 1 and it should take no longer than 4-5 minutes. Now descend from the ledge above the Old Mans Nose and where the reef meets the sand it forms an 'L' shape. The reef runs to the north and the sea grass runs to the west, now re-check your bearing of 310° and continue to the wreck.

Note: If the visibility is not too good and you are intending to swim mid water, beware of the currents which sometimes occur in this area, only a slight current will drift you off course and consequently you will miss the wreck

Return routes when it is time to leave the wreck a compass bearing of 90° will take you back to Sugar Loaf whereas a bearing of 130° will take you back to the reef below the Old Mans Nose. Of course, you can take any compass bearing between the two which will lead you back onto the main reef and your exit point.

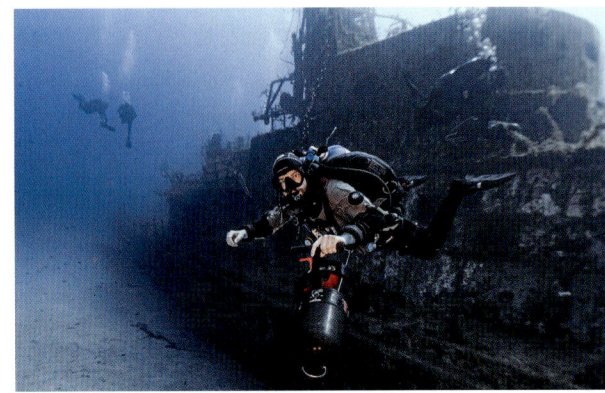

Using a DPV to visit and explore the P29 Patrol Boat.
PHOTO: JON BORG www.jonborg.com

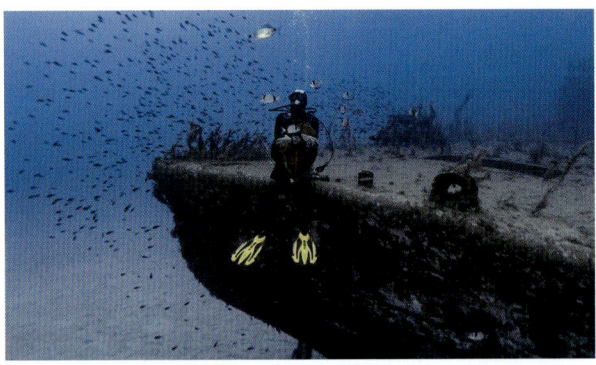

The stern of the P29, your leaving point for the E1 exit.
PHOTOS: JON BORG www.jonborg.com

Below: This wreck is now home for a variety of marine life.

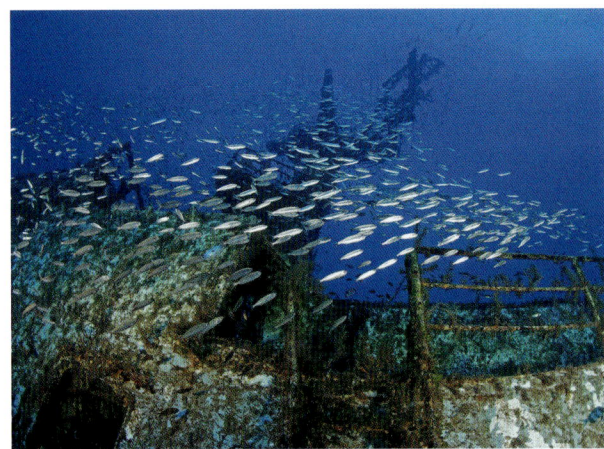

A shoal of Bogues (Boops boops) giving a stunning display.
PHOTO: MAX VALLI - ORANGE SHARK DIVE CENTRE

The gun an added attraction and photo shoot opportunity.
PHOTO: DAN-MARCELLO DI FRANCESCO-ORANGE SHARK

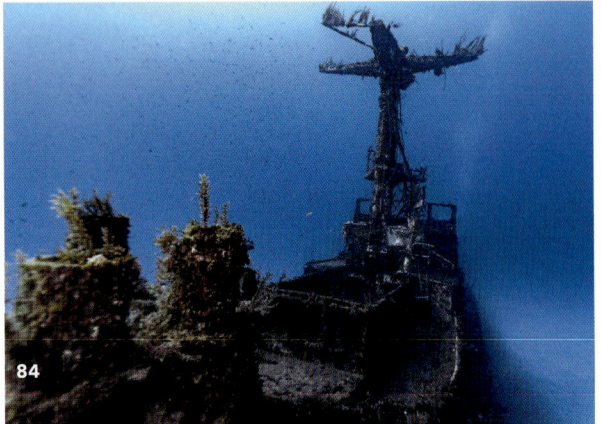

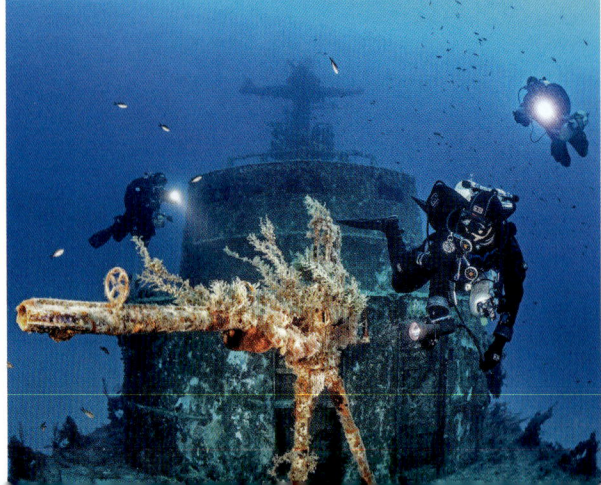

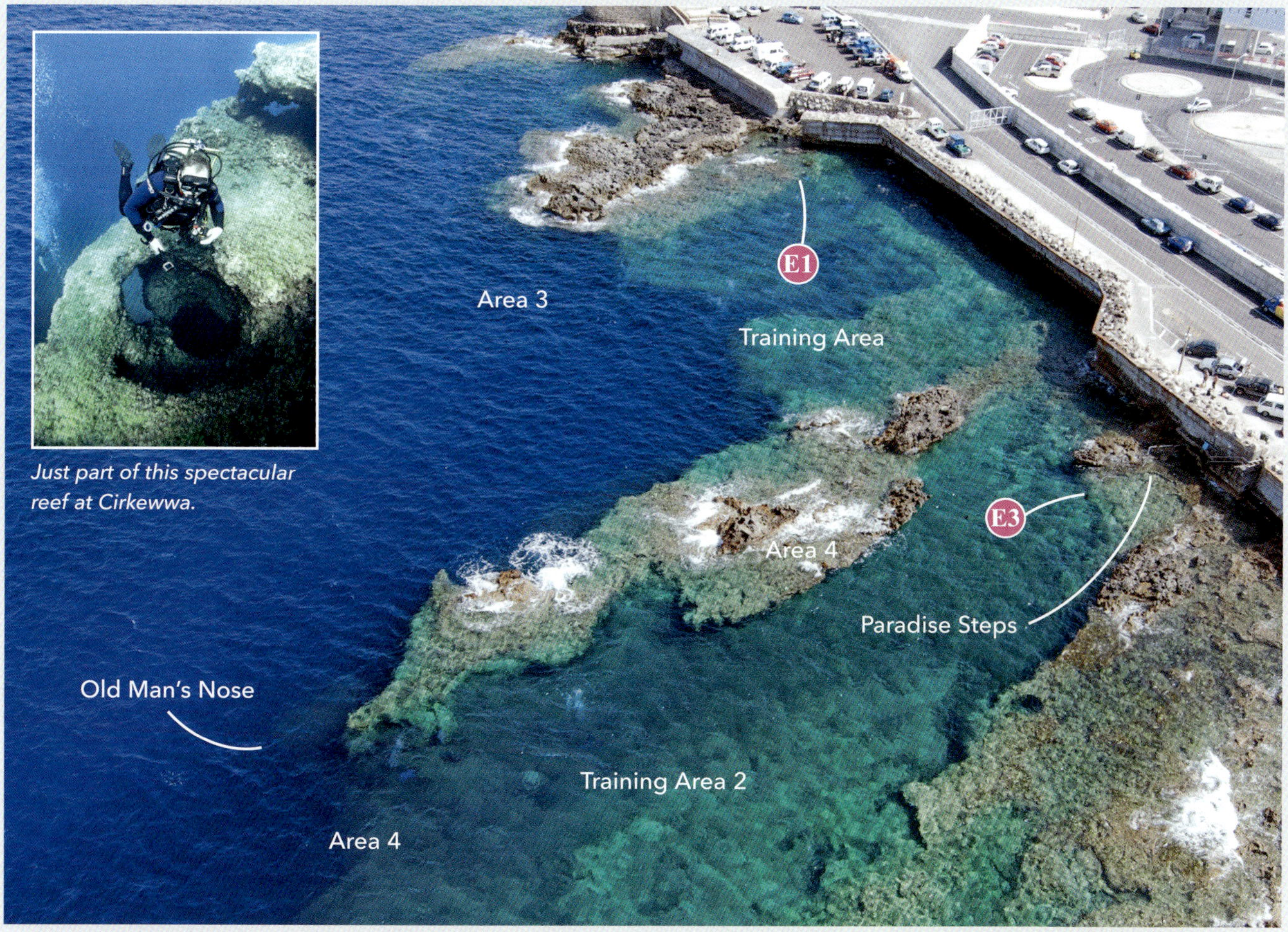

P29 PATROL BOAT - CIRKEWWA MARINE PARK

Just part of this spectacular reef at Cirkewwa.

Area 3
Training Area (E1)
Area 4
Paradise Steps (E3)
Old Man's Nose
Training Area 2
Area 4

PHOTO: PGL AERIAL PHOTOS

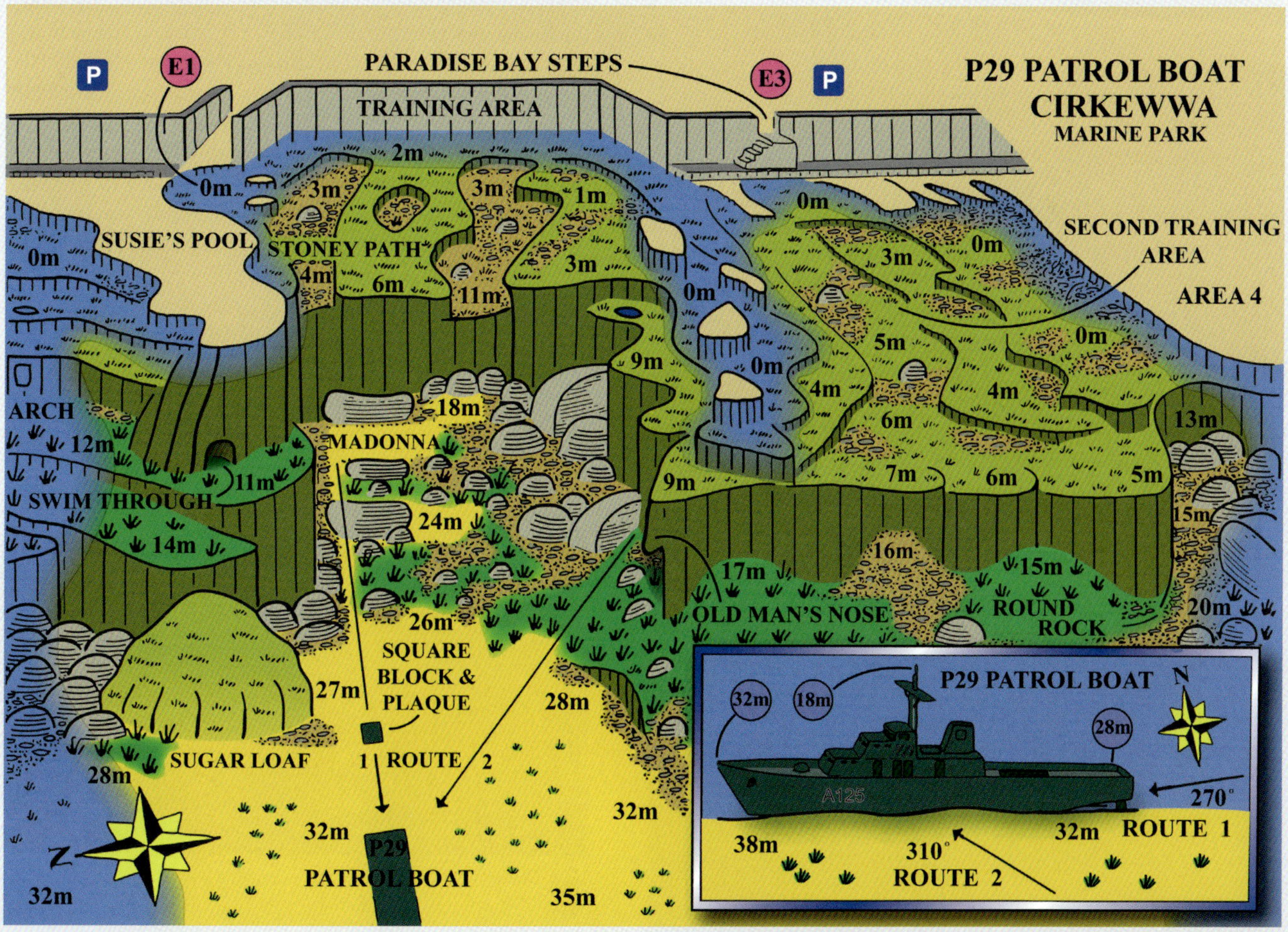

P29 PATROL BOAT CIRKEWWA MARINE PARK

P (E1) PARADISE BAY STEPS TRAINING AREA (E3) P

SECOND TRAINING AREA
AREA 4

SUSIE'S POOL
STONEY PATH
ARCH 12m
SWIM THROUGH 14m
MADONNA
OLD MAN'S NOSE
ROUND ROCK
SUGAR LOAF
SQUARE BLOCK & PLAQUE
ROUTE 1
ROUTE 2
P29 PATROL BOAT

P29 PATROL BOAT
32m / 18m / 28m
A125
38m 270°
310° ROUTE 2 ROUTE 1

PARADISE BAY - CIRKEWWA MARINE PARK

Paradise Bay — Area 5

The long swim is the nickname given to this site by myself, but in reality, it can be completed, taking a leisurely swim, in less than 40 minutes. Your entry point is E4 on the western side of South Quay.

Beware the jetty can be extremely slippery.

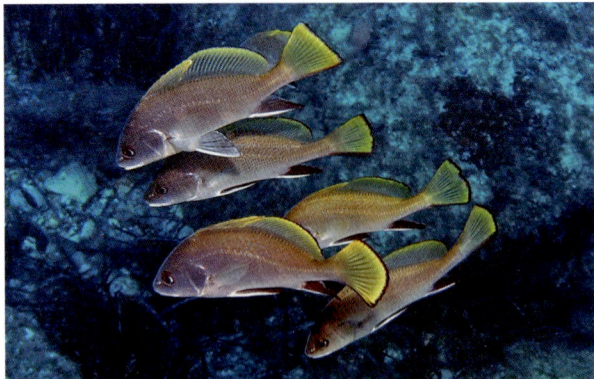

Brown meagres (Sciaena umbra) a shoal of these colourful fish.   PHOTO: PATRICK SCHEMBRI - WALRUS DIVING CLUB

There is no exit point at the quay or throughout most of the route, however, a short distance from the quay, a little cove where you could exit the water in an emergency, this would involve walking over a very uneven surface. I suggest you take your vehicle to E4 unload, then park it near your exit point E3, returning to your buddies on foot.

THE DIVE   Minimum time - 45 mins

Below your entry point E4 the depth at the side of the quay is 4m. When you are under water just follow the reef in a westerly direction keeping it on your right-hand side. After a short distance you have a choice to stay on the ledge at 10m or go down to the next level at 15/18m. If you decide to stay at 10m after some 6/8 minutes you will find a curve in the reef, inside this area is an arch, good for photography.

If you went to the lower reef, it will take you 10/12 minutes or one minute from the arch to the large boulder right up against the main reef, it is possible to swim under it but the entrance is hidden by smaller boulders.

Once through the other side you can take one of two routes: the first one with a maximum depth of 32m, the second has a maximum depth of 20m. The first option is to follow a compass bearing of 270° down to an area of large boulders, with a maximum depth on the sand of 32m. Once you have run out of bottom time or you just want to move on, take an easterly compass bearing, heading back up the reef, taking your time to explore, when a depth of 20m is reached you should be between Valley Way and Round Rock.

Alternatively, continue round the reef keeping it on your right, where the seabed rises to 16m, here you will find Chris's Rock; this smallish rock resting on stones makes a great hiding place for marine life, we once found a nice cuttlefish here. From here move on along the base of the reef to a depth of 19m which is the start of Valley Way a narrow route between the main reef and boulders. In this area there are many hiding places for marine life such as Morays, Groupers, Octopuses and large Scorpion fish. When you reach 11m, bear left between two rocks, once through these looking down and slightly to your left you will see a stony seabed at 19m and the very large overhang at the base of Round Rock, explore this area and then ascend Round Rock onto the ridge at 9m and head into the second training area and E3.

Below: To the right of the diver is the large boulder which you can safely swim underneath.

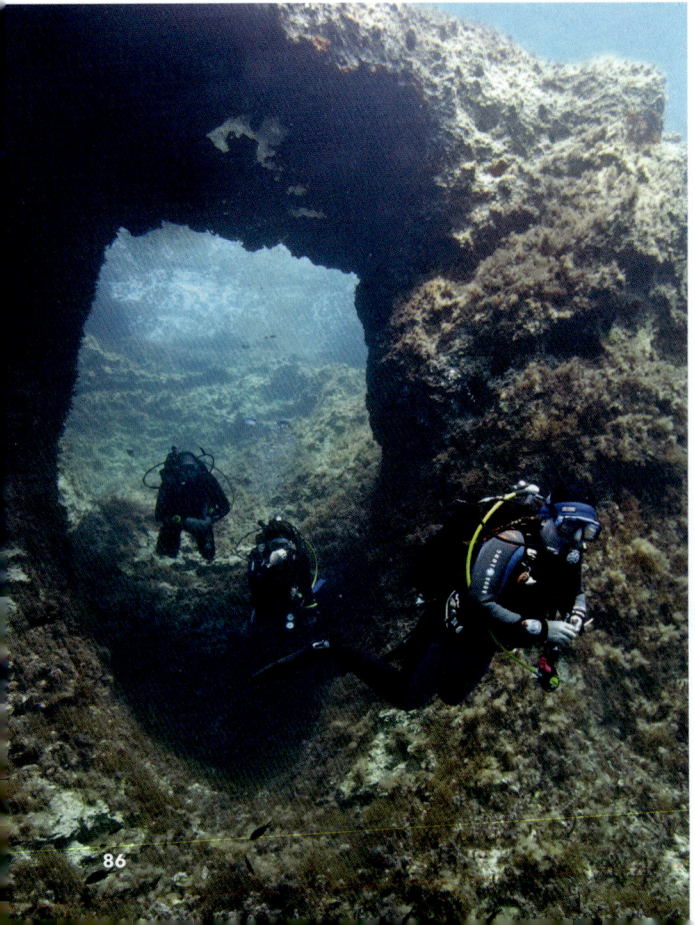

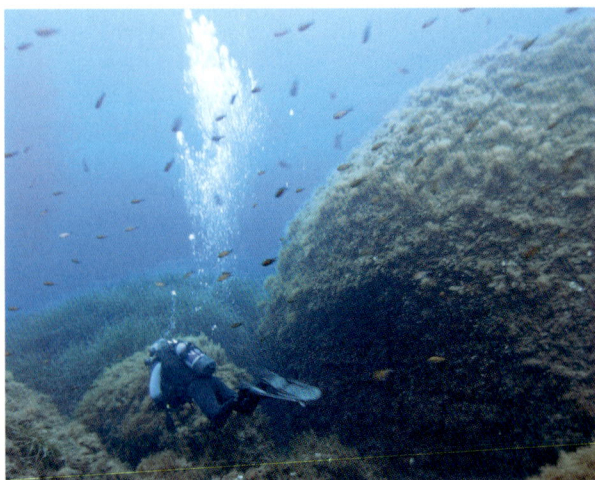

Left: Bens Arch also known as Paradise Arch.

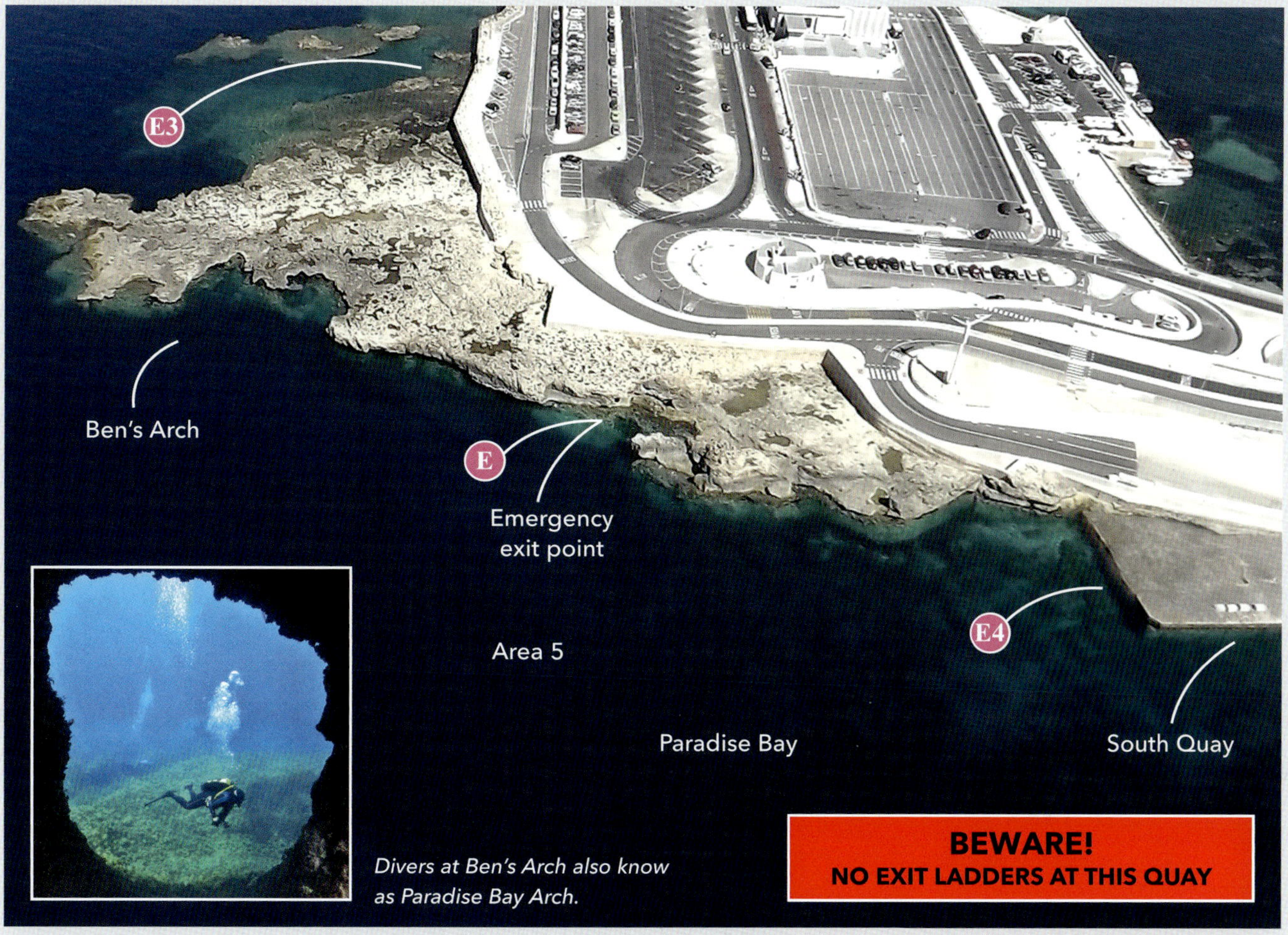

PARADISE BAY - CIRKEWWA MARINE PARK

- Ben's Arch
- E3
- E
- Emergency exit point
- Area 5
- Paradise Bay
- E4
- South Quay

BEWARE! NO EXIT LADDERS AT THIS QUAY

Divers at Ben's Arch also know as Paradise Bay Arch.

PHOTO: PGL AERIAL PHOTOS

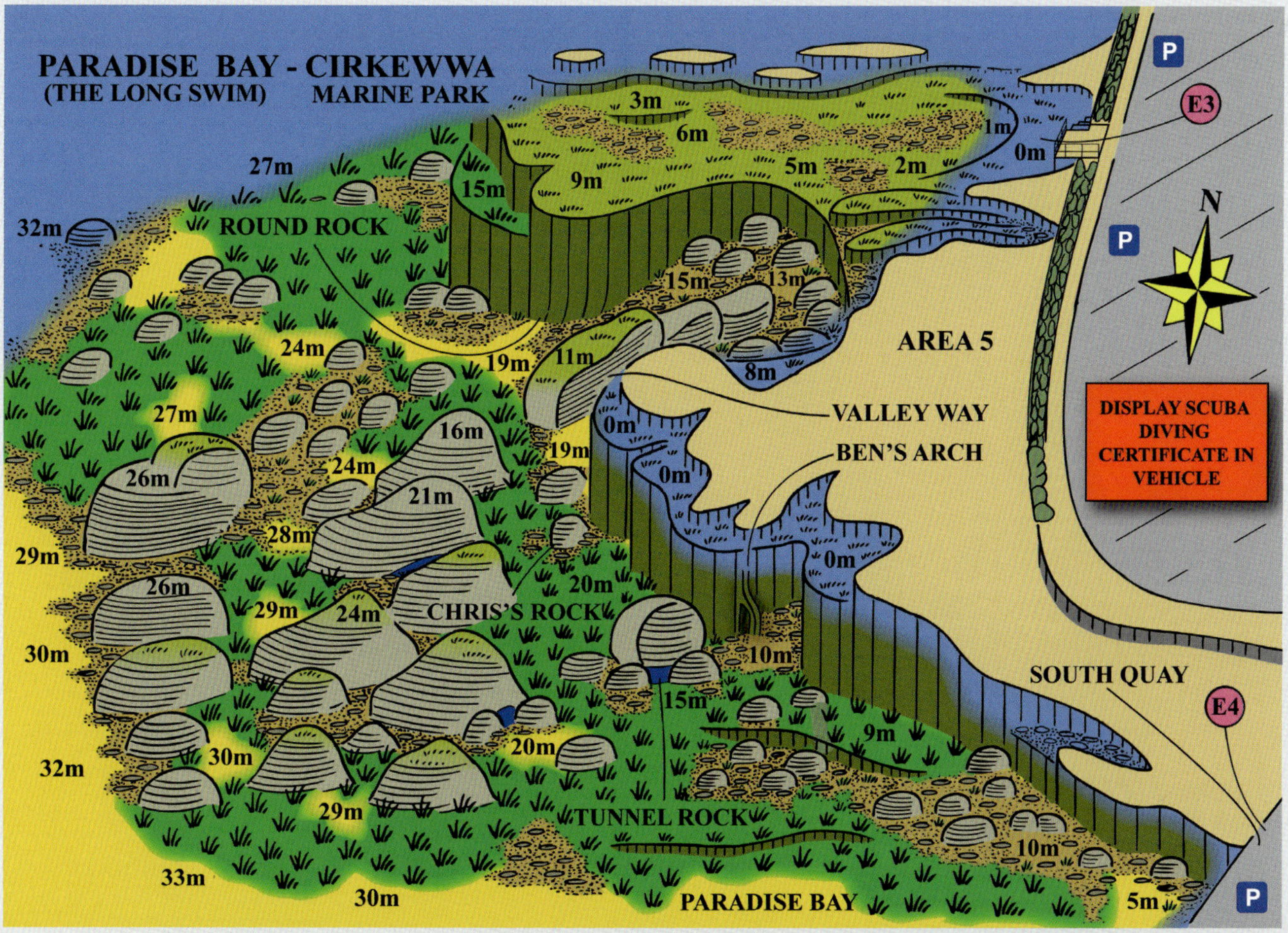

PARADISE BAY - CIRKEWWA (THE LONG SWIM) MARINE PARK

Depths marked: 3m, 6m, 1m, 0m, 5m, 2m, 27m, 15m, 9m, 32m, ROUND ROCK, 15m, 3m, 24m, 19m, 11m, 8m, 27m, 16m, 0m, AREA 5, 26m, 24m, 21m, 0m, VALLEY WAY, BEN'S ARCH, 28m, 19m, 29m, 26m, 24m, 20m, 0m, 30m, CHRIS'S ROCK, 10m, SOUTH QUAY, E4, 32m, 15m, 9m, 30m, 20m, 29m, TUNNEL ROCK, 10m, 33m, 30m, PARADISE BAY, 5m

E3, P, N, P

DISPLAY SCUBA DIVING CERTIFICATE IN VEHICLE

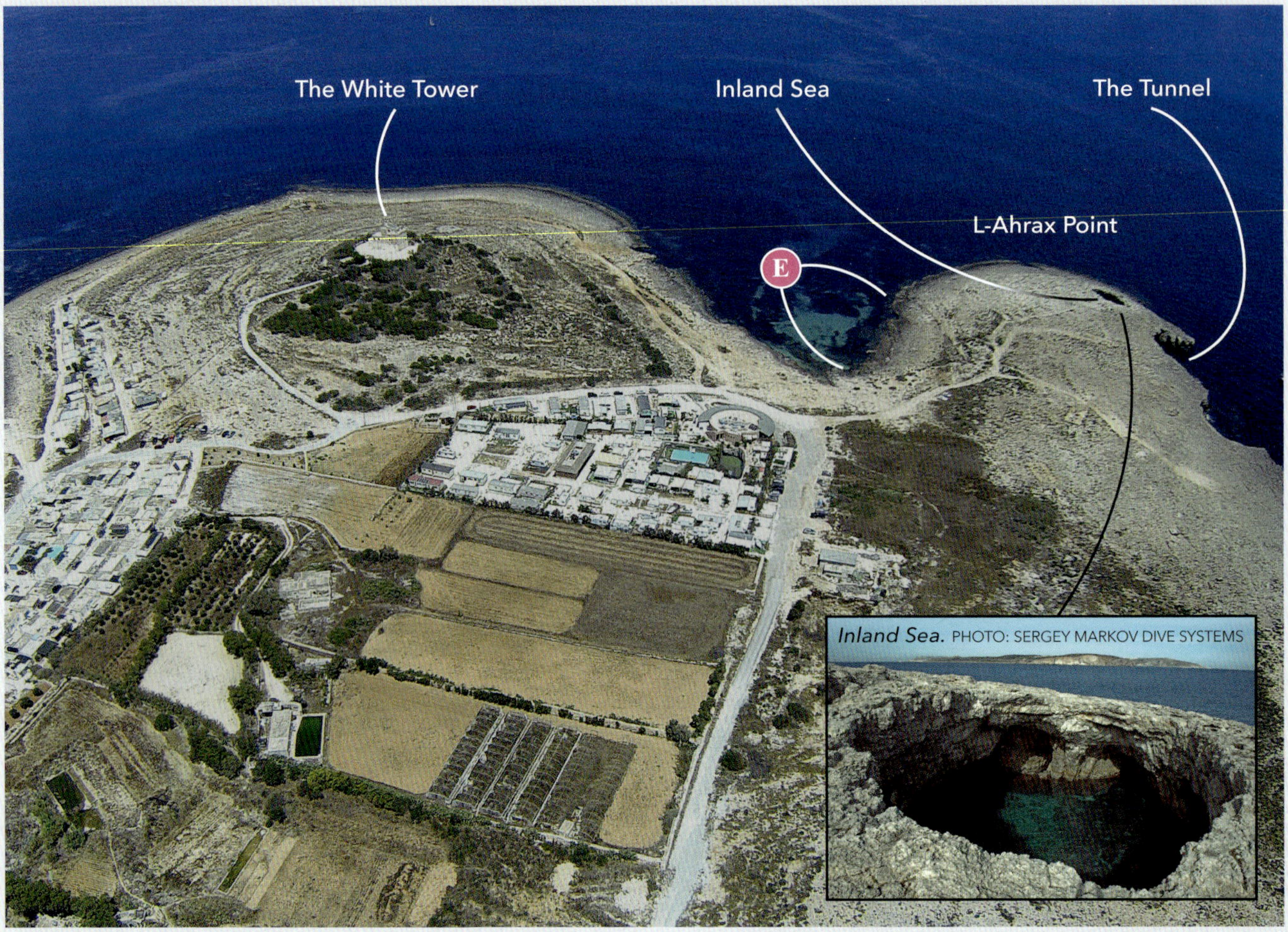

L-AHRAX POINT - SLUGS BAY - MELLIEHA

Labels on aerial photo: The White Tower, Inland Sea, The Tunnel, L-Ahrax Point

Inland Sea. PHOTO: SERGEY MARKOV DIVE SYSTEMS

PHOTO: PGL AERIAL PHOTOS

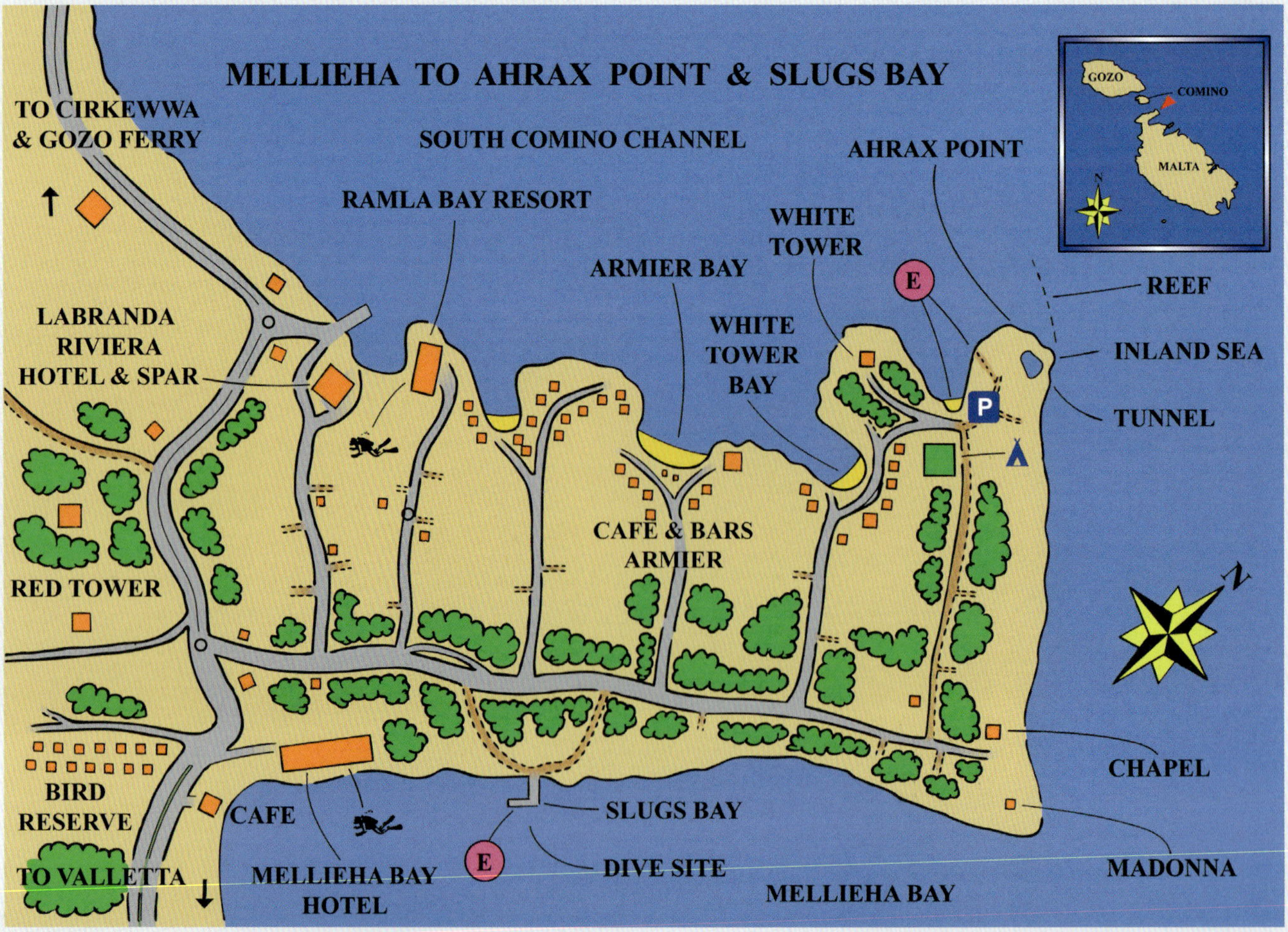

MELLIEHA TO AHRAX POINT & SLUGS BAY

Map labels:
- TO CIRKEWWA & GOZO FERRY
- SOUTH COMINO CHANNEL
- RAMLA BAY RESORT
- AHRAX POINT
- WHITE TOWER
- ARMIER BAY
- REEF
- WHITE TOWER BAY
- INLAND SEA
- LABRANDA RIVIERA HOTEL & SPAR
- TUNNEL
- RED TOWER
- CAFE & BARS ARMIER
- BIRD RESERVE
- CAFE
- CHAPEL
- MELLIEHA BAY HOTEL
- SLUGS BAY DIVE SITE
- MADONNA
- TO VALLETTA
- MELLIEHA BAY

Inset: GOZO, COMINO, MALTA

L-Ahrax Point - Reef Tunnel & Inland Sea

To reach L-Ahrax Point follow the road to Cirkewwa past Mellieha Bay and the sandy beach continue up the hill to the roundabout and turn right. Follow this road for about 2km and take the fifth or sixth turning on the left. Both these roads will lead you down to the campsite and your parking place. **See local map.** Entry point E1 is directly in front of you. For E2 continue along a track by the right-hand side of the bay, at the end of the track is a concrete pad, E2 is a short walk from here. **See Dive Site plan.** This dive site is often done to as a boat dive, but if that is not possible and you have the time and energy, this is an enjoyable and rewarding dive. **Beware of small boats around this Headland.**

This away from the madding crowd dive site is situated on the most northerly point of Malta, and is definitely worth a visit, if you decide to dive here remember that all amenities are some distance away. There are a number of ways to dive this site but it could be divided into two main areas, using both entry points, E1 and E2.

South Reef Tunnel and Inland Sea, maximum depth on the reef is 12m over the ledge depths of 22m can be reached; the tunnel is reasonably shallow at 8m.

North reef, which is reasonably level with a maximum depth of 10m, once over the edge you have a drop off down to 23m, away from the reef depths of 30m plus can be reached.

The best time to dive this site is with the sun directly on the reef, later in the day the reef will be in the shade and all the bright colours will have disappeared. The coast line around the headland is very rugged which makes it almost impossible to exit and even more difficult to walk on with diving equipment. There is one small area, which is suitable for an emergency exit if required. {see plan}. You can follow one of my dive plans or you can plan your own to reach the Tunnel and Inland Sea.

Divers in the tunnel leading to the Inland Sea.

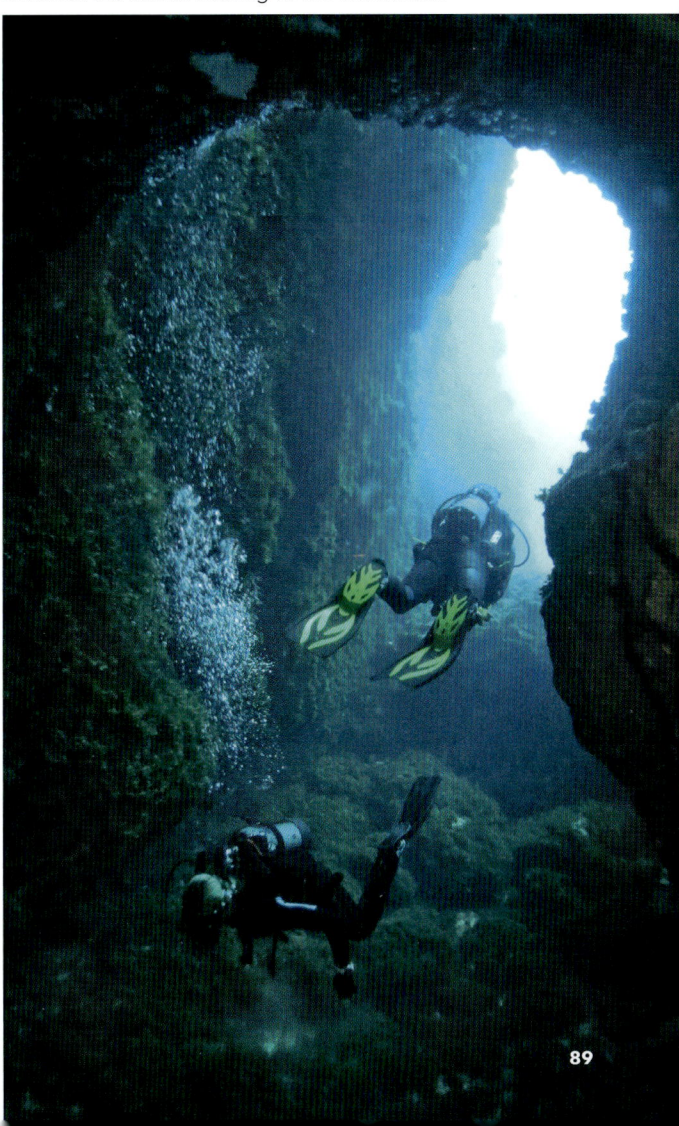

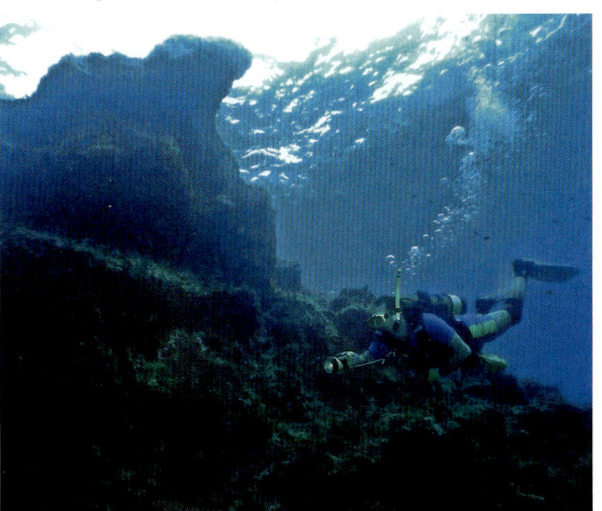

The drop off point just outside the tunnel, if boat diving this site. PHOTO: MAX VALLI - ORANGE SHARK DIVE CENTRE

Below: Eagle Rock, it's head points towards the tunnel.

Reef Tunnel & Inland Sea

THE DIVE — Minimum time - 50 mins

Using entry/exit point E1 from here surface swim following the coastline all the way round until it meets the main reef with its drop off to 22m plus. Of course, you can descend at any time you wish to, this distance of approximately 250 meters will possibly take you some 20 minutes. At this point you will need to descend unless you have already done so, here the depth will be approximately 6m, keeping the coastline reef to your right and head in a southerly direction for about 6 minutes you will come to a distinct corner where the coastline reef now runs in a southwesterly direction, continue to follow its line. The average depth in this area will be 12m. Within 2 minutes you will be able to see up on your left a rock shaped like an eagle's head, the entrance to the tunnel, which leads to the Inland Sea, is on your right. You will be unable to see straight through the tunnel, as there is a slight bend in it, the depth inside is 8m. The floor of the tunnel is covered in small rocks and they are in turn covered in red seaweed, these hard petal-like flowers remind me of roses.

When you leave the tunnel return to the distinct corner, now head in a north westerly direction until you reach the drop off, you should pass a lone rock right on the edge of the drop off. Now follow the ridge along in a northerly direction until it turns and heads west, continue to where the reef meets the coastline. Continue to follow the edge until you meet the main coastline reef at 6m, from here it is approximately 250 meters to your exit point, this could take you as long as 15/20 minutes, just keep the reef on your left.

If you have the air, take your time and explore this shallow reef. On your way back you will pass a small quarry with a depth of 10m with a little cove at the rear and inside there is a small arch. Now follow the reef all the way round until you reach many little sandy gullies here the water is very shallow, if you wish you could surface and swim to your exit point E1.

Facilities like a telephone and café are available when the camp site is open, otherwise there are no amenities within this area, the nearest telephone and café are some distance away (see plan).

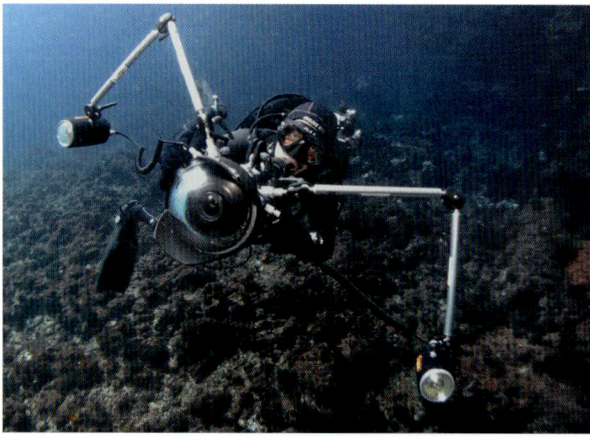

An excellent dive site to try your photo skills.

Below: A shoal of barracuda (Sphyraena sphyraene).

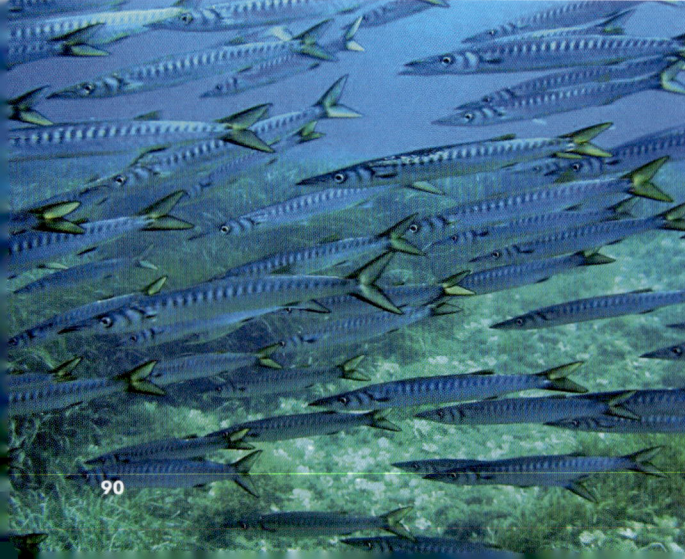

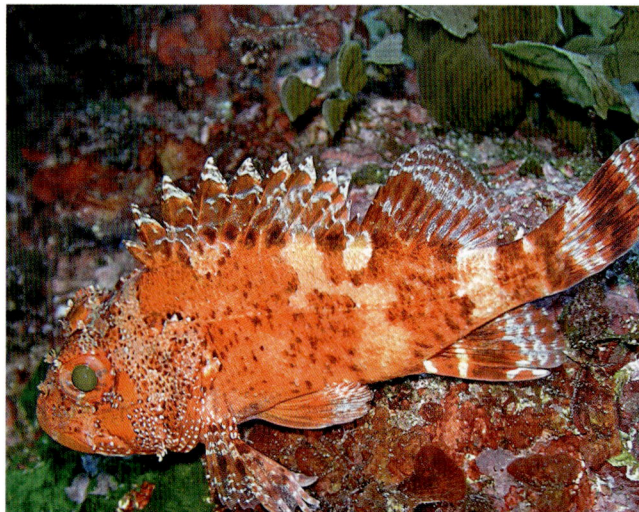

Red scorpion fish. PHOTO: SHARON FORDER

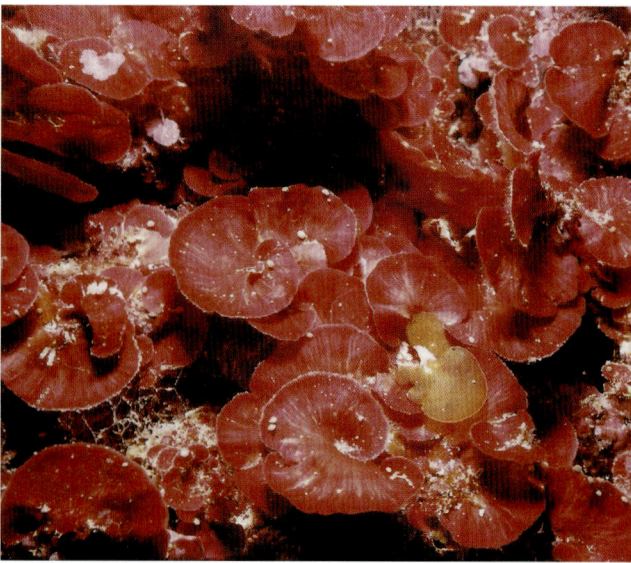

Sea rose coral covers many areas of this Inland Sea.

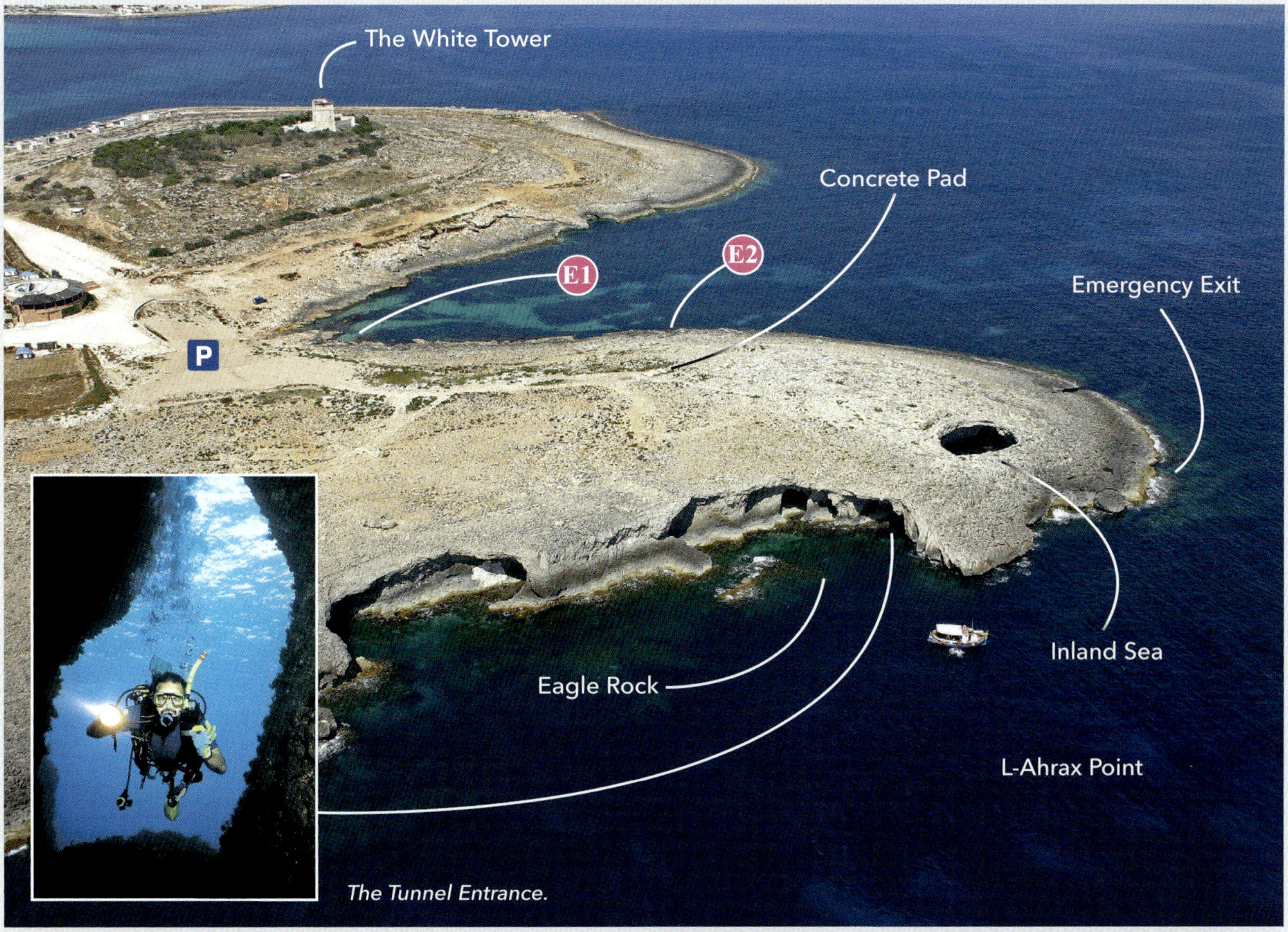

L-AHRAX POINT - REEF TUNNEL INLAND SEA

- The White Tower
- Concrete Pad
- E1
- E2
- Emergency Exit
- Eagle Rock
- Inland Sea
- L-Ahrax Point
- The Tunnel Entrance.

PHOTO: PGL AERIAL PHOTOS

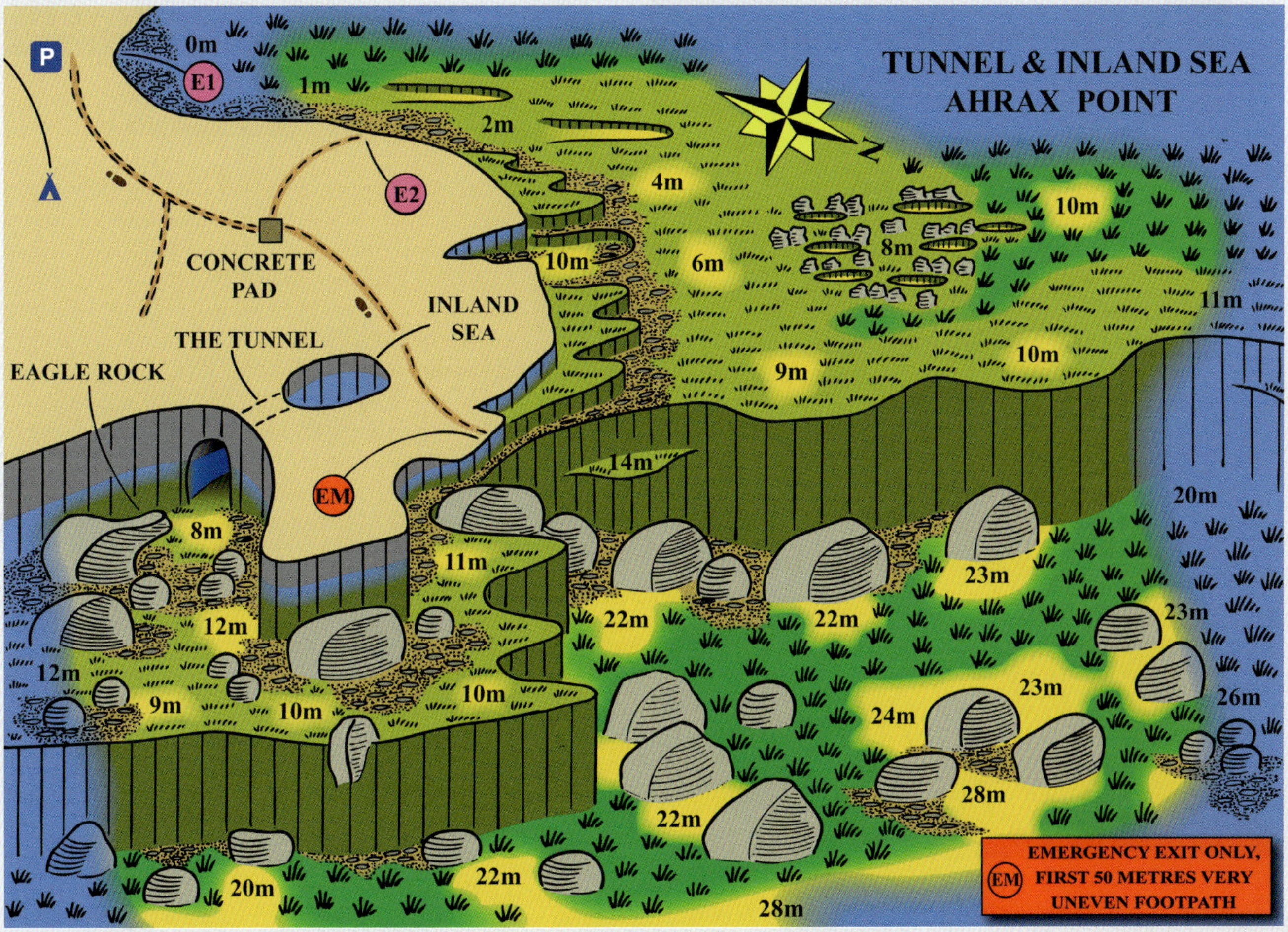

TUNNEL & INLAND SEA AHRAX POINT

- EAGLE ROCK
- CONCRETE PAD
- THE TUNNEL
- INLAND SEA
- E1
- E2
- EM

EMERGENCY EXIT ONLY, FIRST 50 METRES VERY UNEVEN FOOTPATH

Slugs Bay - Marfa Ridge East - Mellieha Bay

To reach Slugs Bay the directions are the same as for Ahrax Point, but after turning right at the top of the hill continue for just under 1 km. When you have passed the turning to Armier, continue round a slight bend and then on your right-hand side you will find an entrance to a track, which will lead you down to Slugs Bay. Normally a 4x4 will be required for the 400-metre drive, due to the condition of the track. **When walking on the jetty take care, for if it is wet it can be extremely slippery.**

The name of this dive site does not do justice to this peaceful pretty area on the north side of Mellieha Bay, with its jetty and secluded cove. Only disturbed by walkers during the spring months admiring the many colourful wild flowers. The dive area consists of rocks, sea grass sandy areas with a maximum depth of 12m. To the east of the dive site in an area of small shingle/sand, where fossilized shark's teeth have been found, remember that it is illegal to remove certain items from under the water.

This is not a popular dive site, due to the conditions of the track, especially after heavy rainfall, but if you have a 4x4 that's great. It is a site used mainly when sea conditions do not permit diving elsewhere on the island, the bay is protected from the north northwesterly seas.

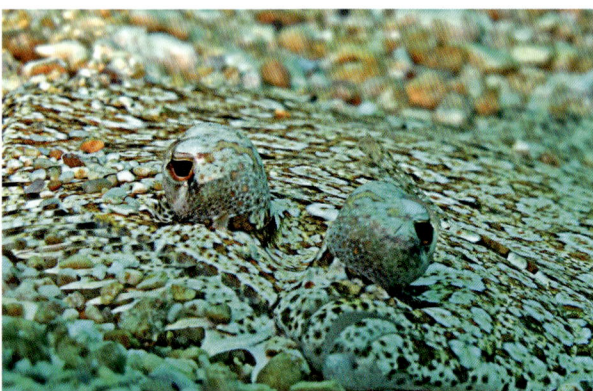

The eyes of a turbot (Psetta maxima) so very well camouflaged. PHOTO: JOE FORMOSA

Great dive site for your first dive or navigation.
PHOTO: SERGEY MARKOV - DIVE SYSTEMS

THE DIVE — Minimum time - 50 mins

This dive site is good for training new divers or to test your skills in navigation. The way I normally dive this area is to enter the water from the outer part of the jetty, entry point E1. Once on the bottom head out over the posidonia grass and sandy areas with a compass bearing of 140° for approximately 5 minutes, now turning left and a compass bearing of 50° for a further 8/10 minutes. Where you will find a small reef, then an area of shingle, this is where shark teeth have been found. Now follow the reef all the way round to your left until you have a compass bearing of 270°, this will take you towards the shore. Once you have explored this area and it is time to return, 180° will take you back over the little reef and to the sandy areas surrounded by posidonia grass, this should take 8/10 minutes. Then for the 3 minutes use a compass bearing of 230° then a bearing of 270° will take you towards the jetty or into the cove and your exit points E1 E2. Maybe you could plan your own dive here and discover how good you are with the compass.

There are no facilities here at all and the nearest services are some distance away at Mellieha.

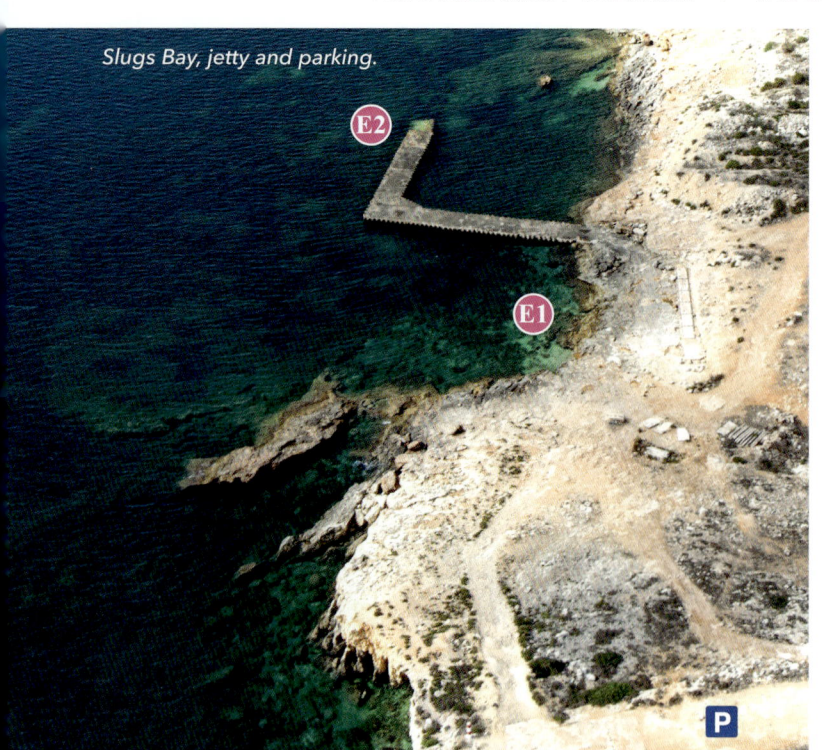

Slugs Bay, jetty and parking.

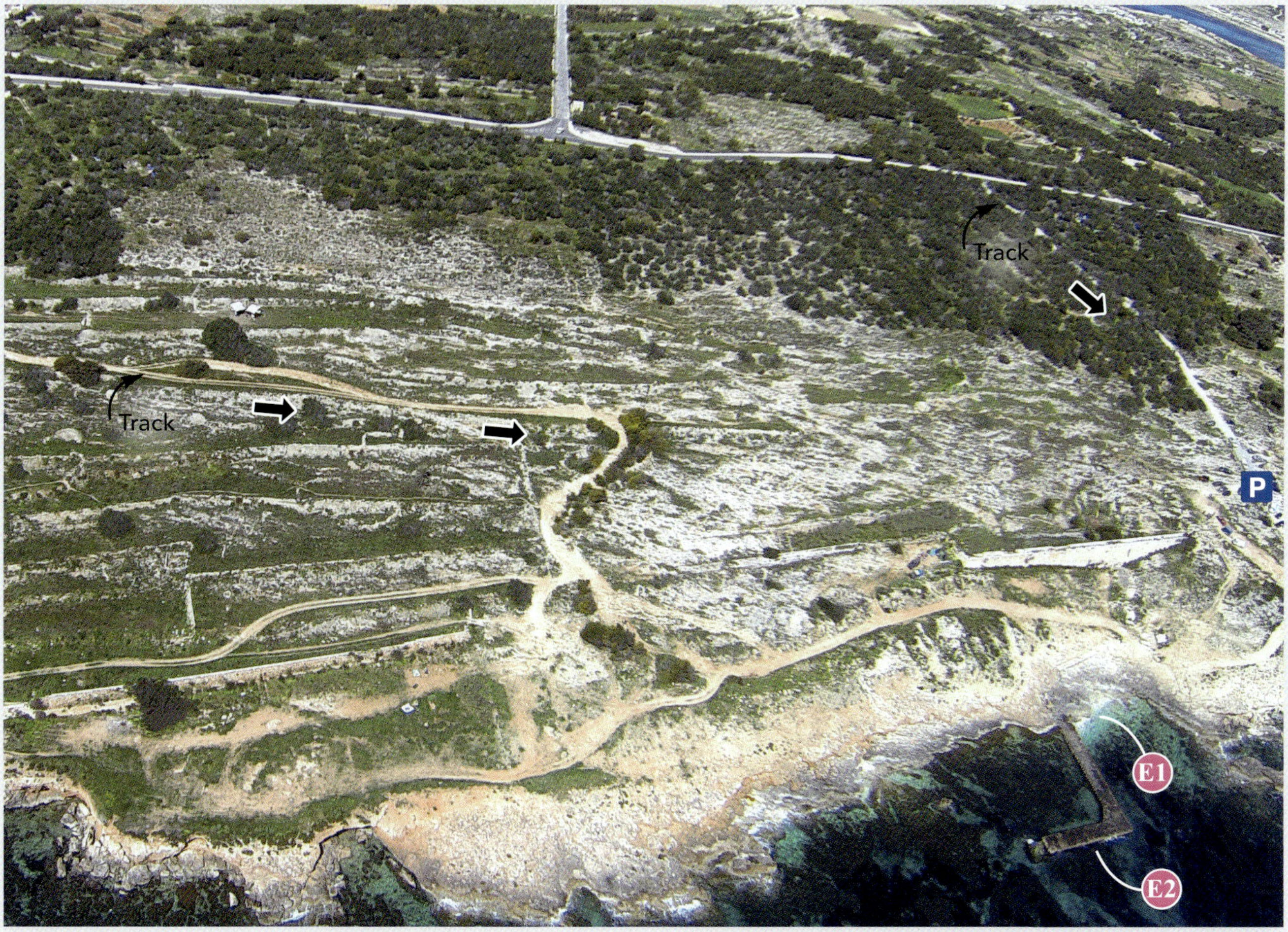

Track
Track
P
E1
E2

PHOTO: PGL AERIAL PHOTOS

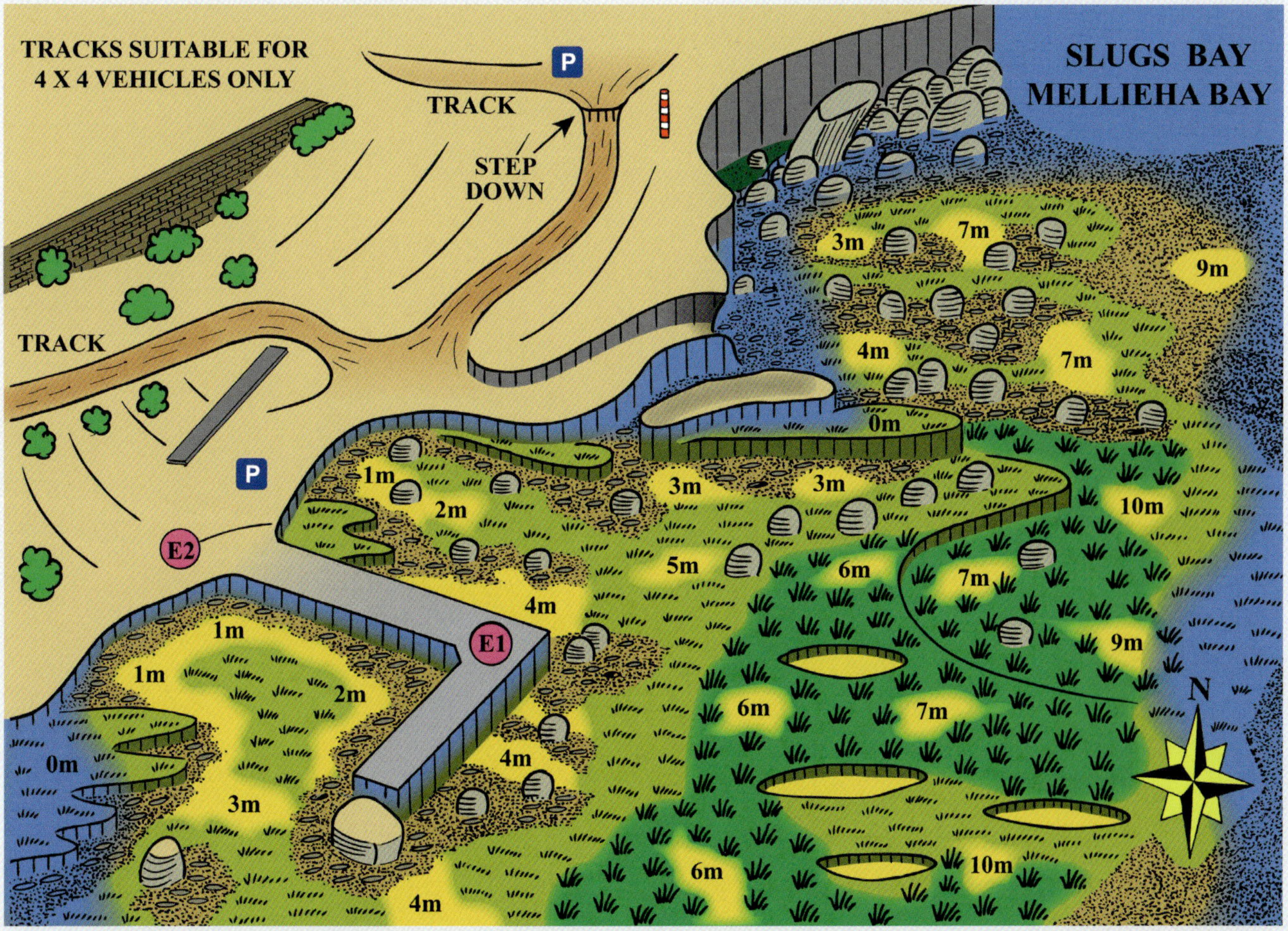
TRACKS SUITABLE FOR
4 X 4 VEHICLES ONLY
P
TRACK
STEP
DOWN
SLUGS BAY
MELLIEHA BAY
TRACK
P
E2
E1
3m
7m
9m
4m
7m
0m
1m
2m
3m
3m
10m
5m
6m
7m
4m
9m
1m
1m
2m
N
0m
6m
7m
4m
3m
6m
10m
4m

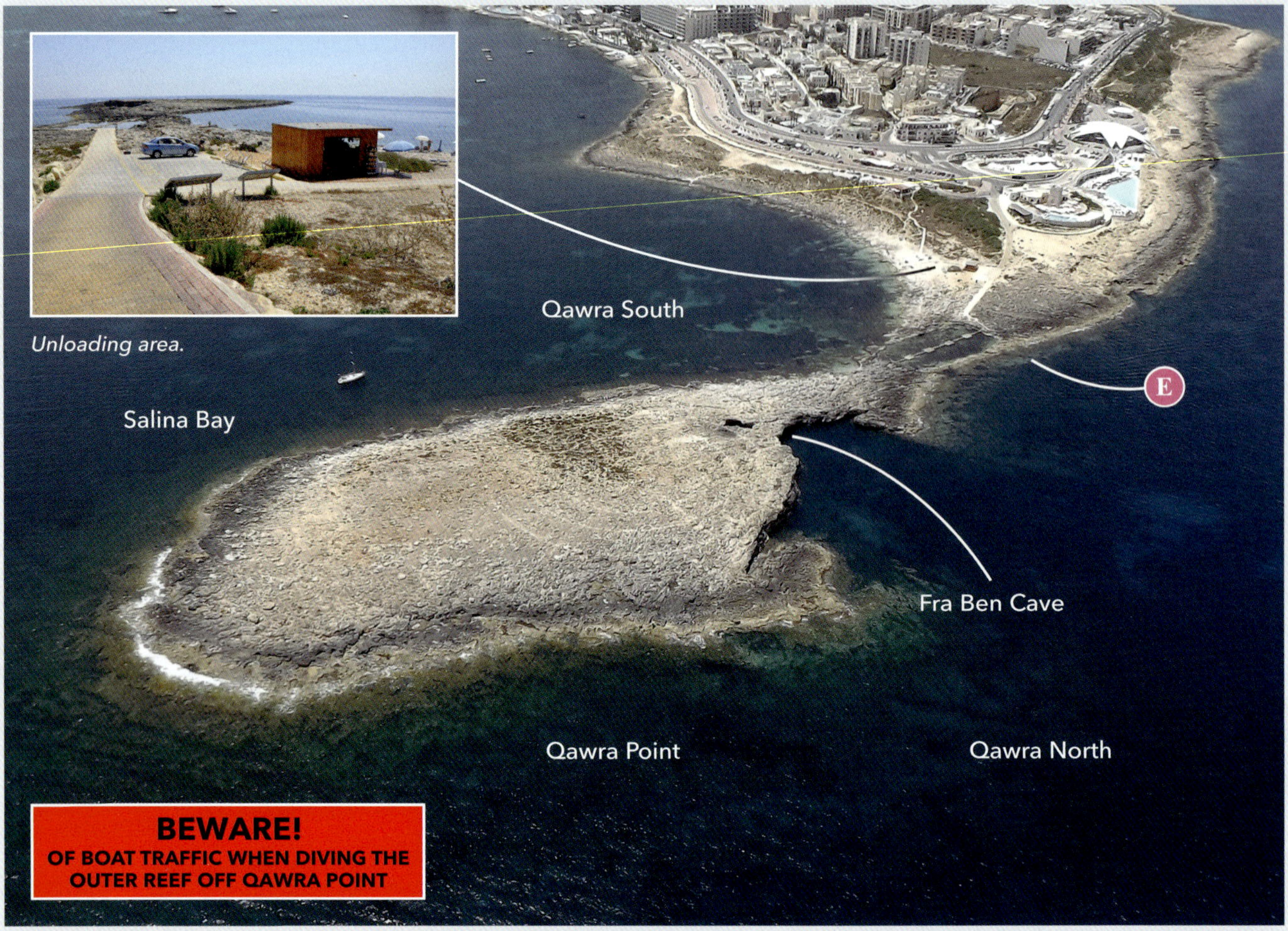

QAWRA POINT - QAWRA

Unloading area.

Salina Bay

Qawra South

Fra Ben Cave

Qawra Point

Qawra North

E

BEWARE!
OF BOAT TRAFFIC WHEN DIVING THE OUTER REEF OFF QAWRA POINT

PHOTO: PGL AERIAL PHOTOS

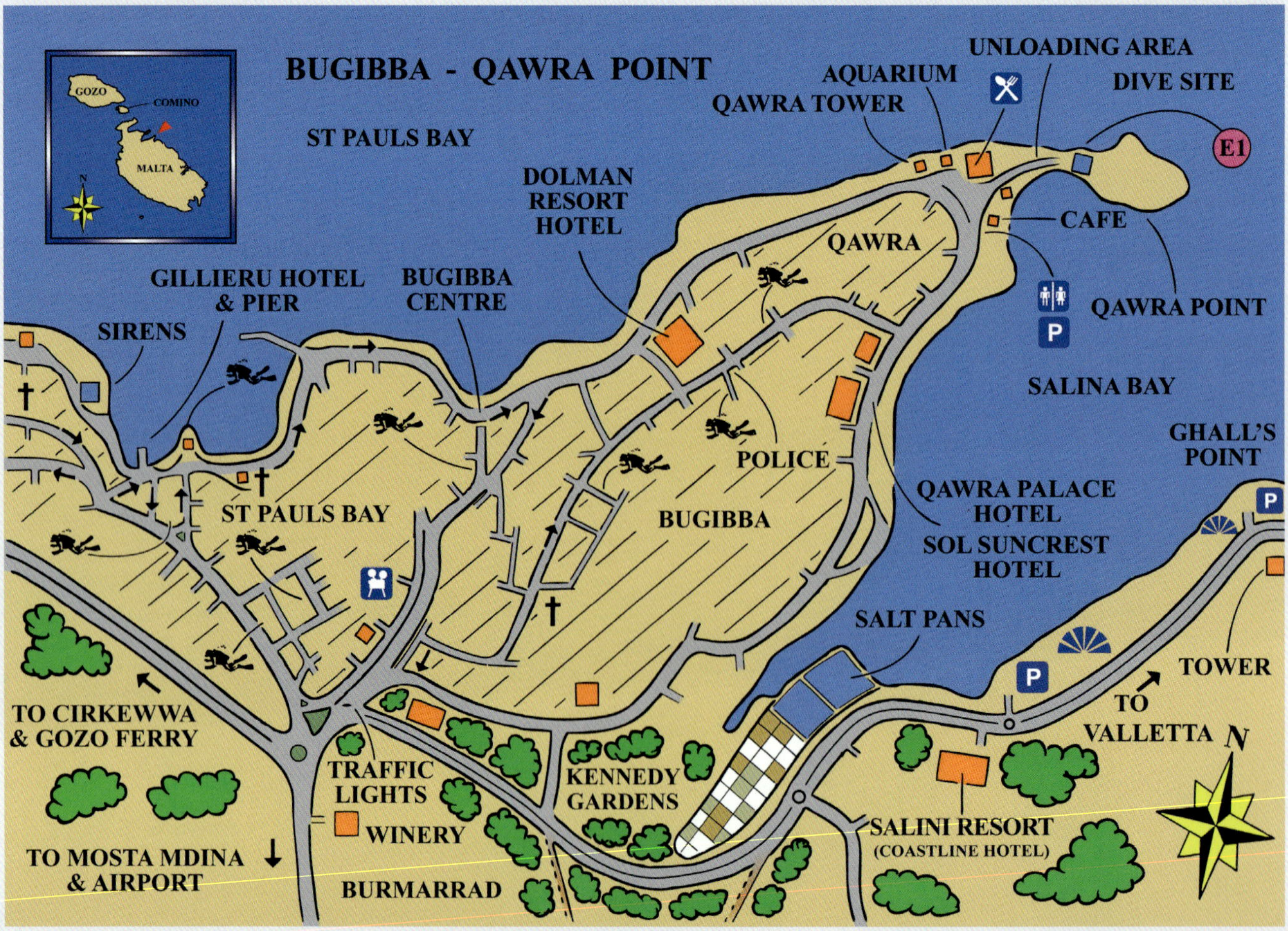

BUGIBBA - QAWRA POINT

GOZO, COMINO, MALTA

ST PAULS BAY

DOLMAN RESORT HOTEL

AQUARIUM
QAWRA TOWER

UNLOADING AREA
DIVE SITE

E1

CAFE

QAWRA

QAWRA POINT

GILLIERU HOTEL & PIER

BUGIBBA CENTRE

SIRENS

SALINA BAY

ST PAULS BAY

POLICE

BUGIBBA

GHALL'S POINT

QAWRA PALACE HOTEL
SOL SUNCREST HOTEL

SALT PANS

TOWER

TO CIRKEWWA & GOZO FERRY

TRAFFIC LIGHTS
WINERY

KENNEDY GARDENS

TO VALLETTA

TO MOSTA MDINA & AIRPORT

BURMARRAD

SALINI RESORT (COASTLINE HOTEL)

N

Qawra Point Reefs & Cave - Qawra

This dive site is situated very close to the busy resort of Bugibba / St Pauls Bay on a peninsular of land on the north coast called Qawra Point. To find this site you need to follow the eastern coastal road through Bugibba to Qawra, passing the large hotels on the sea front until you reach a long sweeping bend. Turn right and look for the single-track road that leads down to your unloading area. If you do not have a pass or there are no parking spaces, unload and park at the top. The north side of Qawra Point is the area for diving, the south side is normally use for novice training and try dives.

There are a number of ways you could dive this site; I have selected three. Just off the north shore opposite the pool and your entry point, is a large area with average depths of 2/8m, this large inshore area is an excellent place to finish your dive, a second dive, or visit the cave, here you will often find thousands of glass fish. Once through the cave you will find yourself in a small inland sea, in which you can surface and snorkel around a central rock.

The last two dives suggested are deeper, 30m plus, and are suitable for experienced divers only. Sometimes due to northerly winds it is not possible to dive this site as the entry/exit point is surrounded by jagged rocks and therefore requires calm sea conditions.

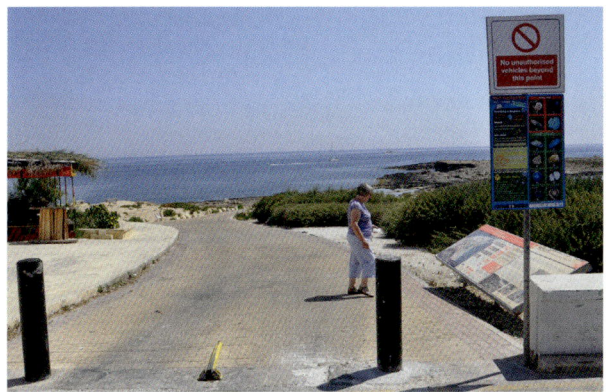

The entrance for the road leading to the unloading area.

THE DIVE — Minimum time - 40 mins

Dive 1 which is suitable for all grades of divers. Once you have entered the water head in an easterly direction, this will take you over an area covered by short marine growth, posidonia grass and many small gullies, with an average of depth of 6m to the first point on the headland. Once you have rounded the corner head into the small bay keeping the reef on your right-hand side, this will lead you to the cave and small inland sea, be careful not to miss the entrance.

When leaving this area, and you have enough air, turn right and head in a northerly direction, just before the end of the bay you will find an area with rough rocks and boulders, they are covered in coral and marine life and if you have camera a good opportunity for macro photography. Remember you are now 15 to 20 minutes away from your entry point. When it is time to head back follow the reef in a south westerly direction not exceeding a depth of 8 to 9m. When you wish to reach the shore line and your exit point take a southerly compass bearing.

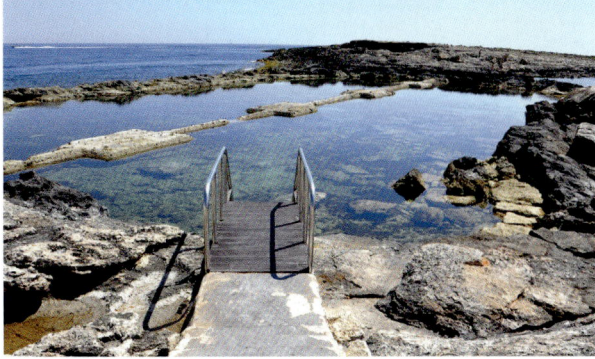

Once used for target practise by British planes, The Pool.

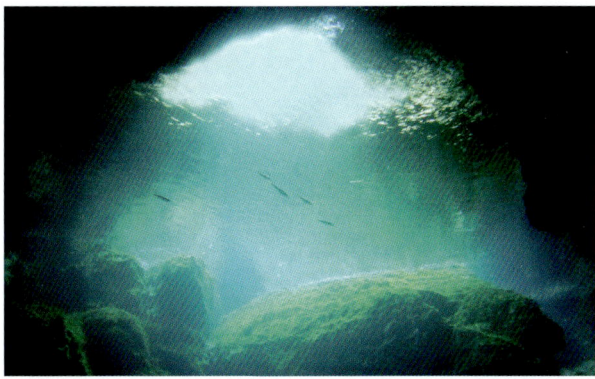

Fra Ben Cave with its blow hole.

BELOW: A diver in the entrance to the cave.
PHOTO: ARKADIUSZ SREBNIK POLANDDIVING PHOTO

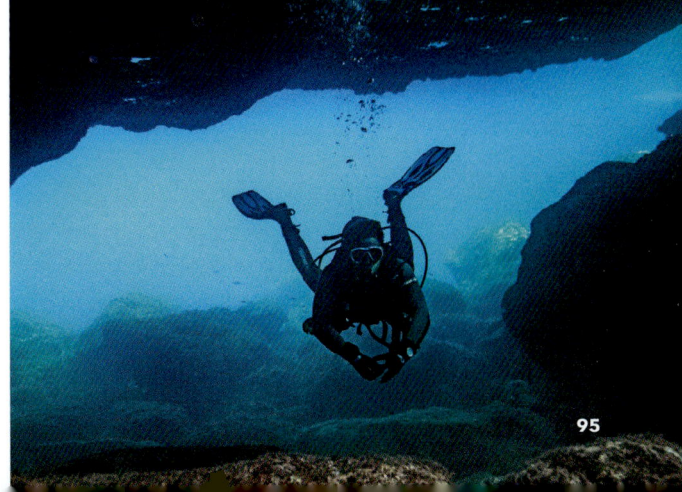

THE DIVE — Minimum time - 50 mins

Dive 2 will take you to 30m plus. From the entry point surface swim out for 8 to 10 minutes on a compass bearing of 330° you can of course go under water but you will pass over mostly sea grass and use valuable dive time. Now descend to the sea bed if your depth is 28m or less continue down and over the reef to the bottom, if your depth is 32m or more head south back to the base of the reef.

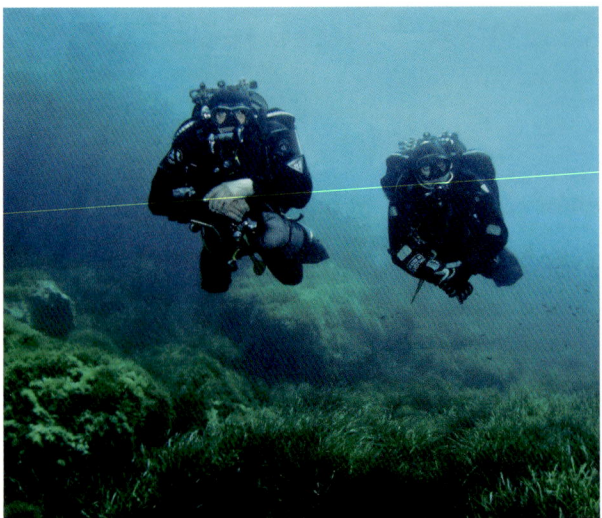

The area outside of Fra Ben Cave depths 6-11m.

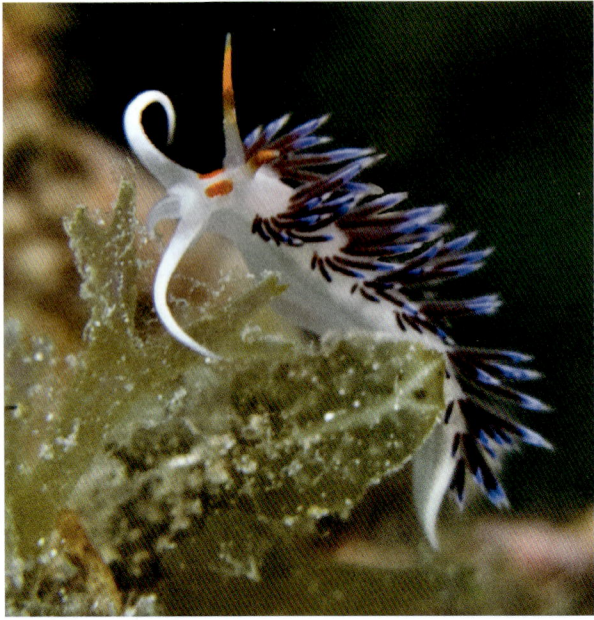

Blue and white nudibranch. PHOTO: SHARON FORDER

Below: The small arch at 15m can you find it?
PHOTO: ARKADIUSZ SREBNIK POLANDDIVING PHOTO

Follow the line where the reef meets the sand in an easterly direction, your depth will gradually increase to 36m, this should take you approximately 10 minutes. Here you will see a number small jagged rocks dotted around in the sand.

This is possibly a good time to head south up over the reef to shallower depths, here the seabed is covered in sea grass with small areas of sand. Now look for the larger areas of sand at a depth of 19m and the small arch (see plan) Continue on, turning east when you reach the reef, depth 15m, this will take you on to another area of sand, cross the sand to the other side still keeping the reef on your right. In a small corner of the reef there is a plaque in memory of four Maltese divers who lost their lives in a tragic accident. Continue up over the drop off where you will find a small ledge, keeping this on your right, it will lead you towards the cave. Take your time to explore both the cave and the small inland sea. When it is time to return, head out of the cave, keep the reef on your left, at its end head south west parallel with the shore line and towards your exit point, maybe if you have left some marker stones it will be easier for you to find.

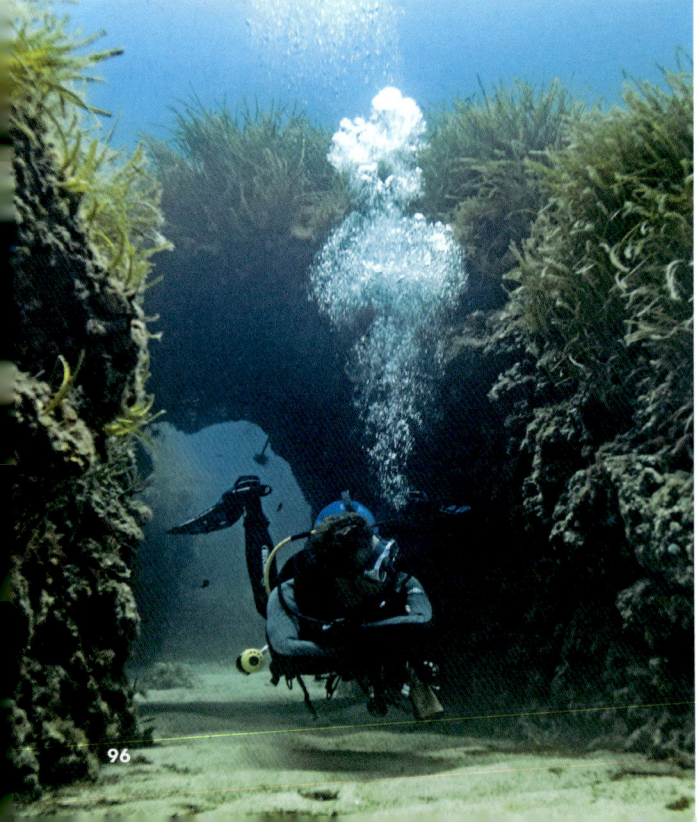

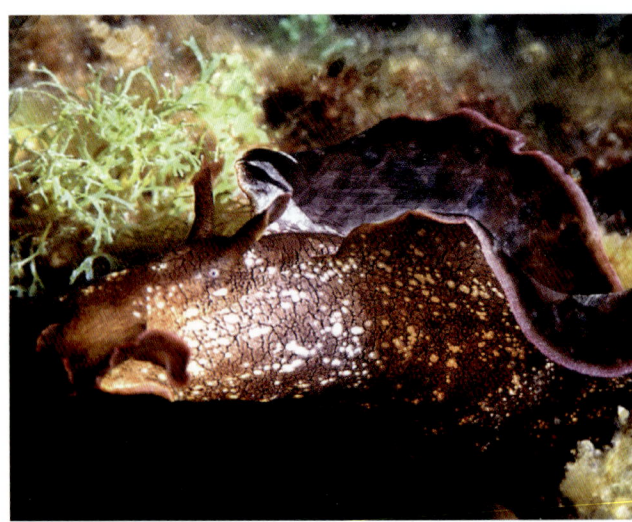

This cute sea hare found on rocky algae rich sea beds.

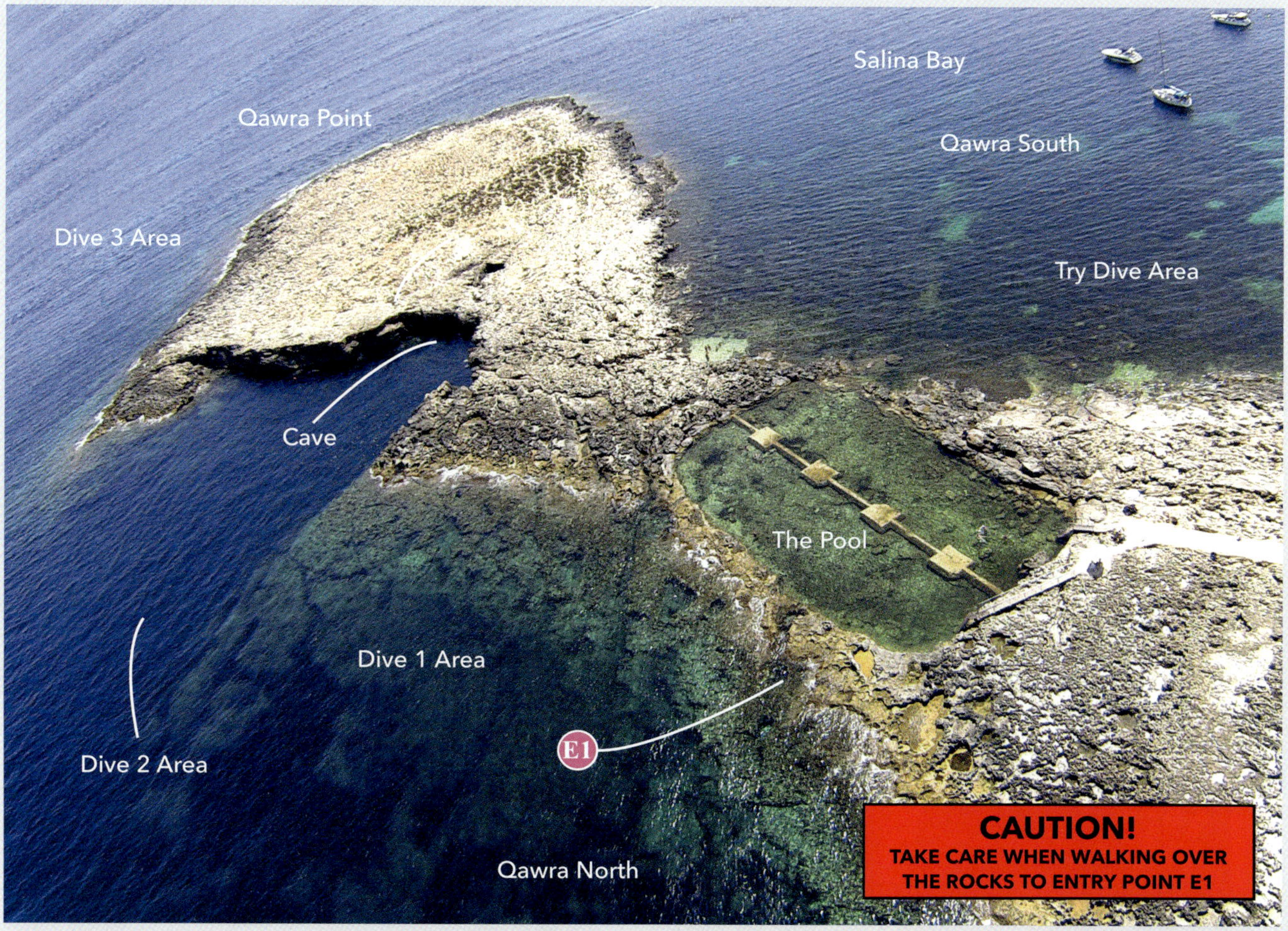

QAWRA POINT - REEFS & CAVE - QAWRA

Aerial photo labels:
- Dive 3 Area
- Qawra Point
- Salina Bay
- Qawra South
- Try Dive Area
- Cave
- The Pool
- Dive 1 Area
- Dive 2 Area
- E1
- Qawra North

CAUTION! TAKE CARE WHEN WALKING OVER THE ROCKS TO ENTRY POINT E1

PHOTO: PGL AERIAL PHOTOS

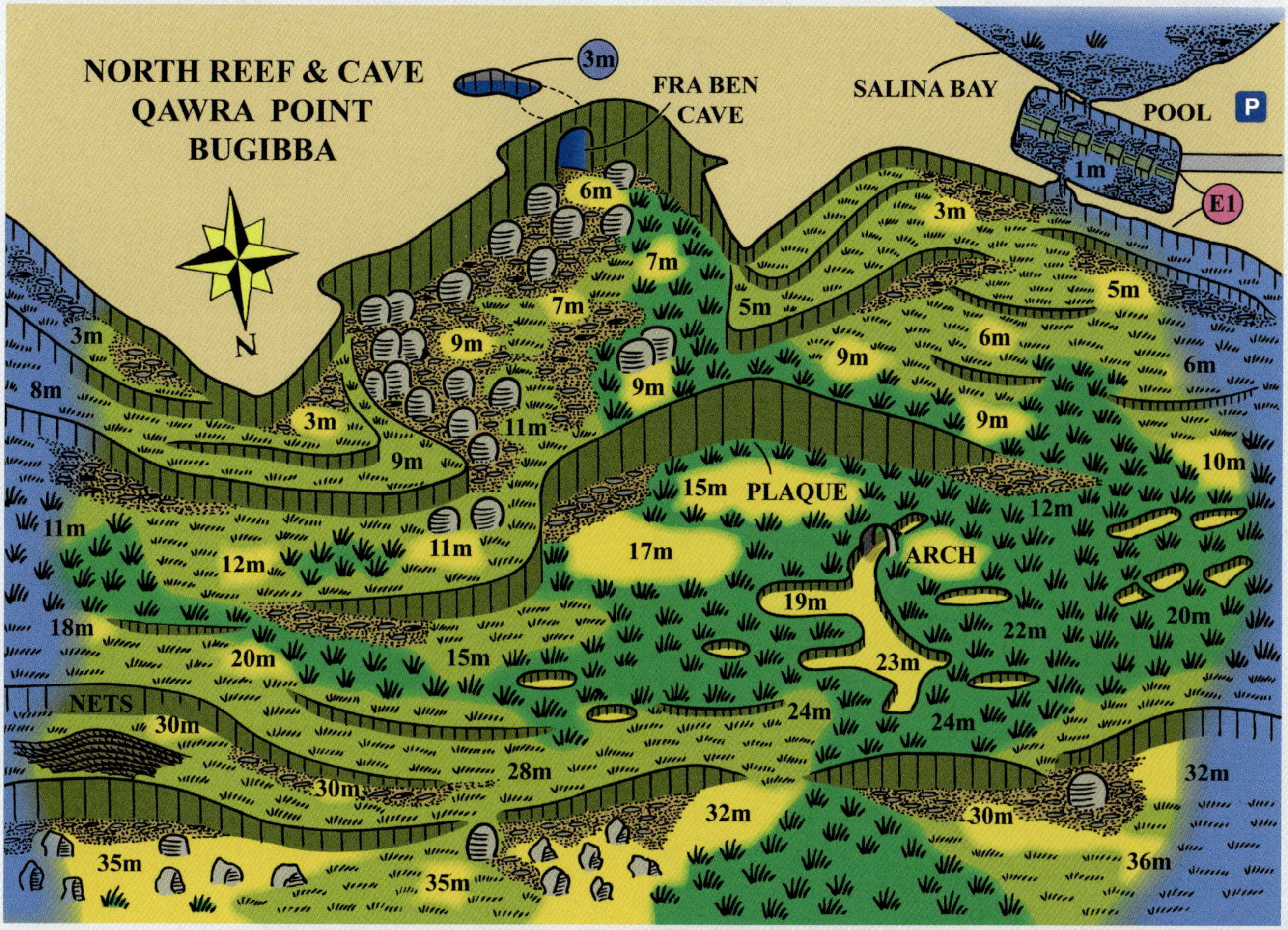

NORTH REEF & CAVE QAWRA POINT BUGIBBA

Map labels:
- FRA BEN CAVE
- SALINA BAY
- POOL
- P
- E1
- N
- 3m, 6m, 7m, 7m, 9m, 9m, 11m, 3m, 9m, 11m, 3m, 8m, 11m, 12m, 18m, 20m, 15m, 11m, 1m, 3m, 5m, 6m, 9m, 5m, 6m, 9m, 10m, 12m, 15m PLAQUE, 17m, 19m, ARCH, 22m, 20m, 23m, 24m, 24m, 32m, NETS, 30m, 30m, 28m, 32m, 30m, 36m, 35m, 35m

THE DIVE
Minimum time - 60 mins

Dive 3 This is a long dive with a depth of 36m, from your entry, surface swim in an easterly direction to the furthest point of headland. Continue out until the shallow reef below you almost disappears, this will take 10/15 minutes. Descend, once on the seabed, continue down and over the reef to 30m where you will find a large old heavy fishing net, here the reef drops to sand at 35m plus. If your surface swim was too far and you are unable to see the reef on your descent, head in a southerly direction, back to the reef.

Now follow the main reef in an easterly direction, within a few minutes the reef will bear round to the right and head in a southerly direction, continue with the reef on your right. This area of sand between two reefs approx. 30 meters wide comes to a dead end.

At the end ascend the reef up to the posidonia grass, where your depth will be 22m from this point it will take you some 10 to 15 minutes to reach a depth of 9m and further 25 minutes to your exit point. Now continue on a south south-westerly direction over the sea grass slowly ascending, once you have reached a depth of 9m or less head in a westerly direction. When you have passed the area where the cave is and rounded the point at 5m take a south-westerly bearing towards your exit point.

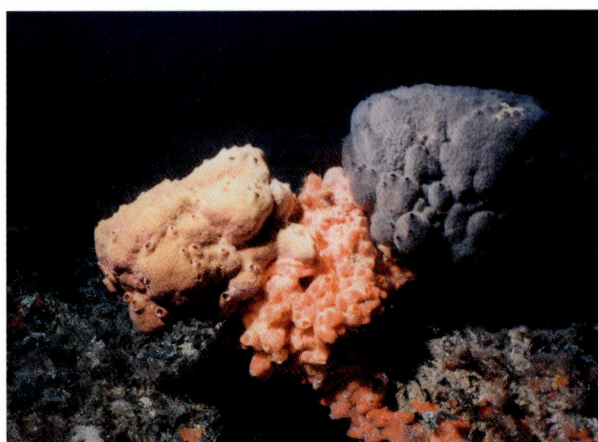
Bath sponges (Spongia officinalis) also found here.

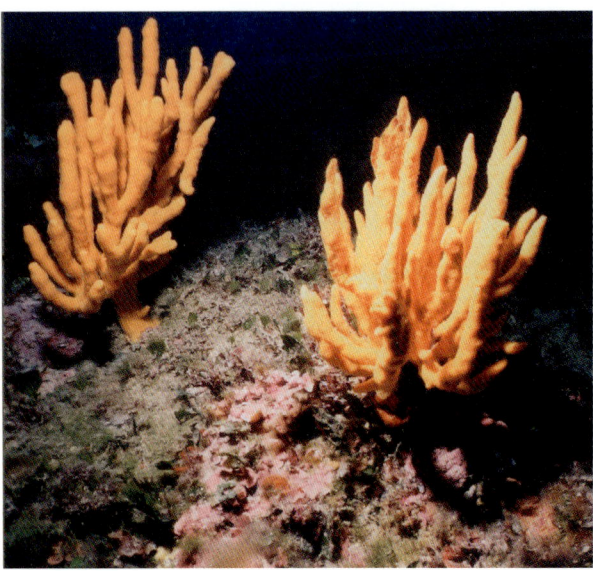
Tree sponges (Asinella polypoides) found here.

Below: One of the many caves found off Qawra Point.
PHOTO: ARKADIUSZ SREBNIK POLANDDIVING PHOTO

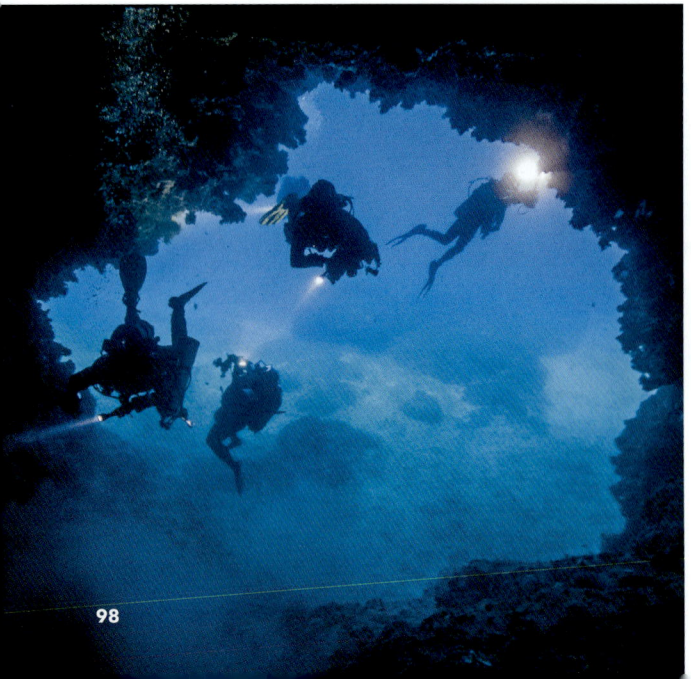

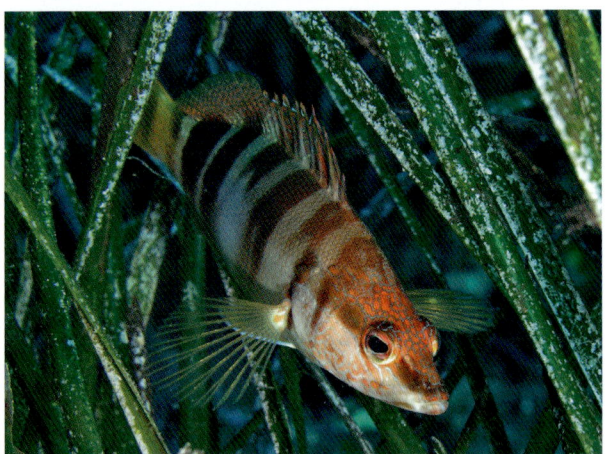
Painted comber (Serranus scriba) hiding in the sea grass.
PHOTO: SHARON FORDER

St. Pauls Shipwreck

St Paul's islands can clearly be seen from Qawra point and the history of the shipwreck is as follows; According to the Acts of Apostles, St Paul and St Luke were on their way to Rome to be tried as political rebels when their ship foundered on the rocks of Malta. The actual site of the shipwreck is generally thought to have been one of the islets to the north of St Paul's Bay. It was here at Qawra Point where the MV *Hephaestus* ran aground on the 10th February 2018 this is the day, each year the Maltese people celebrate the coming of St Paul. In 2022 the MV *Hephaestus* was scuttled off Xatt L-Ahmar Gozo, as an artificial reef.

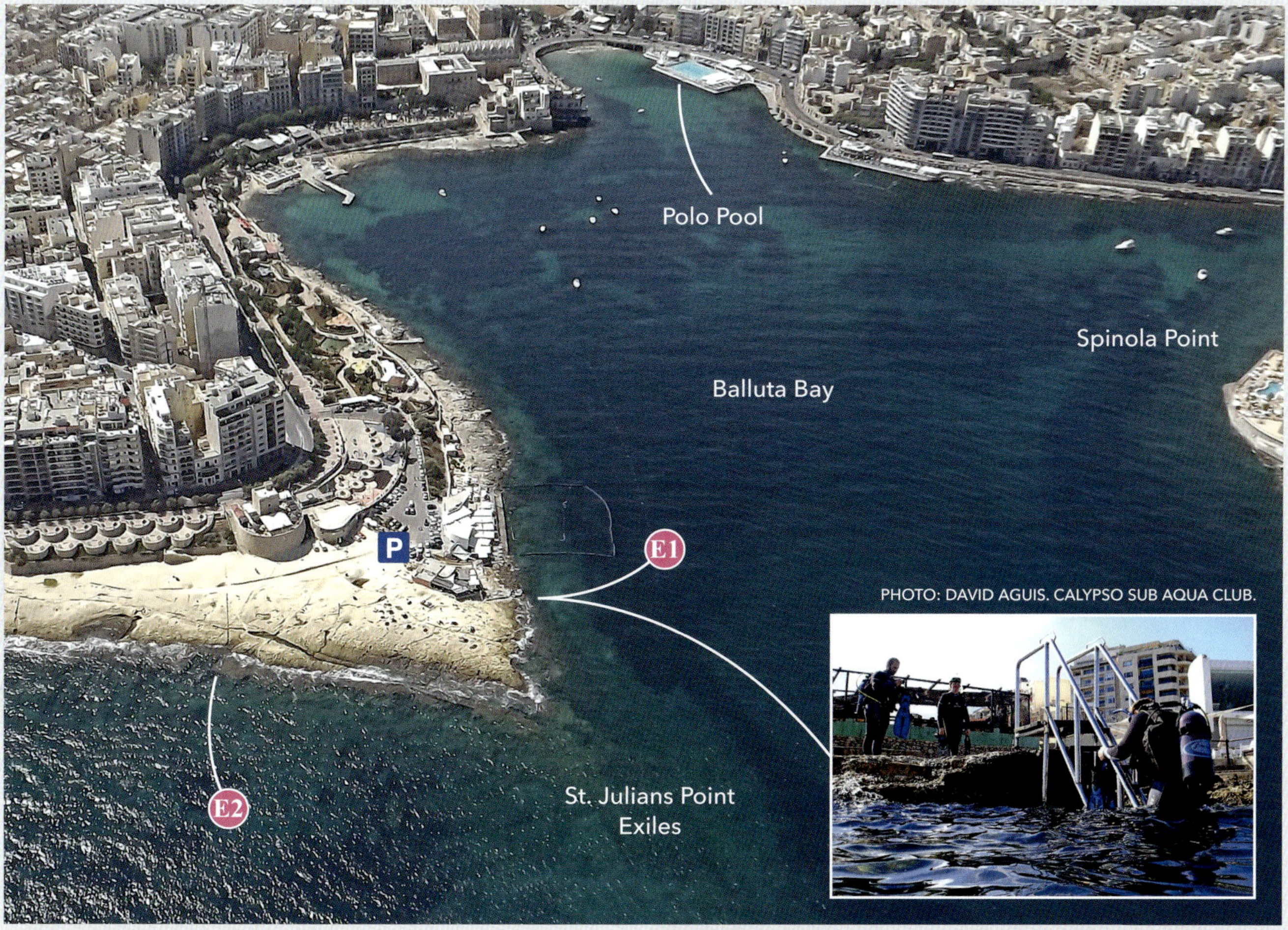

SLIEMA - ST. JULIANS - PACEVILLE

Polo Pool
Spinola Point
Balluta Bay
St. Julians Point
Exiles

PHOTO: DAVID AGUIS. CALYPSO SUB AQUA CLUB.
PHOTO: PGL AERIAL PHOTOS

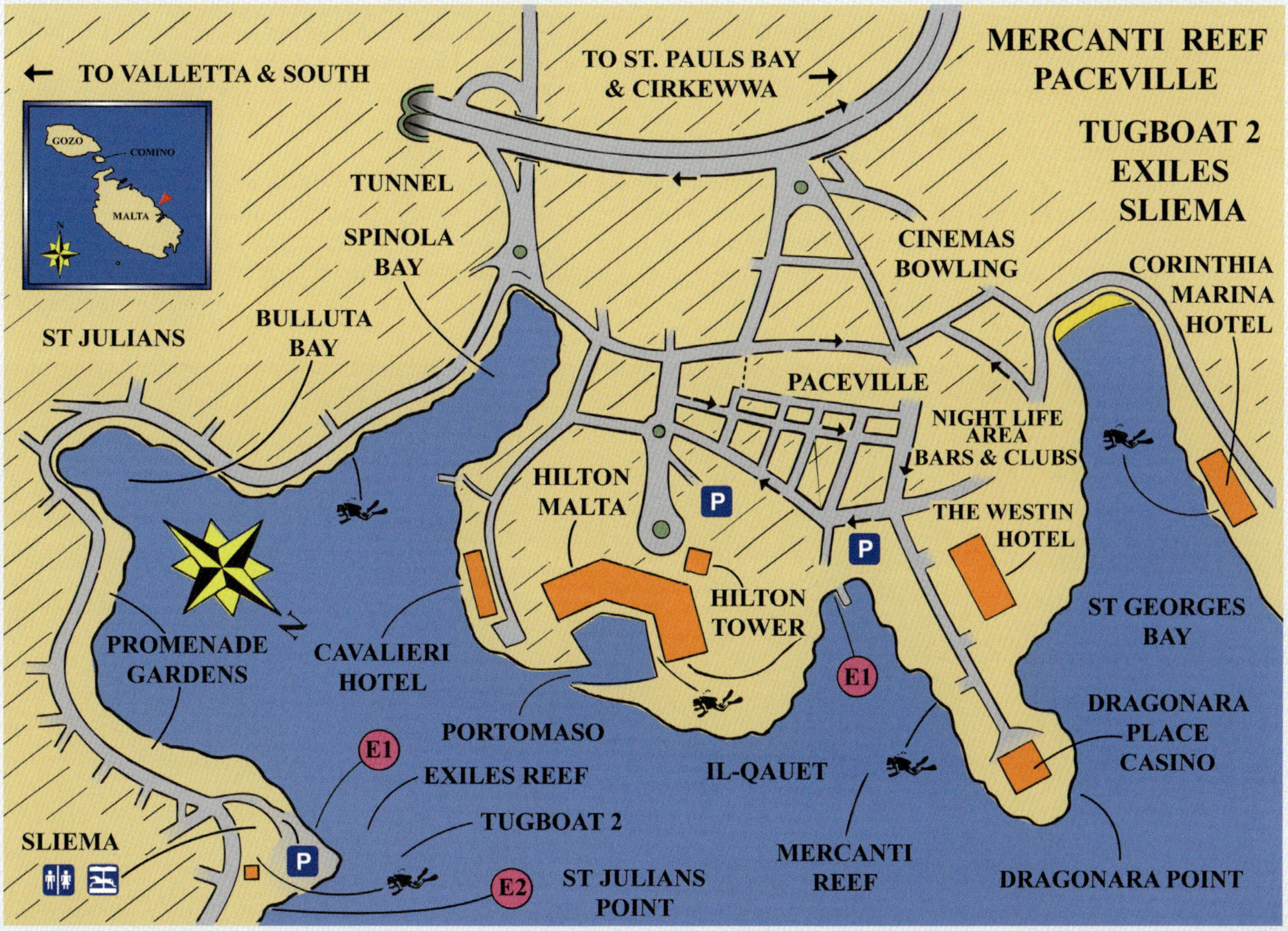

MERCANTI REEF
PACEVILLE
TUGBOAT 2
EXILES
SLIEMA

TO VALLETTA & SOUTH
TO ST. PAULS BAY & CIRKEWWA
TUNNEL
SPINOLA BAY
CINEMAS BOWLING
CORINTHIA MARINA HOTEL
ST JULIANS
BULLUTA BAY
PACEVILLE
NIGHT LIFE AREA BARS & CLUBS
HILTON MALTA
THE WESTIN HOTEL
ST GEORGES BAY
PROMENADE GARDENS
CAVALIERI HOTEL
HILTON TOWER
DRAGONARA PLACE CASINO
PORTOMASO
EXILES REEF
IL-QAUET
TUGBOAT 2
MERCANTI REEF
DRAGONARA POINT
SLIEMA
ST JULIANS POINT

Mercanti Reef - Paceville

This unique dive site with its entry point almost in the heart of Malta's main night life area, is situated on the south side of Dragonara Point, where the Dragonara Palace Casino is situated. (Il-Qaliet). To find this site, head towards the Hilton Tower the parking and entry point are situated on the north side of this building. Most of the streets within this area are one way so follow the local map. There is a large car park near your entry point, unless you are prepared to come early may I suggest late afternoon or weekends would be a good idea, as parking here during the week is very difficult.

THE DIVE — Minimum time - 60 mins

From your entry point E1or E2 you have just over a 250-metre surface swim, less if you are able to use the beach front on Dragonara Point (hotel property) as this is slightly closer to the reef.

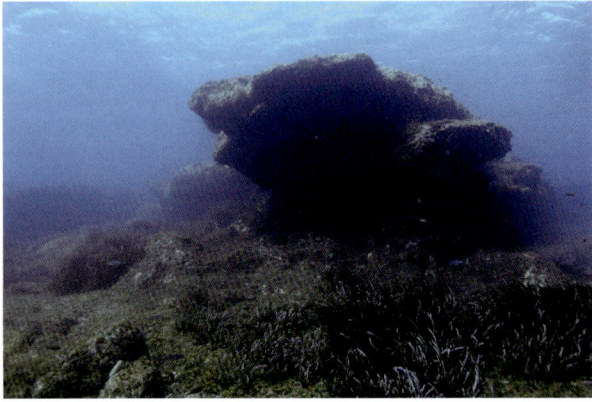

Mercanti Reef south. PHOTO: DIVEWISE DIVE CENTRE

When you reach the reef, descend, below the marker post is a small shallow valley of stones which run out in the direction of your route back to your exit point.
Now head north until you reach a large area of flat rock with gullies running out in a westerly direction, after exploring this area, head back past the marker post. Now follow the reef in a southerly direction keeping it on your left-hand side for some 6 minutes, in front of you will be a large rock, it looks a bit like a blackberry, **you now have two choices.**

Choice 1 you can continue all the way along the reef round the end and continue up the other side, you are now heading north. Along the back of the reef the sea bed is much flatter. Now you should keep close to the reef due to any boat traffic.
When you are 20 minutes into your dive turn and retrace your steps to the small stony valley, below the marker post, maximum depth so far is 10m. From here to your exit will take you some 20 minutes with on a compass bearing of 250°. This dive will test your navigational skills.

Choice 2 go on the inside between the reef and Blackberry rock, now take a bearing of 200/210° to the southern end of the inshore reef exploring the rugged east side before returning to the end, then head in a northerly direction so that the inner reef is on your left and when the visibility is good you will see the main reef on your right. Follow this to the end of the valley here, if you have taken the time to explore, you could be 40 minutes into your dive, **for your return route see Choice 1.**

There are far too many small overhangs fissures and places to explore to be indicated on this small map, this is an excellent dive and should not be rushed. The marine life here is plentiful, so take your camera.

Left: This large moray (Muraen Helena) has a home here. PHOTO: VERONICA BUSUTTIL

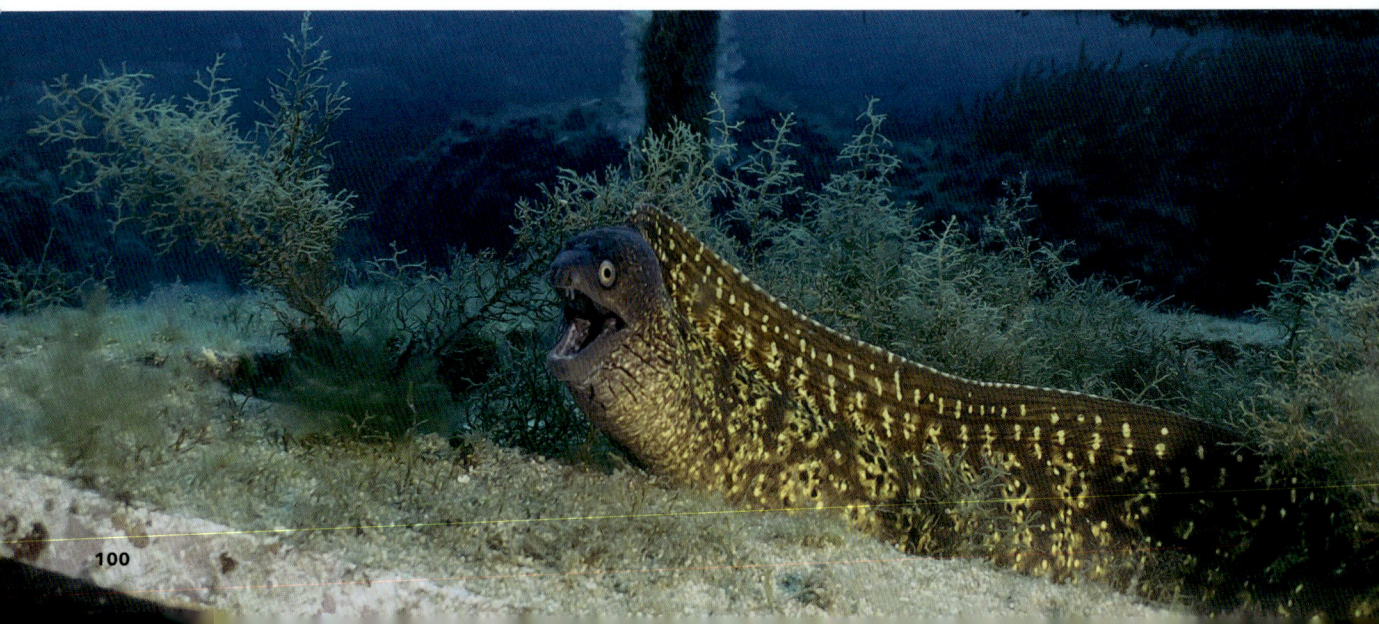

Dragonara Point
St. George's Bay
Il-Qaliet
P
E1
E2
Reef Marker
Mercanti Reef

Conger. PHOTO: Joe Formosa

Male rainbow wrasse.

PHOTO: PGL AERIAL PHOTOS

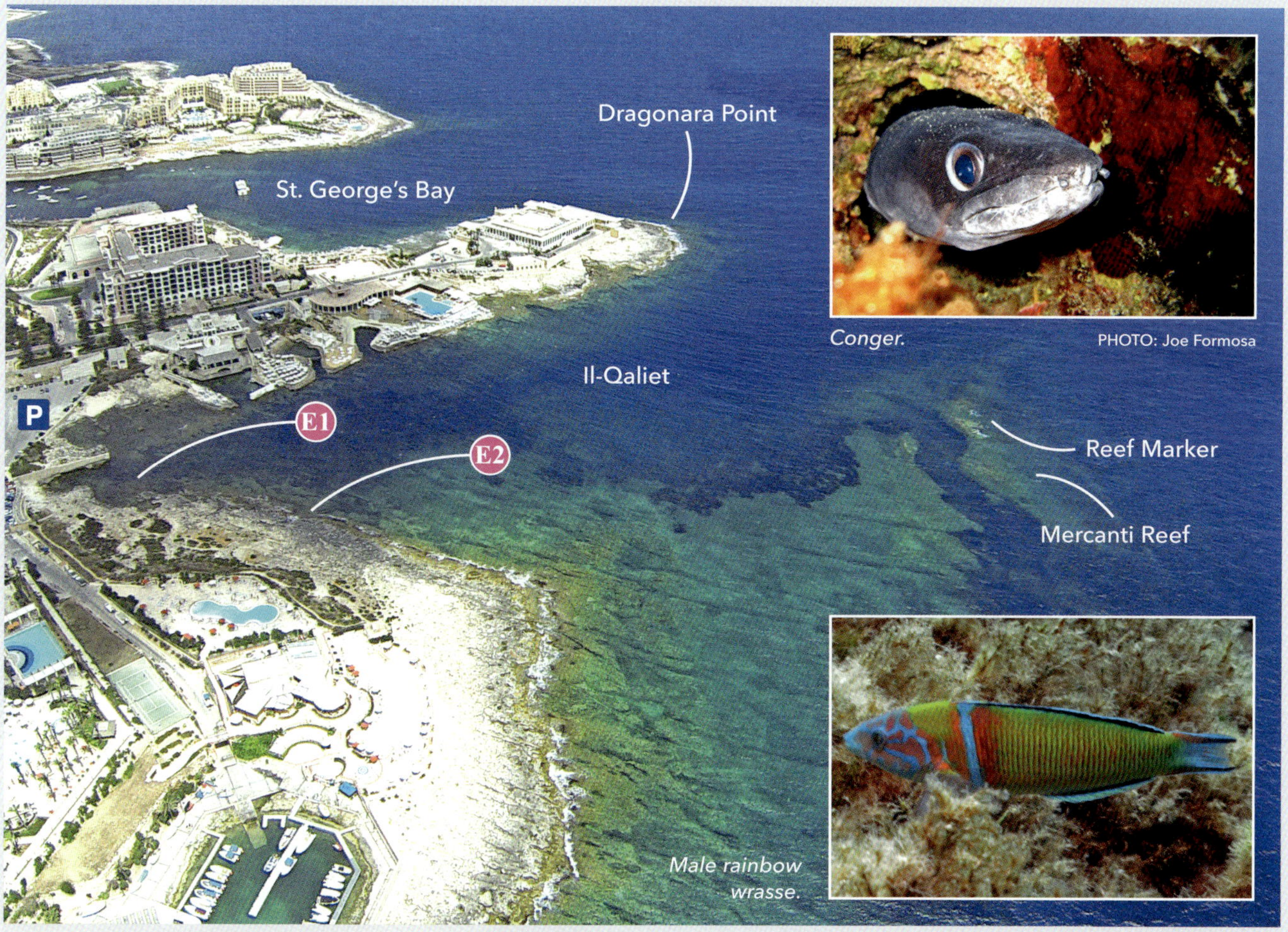

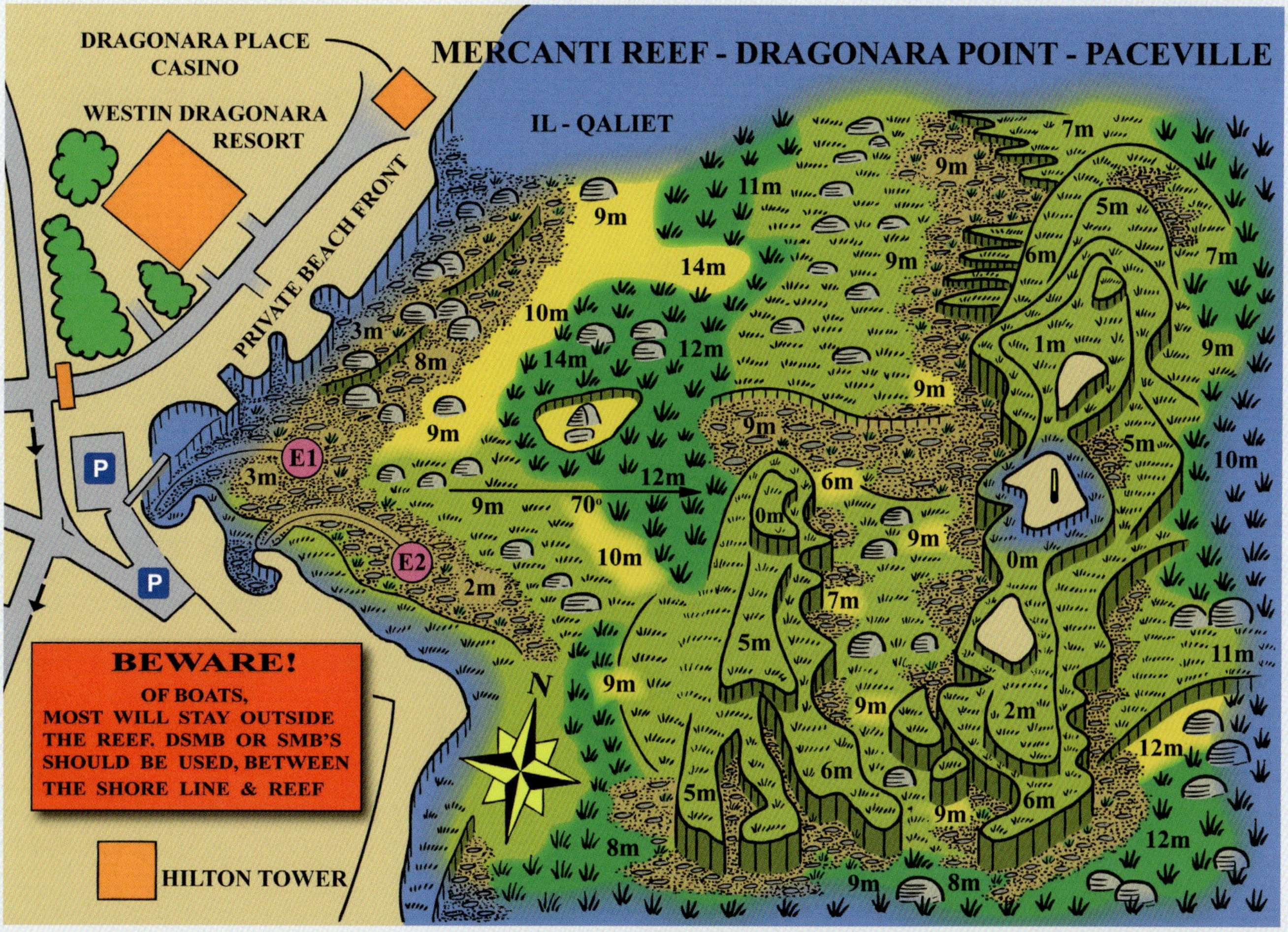
MERCANTI REEF - DRAGONARA POINT - PACEVILLE
DRAGONARA PLACE CASINO
WESTIN DRAGONARA RESORT
PRIVATE BEACH FRONT
IL - QALIET
P
P
E1
E2
N
70°
3m
8m
9m
10m
14m
12m
11m
14m
9m
3m
2m
9m
12m
10m
7m
9m
6m
0m
5m
7m
9m
6m
5m
8m
9m
8m
9m
1m
5m
0m
2m
6m
9m
12m
11m
10m
9m
7m
5m
7m
BEWARE!
OF BOATS,
MOST WILL STAY OUTSIDE
THE REEF. DSMB OR SMB'S
SHOULD BE USED, BETWEEN
THE SHORE LINE & REEF
HILTON TOWER

Tugboat 2 - Exiles - St. Julians Point - Sliema

This dive site is off the coastal road in Sliema close to St. Julians tower. From St. Julians pass the water polo pool and in about 600 metres, before a right-hand bend, turn left down a narrow road to a car park. From Sliema centre follow the coast road past Fortizza, now look out for the St Julians Tower on your right, just before a left-hand bend with a central barrier, immediately after this, turn right down the narrow road to your dive site. **Parking here can be a problem especially on week days, you may have to wait for a space.**

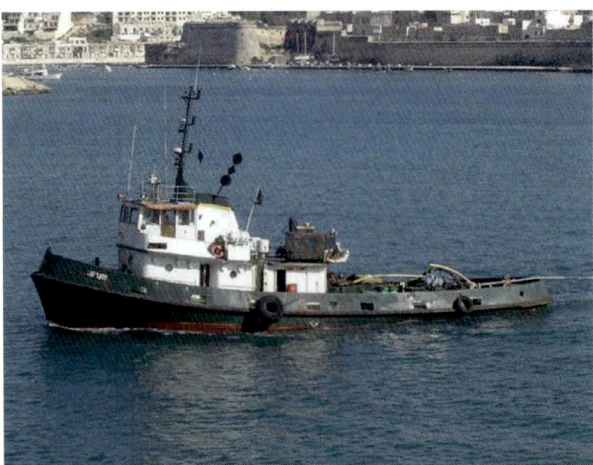

Tugboat 2 working in Grand Harbour.

This dive site is for divers of all experience, with its gently sloping reef, gullies and overhangs to explore. Edged by areas of sand, where there is an abundance of marine life. At the end of the reef is the wreck of Tugboat 2 at 22m, a great area for training in navigational skills, or you quite simply want a change.

Below: The edge of the reef with its groupers.
PHOTO: LELI SCERRI CALYPSO BS-AC

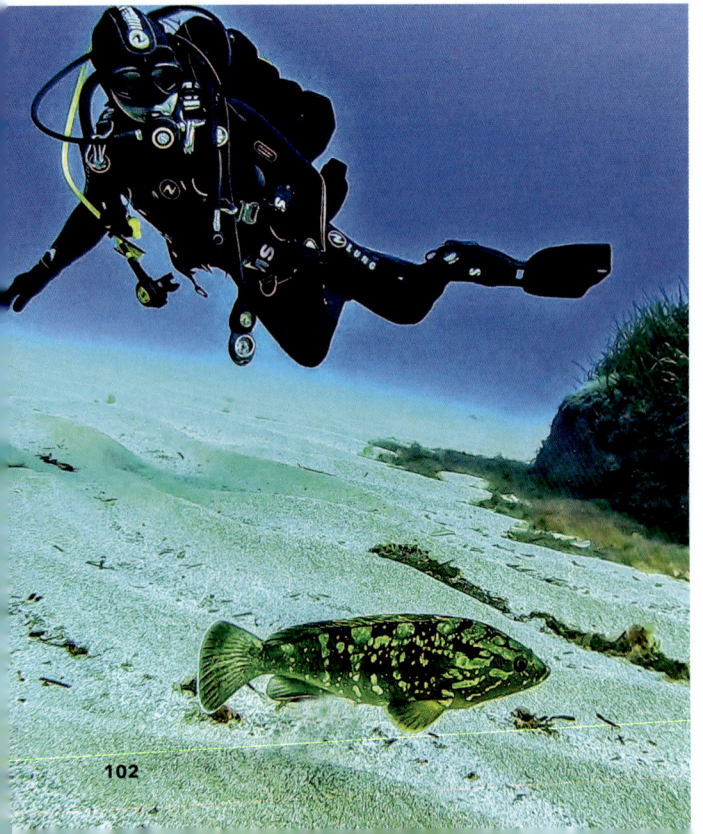

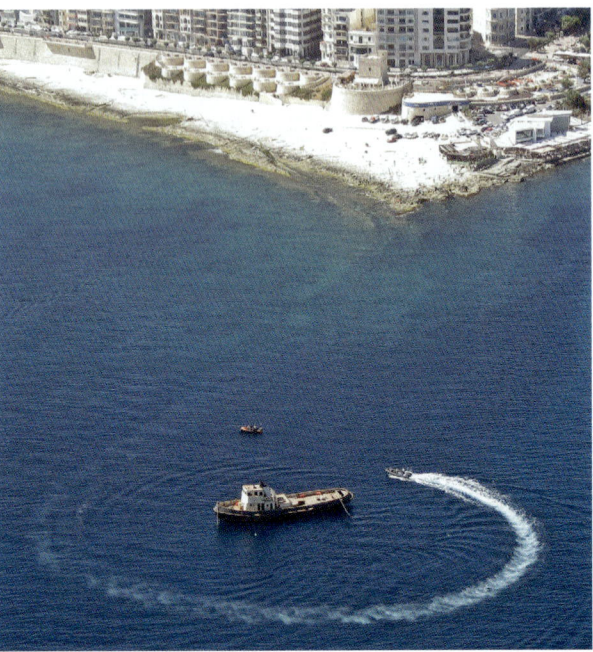

The sinking. PHOTO: LUCA PAPARELLA ITALIAN AIR FORCE

Tugboat 2 - Tuo Lun Er Hao

Tugboat Number 2 was built in Malta in 1975 for the Chinese Government, named, *Tuo Lun Er Hao* and registered in Tientsin China. With her sister *Tugboat Tuo Lun Yi Hao* worked together on the China Dock 6 project in French Creek, Grand Harbour. In 2000 she was purchased by Bezzina Marine Services Ltd, working in their shipyards, until being laid up. Her sister ship, now named 'Anni' is still working and was present at the scuttling. Tugboat 2 has a gross weight of 141 tons, a length of 30 metres, a beam 7.5 metres and a height of 9.5 metres. The Professional Diving Schools Association with the Maltese Tourism Authority requested planning permission to scuttle the ship. Once planning permission had been granted, she was made environmentally friendly and was scuttled as a diver attraction on the 20th June 2013.

She just adds to the excellent variety of diving in the Maltese Islands. This wreck will allow divers with a qualification to this depth to visit a wreck and see for themselves how the marine life gradually moves in. Originally, she was sitting upright on the sand at 22m, but during the winter of 2016/17 a huge storm moved her nearer the reef, still upright slid at a depth of 22m.

There are a number of ways in which to reach the wreck of Tugboat 2, but I am going to suggest two, both using entry point E1, your travel time to the wreck could take you between 12 and 20 minutes depending on your dive plan. While exploring the wreck, take time to stop and examine the rocks that the Tugboat ploughed into, see how cleanly it has split the rock, before bouncing back and coming to rest in an upright position, with the bow on the reef and the stern on the sand. Fish and marine life are taking up residence on the wreck, groupers, octopus and a shoal of saddle bream, have found a home. Unfortunately sand and dead sea grass has covered the engine room floor, please ensure that care is taken and penetration diving procedures are followed.

BEWARE of boat traffic rounding the headland. The yellow Marker Buoys maybe removed during the winter months, always carry a DSMB.

THE DIVE — Minimum time - 50 mins

Choice 1 from entry point E1 descend and take a compass bearing between 300° and 330° this will take you over the short marine growth, then over the sea grass down onto the sand at 12m, time about 3 minutes.

Now keeping the reef on your right follow the reef edge where it meets the sand, for a short while your heading will be 30° in about 2 minutes it will change to a Northerly direction, depth 13m. Continue along the reef edge until you reach a depth of 20m and possibly 17 minutes into your dive, the reef will change direction to 30° and then 60°, on your left sand on your right sea grass, boulders and rocks, look out for 'Heart Rock' from here it is about 40 metres along the edge of the reef to the wreck, Mini Car Rock is about half way. Tugboat 2 rests with the bows into the reef and the stern on the sand. Total time to reach the wreck approximately 19/20 minutes, of course you may be faster than me.

Below: Mini Car Rock only 20 metres from Tugboat 2.

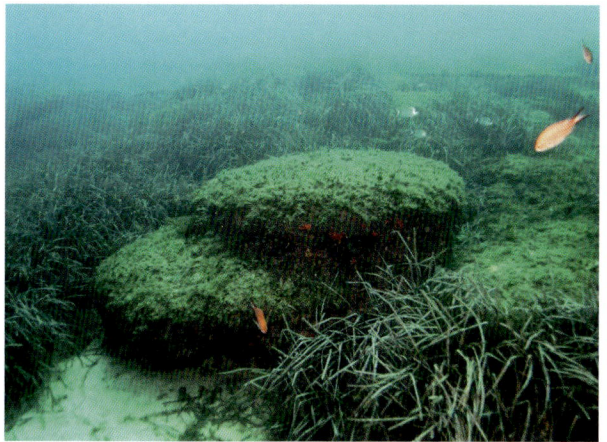

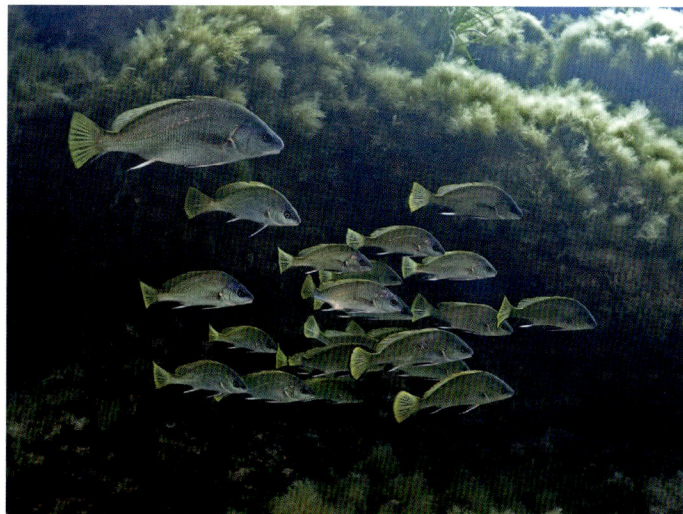

A shoal of brown meagre on this shallow reef.

PHOTOS: SERGEY MARKOV DIVE SYSTEMS DIVE CENTRE

Below: Hiding under a rock is a small octopus.

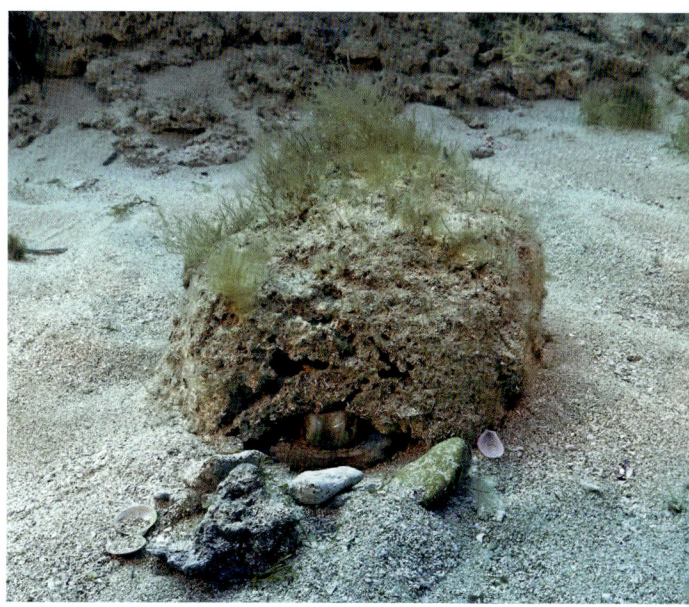

Below: Heart Rock some 30 metres from Tugboat 2.

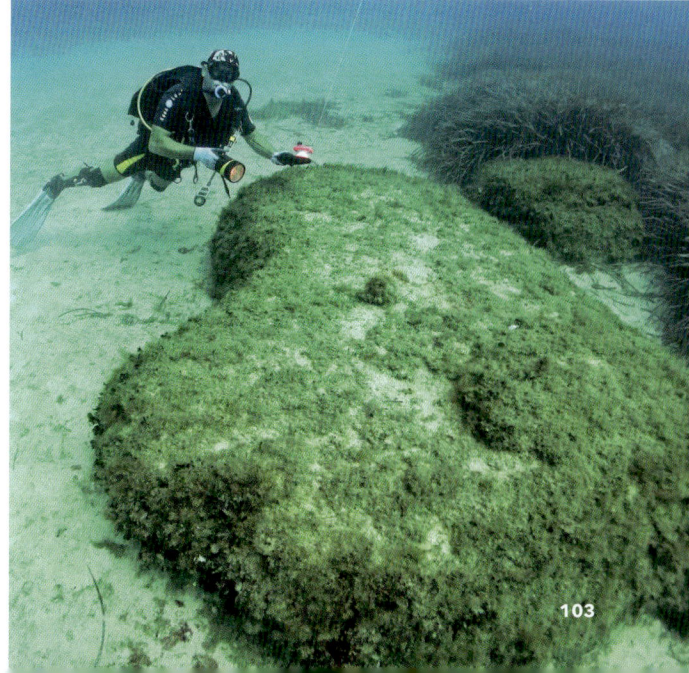

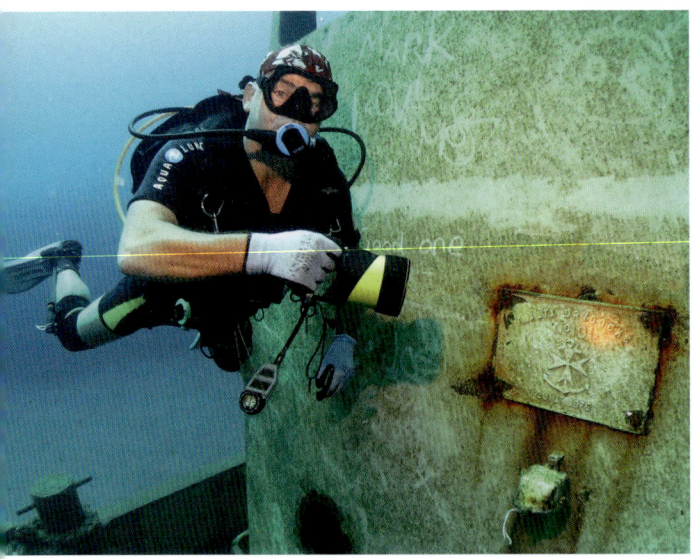

The dated plaque reads Malta Dry Dock No. 101 1975.

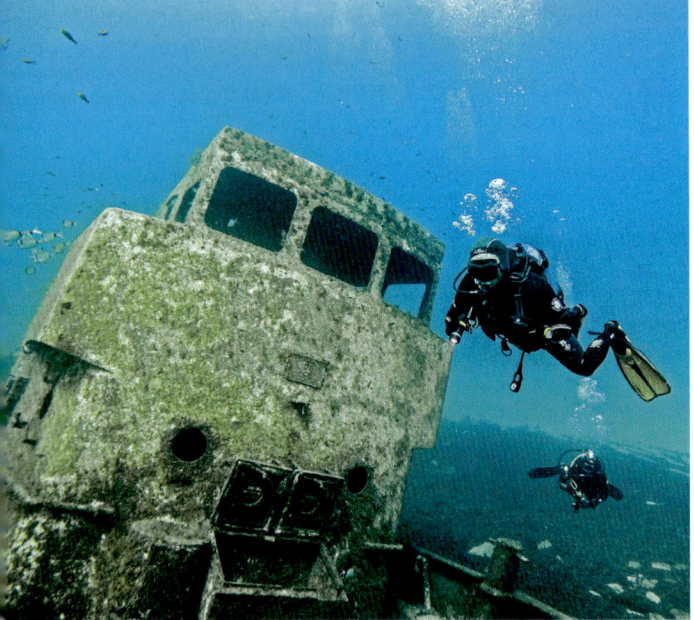

Divers around the bridge of Tugboat 2.
PHOTOS: ARKADIUSZ SREBNIK POLANDDIVINGPHOTOS
Below: The bow of Tugboat 2 resting on the rocks.

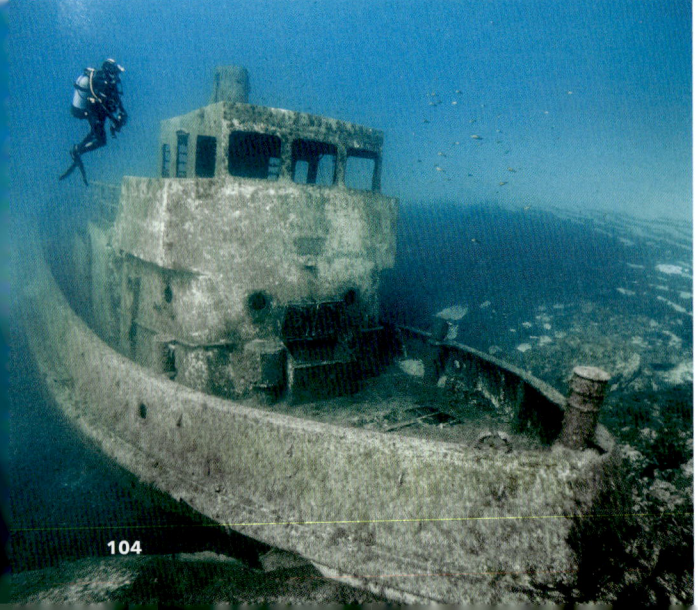

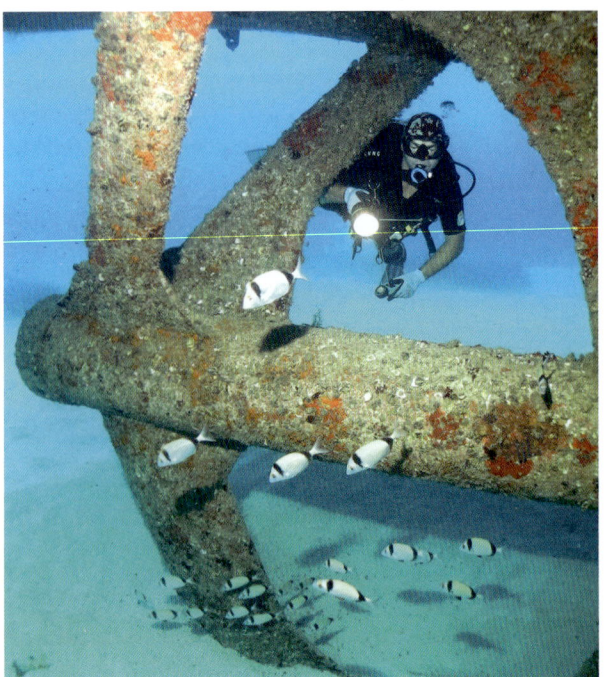

Two-banded sea bream under the stern of Tugboat 2.

Choice 2 from entry point E1 descend and take a compass bearing of north 0° to 330° continue down and over the reef until you reach the sand, basically this way you are cutting off the corner at the start of **choice 1.** Now follow the edge of the reef where it meets the sand, continue all the way to the end and round to Heart Rock, as in **choice 1,** this route could save you 3 to 4 minutes making travel time to the wreck of approximately 16 minutes.

Choice 3 is possibly in my opinion the best way to reach the wreck. From entry point E1, surface swim to the end of St Julians Point, keeping the reef on your right for protection from boat traffic. Now descend to a depth of 5m and take a 360° to 350° compass bearing; it will take you about 12 minutes to reach the end of the reef and if your navigation has been good, Tugboat 2. If not, you should be able to see the six boulders, which include Heart Rock then Mini Car Rock, sometimes not easy to find bearing in mind they are only a metre in height, green and surrounded by Posidonia grass, **see choice 1,** total time to the wreck approximately 14 minutes or less.

Return routes, you have a choice, a compass bearing of 180° will take you to exit E1, a bearing of 130°/140° will take you over the reef to exit E2. If I had air and time, I would normally follow **choice 1 route in reverse,** where the reef meets the sand all the way back to a depth of 12m, or at any time head up over the reef to exit E1.

The reef can have a variety of marine life, groupers, brown meagre, octopus, painted comber, cardinal fish and nudibranchs to name but a few. It is always a good idea to check out on the sand for tun shells, rays, flying gurnards and dabs. Lots to see a great dive even better if you have a camera.

E2
E1
St. Julians Point
Wreck Marker Buoy
The edge of this reef can be spectacular with marine life, which could be your return route.
Note, the Calypso Stones may not be visable due to being covered with sand.

The sinking of Tug Boat 2.
PHOTO: DIVE SYSTEMS DIVE CENTRE

Tug Boat 2.

PHOTO: JOE ABDILLA & PAUL GAUCI

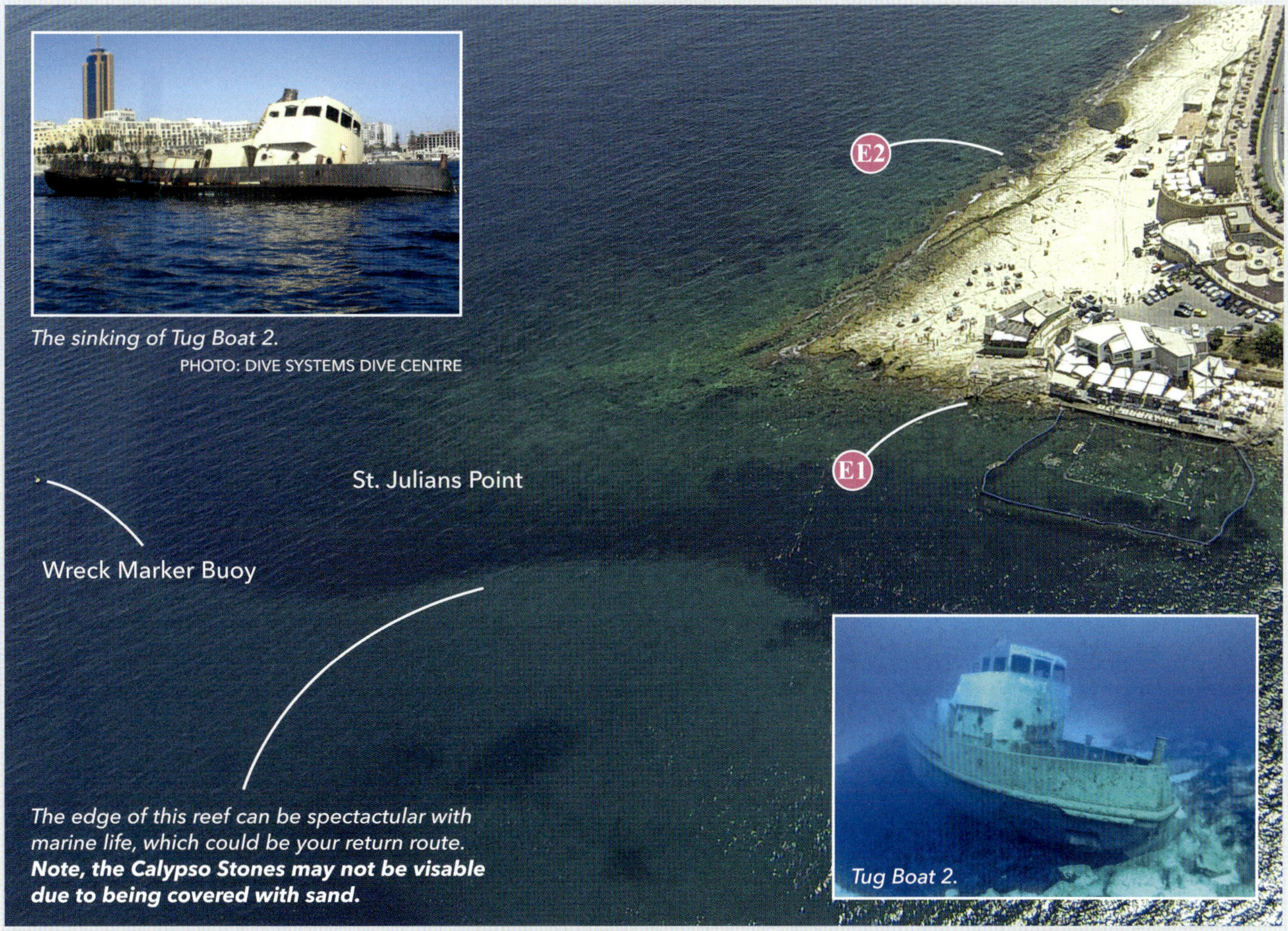

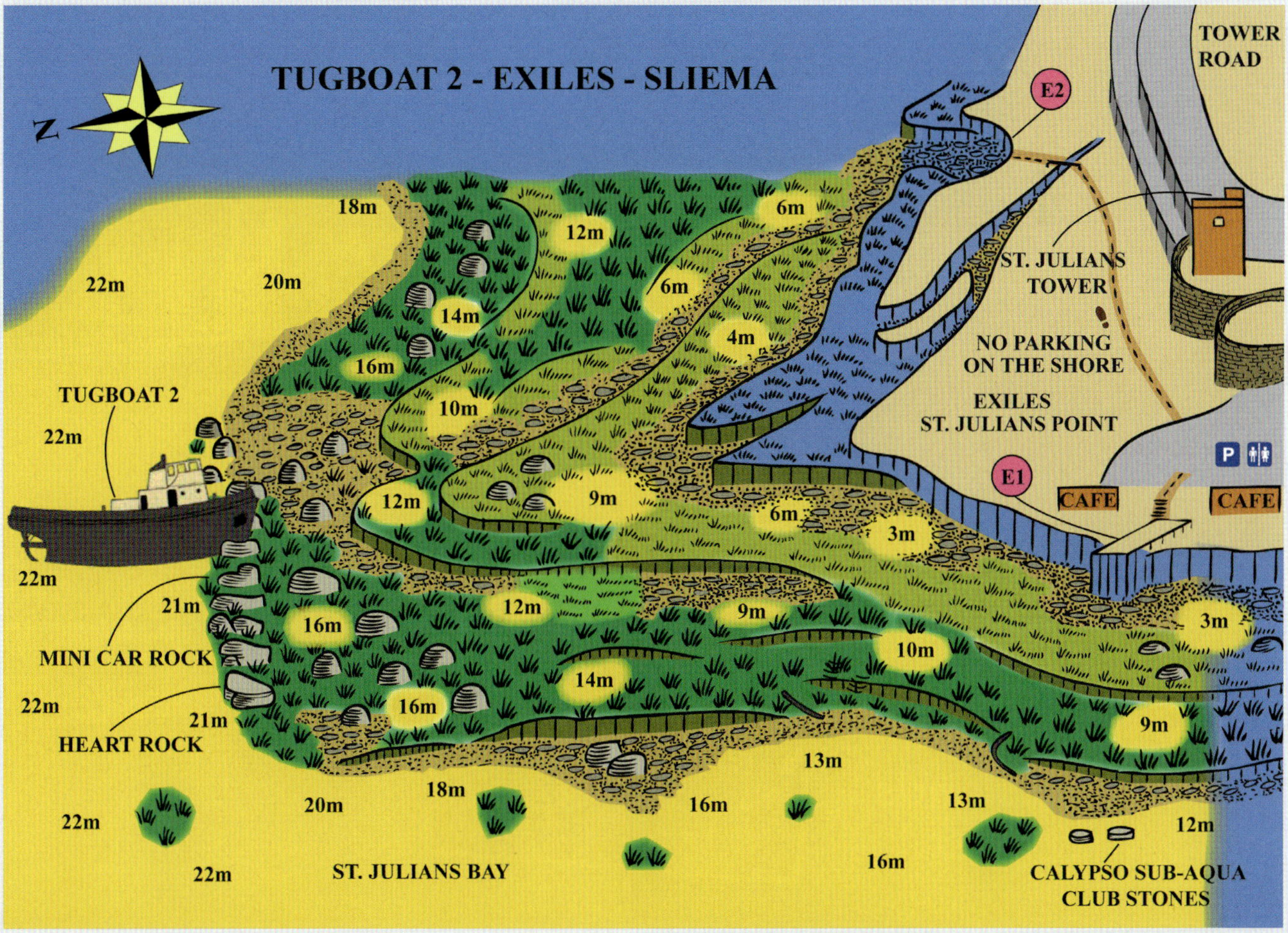
TUGBOAT 2 - EXILES - SLIEMA
N
TOWER ROAD
E2
ST. JULIANS TOWER
NO PARKING ON THE SHORE
EXILES ST. JULIANS POINT
P
E1
CAFE
CAFE
TUGBOAT 2
MINI CAR ROCK
HEART ROCK
ST. JULIANS BAY
CALYPSO SUB-AQUA CLUB STONES
18m
22m
20m
12m
6m
6m
14m
4m
16m
10m
22m
12m
9m
6m
3m
22m
21m
12m
16m
9m
10m
3m
14m
22m
21m
16m
9m
13m
18m
22m
20m
16m
13m
12m
22m
16m

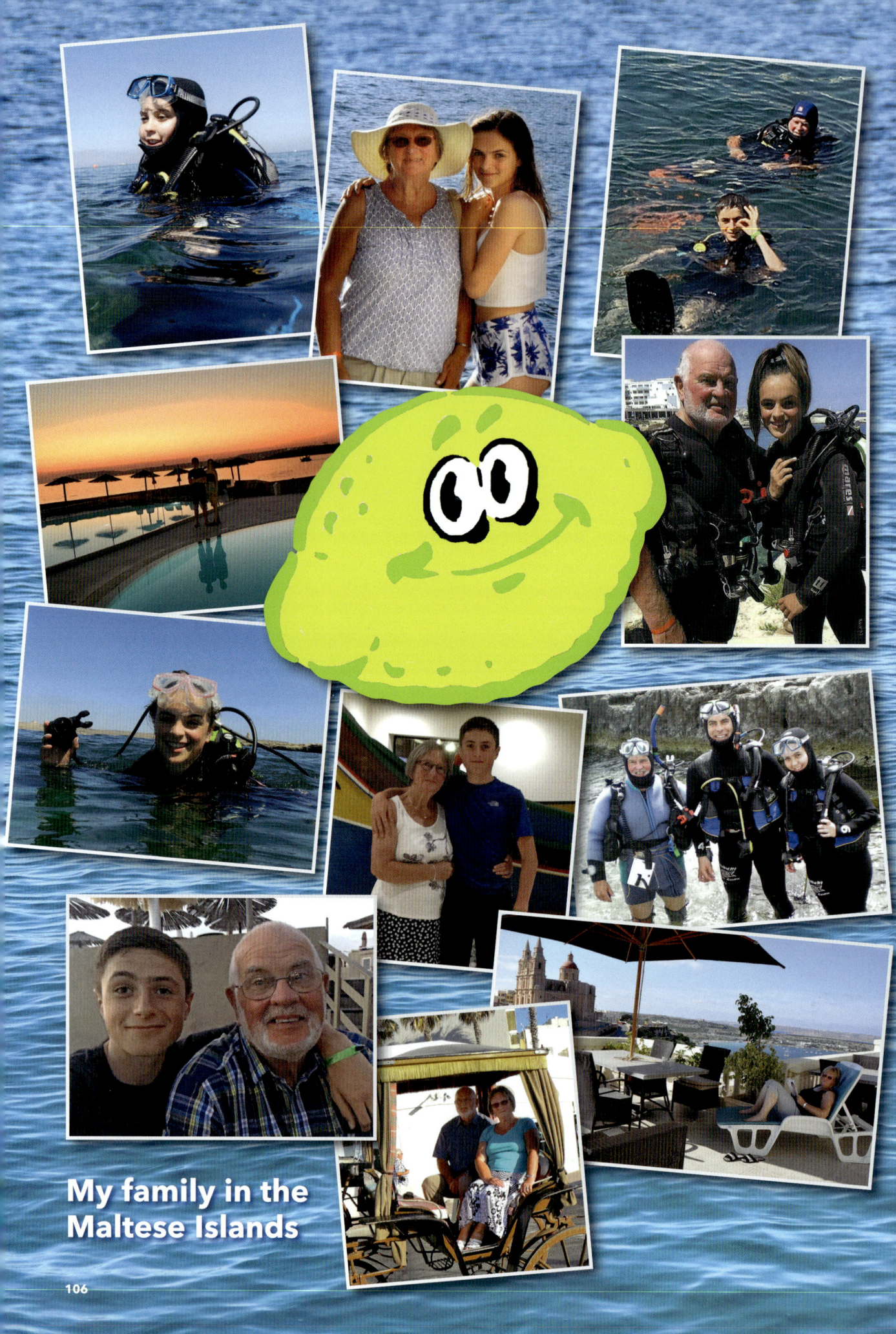

My family in the Maltese Islands

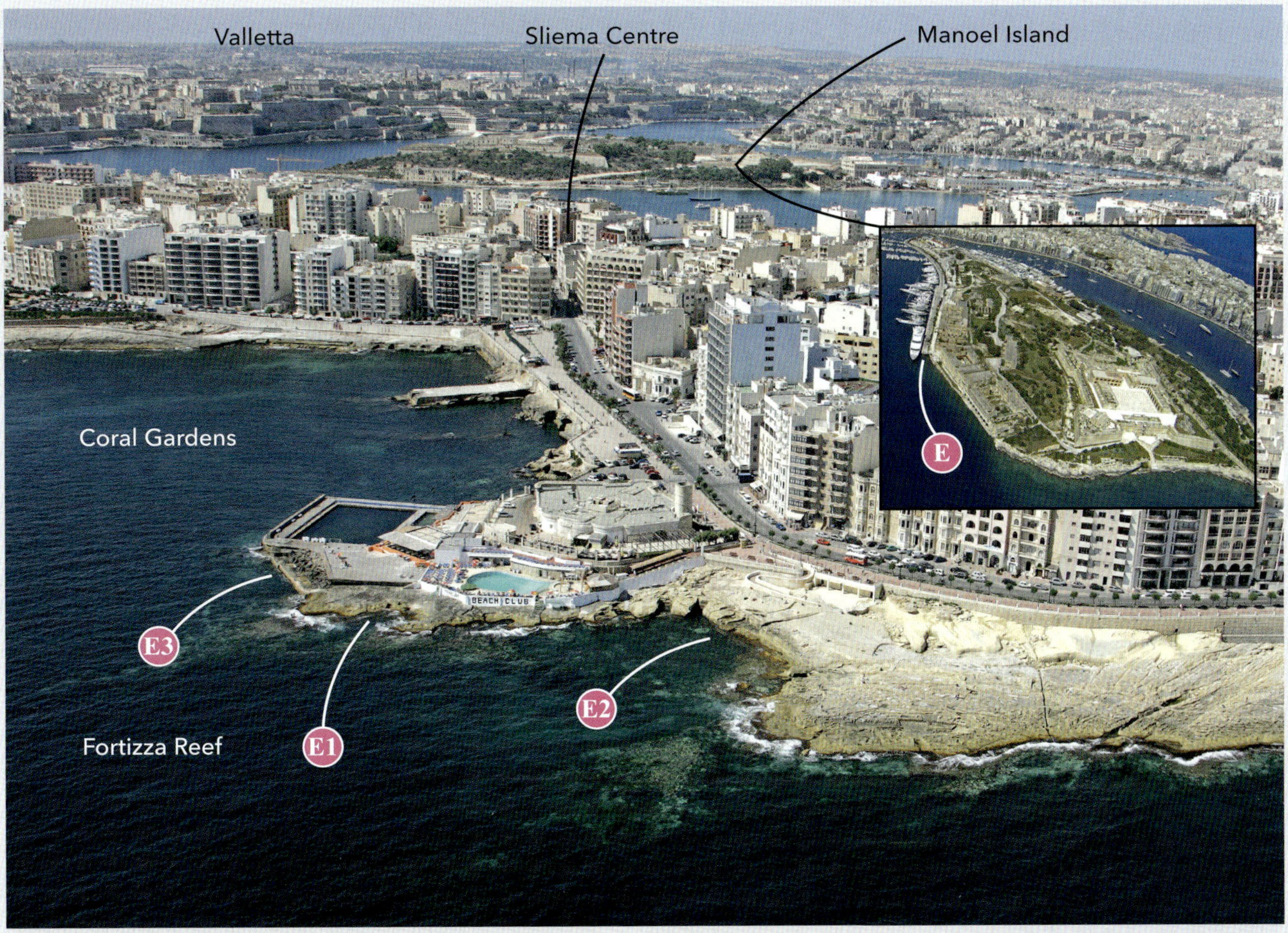

SLIEMA - FORTIZZA - MANOEL ISLAND

Valletta — Sliema Centre — Manoel Island

Coral Gardens

E3 — Fortizza Reef — E1 — E2

E (Manoel Island inset)

PHOTOS: PGL AERIAL PHOTOS

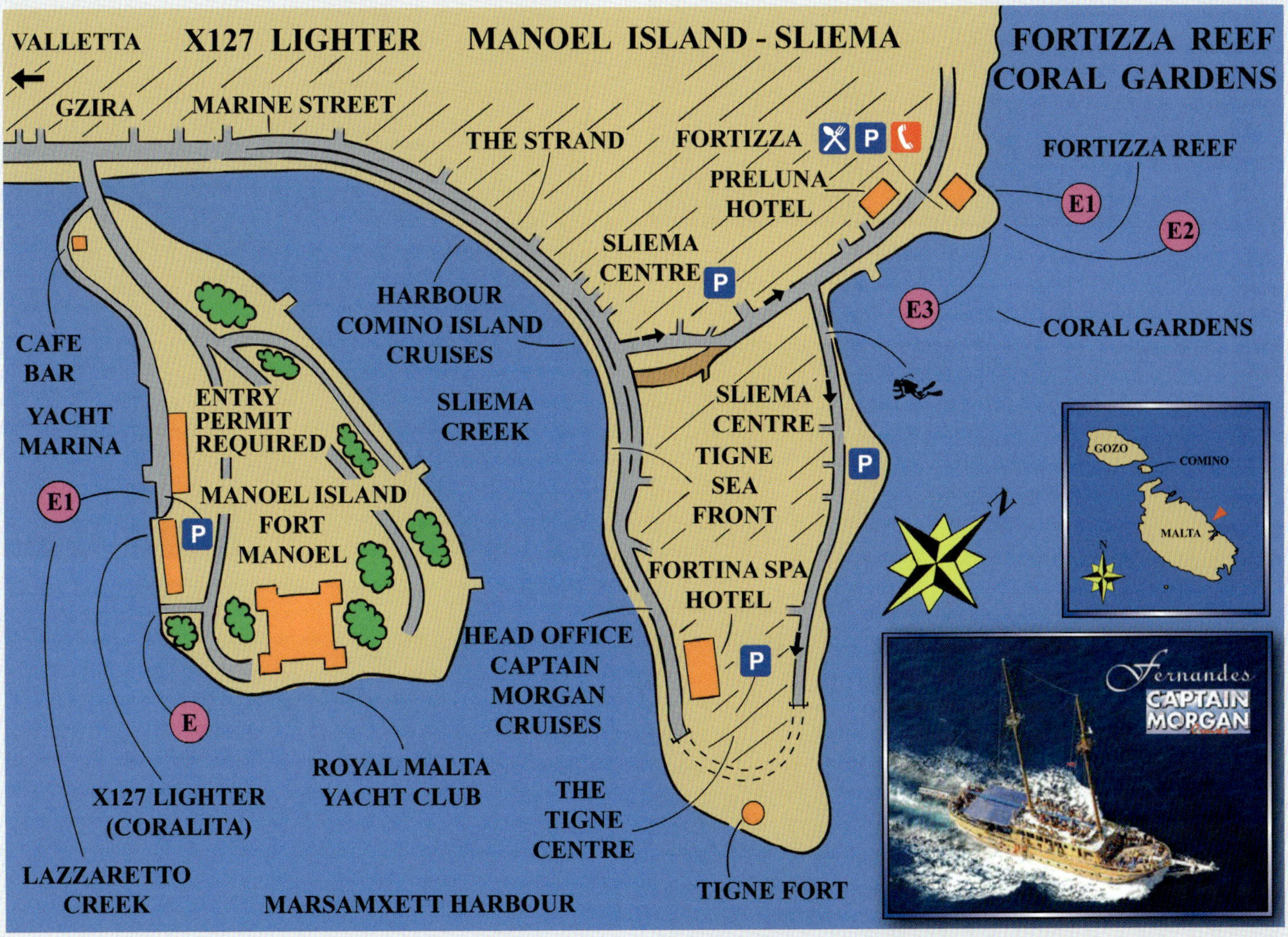

MANOEL ISLAND - SLIEMA / FORTIZZA REEF CORAL GARDENS

- VALLETTA
- X127 LIGHTER
- GZIRA
- MARINE STREET
- THE STRAND
- FORTIZZA
- PRELUNA HOTEL
- SLIEMA CENTRE
- FORTIZZA REEF
- E1
- E2
- E3
- CORAL GARDENS
- CAFE BAR
- YACHT MARINA
- E1
- HARBOUR COMINO ISLAND CRUISES
- ENTRY PERMIT REQUIRED
- SLIEMA CREEK
- MANOEL ISLAND FORT MANOEL
- SLIEMA CENTRE TIGNE SEA FRONT
- FORTINA SPA HOTEL
- HEAD OFFICE CAPTAIN MORGAN CRUISES
- E
- X127 LIGHTER (CORALITA)
- ROYAL MALTA YACHT CLUB
- THE TIGNE CENTRE
- LAZZARETTO CREEK
- MARSAMXETT HARBOUR
- TIGNE FORT

GOZO — COMINO — MALTA

Fernandes CAPTAIN MORGAN

Fortizza Reef - Coral Gardens - Sliema

These dive sites are in the bustling centre of Sliema, with its shops, cafes, bars and seafront promenades. The car park is next to the Fortizza restaurant which is right on the seafront. You may have to wait for a space to park, but availability is better in the afternoons or mornings at weekends. Check out your routes to your entry points E1, E2 or E3, all are reached from the north side of the Fortizza restaurant, see aerial photos. If you are using the Preluna Beach Club to reach your entry point, please ask permission, normally they have no objections.

Fortizza Reef

The depth range is 2m to 16m, with many areas to explore, tunnels, arches, small caves and a surprising amount of marine life, which makes it an excellent area for photography. This site will test your navigational skills to the full, either with a compass or by pilotage. All this adds up to an interesting and enjoyable dive location.

THE DIVE — Minimum time - 45 mins

Using entry E1, which is front of the Preluna Beach Club, enter the water and swim straight out of the little pool and descend to 6m, keep the reef on your left, go to its end where your depth will be 8m. The compass bearing to Mushroom Rock is 35° distance some 60 metres. First, over the sea grass, then short marine growth, from here you should be able to see Mushroom Rock, which looks like a giant mushroom. Drop over the reef on the left of this rock into The Valley, bear left and on your right will be the tunnel, go through, once emerging the other side take a compass bearing of 60° you will pass three distinct rocks on your left in the reef.

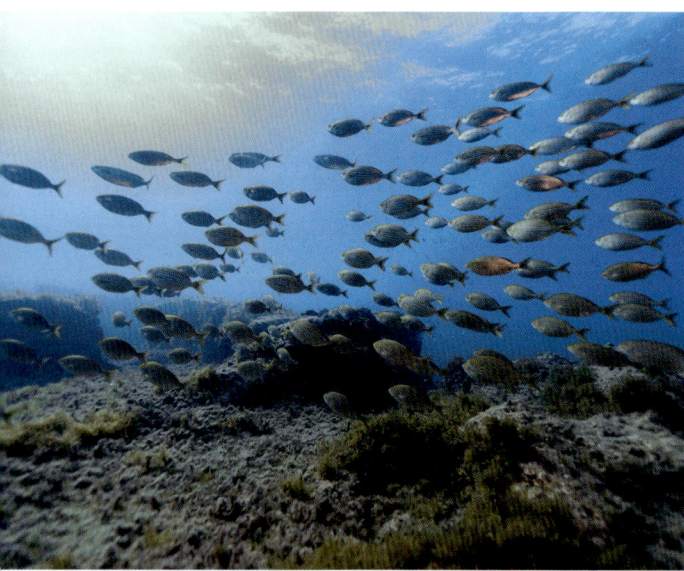

A shoal of Salema fish in these shallow waters.

PHOTOS: JON BORG www.jonborg.com

Checking out one of the many tunnels in this dive site.

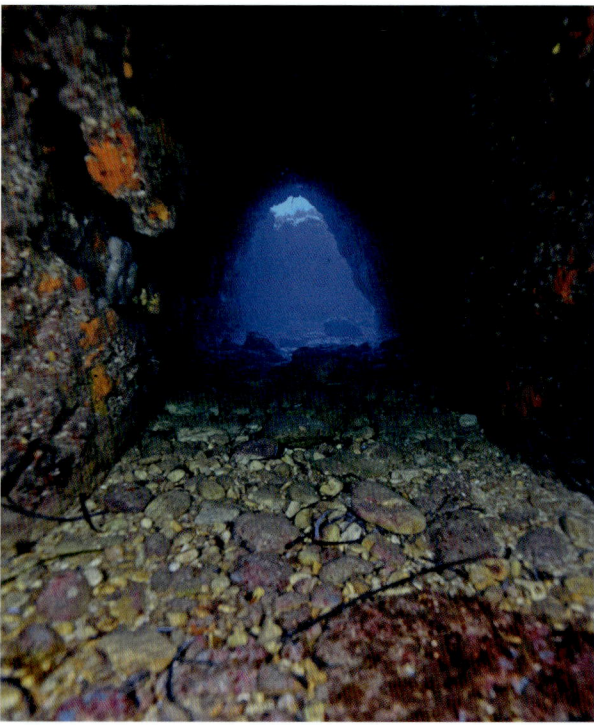

Please respect the corals within these tunnels.

PHOTO: JON BORG www.jonborg.com

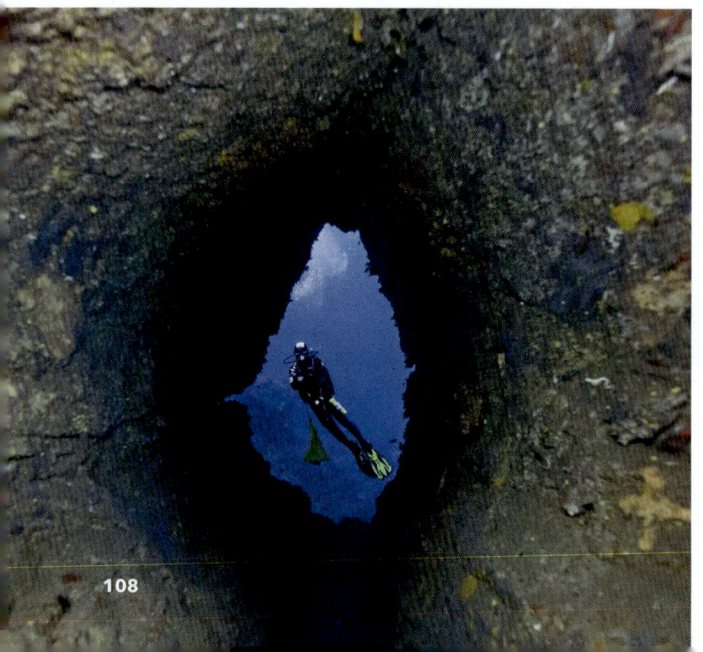

After the third one, bear left into an area covered in sea grass with a reef on each side, continue, after a short distance you will find a cave with a hole in the roof on your left-hand side, depth 14m. return to the third rock and continue with a compass bearing of 60° there are two more bowl areas to explore, if you reach the furthest one your depth will be 16m.

Coral Gardens
PHOTO: JOE WADSWORTH MALTA BLUE DIVING
PHOTO: JON BORG www.jonborg.com
E3
E1
E2
Fortizza Reef

PHOTO: PGL AERIAL PHOTOS

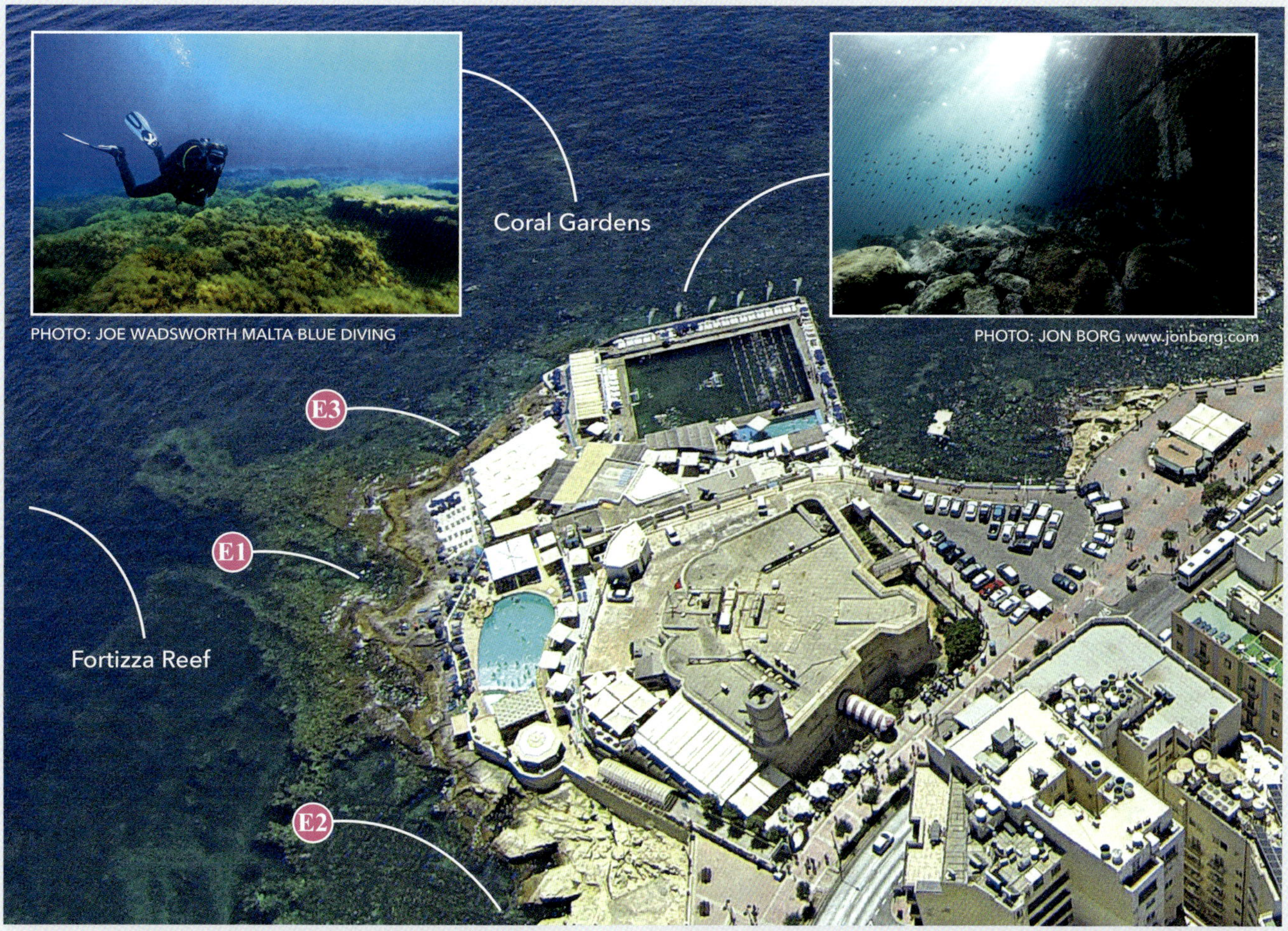

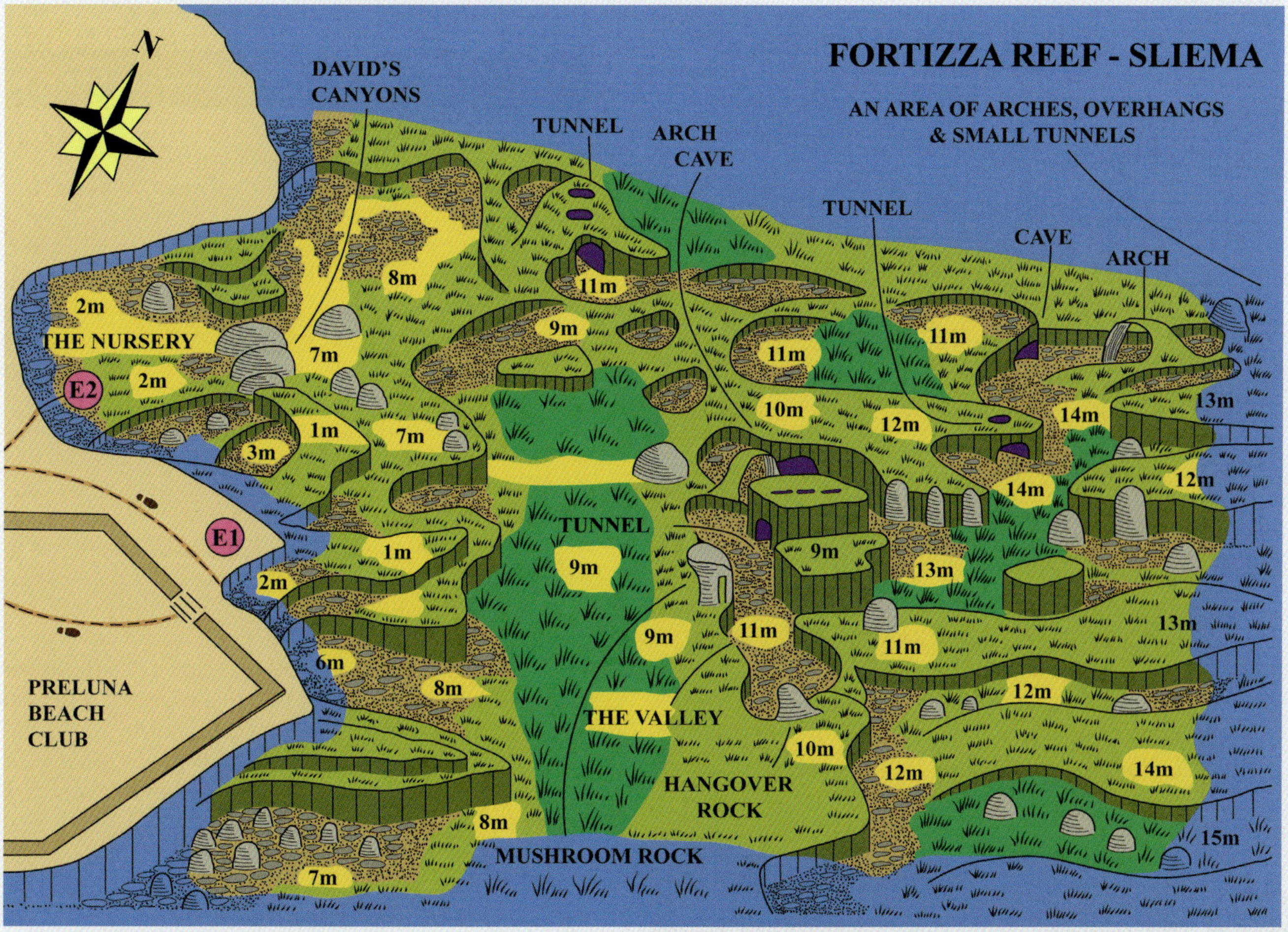
FORTIZZA REEF - SLIEMA
AN AREA OF ARCHES, OVERHANGS & SMALL TUNNELS
N
DAVID'S CANYONS
TUNNEL
ARCH CAVE
TUNNEL
CAVE
ARCH
THE NURSERY
E2
E1
PRELUNA BEACH CLUB
TUNNEL
THE VALLEY
HANGOVER ROCK
MUSHROOM ROCK
2m
2m
3m
1m
7m
7m
8m
11m
9m
11m
11m
10m
12m
14m
13m
12m
14m
9m
13m
1m
2m
9m
9m
11m
11m
13m
6m
8m
12m
10m
12m
14m
8m
7m
15m

CORAL GARDENS - SLIEMA

Your return Route to exit points E1 or E2.

May I suggest you now turn round and head for your exit point, approximate time 20 minutes. Your return route is to follow the opposite side of the valley back to Mushroom Rock and then use the same route back to your chosen exit point. This is my dive plan, but of course with so many areas to visit you could plan your own dive.

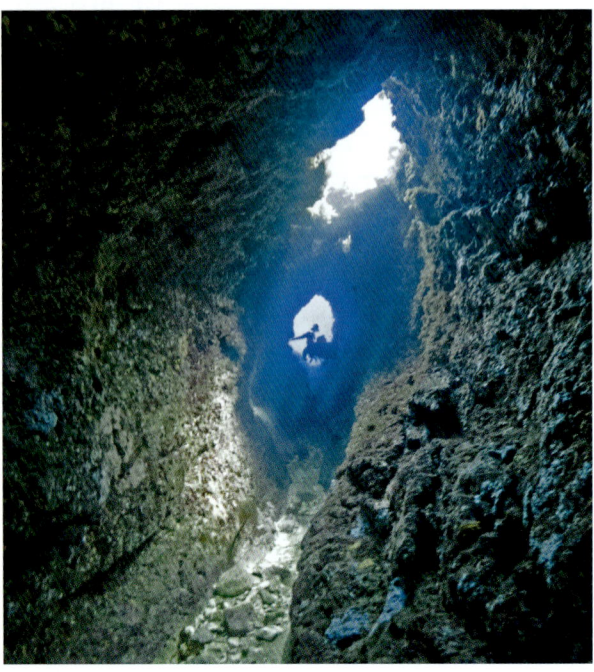

PHOTO: ARKADIUSZ SREBNIK POLANDDIVINGPHOTO
The underwater world of tunnels, arches and small caves.
BELOW PHOTO: JON BORG www.jonborg.com

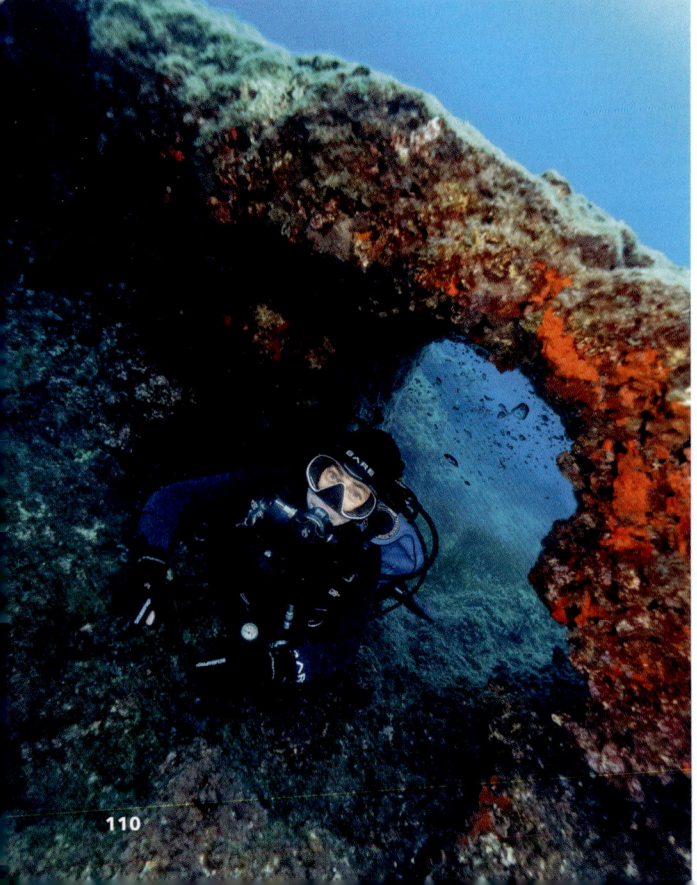

Coral Gardens

Using E3, see aerial photos, the route to your entry point and the dive site will test your navigational skills, the latter is much easier when the visibility is good, you could of course use a dive guide in order not to miss the places of interest in this extraordinary dive location.

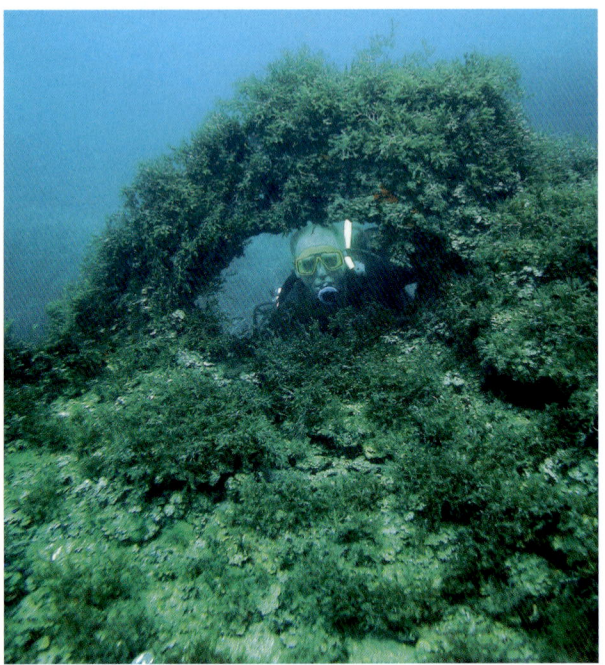

A small arch formed by the sea over many years.

THE DIVE — Minimum time - 55 mins

From your entry point take a compass bearing of 60° over the sea grass within two to three minutes you should reach Overhang Rock with its distinct little cove. Turn right into this narrow valley, turning left would lead you to Mushroom Rock. Keeping the reef on your right-hand side you will pass three little tunnels, once you have explored, cross over to the other side and continue down the valley to a depth of 13m, on your right are the Coral Gardens your direction should be north easterly. There are many small unusual shaped rocks covered in coral on this plateau. From the end of this valley take a compass bearing of 150° this will lead you over a reef at 11m. You are now entering the area of the limestone reef; good buoyancy is essential and take extra care as you admire this unique underwater landscape. Around this area of pinnacle rocks the depth is 14m, this is possibly the deepest part of your dive. **Your return route to all exits** will take you in a westerly direction into Boulder Canyon, then head north west into Scorpionfish Valley. At the end of the valley head 270° to your exit point. Of course, there are many dive permutations for this interesting area, I have chosen probably the most popular one.

It has taken millions of years for the canyon system to form, fragile windows and caves have formed and in turn provided unique ecosystems within themselves. Please avoid the temptation of swimming through the windows in the limestone reefs, good buoyancy is required at all times.
Coral Gardens
E3
E1
E2

A look into a tunnel.
PHOTO: JON BORG www.jonborg.com

Entry Point E1.

PHOTO: PGL AERIAL PHOTOS

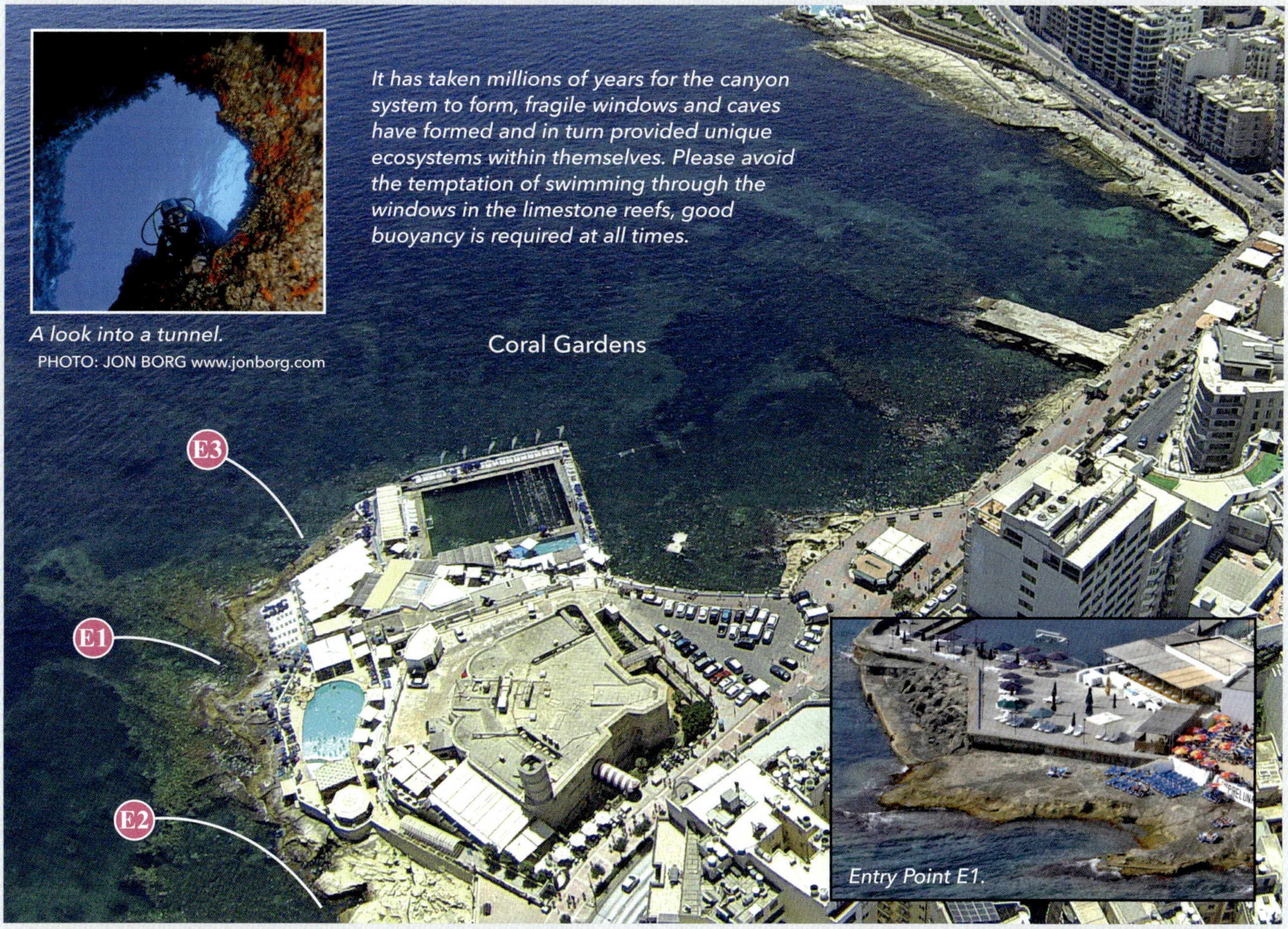

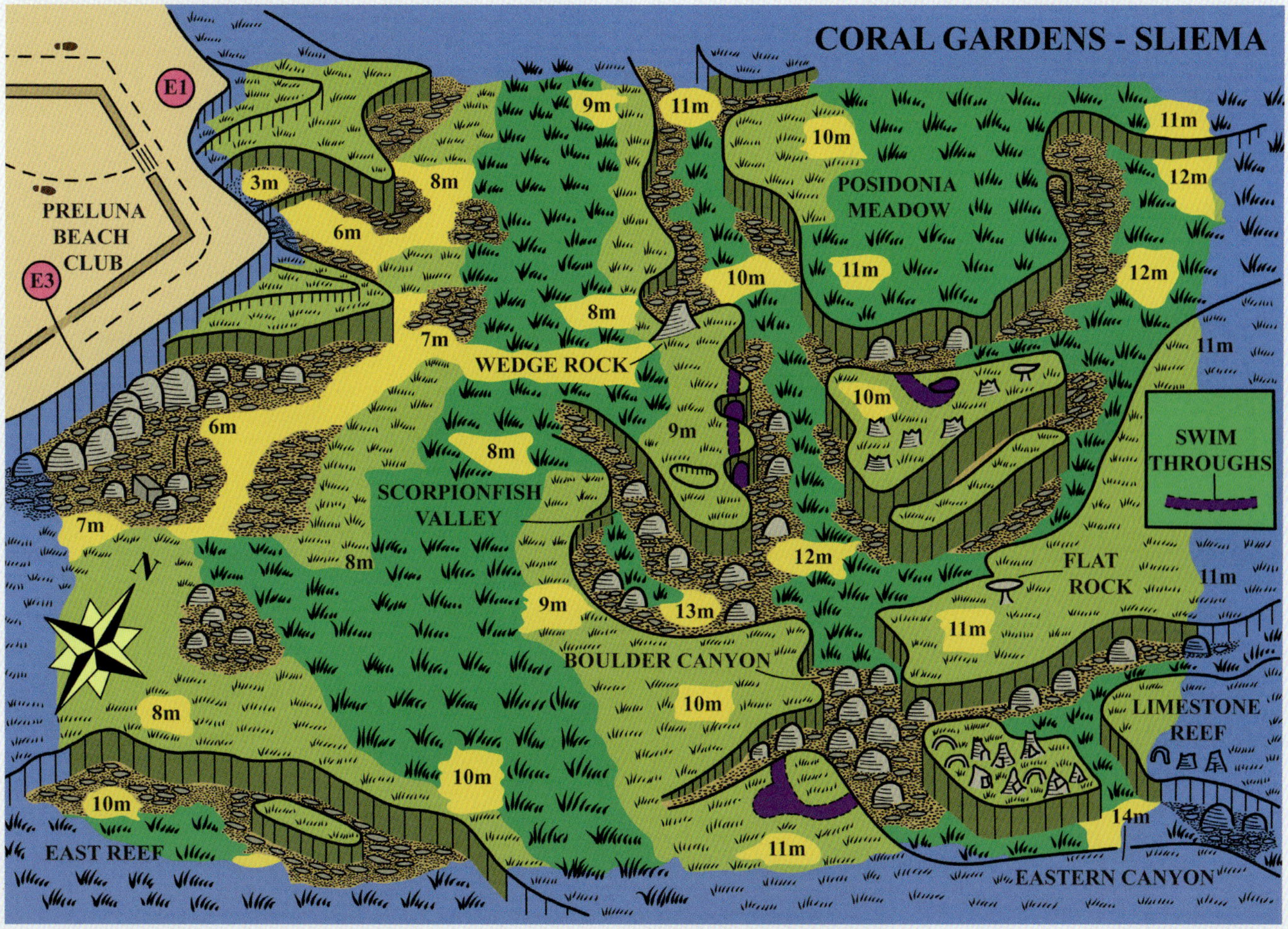
CORAL GARDENS - SLIEMA
E1
E3
PRELUNA BEACH CLUB
3m
6m
7m
8m
9m
10m
11m
12m
13m
14m
WEDGE ROCK
POSIDONIA MEADOW
SCORPIONFISH VALLEY
BOULDER CANYON
FLAT ROCK
LIMESTONE REEF
EAST REEF
EASTERN CANYON
SWIM THROUGHS
N

The *X127* Water Lighter (Coralita) Manoel Island

Manoel Island is situated on the coastal road between Sliema and Valletta see local plan. **Before diving this site consult with your Dive Centre, you will need a swipe card for the barrier.** Once over the little bridge, turn right, where there is a barrier. This road runs alongside the water's edge, your entry point is at the end of the road. **This is private property and whilst here please have respect for resident boat owners.**

Walter Pollock of James Pollock & Sons was asked to build 200 landing craft for the 1915 Dardanelles landings in the Gallipoli campaign during World War 1, these would be *X Lighters*.

The hull construction would be based on the river Thames barges, each would weigh 135 tons, 35 meters in length, a beam of 6.5 metres, a drop-down ramp and a crew of 12 men.

They would be built in 30 ship yards in England and Scotland, this *X127* was built by Goole Shipbuilding and Repairs Co. Beverly, Yorkshire she was fitted with a Campbell 80 BHP engine with twin props. Converted to carry water and fitted with a Tangye engine to pump the water out of the hull to the reservoirs on shore.

These vessels were towed the 3,000 miles from the River Humber via Plymouth to the large harbour of Mudros on the Agean island of Lemnos, this took 25 days. At Cape Hellas on the Gallipoli peninsular two reservoirs were built; the Water Lighters would have to transferred water from the ships to the beach reservoirs. *X127* was involved with the successful withdrawal of troops and horses after what some would say was one of the bloodiest battles in WW1.

After the campaign many of the *Lighters* were sold, 16 went to Malta, the *X127* was one of these. She was converted to carry fuel oil for the tenth Submarine Flotilla, *HMS Talbot* Manoel Island.

On the 6th March 1942 the submarine base was attacked by dive bombers, during this attack the *P36* and *P39* were damaged. The *X127* was hit, caught fire, and sunk shortly afterwards. She remains in the same position today, upright with her bow at 5m and the stern at 22m.

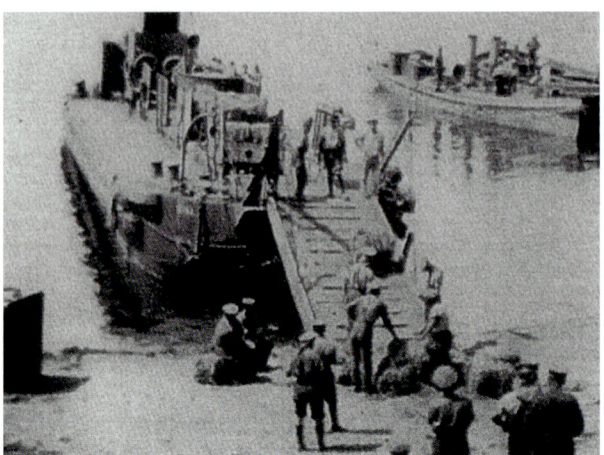

A Water Lighter on the beach in Turkey 1916.

PHOTOS: DAVE MALLARD, ISLE OF WIGHT

The submarine base HMS Talbot on Manoel Island.

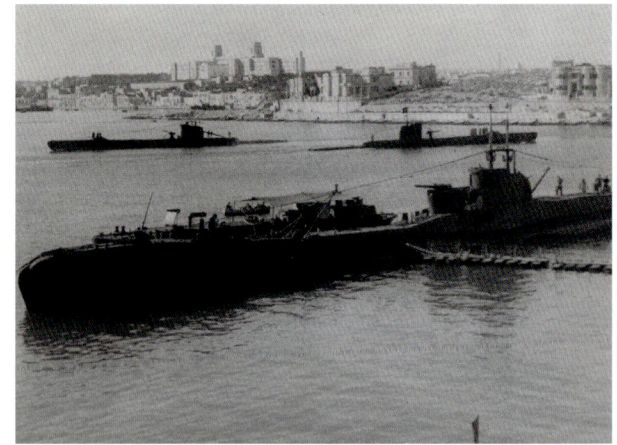

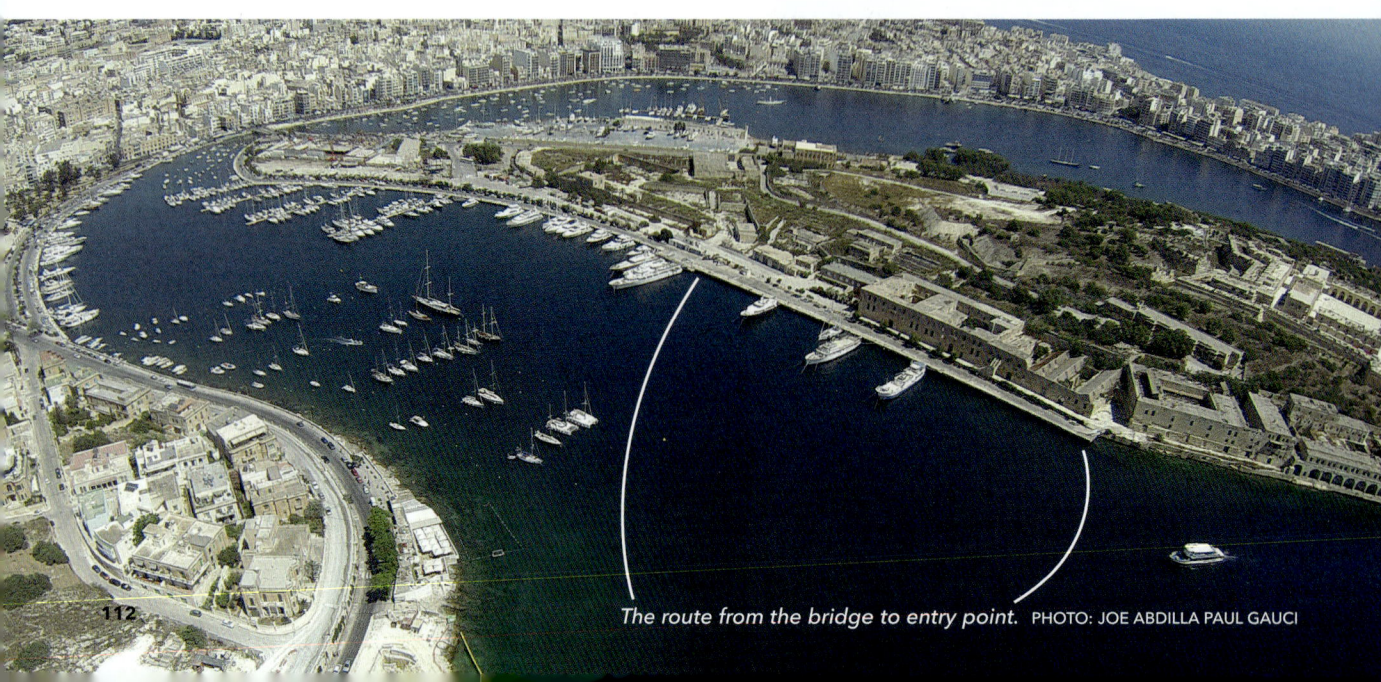

The route from the bridge to entry point. PHOTO: JOE ABDILLA PAUL GAUCI

X127 WATER LIGHTER (CORALITA) - MANOEL ISLAND

The research into this wreck started in 2003 by David Mallard from the Isle of Wight. Originally known as the *Coralita*, it seemed possible that it was the *Lighter X131*, photographs of the fishing trawler *Coral* together with the *X131* in dry dock No.3, Grand Harbour; both vessels were damaged in an air raid on 21st April 1942. The name *Coralita* may have originated from this trawler, but found no evidence to support this. Further research ruled out the X131, and in 2006 he found the vital information proving what everyone has always known that the *Coralita*, was actually the *Lighter X127*. Listed by Lloyds as Wreck No. 37379

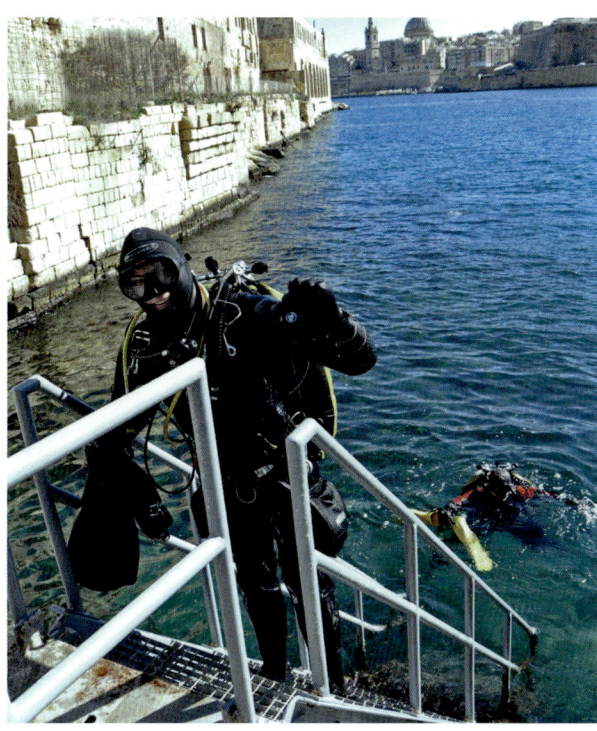

The excellent entry steps at this dive site.

THE DIVE — Minimum time - 35 mins

Once in the water, descend and head in an easterly direction at a depth of 8/9m staying at this depth until you reach the wreck. Starting at the spoon shaped bow, a fitting for the mast and on each side fairleads and towing bollards. Moving down the starboard side passing over the chain locker, on your right on the small upper structure are two hatches, inside is one of the two Tangye water pumps, **just look, do not enter.**

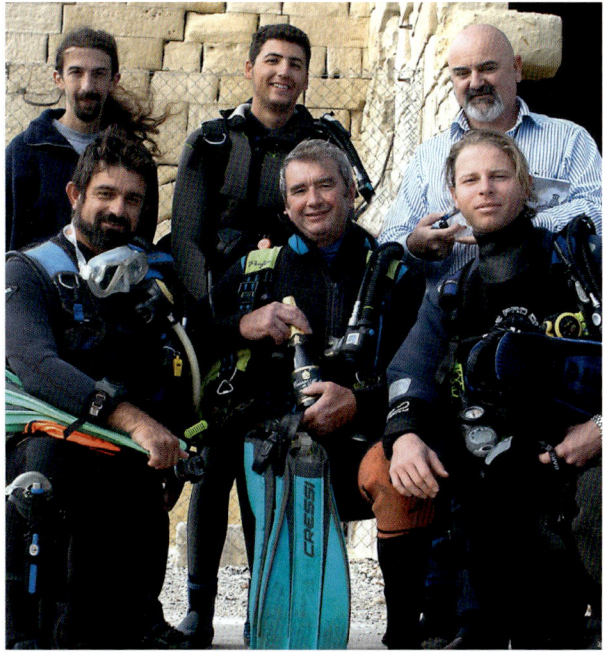

British diver Dave Mallard centre front completed four years of research helped by four divers from Malta. Front left Antonio Anastasi right Patrick Milton. Back row, Rupert Mifsud, Danial B Carsdona, Martin Vella, Dec.2004.

Bottom photos: Almost touching the sea wall, the bows of the X127 lighter just 6m below the surface.

PHOTOS: ARKADIUSZ SREBNIK POLANDDIVINGPHOTO

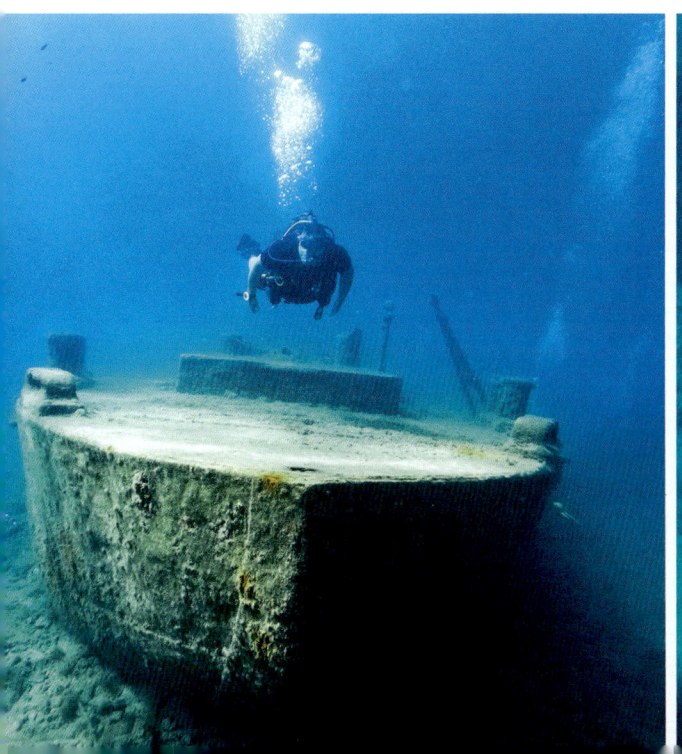
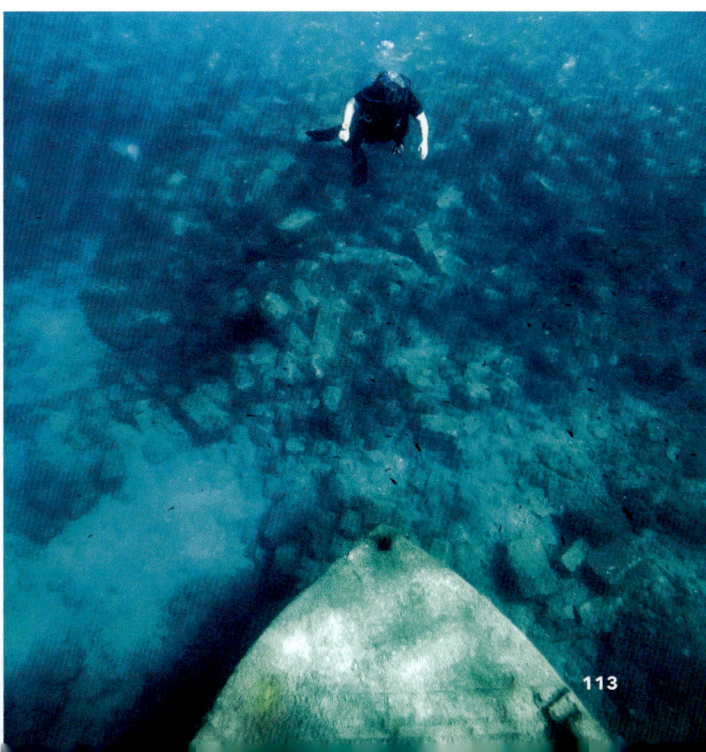

X127 WATER LIGHTER (CORALITA) - MANOEL ISLAND

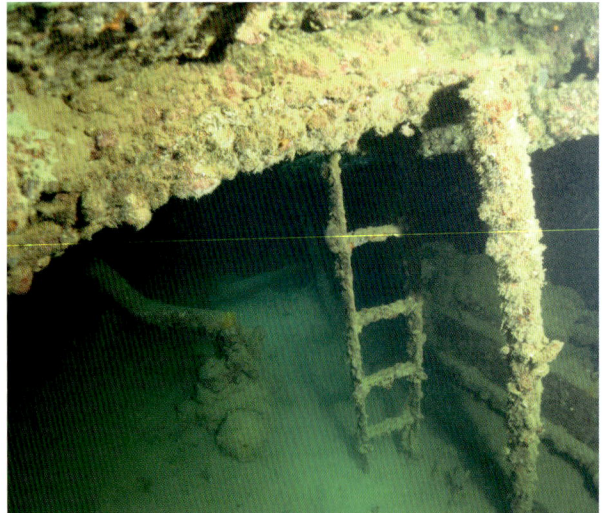

*The ladder into the pump room, **do not enter!***

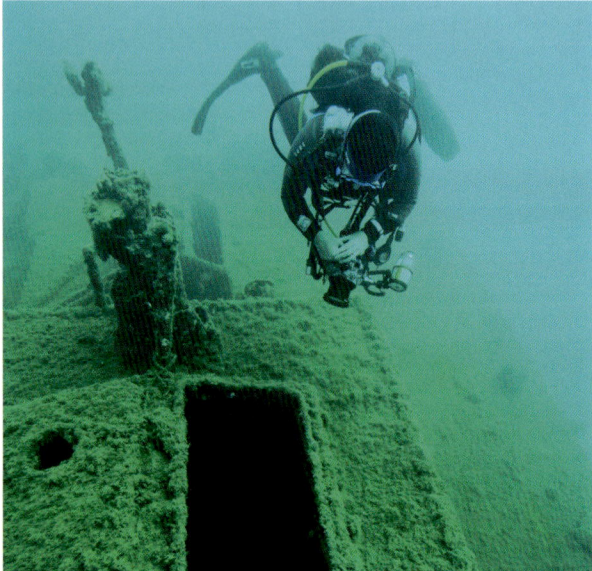

The accommodation hatch for the 12 crew

Below: The stern quadrant rudder at 22m.

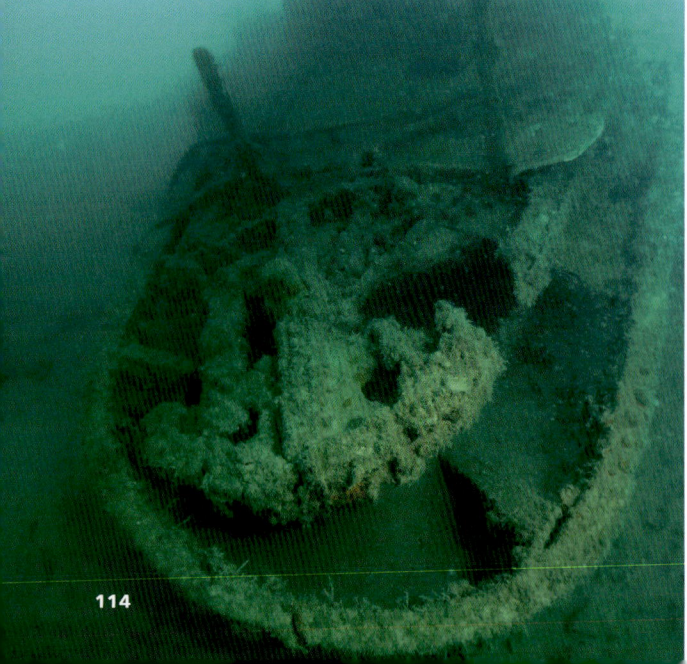

The next four hatches are for the water tanks, on deck is the gun platform, although a gun was never fitted. Further down is the steering pedestal and the compass plate, around the front of this is what remains of the bullet proof screen.

Next are the living quarters, the scuttle entrance with a ladder and the large skylight. Moving down to the stern you will pass the engine room, from here you will be able to see the quadrant rudder, unfortunately the rudder and props are covered with silt. The steering chains run along the deck on both sides of the engine room.

The flag pole fitting, rear fairleads and towing bollards can be seen and looking in the engine room doorway you can see the twin cylinders of the Campbell engine with the flywheel in front, the weight of the engine is 5.5 tons. Fitted to the engine room walls are four sixty-gallon water tanks, on the port side of the engine room are the brackets for the spare anchor. Moving up and along the portside deck, is the much visible bomb damage, showing the damaged hull plating with bent and twisted metal. Continue along the wreck where you will find further damage possibly caused by the submarine P39 being pushed up against the Lighter, when the three bombs were dropped alongside.

Your return route, moving away from the bow in a westerly direction staying reasonably close to the wall, as you do not want to miss your exit steps, as this would lead you into the area where large boats are moored. While exploring this wall and reef, keep a lookout for the marine life which frequent this area.

Remember this is a busy harbour.

Your exit steps, a handy place for early training.

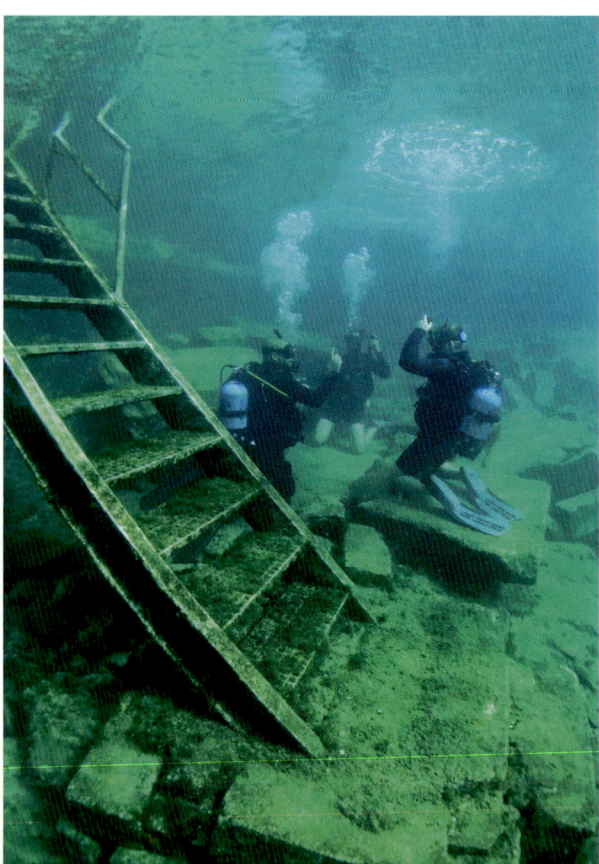

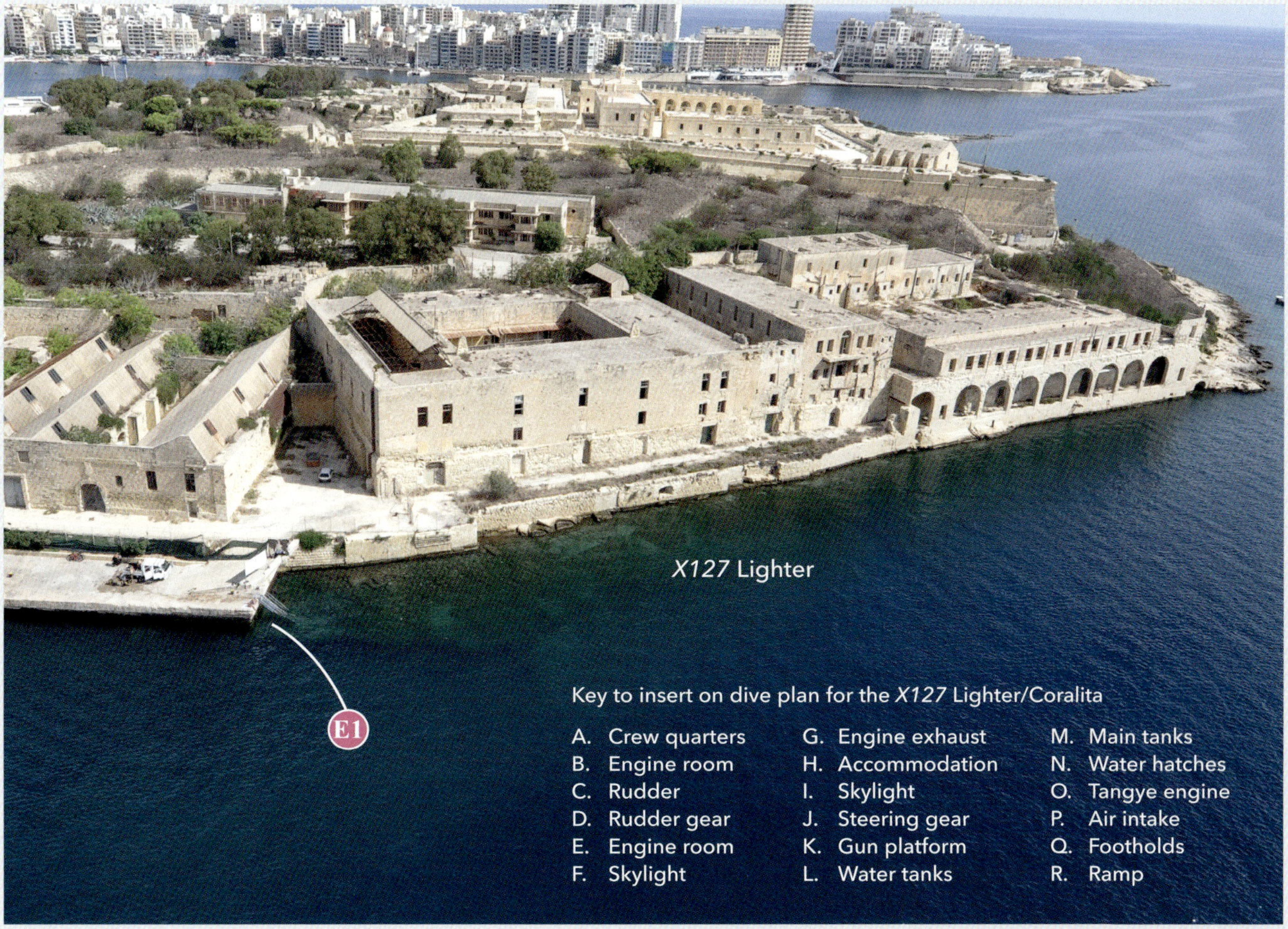

X127 WATER LIGHTER (CORALITA) - MANOEL ISLAND

X127 Lighter

Key to insert on dive plan for the *X127* Lighter/Coralita

- A. Crew quarters
- B. Engine room
- C. Rudder
- D. Rudder gear
- E. Engine room
- F. Skylight
- G. Engine exhaust
- H. Accommodation
- I. Skylight
- J. Steering gear
- K. Gun platform
- L. Water tanks
- M. Main tanks
- N. Water hatches
- O. Tangye engine
- P. Air intake
- Q. Footholds
- R. Ramp

PHOTO: PGL AERIAL PHOTOS

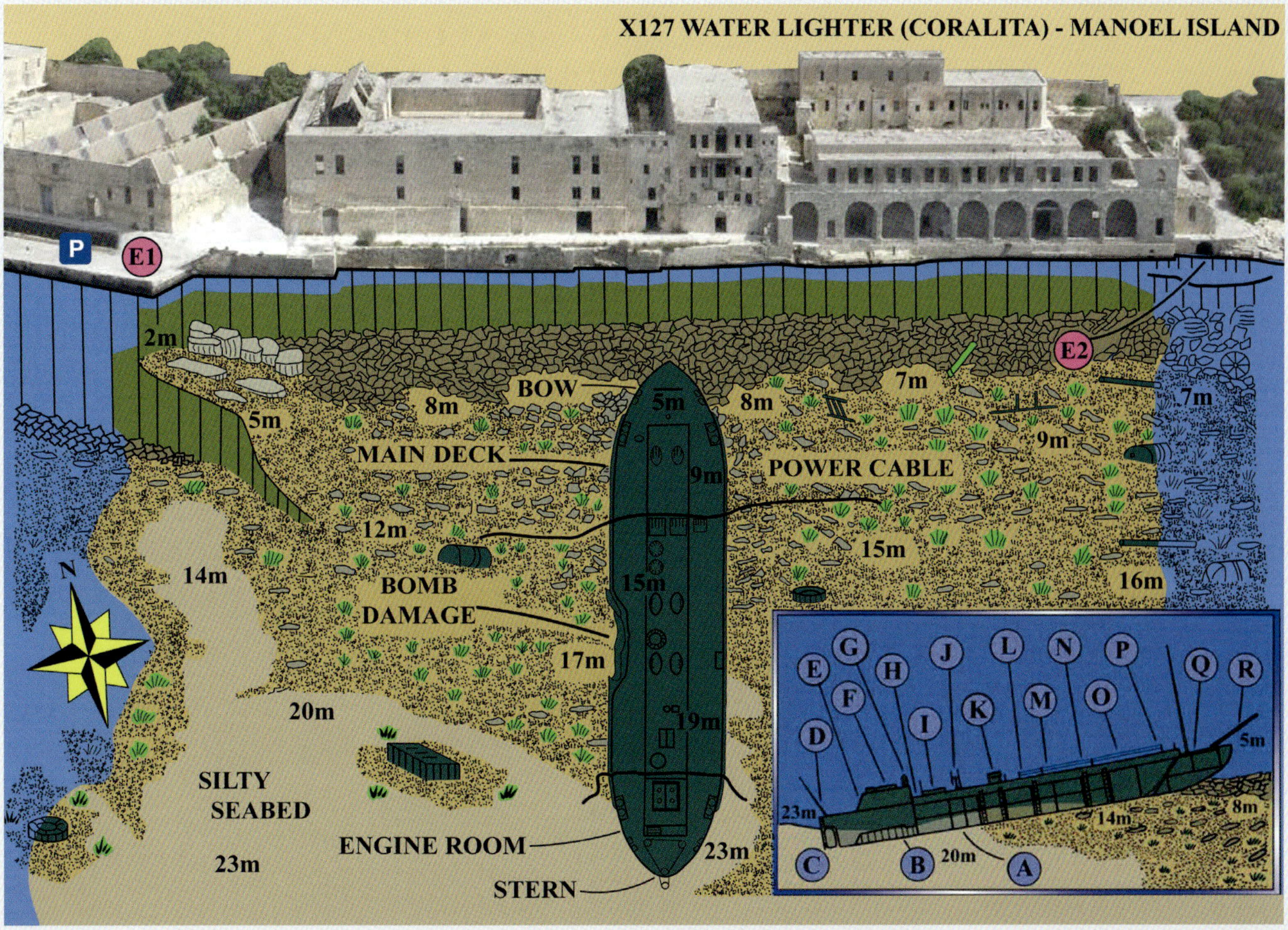

X127 WATER LIGHTER (CORALITA) - MANOEL ISLAND

BOW
MAIN DECK
POWER CABLE
BOMB DAMAGE
SILTY SEABED
ENGINE ROOM
STERN

2m, 8m, 5m, 8m, 7m, 7m, 5m, 9m, 9m, 12m, 15m, 16m, 14m, 15m, 17m, 20m, 19m, 23m, 23m

5m, 14m, 8m, 23m, 20m

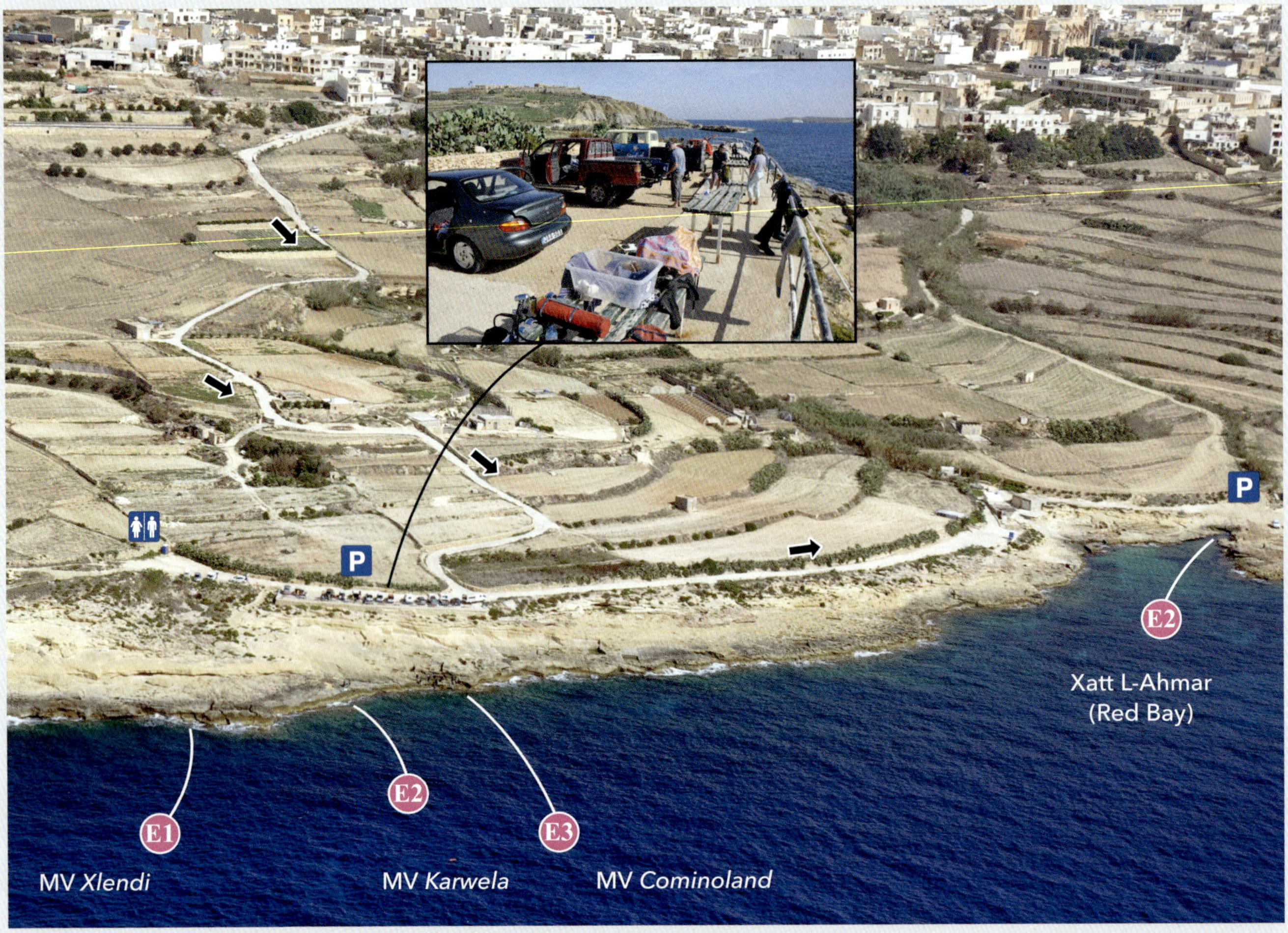

GHANJSIELEM TO XATT L-AHMAR (RED BAY)

Photo: PGL Aerial Photos

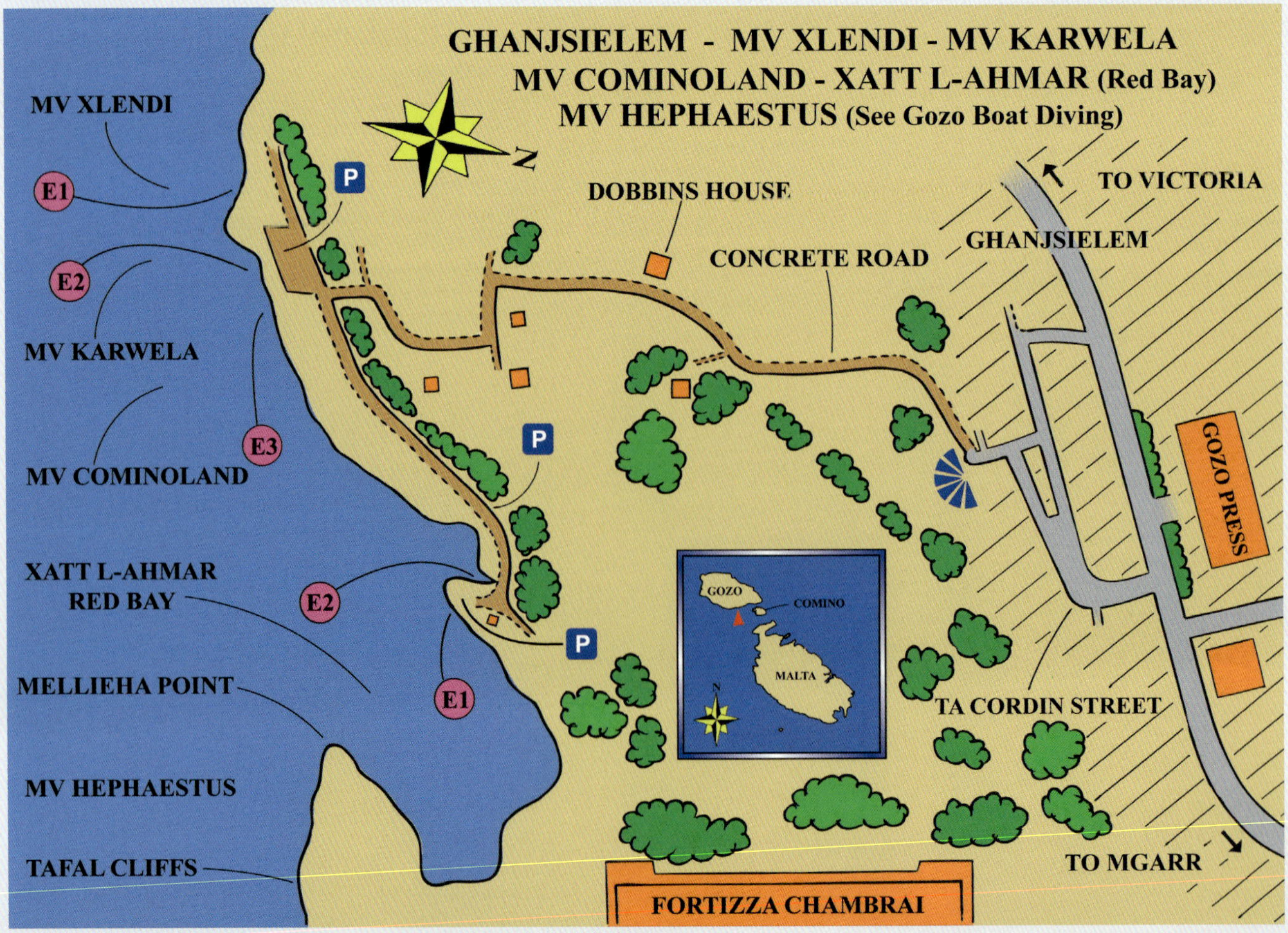

- MV Xlendi — E1
- MV Karwela — E2
- MV Cominoland — E3
- Xatt L-Ahmar (Red Bay) — E2

GHANJSIELEM - MV XLENDI - MV KARWELA
MV COMINOLAND - XATT L-AHMAR (Red Bay)
MV HEPHAESTUS (See Gozo Boat Diving)

- MV XLENDI — E1
- MV KARWELA — E2
- MV COMINOLAND — E3
- XATT L-AHMAR RED BAY — E2
- MELLIEHA POINT — E1
- MV HEPHAESTUS
- TAFAL CLIFFS

DOBBINS HOUSE
CONCRETE ROAD
TO VICTORIA
GHANJSIELEM
GOZO PRESS
TA CORDIN STREET
TO MGARR
FORTIZZA CHAMBRAI

Xatt L-Ahmar - *MV's Xlendi - Karwela - Cominoland*

At the village of Ghanjsielem, turn off the main road, from Mgarr to Victoria, from here the dive sites are some 800 metres. See my local map to the viewpoint and welcome mosaic. The single concrete track winds it way down to the sea front, here turn right for the MV's *Karwela, Cominoland, Xlendi* and left for Xatt L'Ahmar (Red Bay) see aerial photograph. During the summer a one-way system operates for part of this route. The MV *Hephaestus* is in the Gozo Boat Diving section of this book, as I consider it to be a boat dive, although it can be done from Xatt L-Ahmar as a shore dive, with good weather conditions, by experienced divers, maybe using a Diver Propulsion Vehicles.

MV Xlendi

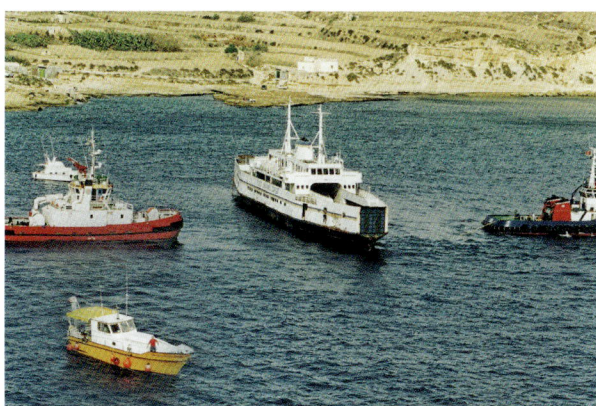

MV Xlendi just before sinking off Xatt L-Ahmar.

This car ferry was built in Denmark by Helsingar, with a gross weight of 1123 tons and a length of 77 metres. On the 12th November 1999, the Gozo ferry boat Xlendi was scuttled off the south coast of Gozo as an artificial reef. Unfortunately, on the way down she struck part of the reef and landed upside down on a sandy seabed at 42m at a slight angle, resting partly on the funnel and the upper structure. After a few days the funnel and the upper structure collapsed and she went totally upside-down, she now lies on a sandy seabed at 42m, with her hull at 36m in depth. The hull is now collapsing inwards due to the weight of the engines now hanging on it.

This is still an excellent dive, with the *Xlendi* and a reef to explore at the end of your dive.

Below: MV Xlendi descending below the waves.

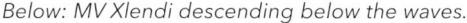
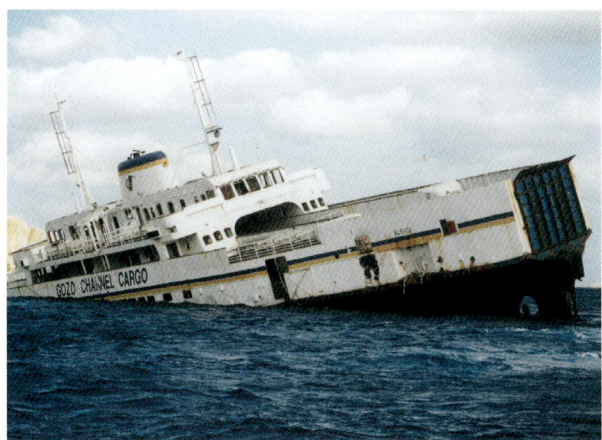

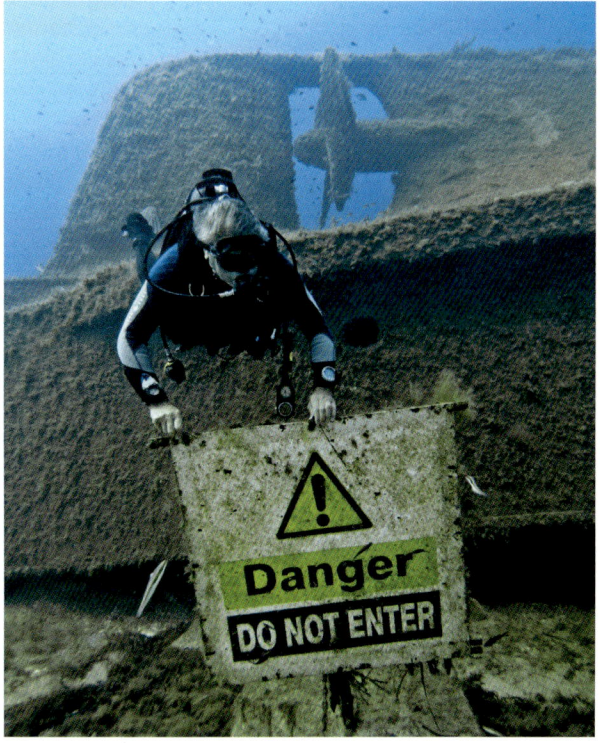

Do NOT enter this wreck, it is prohibited.

Below: This upturned wreck on the sand at 42m plus.

PHOTO: ARKADIUSZ SREBNIK POLANDDIVINGPHOTO

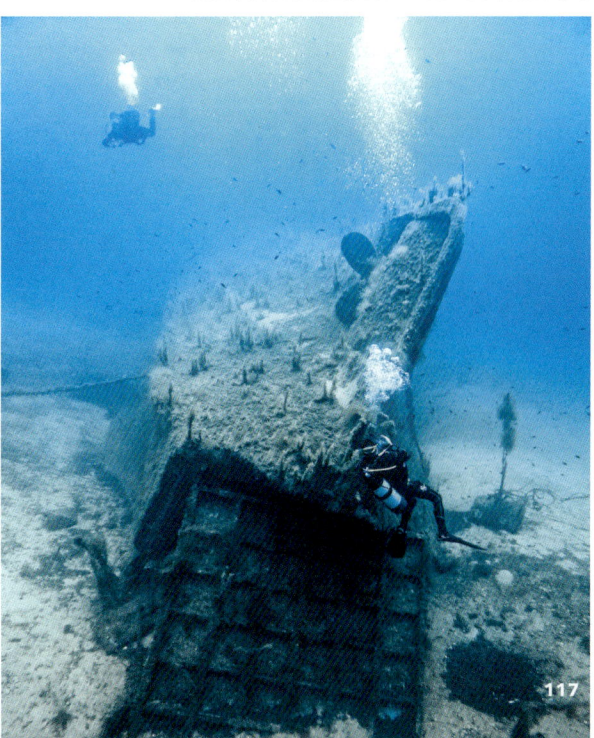

THE DIVE — Minimum time - 45 mins

Check your entry and exit points, for if you decide to use the westerly entry point E1, to exit from here is not possible, you will have to exit from the easterly exit points, E2 or E3. The route to your entry points starts at the westerly end of the car park, down the steps, continue to the water's edge, bear right to E2 and left to E1. If you use E2 once you have entered the water, surface swim round the headland to the other side, below E1. From here your compass bearing to the Xlendi is 200° and approximately 60 metres in distance.

Descend just deep enough to keep the reef in sight. Staying above the reef, will not only help to guide you down to the upturned hull of the wreck, but will also give a better bottom time, this should take you about 4/6 minutes. Follow your dive plan whilst on the wreck, check out the two propellers good for a photo shoot.

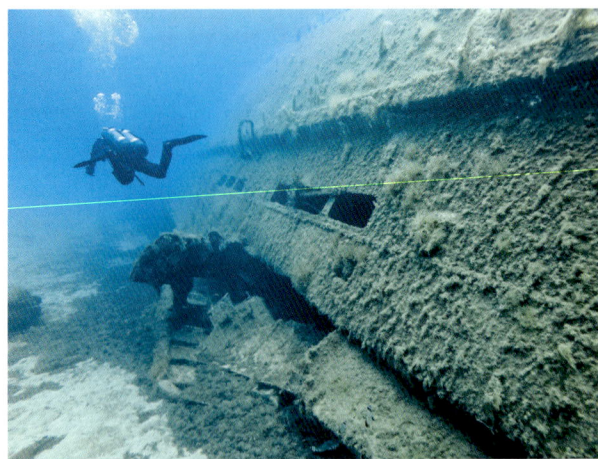
North and reef side of the upturned hull.
PHOTOS: ARKADIUSZ SREBNIK POLANDDIVINGPHOTO
Below: South and seaward side of the hull.

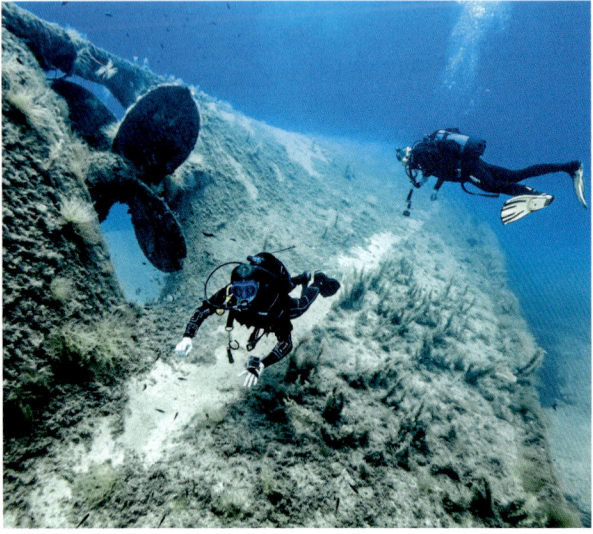
Exploring one of the huge propellers of this ship.
PHOTO: ARKADIUSZ SREBNIK POLANDDIVINGPHOTO

Below: Marine life surrounds the rudder of the ship at 38m.
PHOTO: JON BORG www.jonborg.com

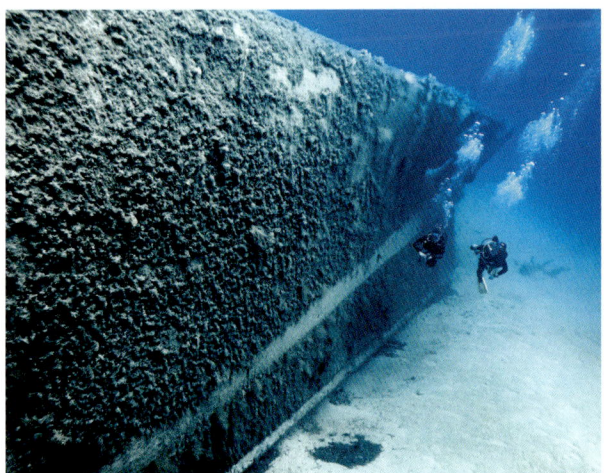

When it is time to leave the wreck do so from the western end as the sandy slope leading to the reef above is much closer. Ascend the reef to your required depth, then follow it in an easterly direction. Were the reef plateau narrows and, on your right, it drops away you will be close to the headland, continue round into a large area of shallower waters depths 6m or less, you are not far from exit points E2 or E3.

BELOW: The Red Mullet have found a new resting place
PHOTO: PETE BULLEN ST ANDREWS DIVE COVE

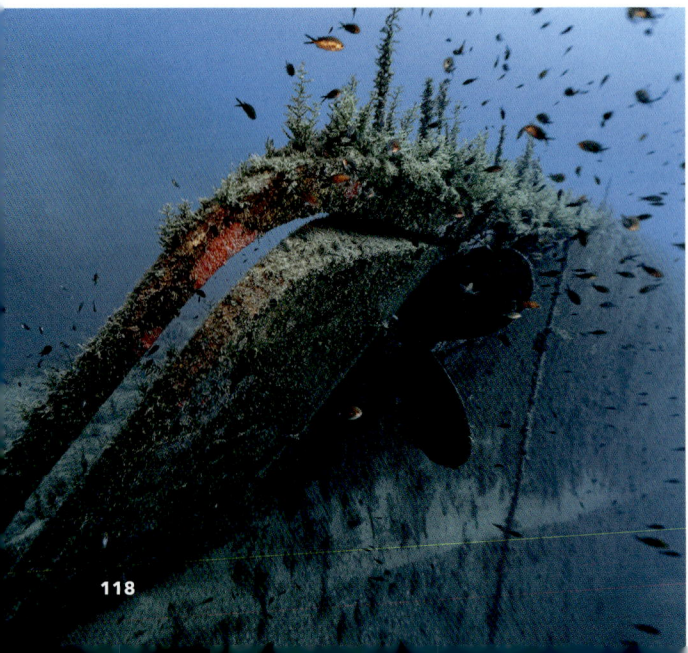

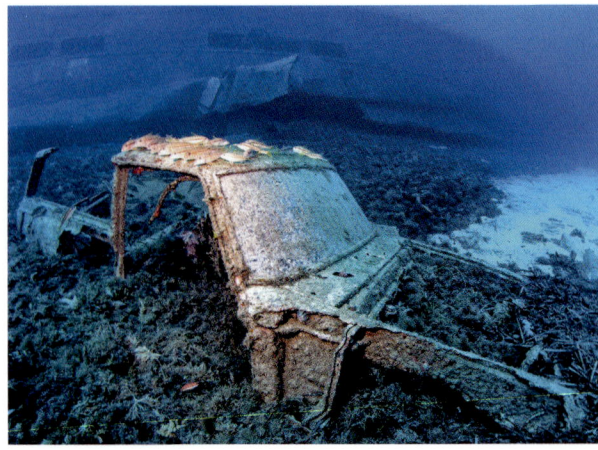

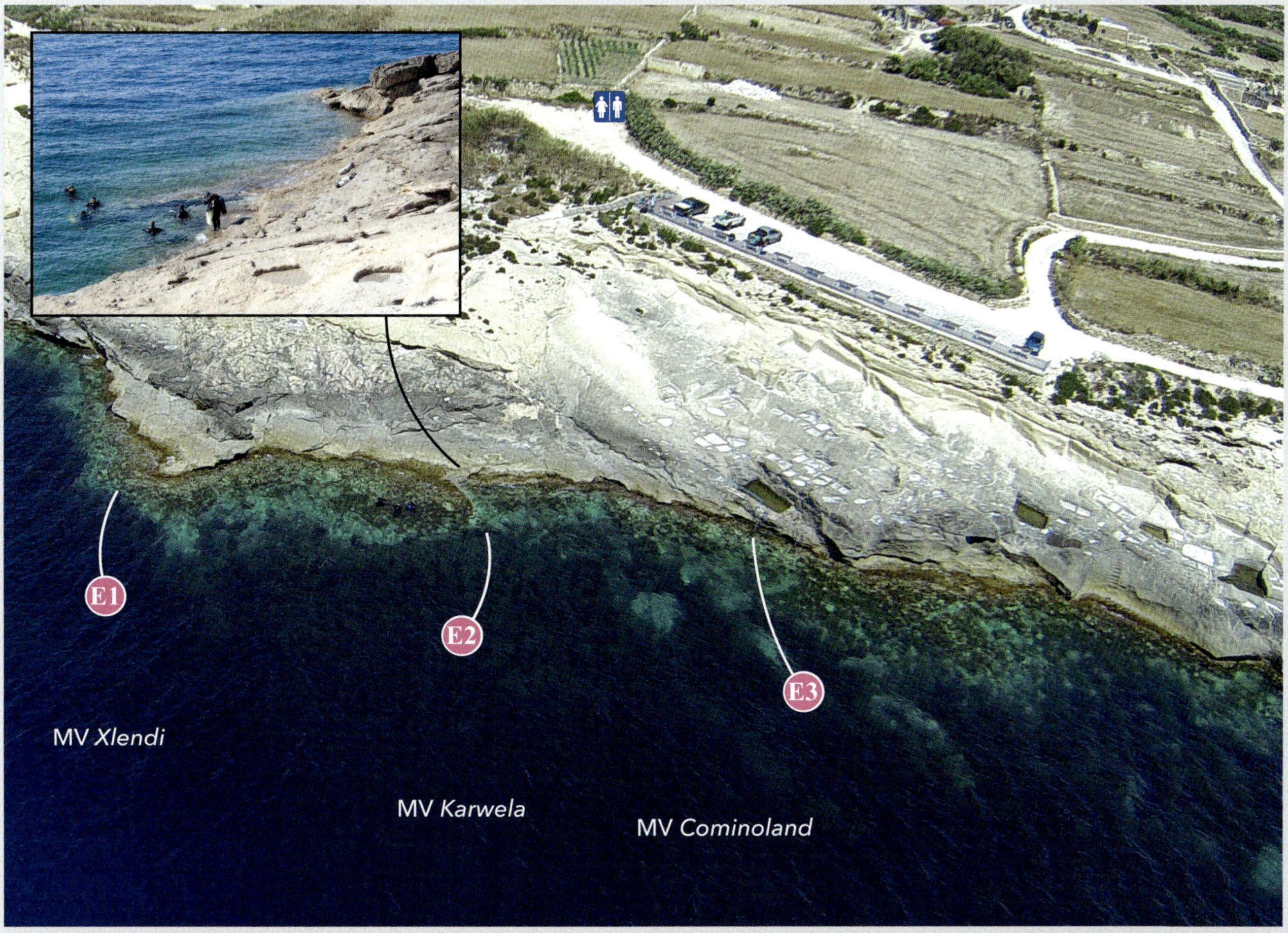

MV *XLENDI* - XATT L-AHMAR

PHOTO: JOE ABDILLA & PAUL GAUCI

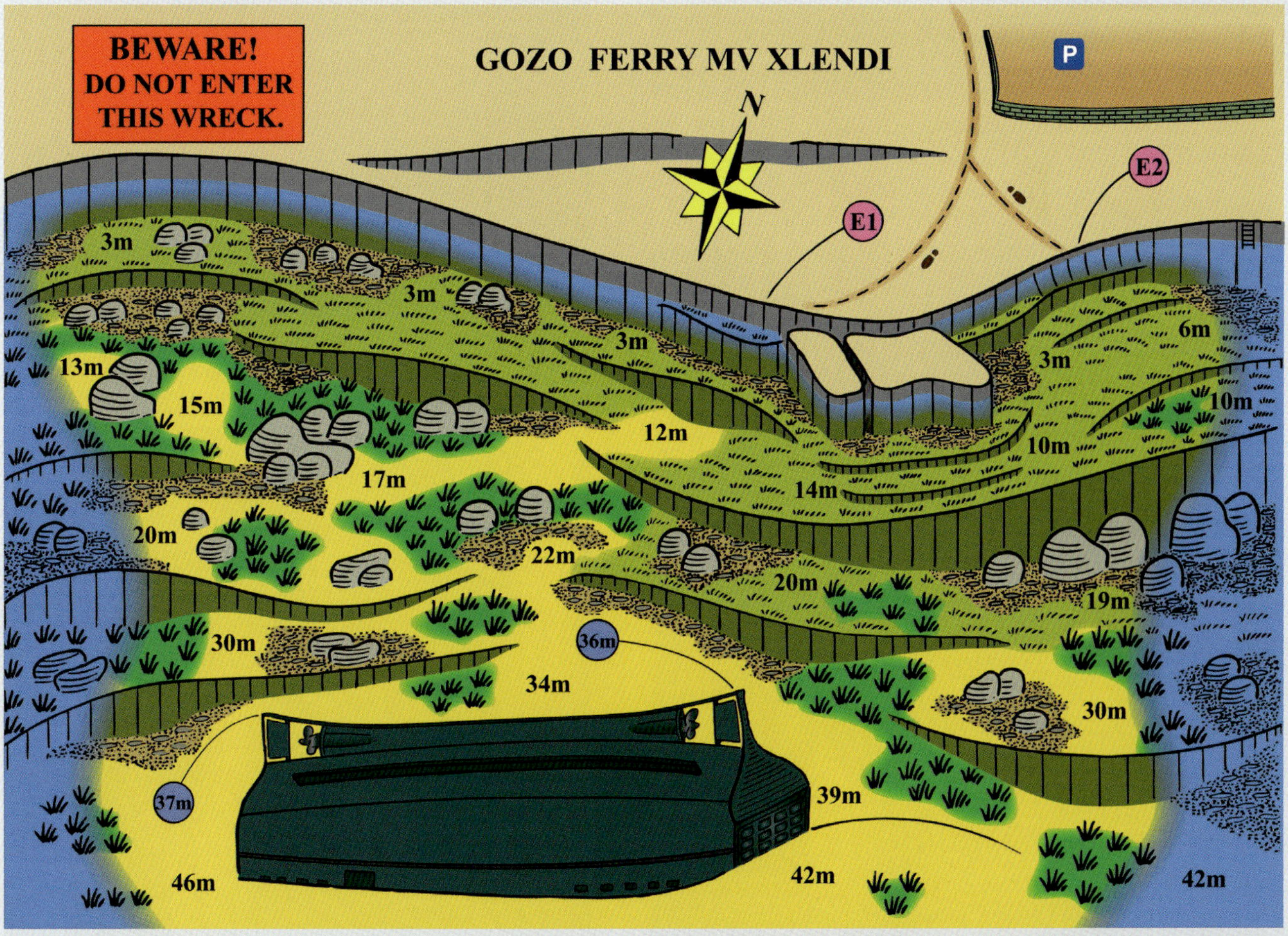

BEWARE! DO NOT ENTER THIS WRECK.

GOZO FERRY MV XLENDI

The scuttling of the two ships
MV *Karwela* & MV *Cominoland*

After being made environmentally safe, on the 12th August 2006 MV *Karwela* and *Cominoland* were towed out of Marsa dockyard. It took over seven hours to reach Gozo. The *Karwela* was sunk at 1600 hrs followed by the *Cominoland* 25 minutes later. With their air-filled blue buoyancy tanks, they sank below the waves and now they both sit upright on the sandy seabed at 42m, some 60 metres apart and in my opinion due to their depths they are separate dives.

MV Karwela

MV *Karwela* was built in West Germany in 1957 by J. L. Meyer of Pepenburg. This passenger ferry has a steel hull, weighs 497 tons, 48 metres in length with a beam of 8 metres. She was first registered in Malta in 1986 and in 1992 she was purchased by Captain Morgan Cruises Malta.

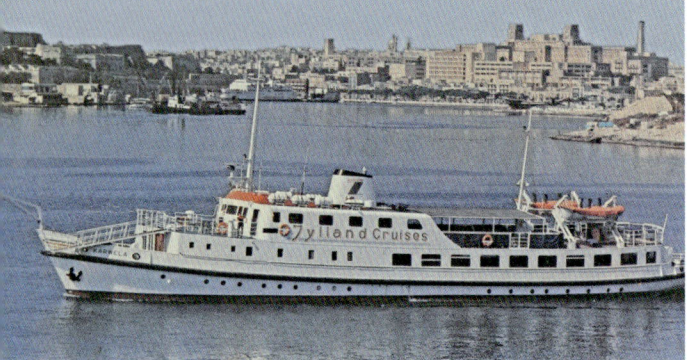

MV Karwela in Marsamxett Harbour in 1900.
PHOTO: GEORGE BRIFFA CAPTAIN MORGAN CRUSIES

Below: A photo by the ships name near the bow.

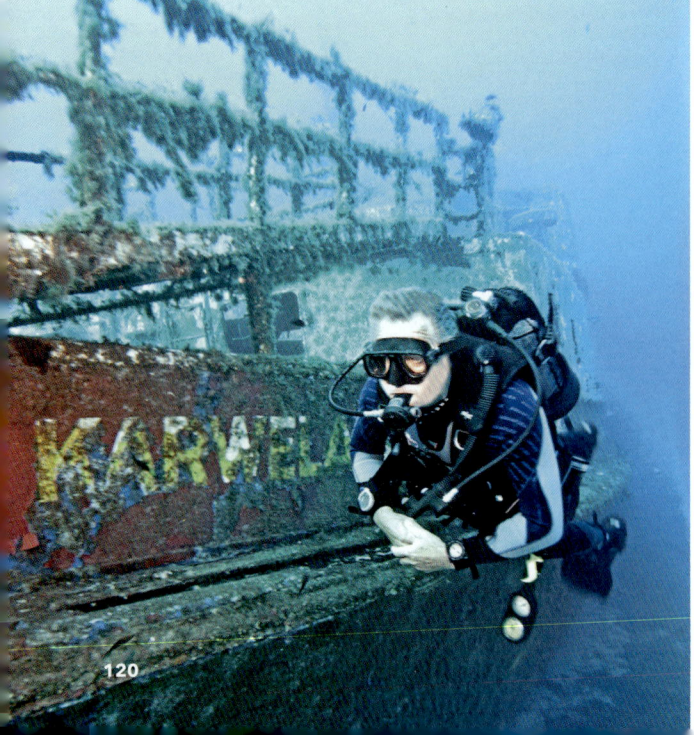

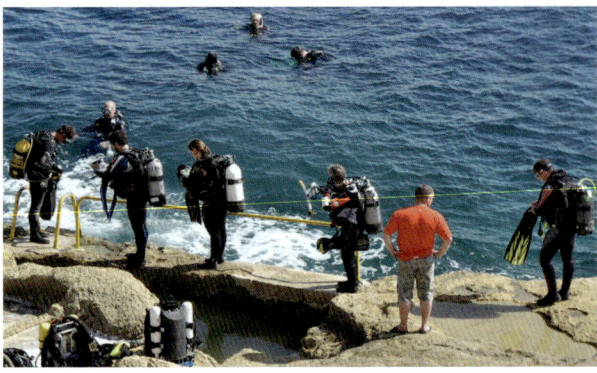

Divers at entry point E3, if no steps exit at E2.

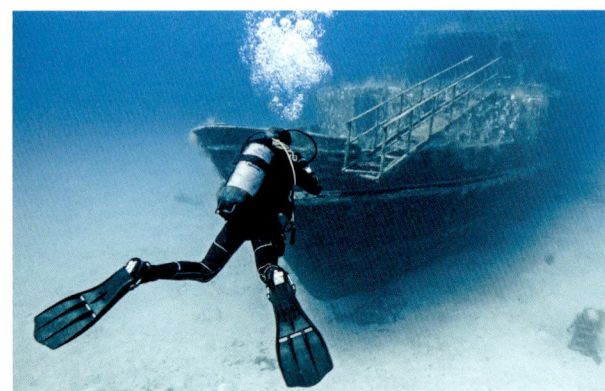

First sighting of the MV Karwela's bows.
PHOTO: ARKADIUSZ SREBNIK POLANDDIVINGPHOTO

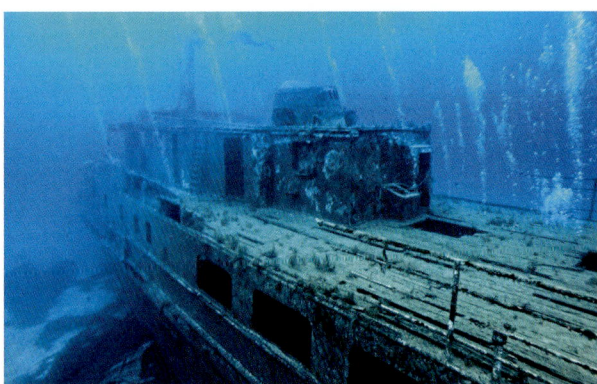

The Port side and main deck of this cruise ship.
PHOTOS: ARKADIUSZ SREBNIK POLANDDIVINGPHOTO

Below: Heading towards the stern of the ship.

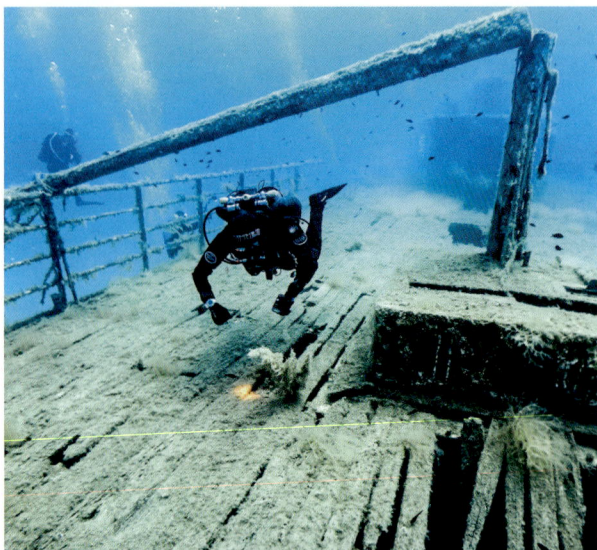

MV KARWELA - XATT L-AHMAR

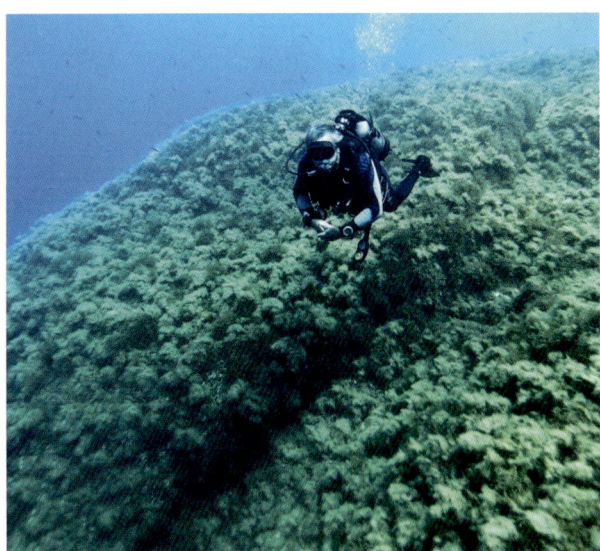
The crack that runs down to the bottom of the reef.

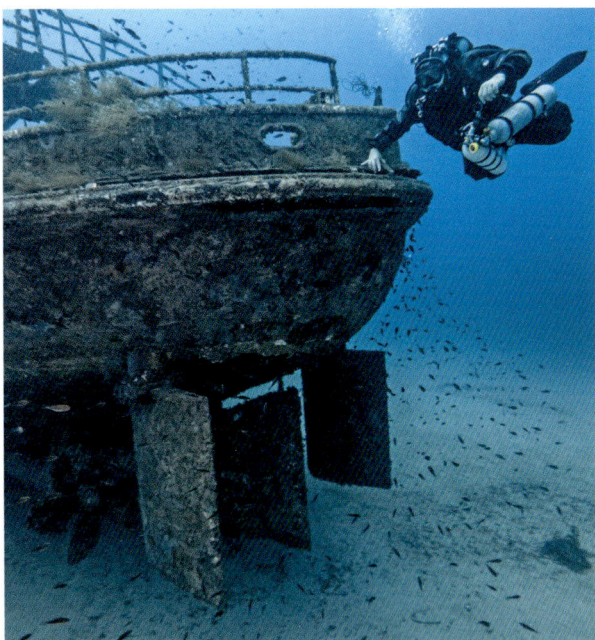
The rudders and propellers of the MV Karwela.
PHOTO: ARKADIUSZ SREBNIK POLANDDIVINGPHOTO

THE DIVE — Minimum time - 40 mins

Using entry points E2 or E3, now surface swim to the east side of the little headland, follow the underwater reef out with a compass bearing of 160° to the drop off, when you can see this drop off, descend to 9m. Now follow the ridge in an easterly direction until you reach the Finger, on your right, there is a crack in the reef which runs down towards sea bed. From this point take a compass bearing of 150° slowly descending to the *Karwela*, the distance from the Finger to the *Karwela* is approximately 40 metres, you will approach her slightly side on.

Explore the wreck and when it is time to leave, head in a northerly direction towards the top of the reef. Take your time to explore the areas of boulders and gullies where the marine life live, whilst doing your safety stop. Work your way in a north westerly direction towards your exit point either E2 or E3.

Below: Above the bridge and forward deck.
PHOTO: ARKADIUSZ SREBNIK POLANDDIVINGPHOTO

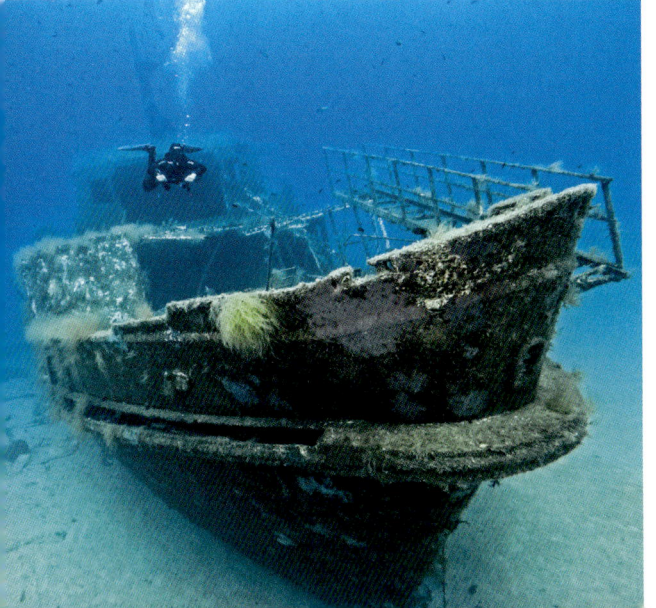

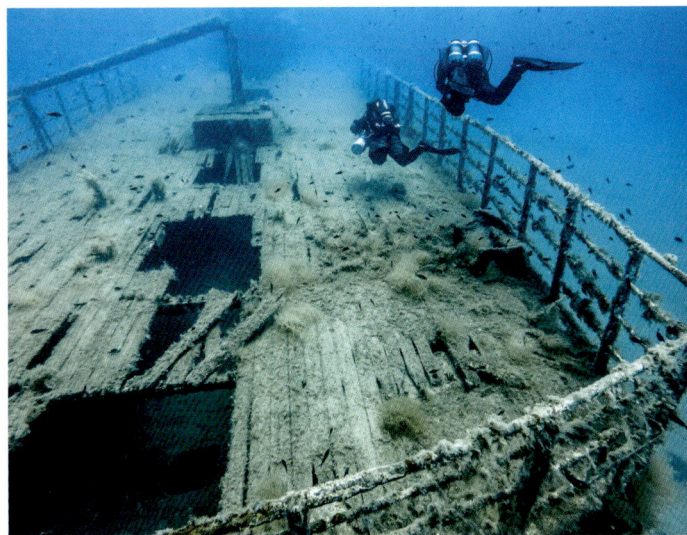
Divers heading away from the stern over the top deck.
PHOTOS: ARKADIUSZ SREBNIK POLANDDIVINGPHOTO
Below: The main staircase to the lower decks.

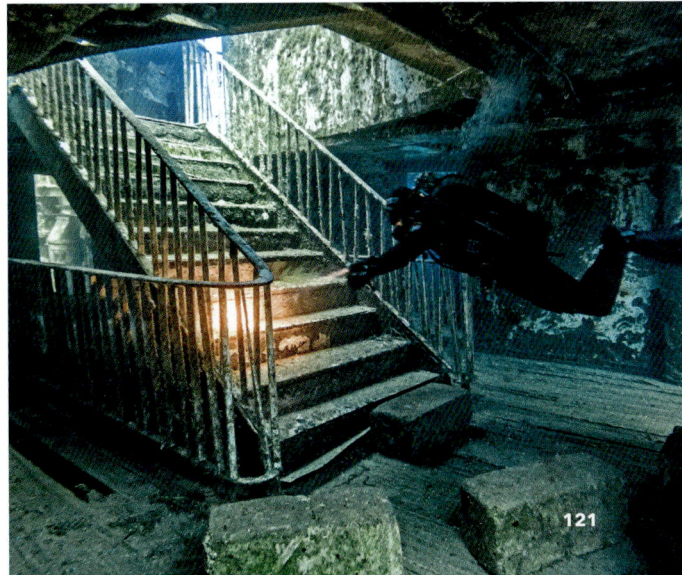

MV Cominoland

Built in Dartmouth England in 1942 by Philip & Son Ltd for the Royal Navy as a minelayer 295-ton ship 34 metres in length and a 8 metre beam. Registered in Malta in 1966 as *Miner Eagle*, in 1976 re-named *Cominoland*, 1980 re-named *Jylland*, purchased by Captain Morgan Cruises, Malta in 1982 and re-named the *Cominoland*.

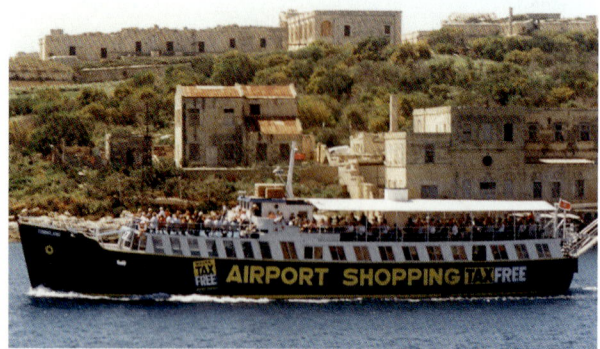

MV Cominoland near Manoel Island in her working days.
PHOTO: GEORGE BRIFFA CAPTAIN MORGAN CRUSIES

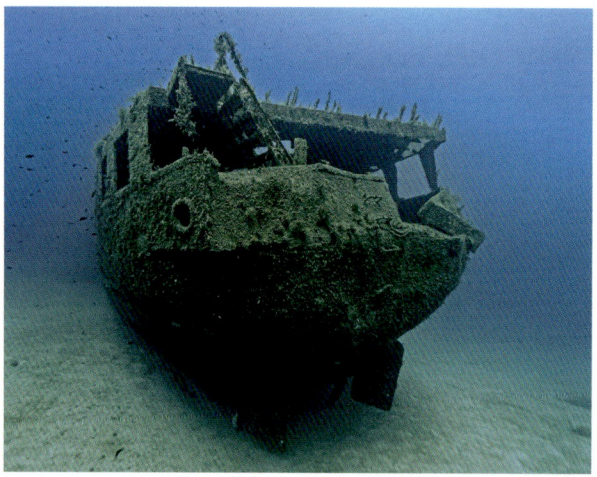

A view of the stern of the MV Cominoland at 42m.
PHOTOS: JON BORG www.jonborg.com
Below: The bow and bridge of the MV Cominoland.

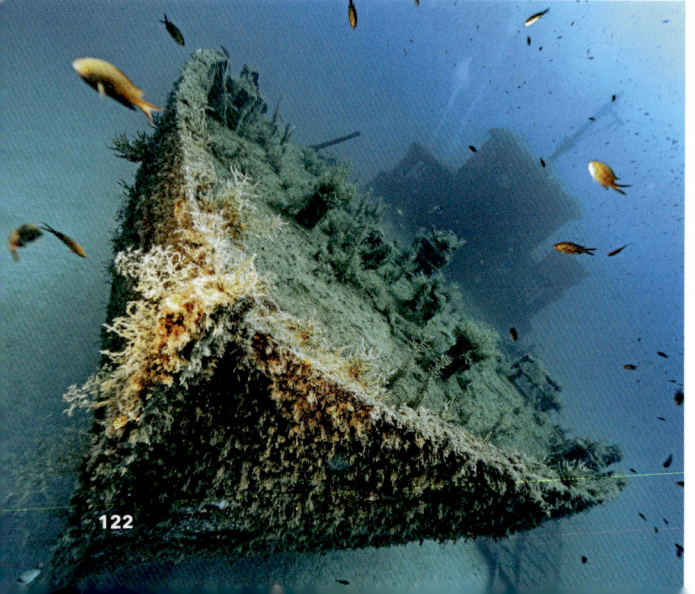

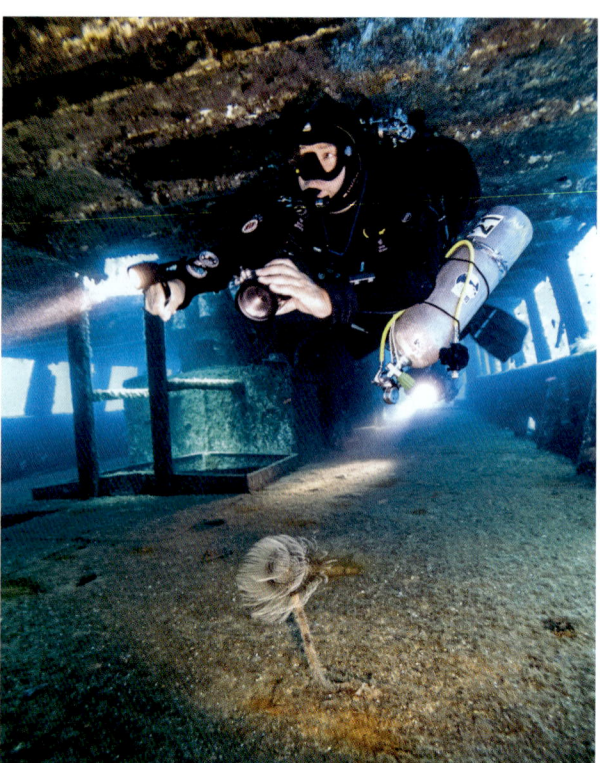

Exploring the inside passenger area of this cruise ship.
PHOTOS: ARKADIUSZ SREBNIK POLANDDIVINGPHOTO

THE DIVE — Minimum time - 45 mins

Using entry points E2 or E3 and once in the water surface swim out heading in a south-easterly direction. While you are still able to see the seabed descend and continue on your course until you come to the edge of the drop off. Follow it along in an easterly direction past the Altar stone to the area of boulders, here you need to descend to the top of the drop off at 25m move on with a compass bearing of 150° towards the *Cominoland* it lies side on to the shore so finding it should be no problem, this should take about 8 minutes into your dive. When it's time to leave the wreck and to return to the reef, **you have two choices.**

Choice 1 from the wreck head north towards the reef, once there stay on your course until you reach your safety stop depth, now turn and head in a westerly direction, this will lead you to an area below your exit points E2 and E3 with depths of 6m and less.

Choice 2 if you wish to return to your exit point via a different route and you have the air then try this, only if the visibility is good and there are no currents. Leave the bows of the *Cominoland* head in a westerly direction 270° slowly ascending whilst moving forward, after you have passed over the *Karwela's* bows, take a bearing of 330° to the top of the Finger, 9m. The distance you have travelled will be 100 metres and will possibly take you 10 minutes to reach this depth. Now head north into a large shallow area of small gullies and short marine growth, where you can explore close to your exit points, E2 and E3 with depths of 6m and less.

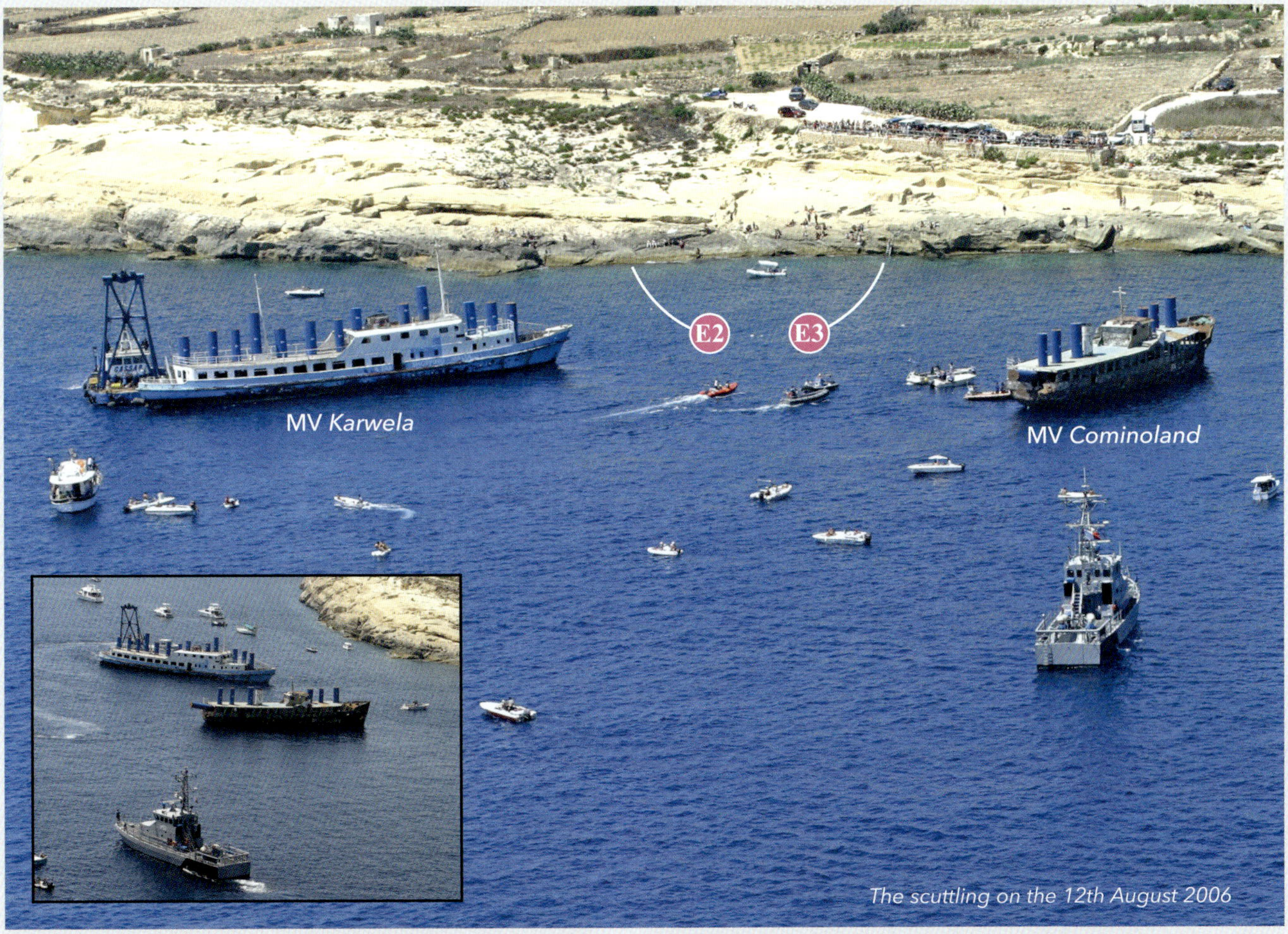

MV KARWELA - MV COMINOLAND - XATT L-AHMAR

The scuttling on the 12th August 2006

PHOTO: PGL AERIAL PHOTOS

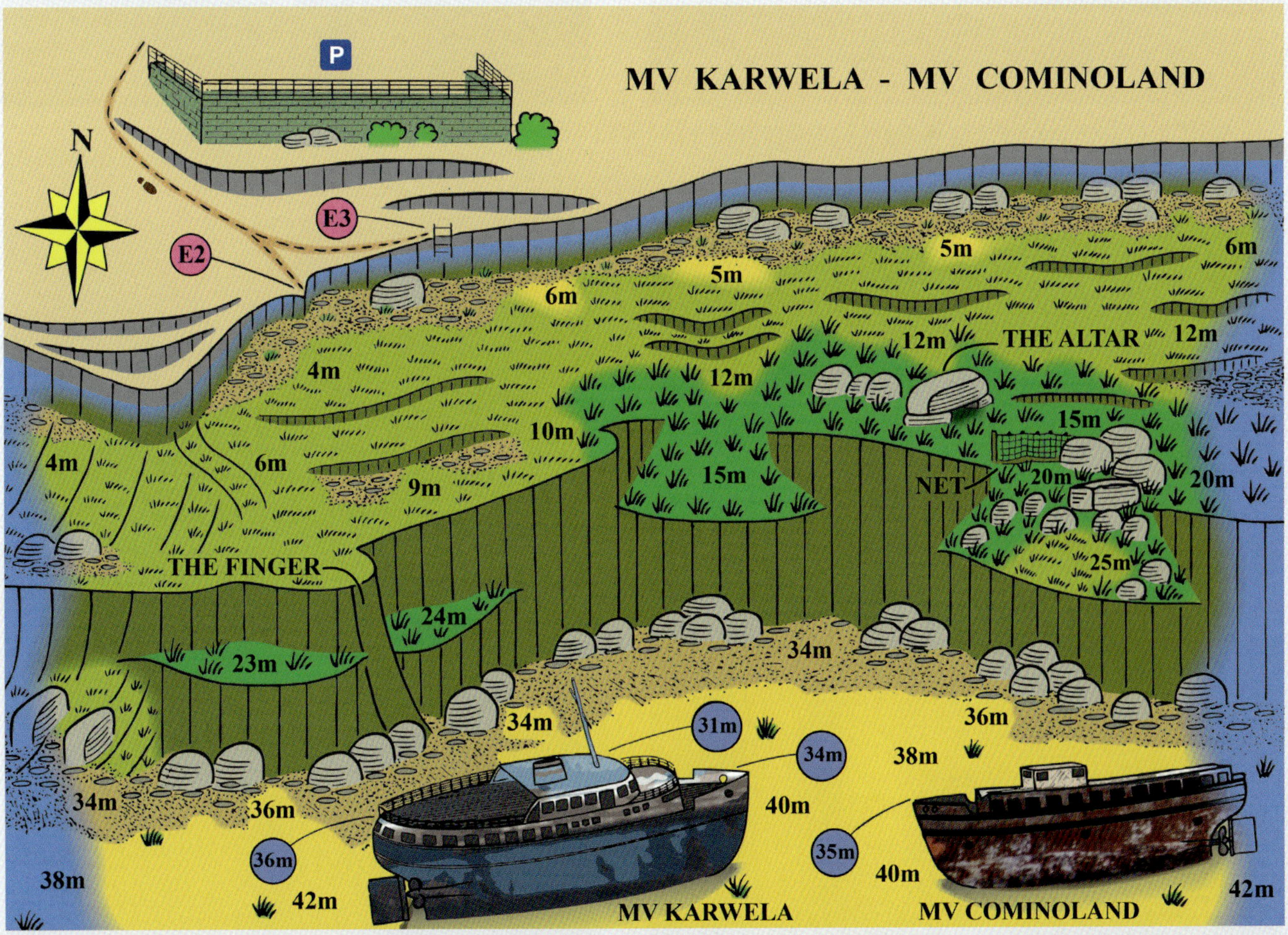

Xatt L-Ahmar (Red Bay)

There are two entry/exit points for this dive site E1 and E2. There are a number of ways to dive this site, I have selected one, but of course you can plan your own dive.

THE DIVE — Minimum time - 50 mins

From entry point E1 on a south westerly bearing surface swim across the bay to the headland on the other side, this will take 8/10 minutes. Pass over the little reef at the end of the headland and descend on the other side to 6/9m then head south over the Posidonia grass to the edge of the drop-off, at 24m, now descend to the sea bed at 35m your dive time should be 8/10 minutes.

Now head west along the bottom of the drop off exploring as you go keeping the reef on your right. Within 2 minutes you will reach the overhang, check out the sponges, corals and marine life. Moving on to the small cave with its sandy bottom, just 3 minutes away. From this point you can head away from the reef and descend to the large boulder at 40m looking out into the blue for passing shoals of amberjacks, barracuda and other marine life. Return to the reef your dive time should be 15/20 minutes.

Keep an eye on your deco, here you can ascend the reef to your required depth or continue along its base, both will lead you towards a gentle sloping reef, with small boulders surrounded by posidonia grass. Continue up the sloping reef, once at the top take a bearing of 20° when you reach a depth of 8/9m your dive time could be 27/30 minutes. Here you can explore the gullies and boulders while doing your safety stop, returning to your exit point E1 or E2. This dive plan of course can be done in reverse.

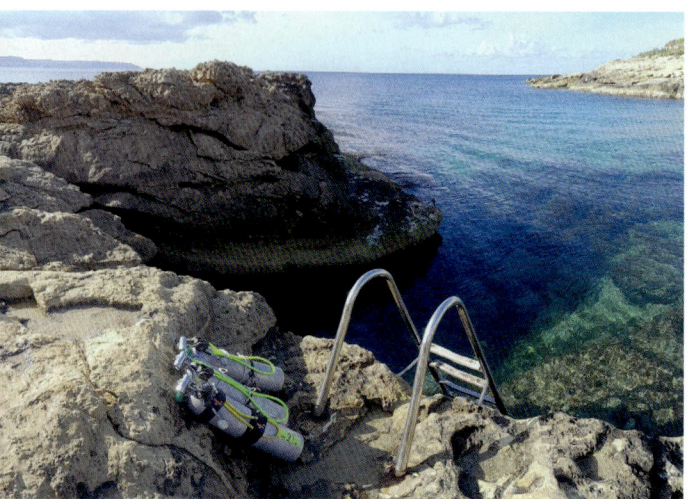

Entry point E2 ok if the ladder is in place, otherwise E1.

Below: Many places to pose for a quality photo.

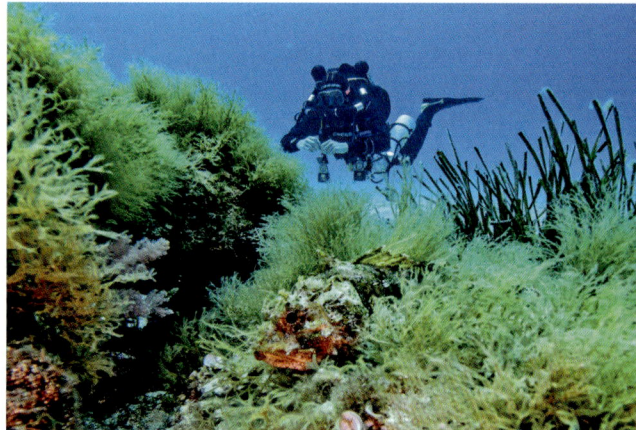

A Scorpion fish almost hidden from the diver.
PHOTO: STEVEN GALICIA www.galicia.be

Below: Many drop-offs surround this small Island.

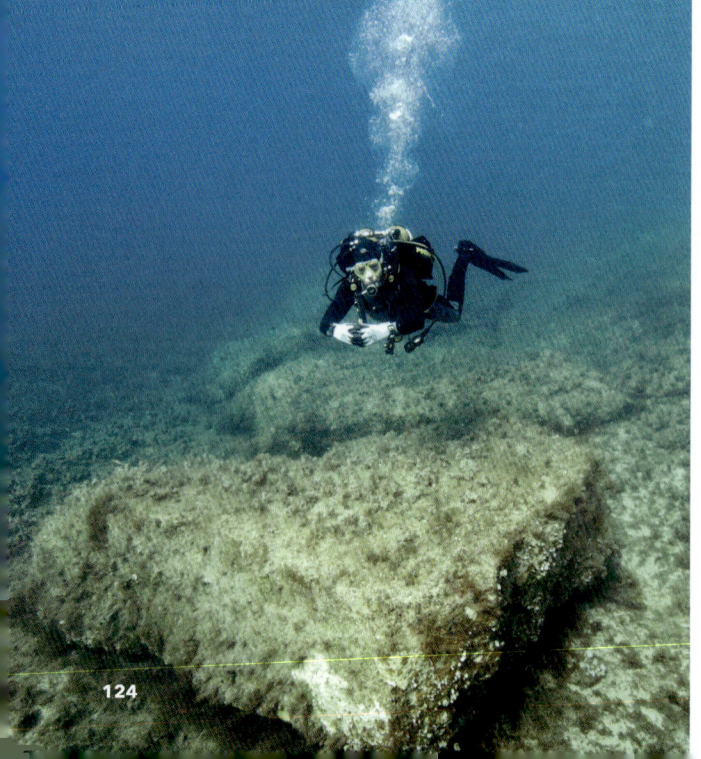

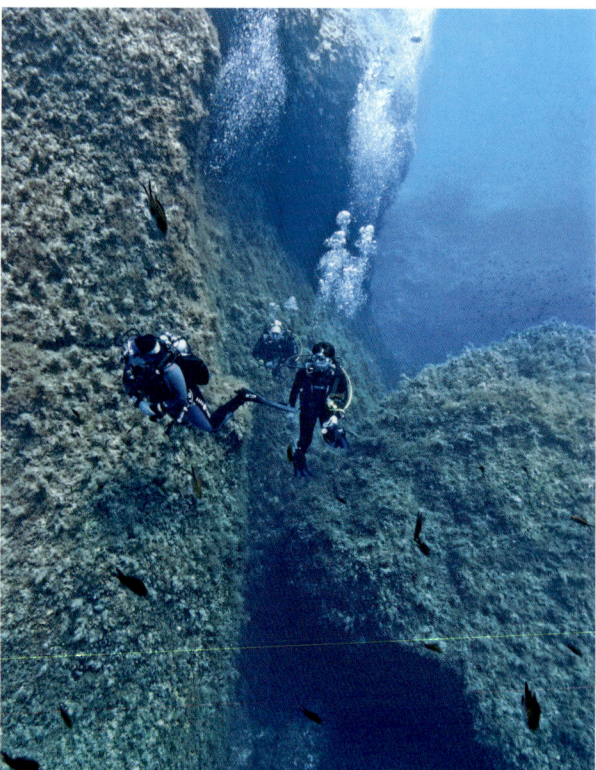

E2
E1
P
Xatt L-Ahmar
(Red Bay)
Mellieha Point
MV *Hephasetus*
PHOTO: MAX VALLI ORANGE SHARK DIVE CENTRE

The MV Hephasetus scuttled off Mellieha Point on the 29th August 2022. For more information on this wreck, go to the Gozo Boat Diving section in this book.

PHOTO: PGL AERIAL PHOTOS

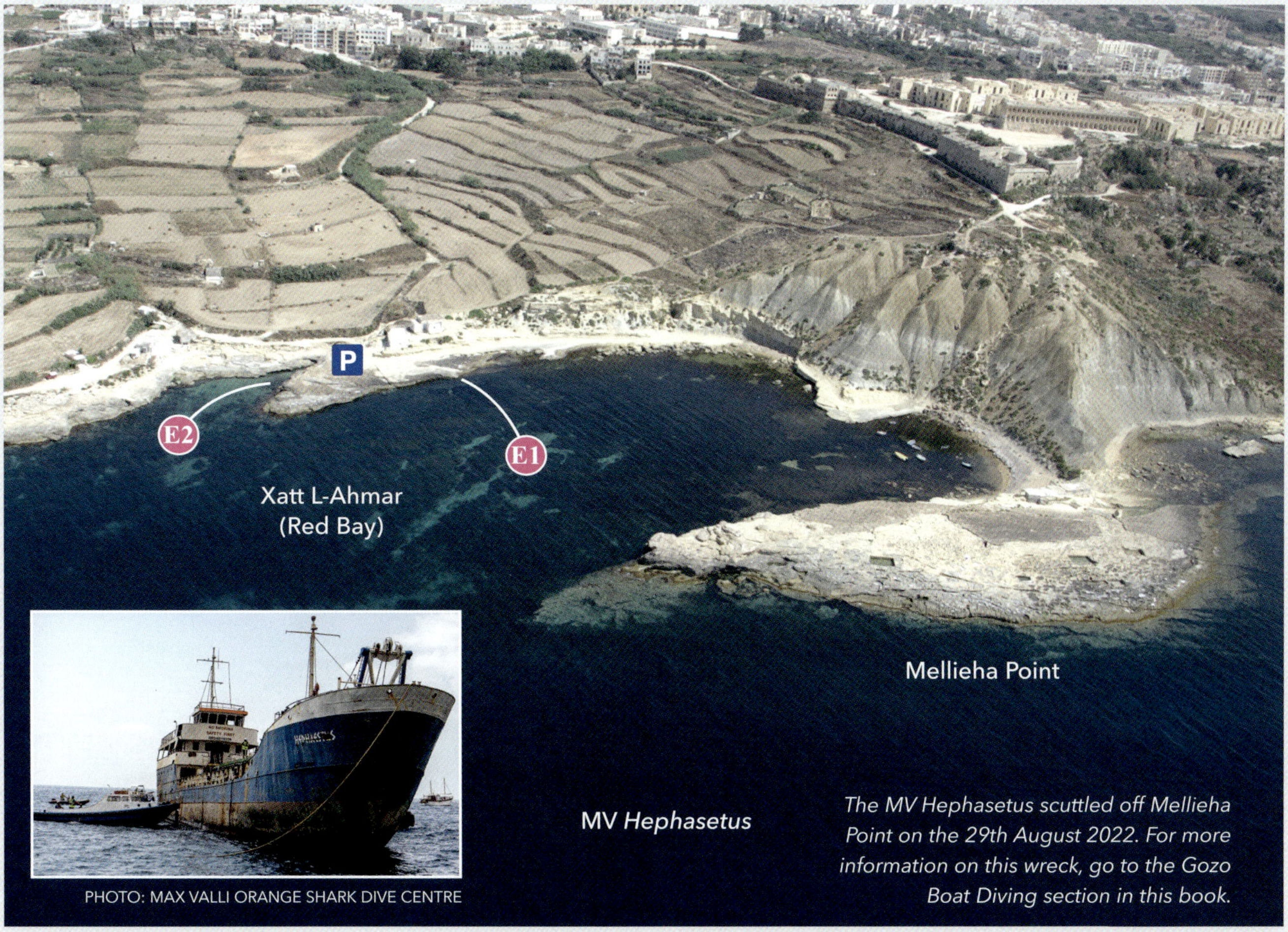

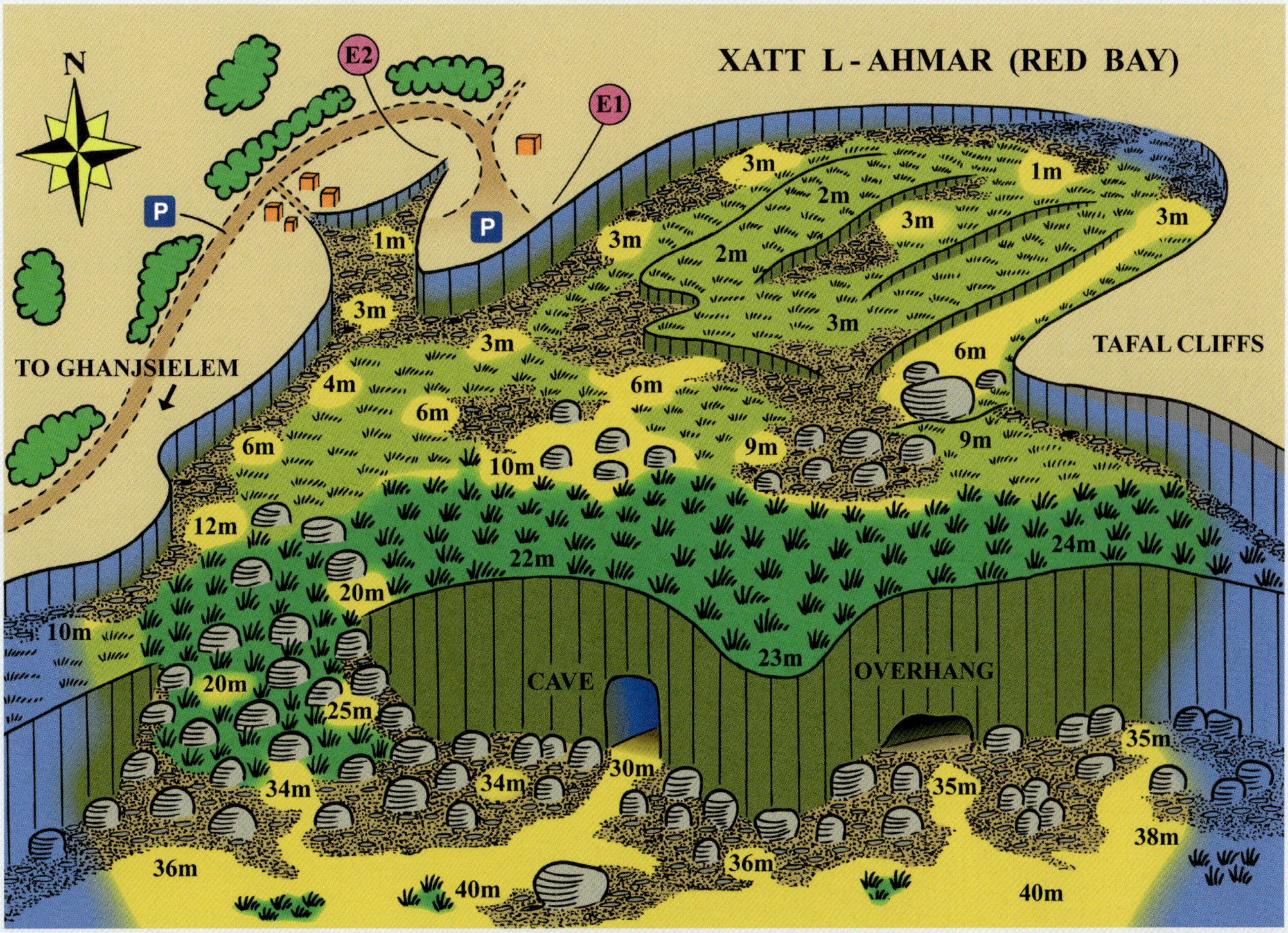
XATT L-AHMAR (RED BAY)
N
E2
E1
P
P
TO GHANJSIELEM
TAFAL CLIFFS
1m
3m
2m
3m
1m
3m
3m
2m
3m
3m
3m
6m
4m
6m
6m
6m
9m
9m
10m
12m
22m
24m
20m
10m
20m
25m
23m
CAVE
OVERHANG
30m
34m
34m
35m
35m
38m
36m
36m
40m
40m

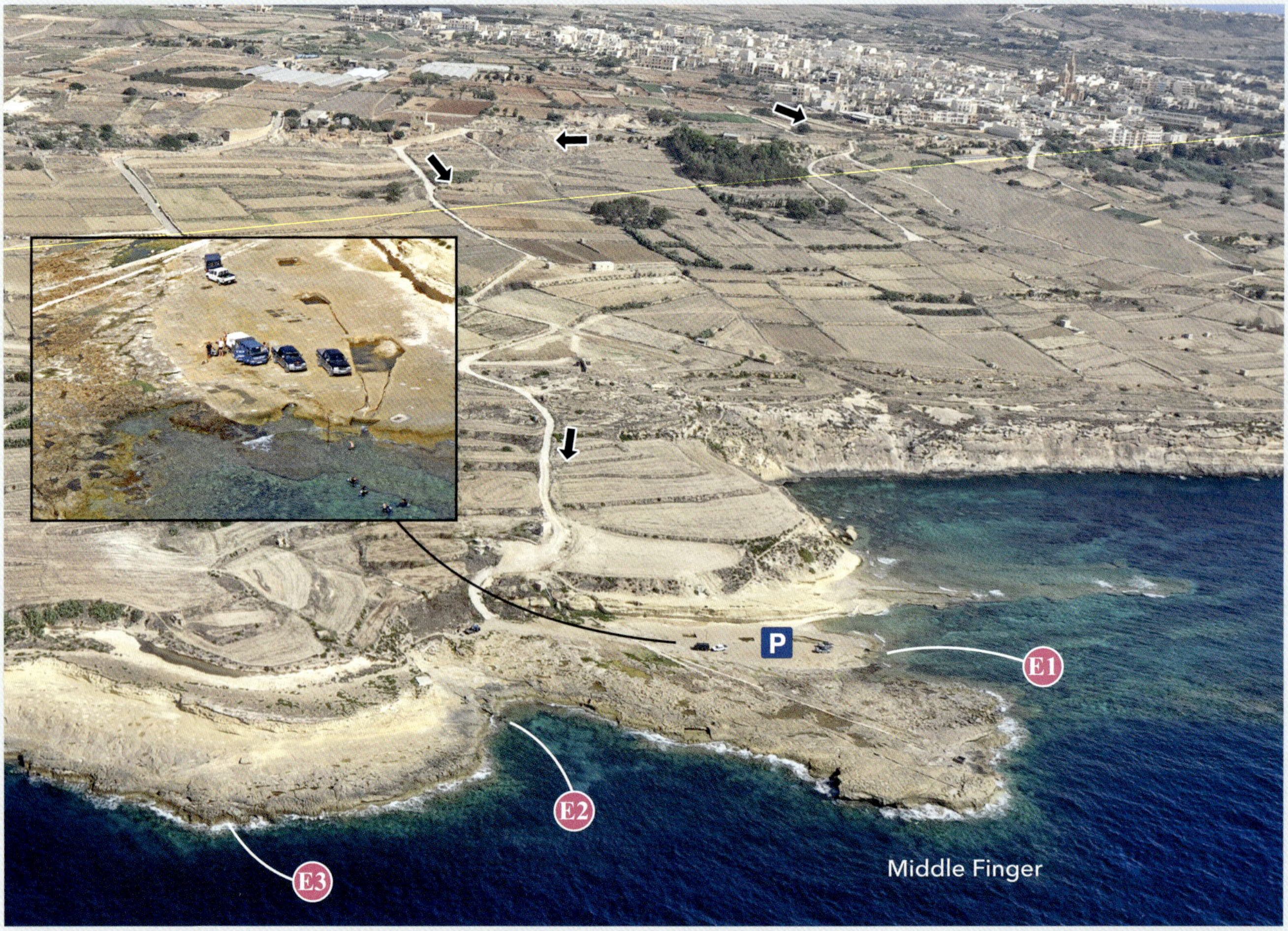

GHANJSIELEM TO RAS IL-HOBZ (MIDDLE FINGER)

PHOTO: PGL AERIAL PHOTOS

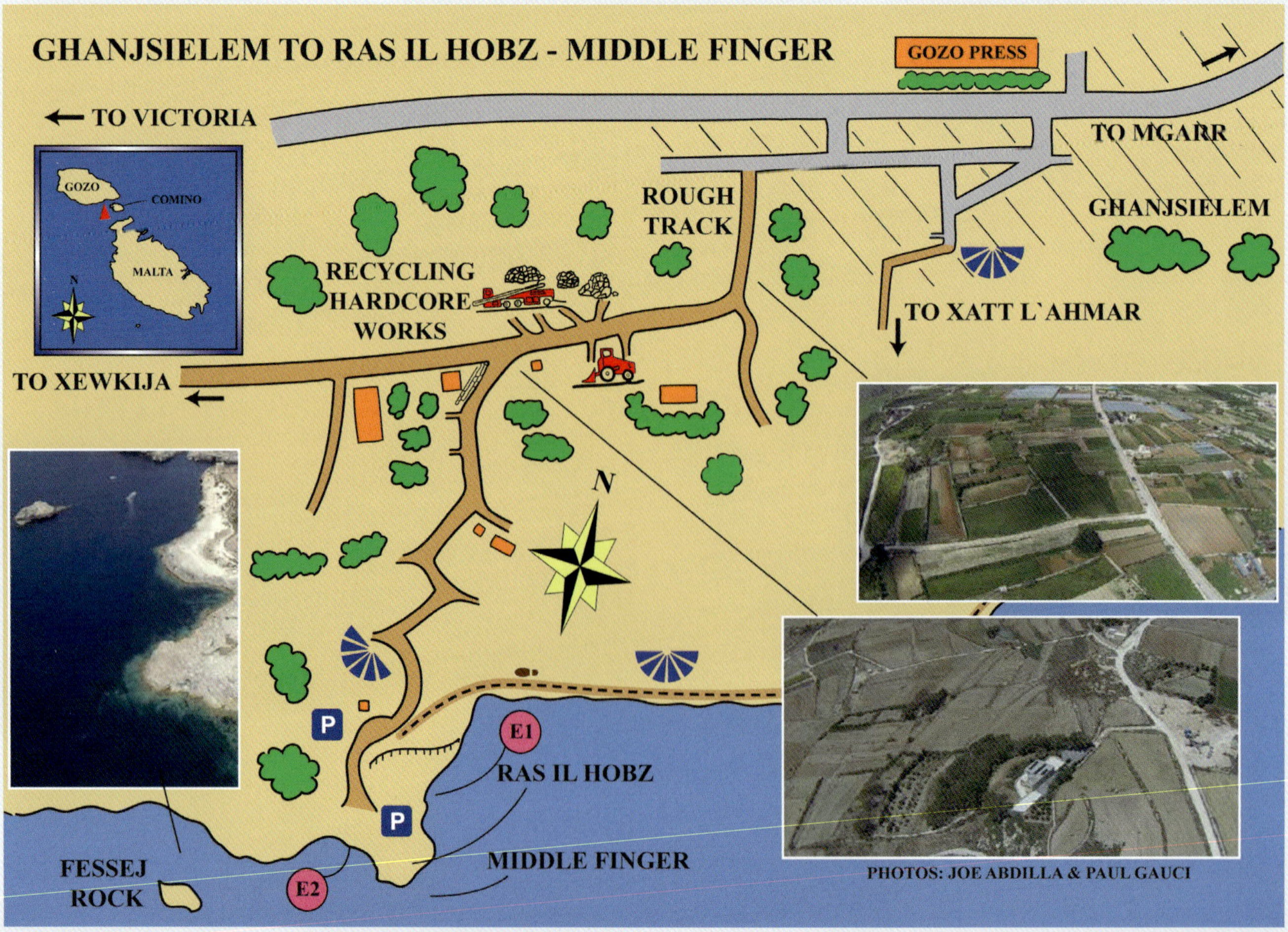

GHANJSIELEM TO RAS IL HOBZ - MIDDLE FINGER

- GOZO PRESS
- TO VICTORIA
- TO MGARR
- GHANJSIELEM
- ROUGH TRACK
- RECYCLING HARDCORE WORKS
- TO XATT L'AHMAR
- TO XEWKIJA
- E1 RAS IL HOBZ
- E2 MIDDLE FINGER
- FESSEJ ROCK

PHOTOS: JOE ABDILLA & PAUL GAUCI

Middle Finger - Ras il-Hobz

Once in Ghanjsielem, turn left if coming from Mgarr, right from Victoria, **see Local Map,** then turn right, next left down a track to Triq Ta-Brieghen, at the bend follow the road round to the right; continue through the rubble recycling area and graveyard for heavy machinery. At the next junction fork left down the hill, on the concrete road. Follow this road until you are just above the parking area. Here there is a short hill down to sea level, may I suggest you check the bottom of this hill for road conditions before taking your vehicle down, unless you have a 4 x 4. The whole distance is approximately 1.5km.

Middle Finger is a unique diving site on the south coast of Gozo and adds to the variety of diving in these Maltese waters. If you gather your fingers together and point them upwards, will give you some idea of the shape of the top of the pinnacles and where it gets its name. They rise up from the seabed to just 9m below the surface and they are only 20 metres from the shore line. The valley between the reef and the shore line, is only 2 metres wide at its narrowest point at a depth of 30m. At the other end, it is 4 metres wide, with a depth of 34m.

To the south western side of the pinnacle out on the sand there is a large anchor at 63m. This is an ideal site for technical diving, for to reach these depths so close to the shore line is not always possible. If your depth is limited, the marine life here is excellent, with shoals of bream, salema fish and bogue to name just a few, these in turn attract fish such as tuna, amberjacks and barracuda. Below 20m you will find a variety of sponges and corals. This is an excellent dive site which I am sure you will enjoy.

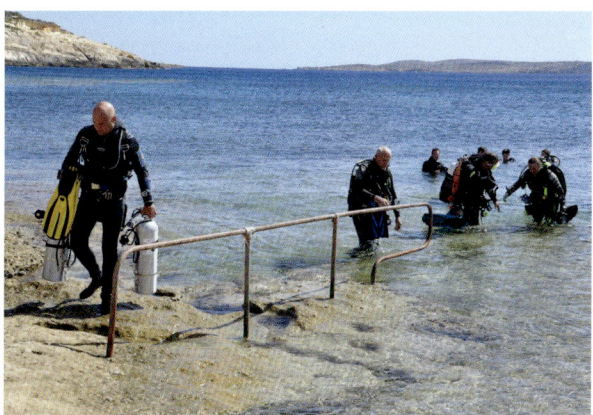

Divers leaving the water at entry exit point E1.

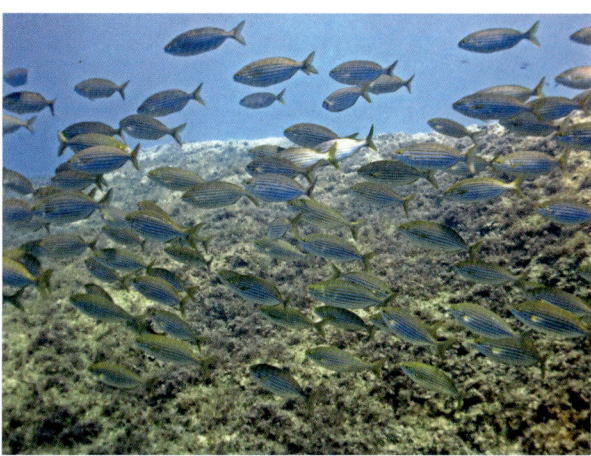

One of the shoals of salema fish around this reef.

Below: The valley between the mainland and pinnacle.
PHOTO: DAVID AGUIS CALYPSO SUB-AQUA CLUB

Below: Divers above the top of the pinnacles at 9m.

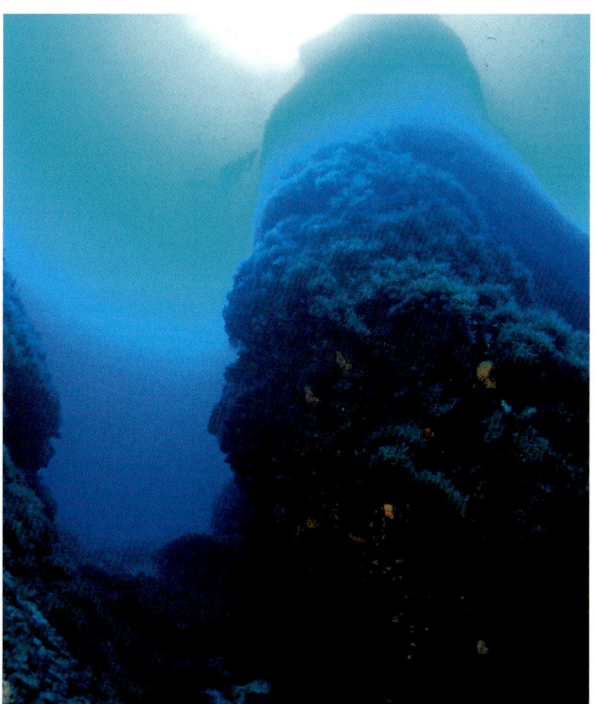

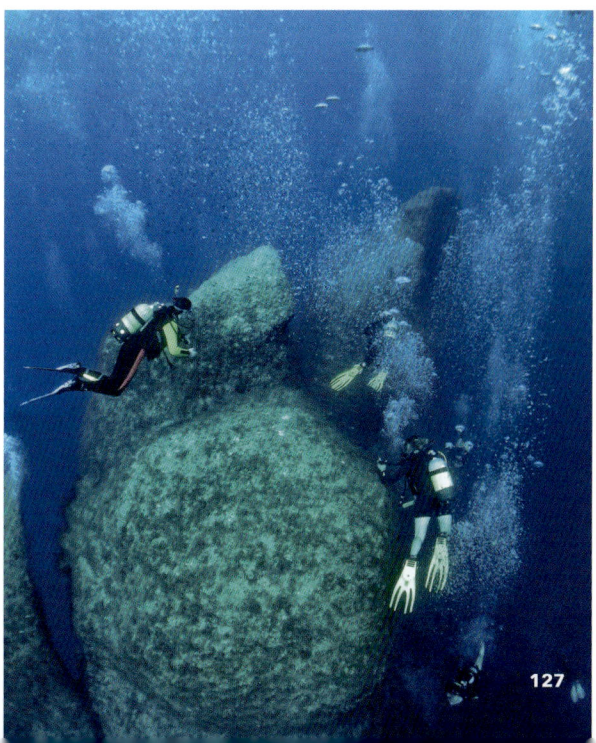

MIDDLE FINGER - RAS IL-HOBZ

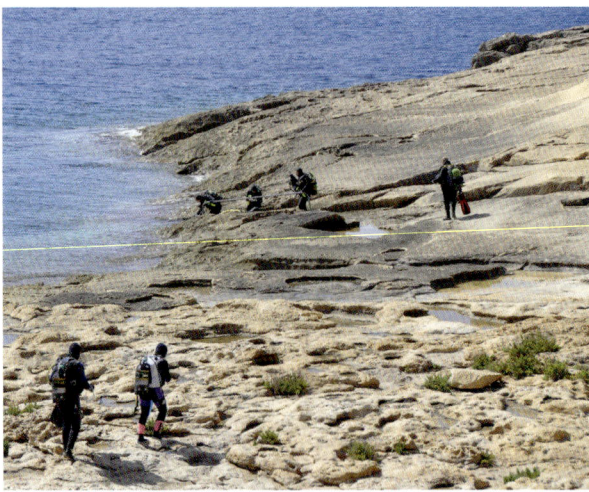

Divers entering the water at entry exit point E2.

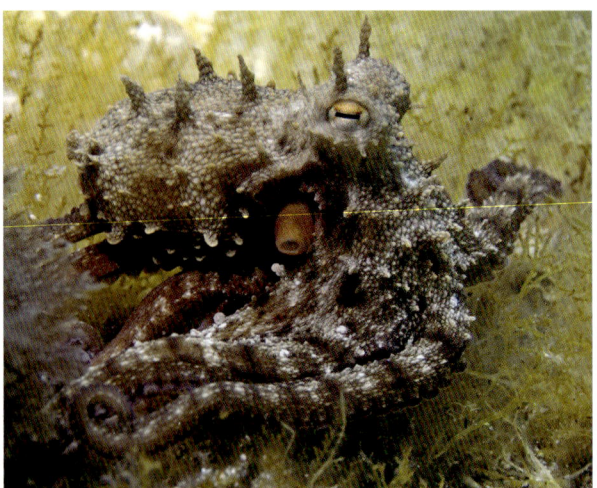

In the shallow waters of this area an octopus out in the open.
PHOTO: SHARON FORDER

THE DIVE — Minimum time - 40 mins

The choice of entry point will probably depend on which side of the sea level area you have parked. Entry point E1 on the eastern side is usually the most popular, maybe due to the larger parking area. In the immediate area of your entry point the reef is only 1 to 2m deep and you will have to go out and around the very shallow areas before heading to the pinnacle. Entry from E2, if you have parked on the western side, here the depth increases reasonably quickly to 5m, but there is not that much difference in distance to the pinnacle, but E1 is slightly shorter.

Your actual dive around the pinnacle will depend on your dive plan and chosen depth, normally ending at the top of Middle Finger: this is an excellent opportunity for a photograph of your buddies at the top of the pinnacles.

Below: A shoal of bogue swim over the pinnacles.

From E1 take a compass bearing of 140° ensuring that you go around the shallow area, once around the shallow reef take a bearing of 230° keeping the main coastline on your right until reaching the drop off. Continue on with the reef on your right at a depth of around 8m, when your compass starts to move towards a westerly direction, move away from shore reef in a southerly direction for some 15 metres and the pinnacle at 9m should come into view.

From E2 follow a compass bearing of 130° keeping the coastline reef on your left, down over a large number of small rocks and boulders until you come to the drop off at 16m, here bear round to the left. If you have decided to swim out at a shallower depth, just keep the main shore line in sight and on your left-hand side. Once your compass bearing starts to give an easterly direction you should be below the headland, move south away from the shore reef, the pinnacle is approximately 15 metres from here.

The huge (3 metres long) anchor at 63m
PHOTO: BRAIN AZZOPARDI ALANTIS DIVING CENTRE

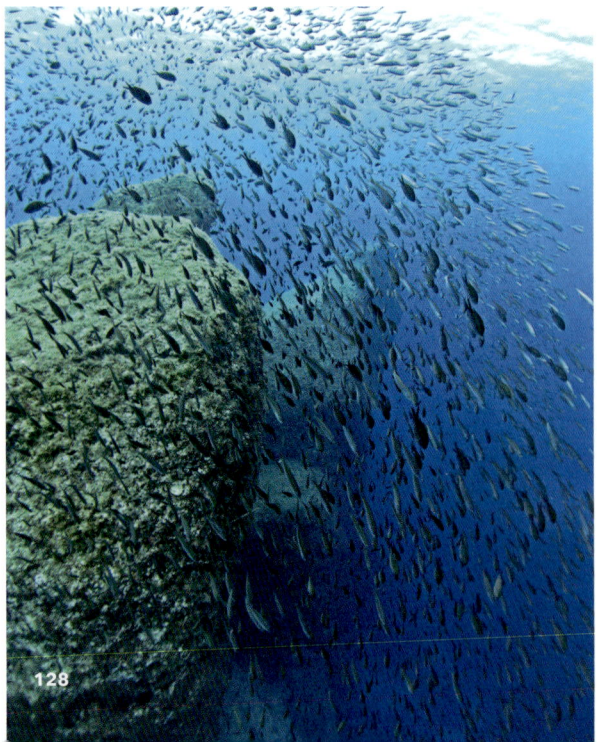

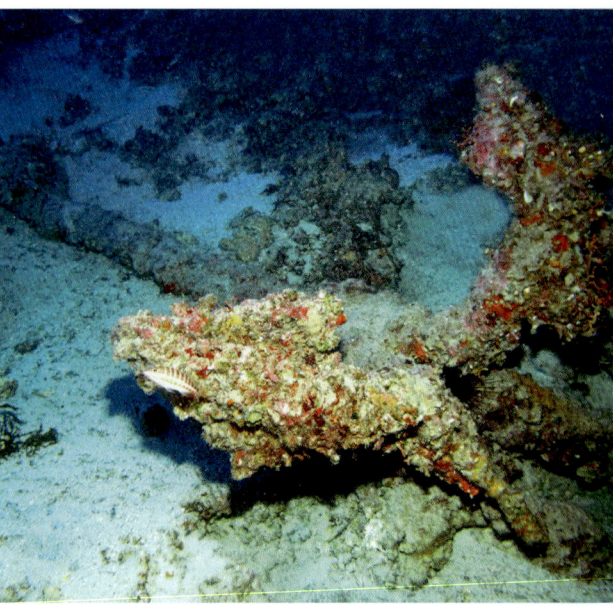

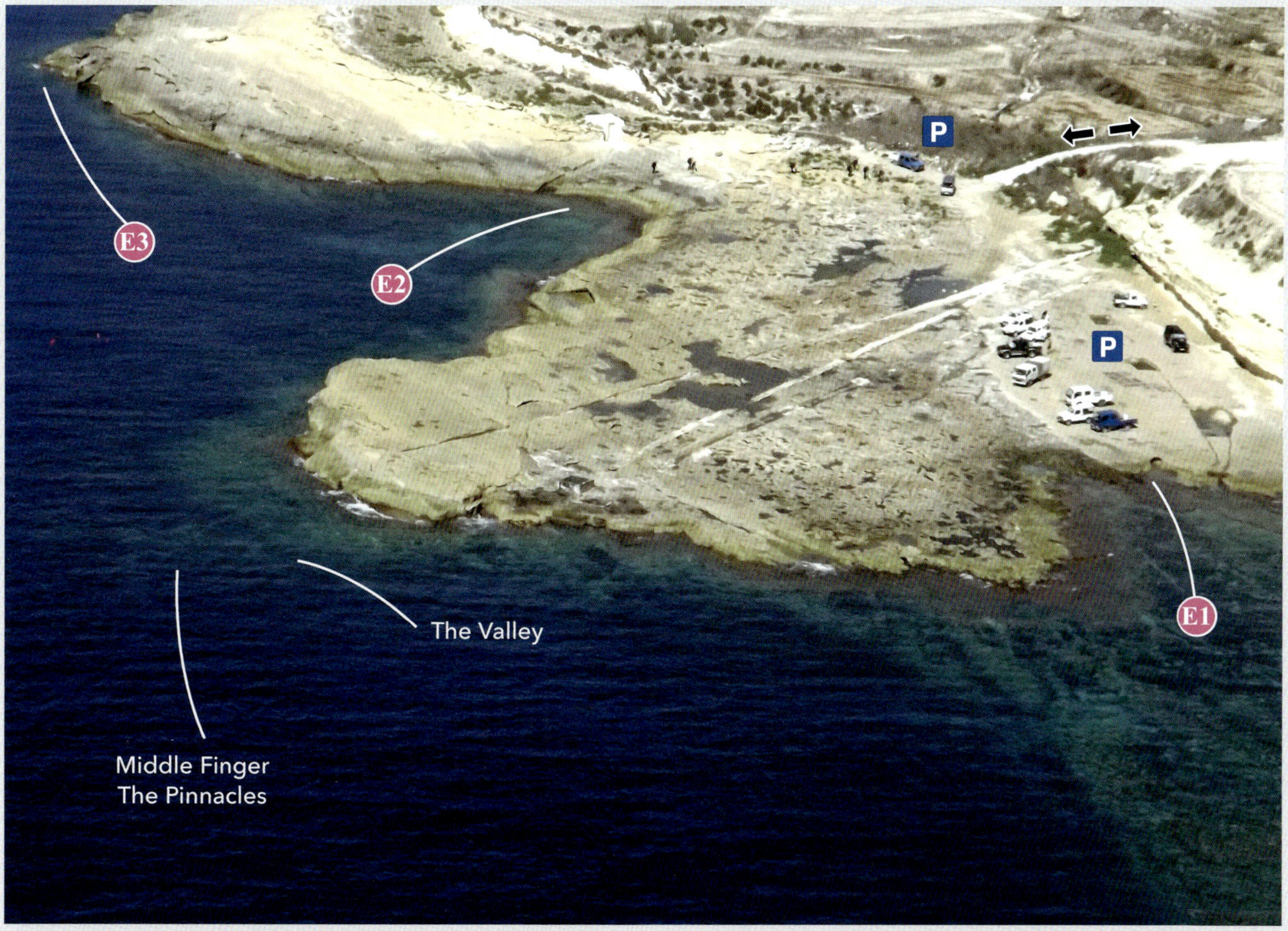

P
P
E3
E2
E1
The Valley
Middle Finger
The Pinnacles

PHOTO: PGL AERIAL PHOTOS

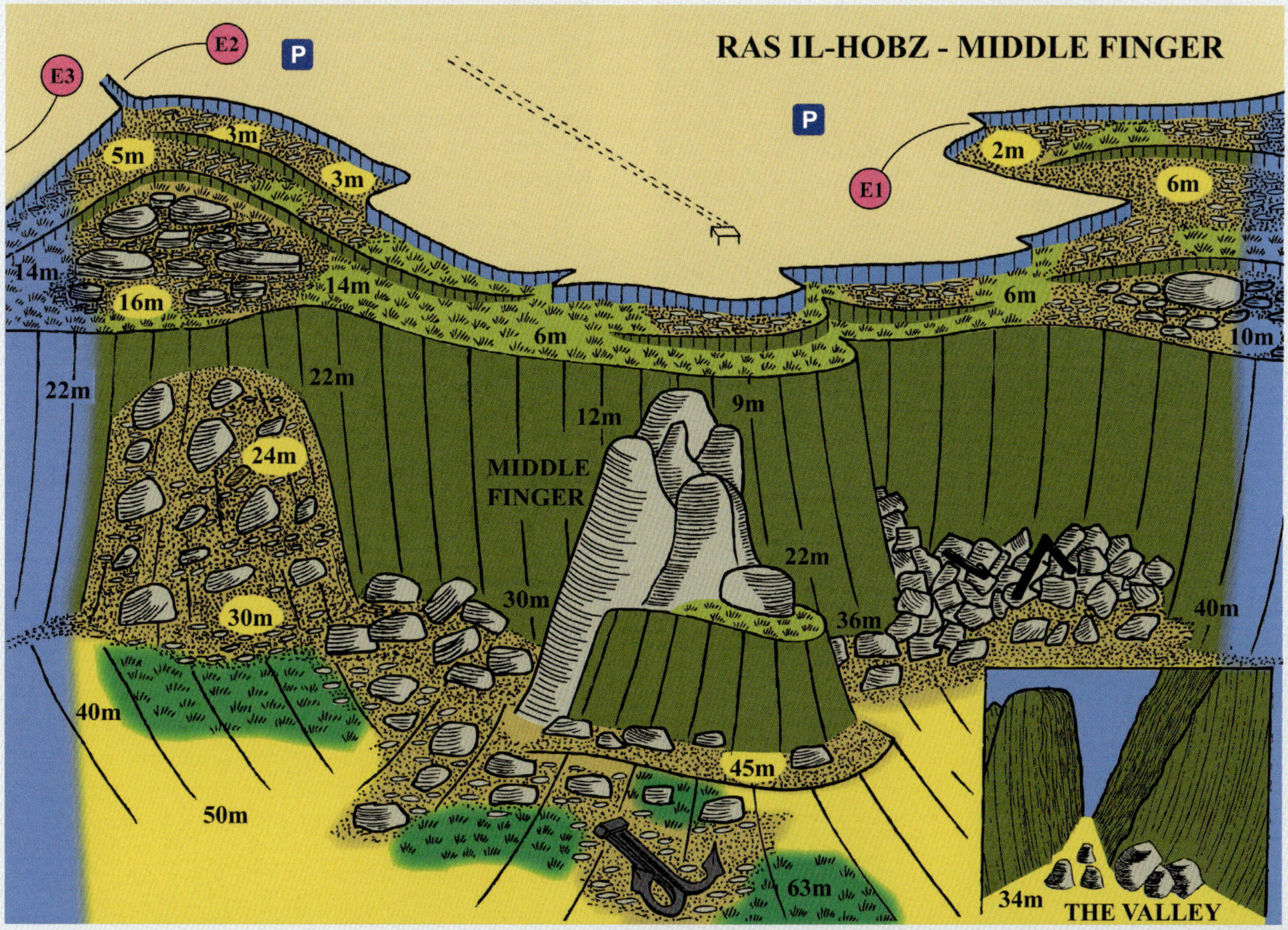
RAS IL-HOBZ - MIDDLE FINGER
E3
E2
P
P
E1
5m
3m
3m
2m
6m
14m
16m
14m
6m
6m
10m
22m
22m
24m
12m
9m
MIDDLE
FINGER
22m
30m
30m
36m
40m
40m
50m
45m
63m
34m
THE VALLEY

MIDDLE FINGER - RAS IL-HOBZ

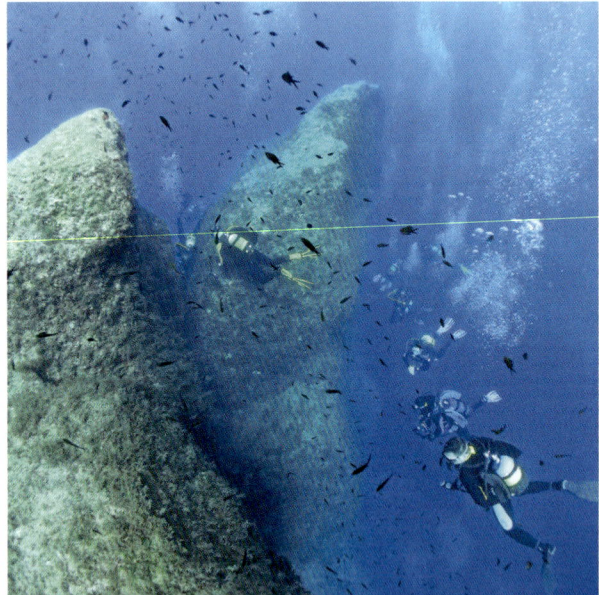

Exploring this very unusual underwater feature.

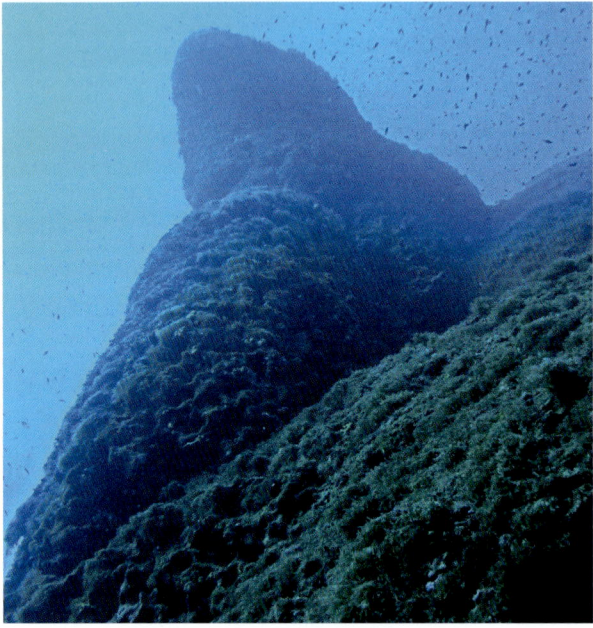

Below: A view of the pinnacle from the open sea.

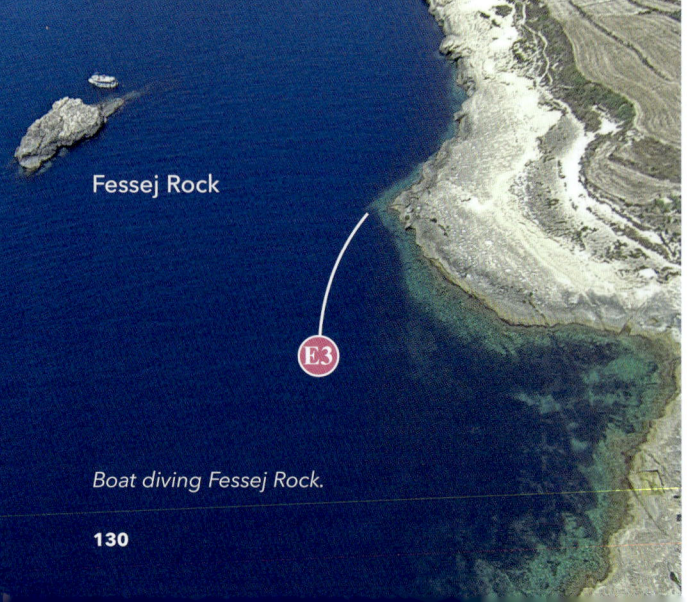

Boat diving Fessej Rock.

Return route: From the pinnacle a north compass bearing will take you back to the main coastline. Your route will depend on which entry point you used, to E1 keep the main reef on your left-hand side. Make sure you give the shallow reef a wide berth for you may run aground! A good idea is to stay at a depth of 3m when you reach the shallow area. For E2 keep the reef on your right-hand side, it will lead you into the bay and your exit point.

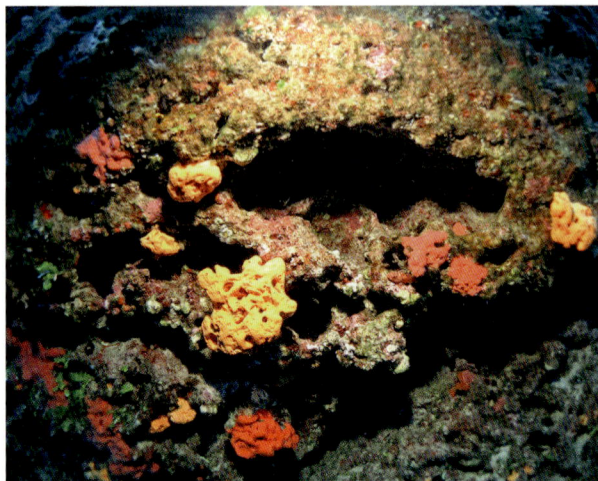

Corals, sponges on the lower parts of this reef.
PHOTO: BRAIN AZZOPARDI ALANTIS DIVING CENTRE

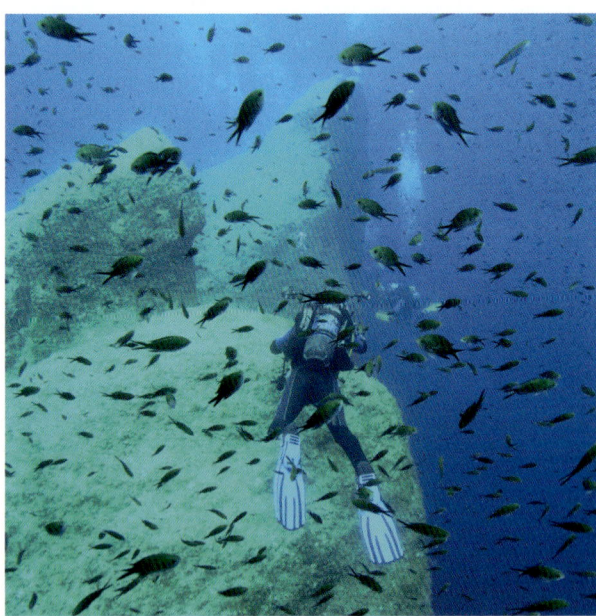

Fantastic photography at the top of the pinnacles.

Fessej Rock: This off shore islet, is normally a boat dive, which will be able to give you cover while diving. This dive site can be found in the Gozo boat diving section of this book.

If shore diving this site, it would be from entry point E3, with a surface swim to Fessei Rock. May I suggest that if you are going to do this dive from the shore, that you use an instructor/guide from one of the local dive centres, as in my opinion it's for experienced divers only.

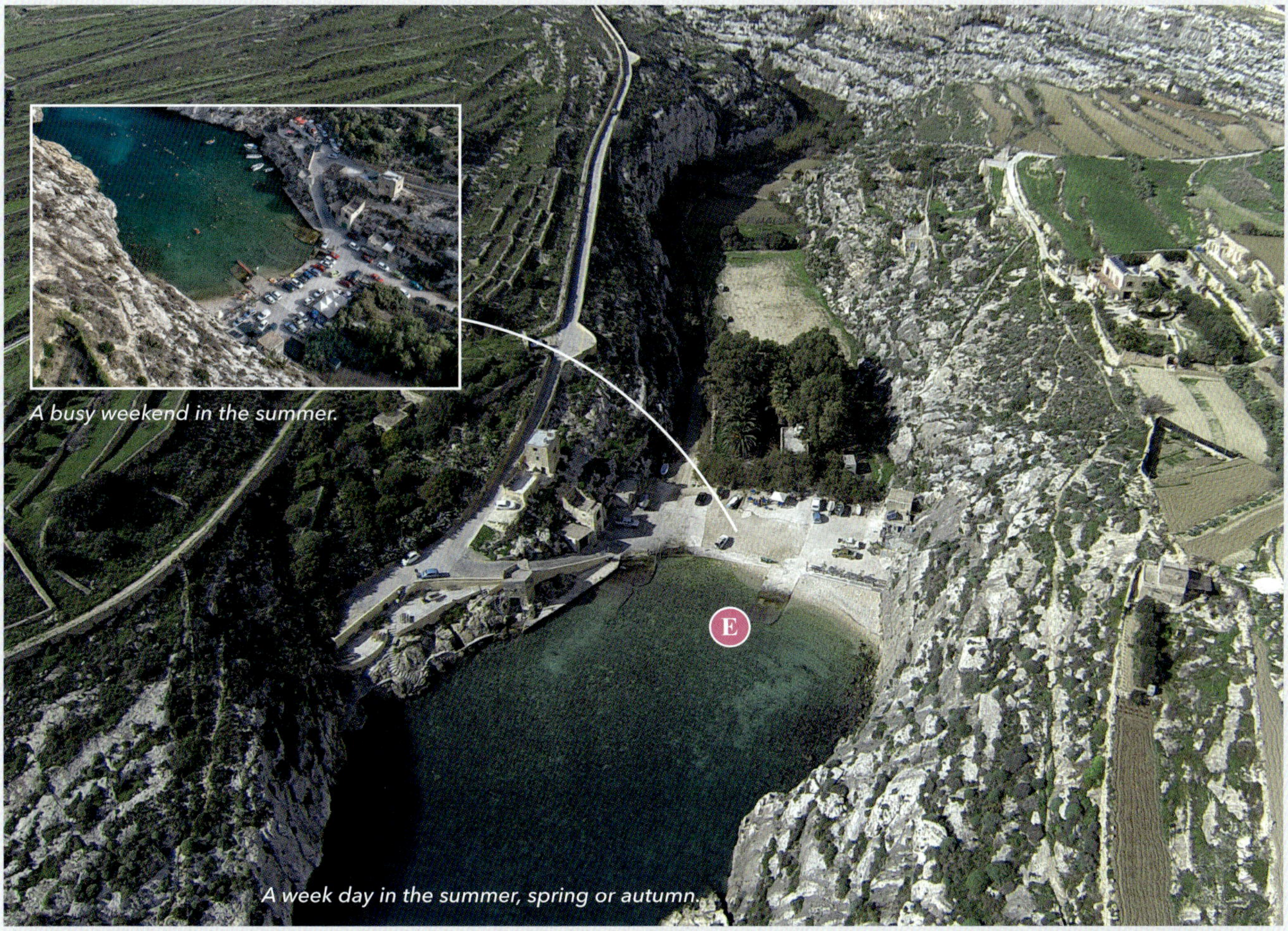

XEWKIJA TO MGARR IX-XINI

A busy weekend in the summer.

A week day in the summer, spring or autumn.

PHOTO: JOE ABDILLA & PAUL GAUCI

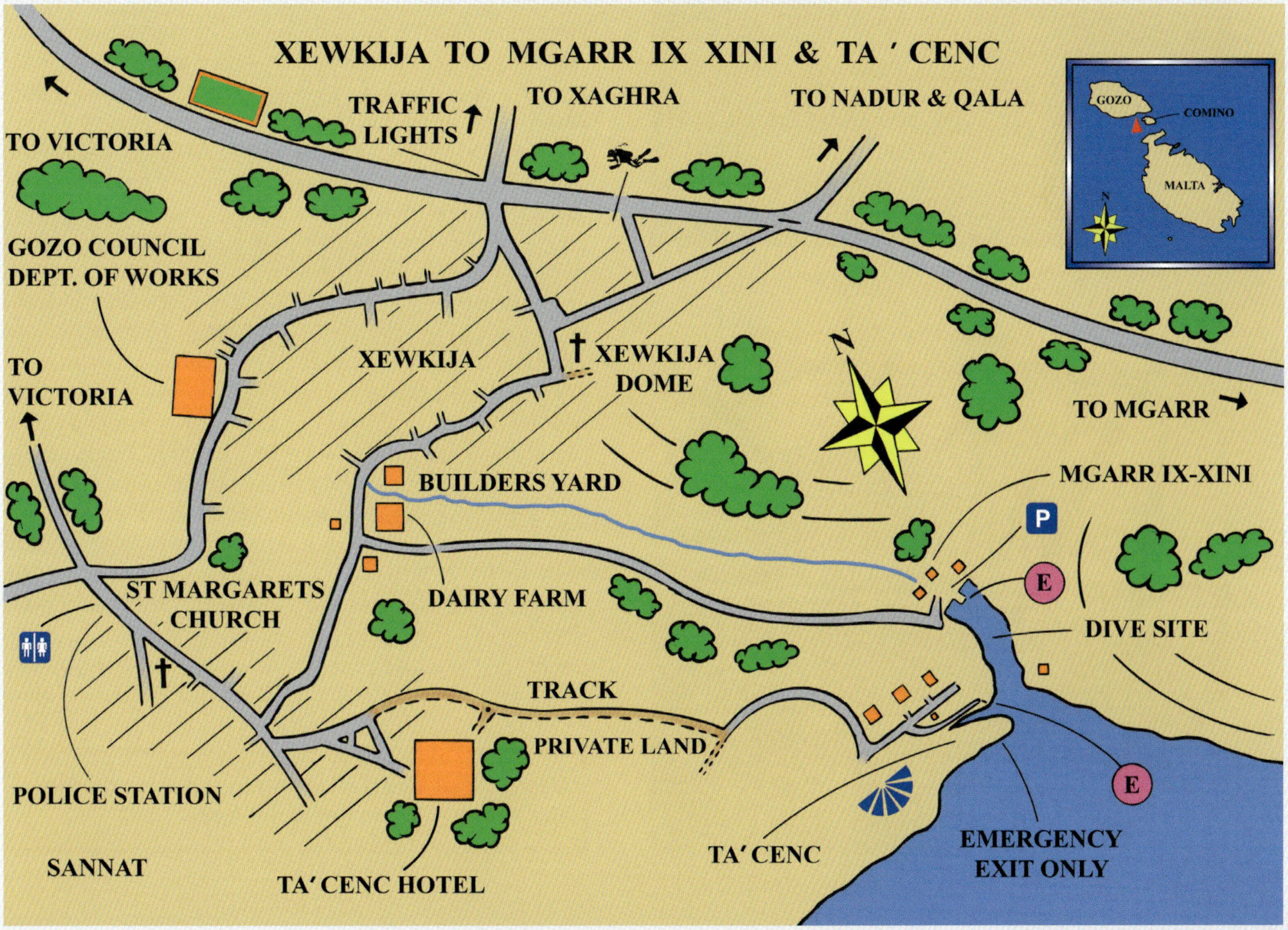

XEWKIJA TO MGARR IX XINI & TA' CENC

- TO VICTORIA
- TRAFFIC LIGHTS
- TO XAGHRA
- TO NADUR & QALA
- GOZO COUNCIL DEPT. OF WORKS
- TO VICTORIA
- XEWKIJA
- XEWKIJA DOME
- TO MGARR
- BUILDERS YARD
- MGARR IX-XINI
- ST MARGARETS CHURCH
- DAIRY FARM
- DIVE SITE
- TRACK
- PRIVATE LAND
- POLICE STATION
- SANNAT
- TA' CENC HOTEL
- TA' CENC
- EMERGENCY EXIT ONLY

GOZO, COMINO, MALTA

Mgarr ix-Xini

There are two routes to this dive site; The best route is from the traffic lights at Xewkija, a distance of some 6 km, see local map. At Sannat, bear left at St. Margarets church, almost at the top of the hill, turn sharp left there is a signpost to Mgarr ix Xini. Follow this road down to the farm buildings at the bottom of the hill; turn right, this single-track road will lead you down to the little hamlet of Mgarr ix Xini, your dive site. Second choice, drive through the old village of Xewkija and the Dome church a distance of approximately 4km. Not an easy route through the old residential area but it is sign posted in places to Mgarr ix Xini. Once at the farm buildings you have to turn left along the single-track road.

This out of the way pretty little inlet is the perfect place for a second dive, training dive, or a night dive. With a gentle sloping bottom and an easy channel to navigate, the inlet runs from north to south. The bottom is mostly sand with some sea grass but this changes to mostly Posidonia grass the deeper and further you go. Remember that there are no exits from the water other than the exit points shown on the plan. Café, toilets are available here during the summer and some weekends in the autumn and spring.

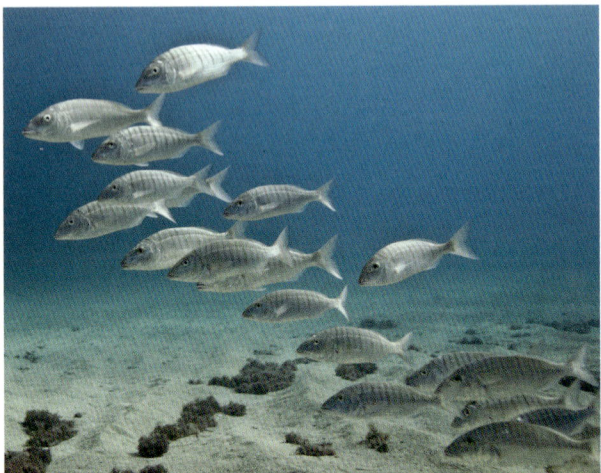
Shoals of striped seabream frequent this inlet.

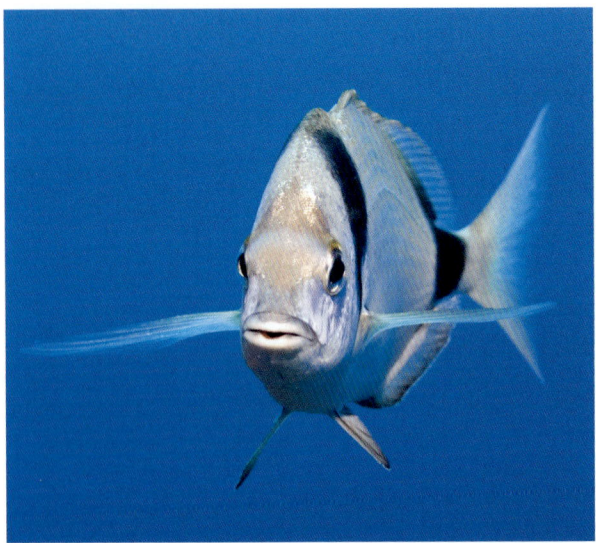
Here's looking at you! a two banded seabream.

PHOTOS: IAN FORDER

A good site to find and photograph the sea horses.

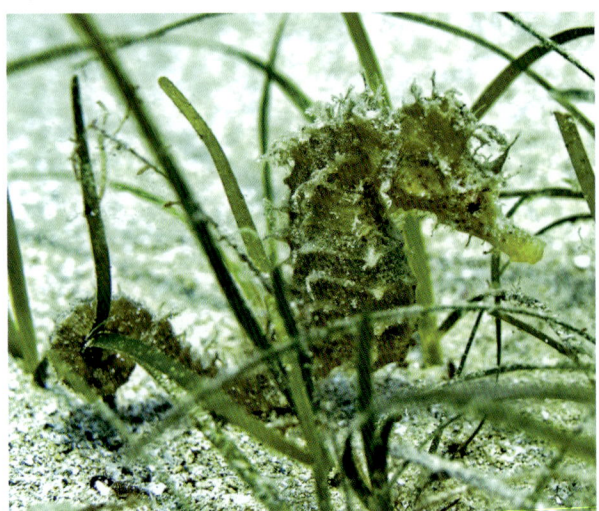

THE DIVE — Minimum time - 50 mins

Once you have entered the water, my dive plan would be to surface swim along the west wall of the channel until the depth below me is about 5m. This is the area where the small boulders end and the sandy area begins. Once on the bottom I would head in a southerly direction following the line where the rock face/coastline meets the sand. The depth gently descends to 10m; here there is a little cave, which narrows at the rear, your time to this point will be approximately 15/20 minutes. To reach the second cave from here will take you a further 10 minutes and down to a depth of 16m. This is quite a large cave, which can be safely entered for it does not go back too far. At this point you are within three to four minutes of the exit point at Ta'Cenc which you could use only in an emergency. Now take a compass bearing of 60° to cross over the inlet to the other side, this will take you about 3 minutes, your return journey from here to E1 is approximately 25 minutes. During the summer this site is a good place to find and maybe photograph seahorses. If you cover the full route, it could take you up to 60 minutes but of course you can make your turning point to suit your own dive plan.

BEWARE of boats mooring in the inlet during the summer it can get quite busy.

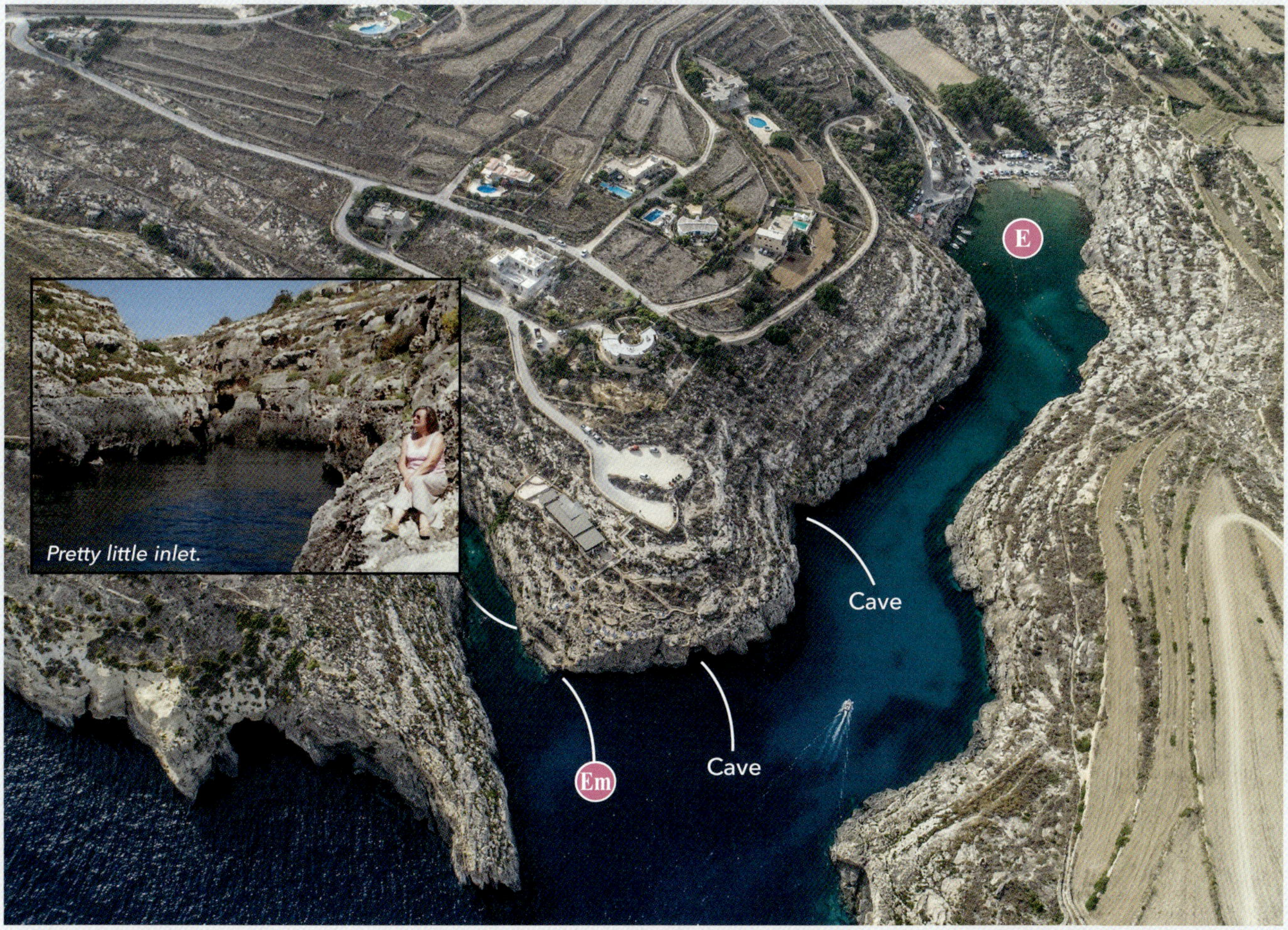

E
Cave
Cave
Em
Pretty little inlet.

PHOTO: PER EIDE STUDIO www.pereide.no

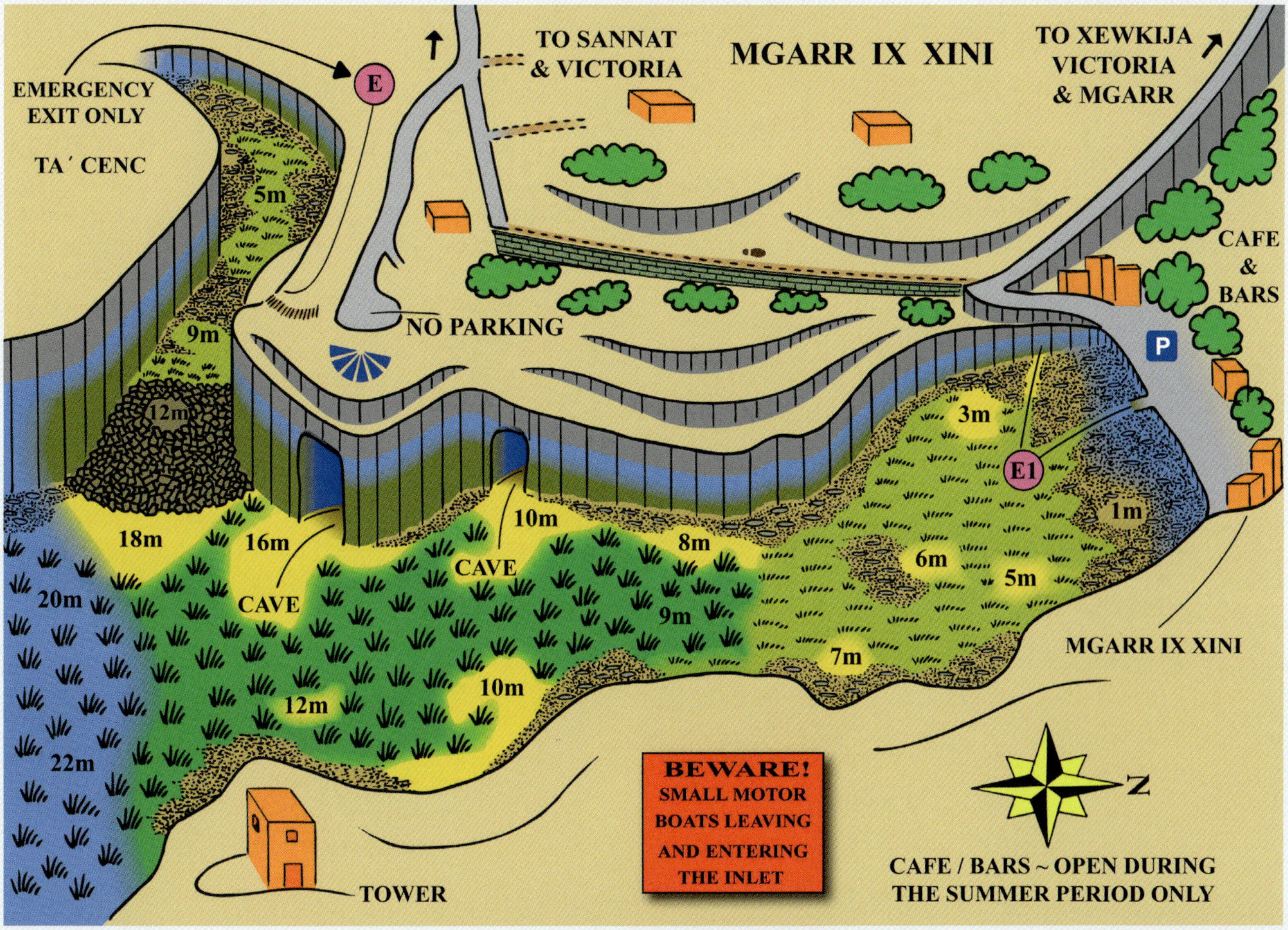
MGARR IX XINI
TO SANNAT & VICTORIA
TO XEWKIJA VICTORIA & MGARR
EMERGENCY EXIT ONLY
TA´ CENC
E
5m
9m
12m
NO PARKING
CAFE & BARS
P
3m
E1
1m
18m
16m
10m
8m
CAVE
CAVE
6m
5m
20m
9m
MGARR IX XINI
7m
10m
12m
22m
BEWARE! SMALL MOTOR BOATS LEAVING AND ENTERING THE INLET
Z
TOWER
CAFE / BARS ~ OPEN DURING THE SUMMER PERIOD ONLY

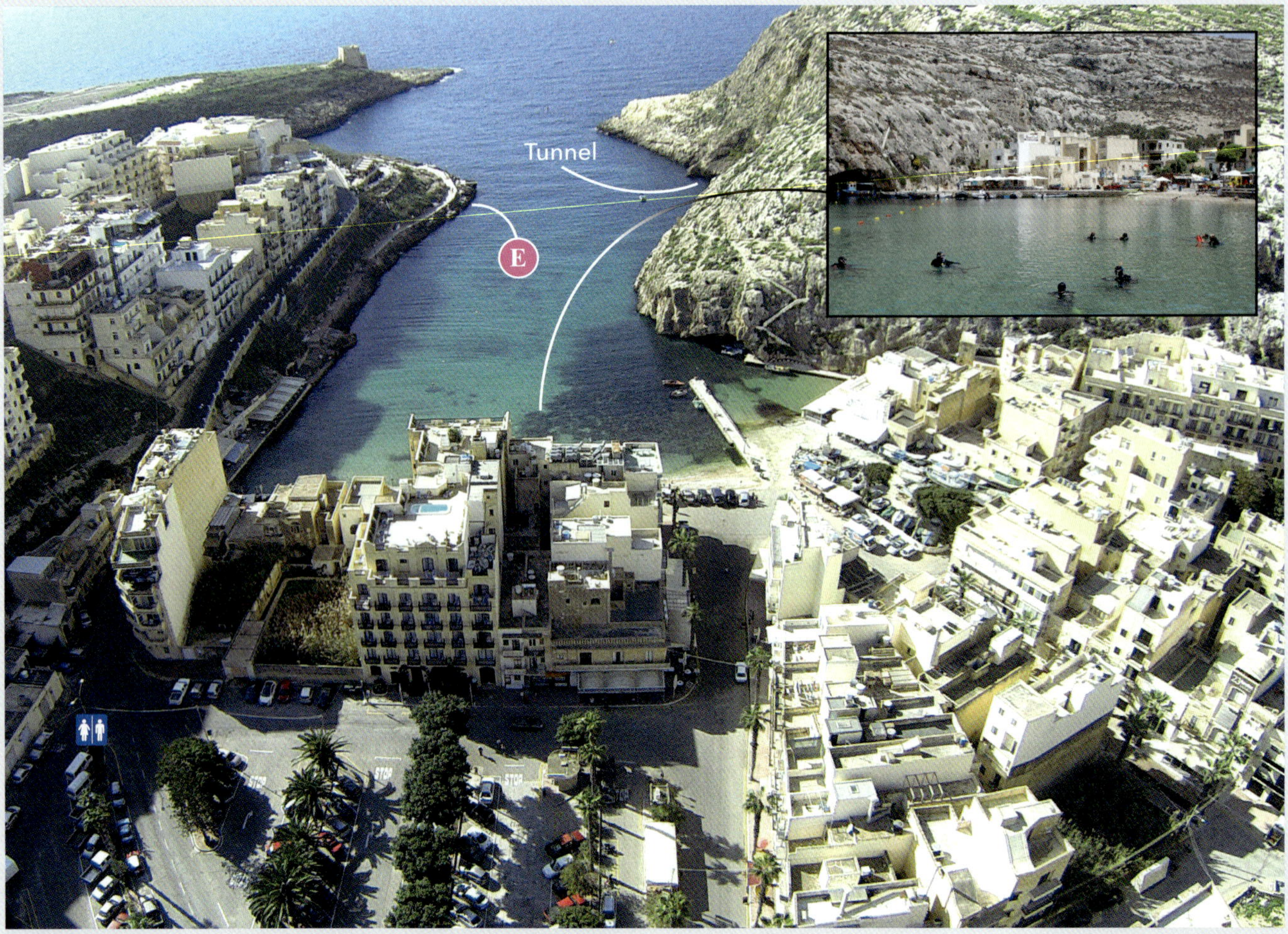

XLENDI & INLET

PHOTO: JOE ABDILLA & PAUL GAUCI

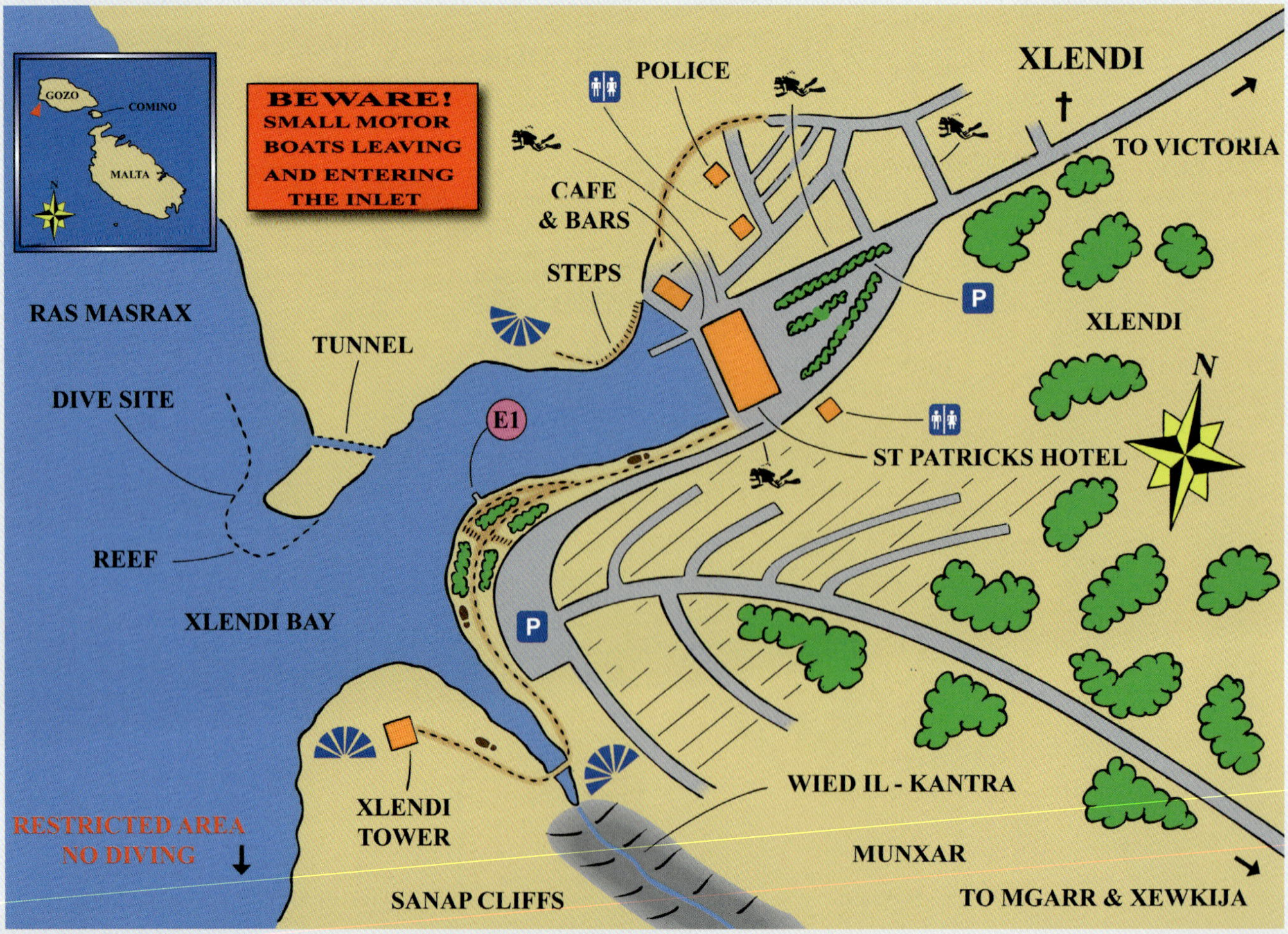

BEWARE! SMALL MOTOR BOATS LEAVING AND ENTERING THE INLET

- POLICE
- XLENDI
- TO VICTORIA
- CAFE & BARS
- STEPS
- XLENDI
- ST PATRICKS HOTEL
- RAS MASRAX
- TUNNEL
- DIVE SITE
- E1
- REEF
- XLENDI BAY
- XLENDI TOWER
- WIED IL - KANTRA
- MUNXAR
- SANAP CLIFFS
- TO MGARR & XEWKIJA
- RESTRICTED AREA NO DIVING
- GOZO
- COMINO
- MALTA

Xlendi Tunnel & Reef - Xlendi

The lovely village of Xlendi is situated on the southwest coast of Gozo, with its large inlet and excellent facilities. There really is only one route to Xlendi and that is from Victoria, a distance of 3 km. When driving through Victoria be careful not to miss the sign posts for Xlendi, as the streets are narrow with many turnings, once you head out of the built-up area the road winds down through a fertile valley. As you enter Xlendi bear left, past the car park, up the hill to your car park. From here you will have a full view of Xlendi inlet, its reef, sea front promenade and the path that leads down to your entry point E1, see local map.

The tunnel is almost opposite your entry point and is some 70-metre in length it runs through the headland with a maximum depth of 8m, you will require a torch at the entrance. The reef just off the headland forms part of the dive plan, see the marker.

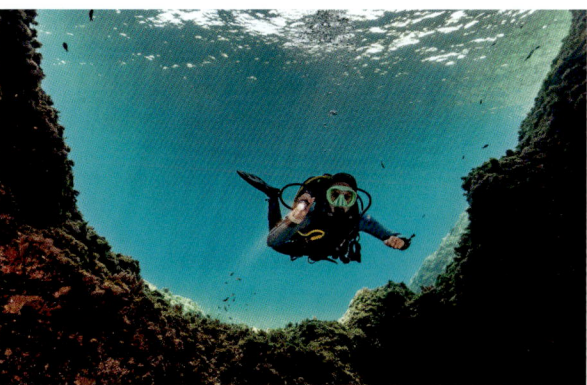

The entrance to this 70 metre long tunnel at 3m.

PHOTO: LEE JELLYMAN RITUAL DIVE CENTRE

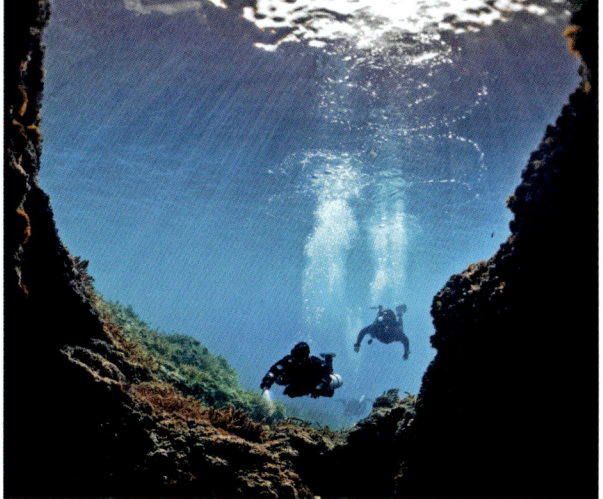

Just inside the tunnel entrance.

PHOTO: LEE JELLYMAN RITUAL DIVE CENTRE

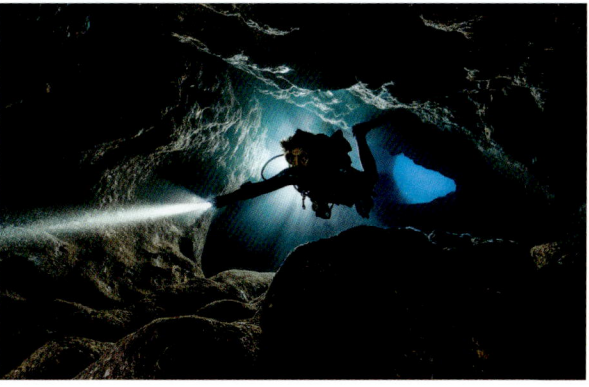

Above / below: A few metres inside the tunnel.

PHOTOS: LEE JELLYMAN RITUAL DIVE CENTRE

THE DIVE — Minimum time - 50 mins

You could rig where you have parked the car and walk down to the entry point E1, which is next to a concrete diving platform. Here you will find steps at the entry/exit point, they will be removed during the winter months. Please take care when entering the water as it is quite shallow close to the shore. To locate the entrance of the tunnel which is below the surface, look for the steep cliffs on the other side of the bay, running down is a formation of rock which looks like a spine, directly below this is the entrance. The bearing from the entry point is 330°, the depth at the entrance to the tunnel is 5m, with a ledge rising to 3m just inside, within a few metres inside there is a large rock in the centre which you will pass on the left, at this point it is quite dark and you will need a torch.

When you have passed this point the depth increases to 8m and from here, normally you can see the exit. From this point in the roof of the tunnel are cracks which allows the light to shine through, with this light and the light from the exit this makes a unique opportunity for some unusual photographs.

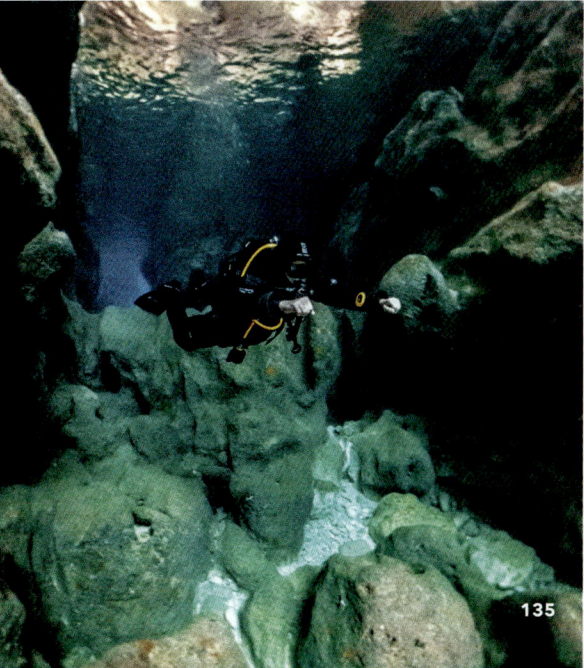

XLENDI TUNNEL & REEF

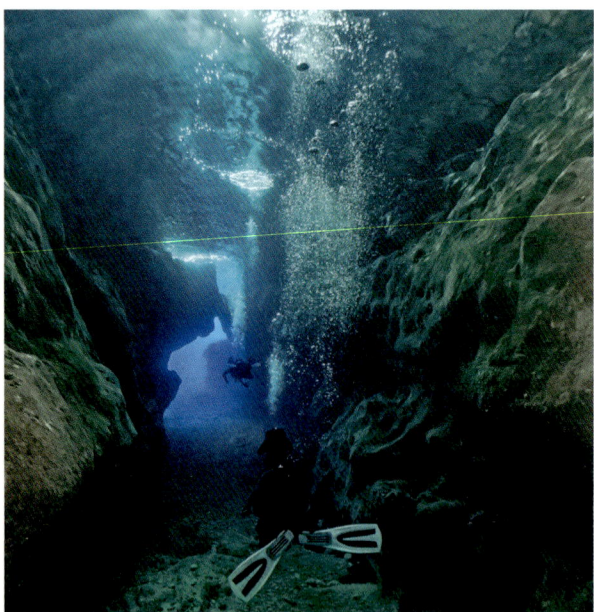

Gently heading to the far side of the tunnel.
PHOTO: LEE JELLYMAN RITUAL DIVE CENTRE

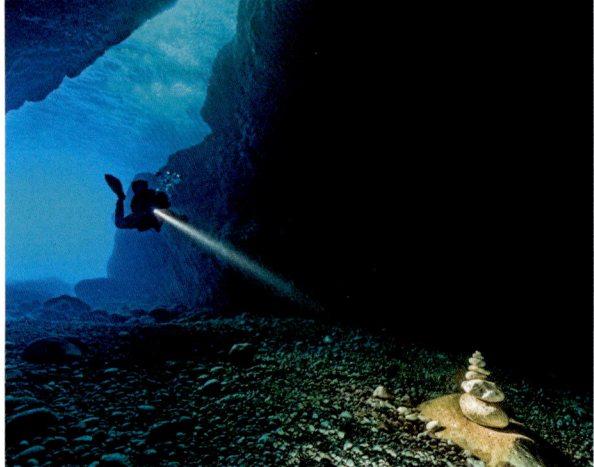

Above / below almost at the far side exit.
PHOTOS: LEE JELLYMAN RITUAL DIVE CENTRE

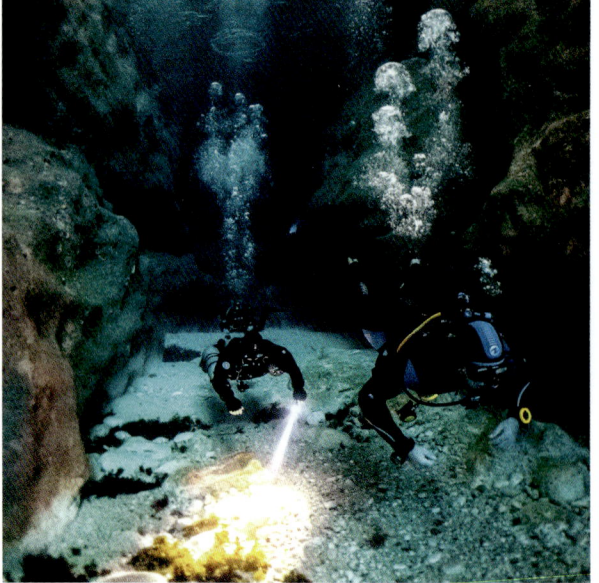

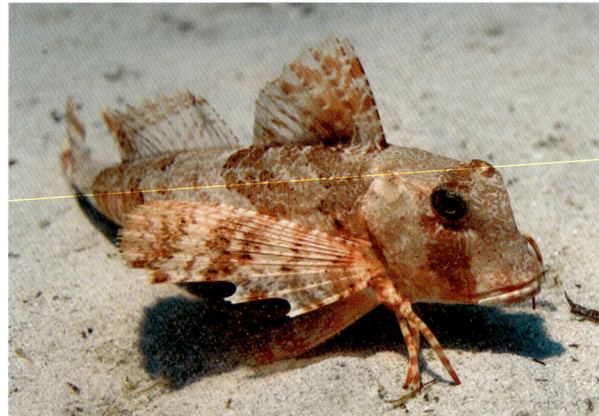

A red gurnard on the sand. PHOTO: SHARON FORDER

Once through the tunnel turn left, you will find that this area is a good place to spot morays and octopus. When it is time to move on, head in a southerly direction, keeping the reef on your left. When you pass the corner of the inner reef there will be an area of Posidonia grass in front of you and providing the visibility is good, you should be able to see the outer reef, if this is not possible, take a compass bearing of 180° and continue over the Posidonia grass until you come to the drop-off, follow it all the way round, keeping it on your left, this route will lead you back into the bay.

You can of course follow the inner reef round which is a much shorter route and has a maximum depth of 12m, unlike the outer reef which has a maximum depth of 25m. Once you are heading in a northerly direction and you reach depths of 8/9m you are in the area where you started the dive and your exit point.

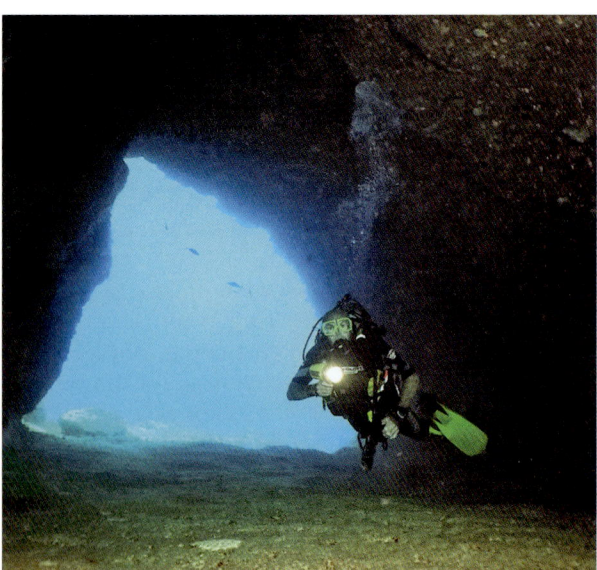

The level seabed at 8m depth near the exit.

Xlendi village is a lovely place with restaurants, cafes and paths with seating along the water's edge, to relax and view the inlet and soak up the sun.

If you fancy a climb, there is a viewpoint on the west side of the bay, an excellent position to take some souvenir photographs of Xlendi.

Xlendi Reef
Tunnel
E
P
A view from the other side.

PHOTO: PGL AERIAL PHOTOS

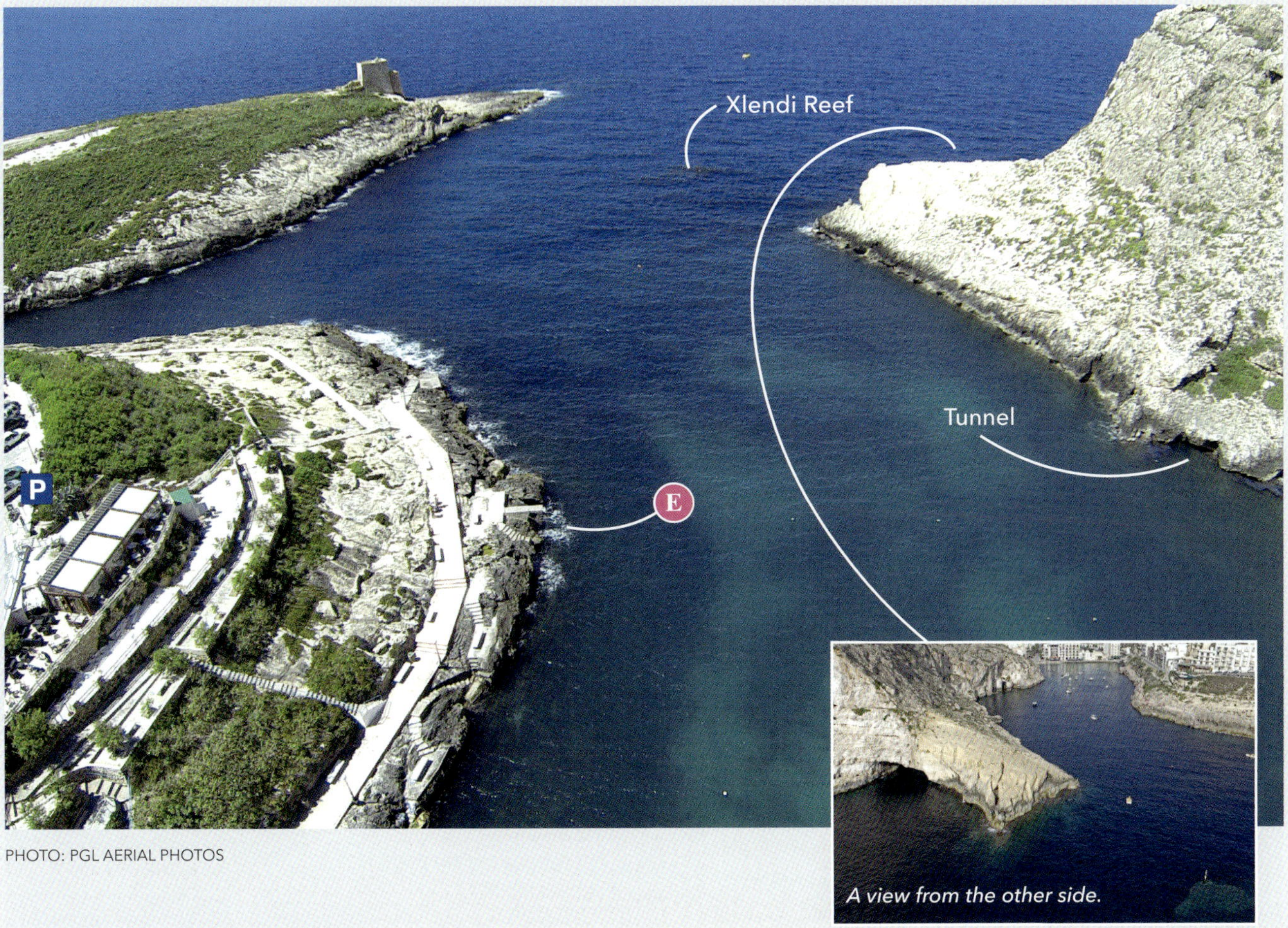

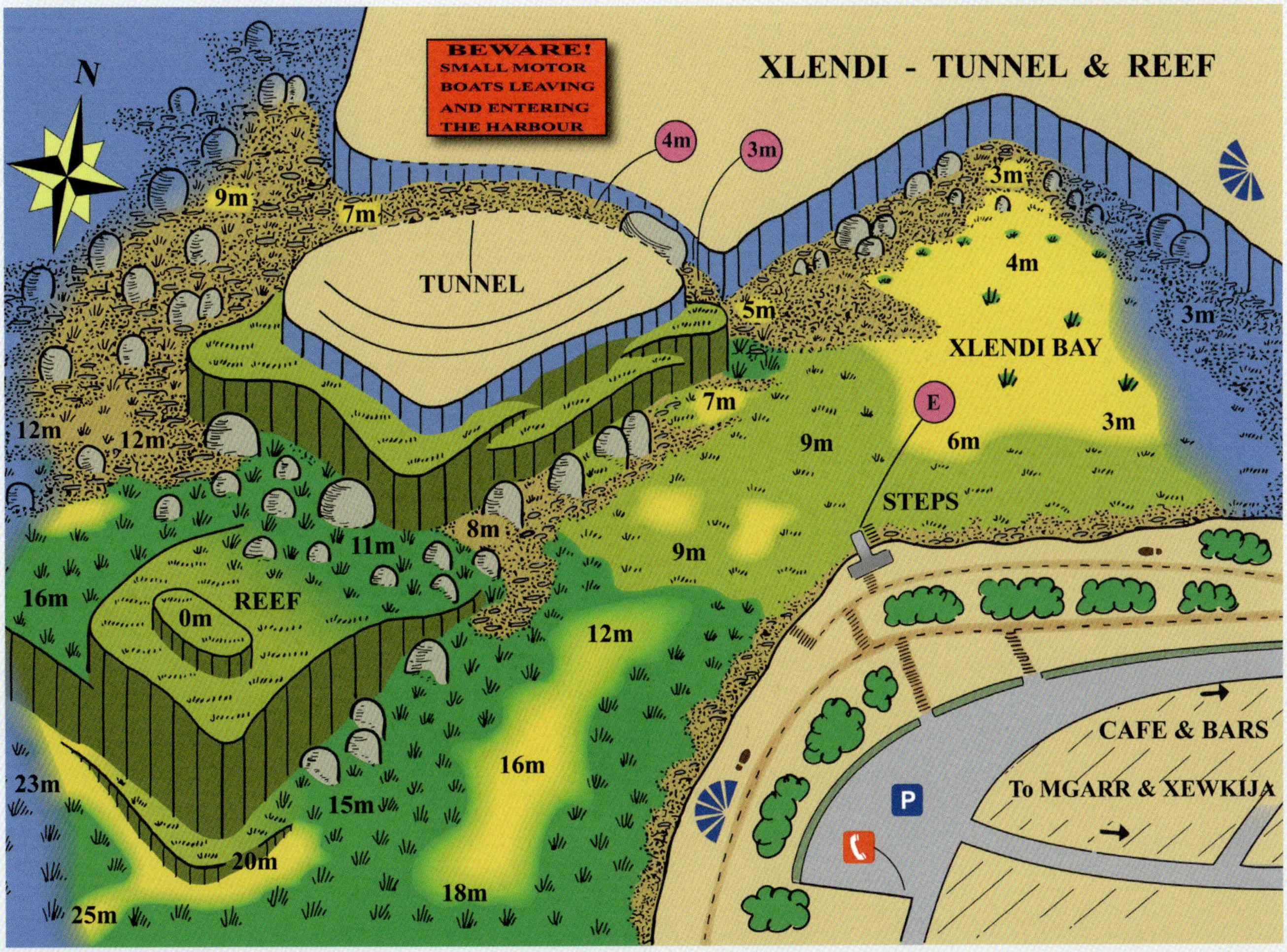
XLENDI - TUNNEL & REEF
N
BEWARE! SMALL MOTOR BOATS LEAVING AND ENTERING THE HARBOUR
4m
3m
9m
7m
TUNNEL
5m
3m
4m
3m
XLENDI BAY
7m
E
12m
12m
9m
6m
3m
STEPS
11m
8m
9m
16m
REEF
0m
12m
CAFE & BARS
23m
16m
P
To MGARR & XEWKIJA
15m
20m
18m
25m

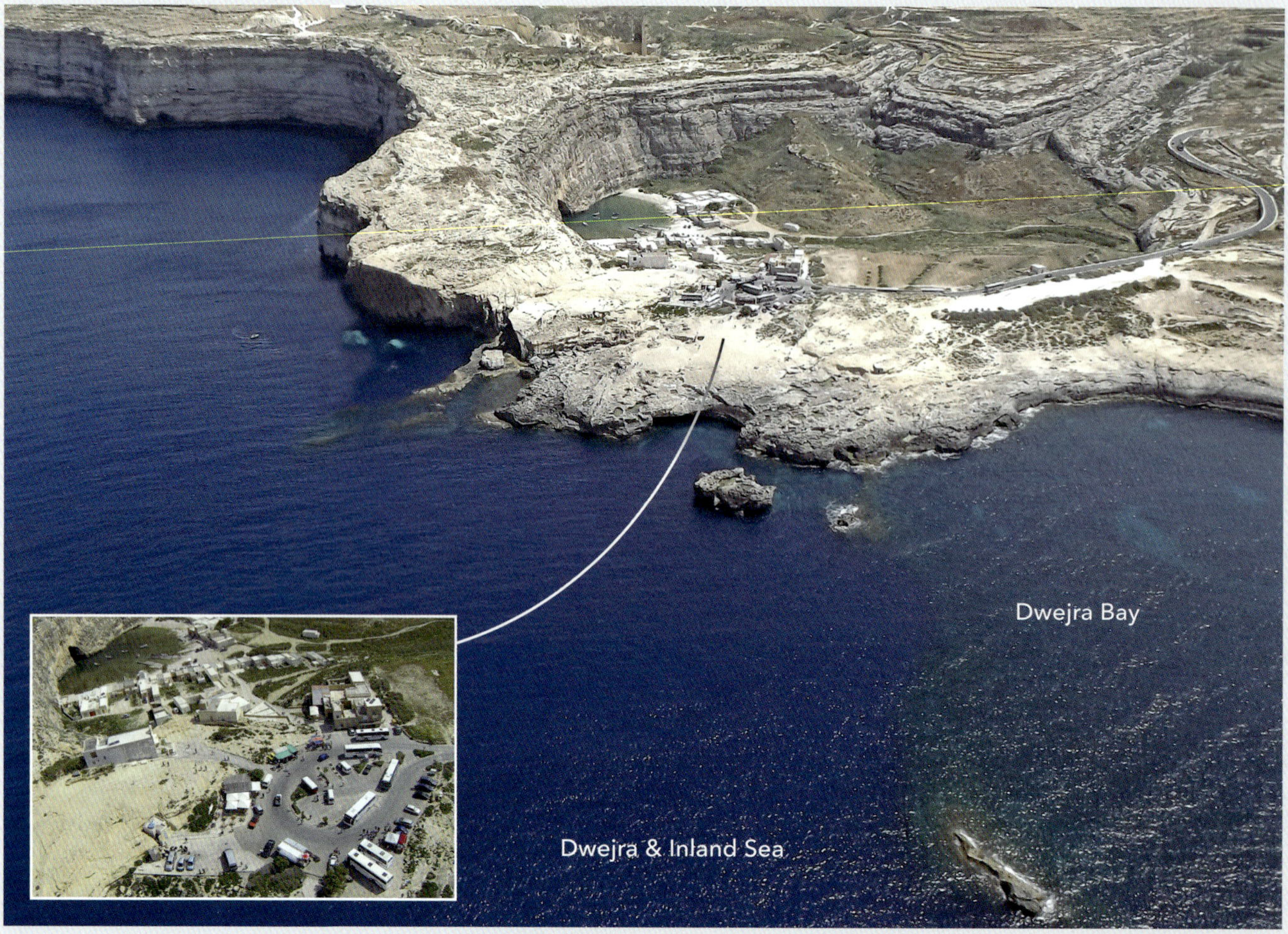

DWEJRA - INLAND SEA

Dwejra Bay

Dwejra & Inland Sea

PHOTO: JOE ABDILLA & PAUL GAUCI

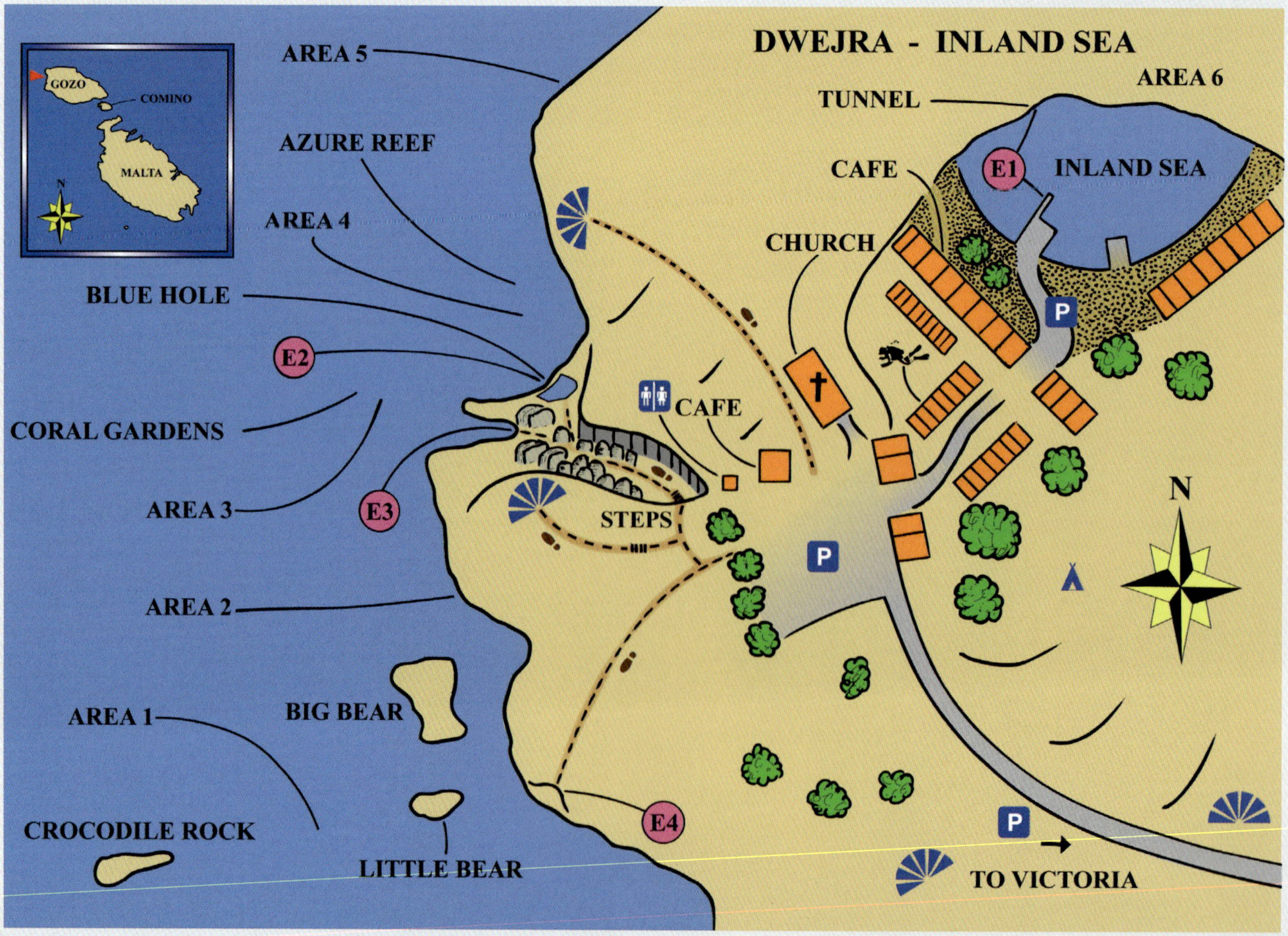

DWEJRA - INLAND SEA

- AREA 5
- AZURE REEF
- AREA 4
- BLUE HOLE
- CORAL GARDENS
- AREA 3
- AREA 2
- AREA 1
- CROCODILE ROCK
- BIG BEAR
- LITTLE BEAR
- TUNNEL
- AREA 6
- CAFE
- E1 INLAND SEA
- CHURCH
- CAFE
- STEPS
- E2
- E3
- E4
- TO VICTORIA

GOZO — COMINO — MALTA

Dwejra - Inland Sea

This proposed World Heritage site at Dwejra normally referred to by divers as the Blue Hole and Inland Sea, is just 5km from Victoria on the west coast of Gozo. Its unique coastline above and below the surface has given pleasure to thousands of tourists and divers. On the 8th March 2017 a storm caused the Azure Window to collapse into the sea, changing the coastal landscape forever, this 28-metre column of rocks has now created a new dramatic underwater reef.

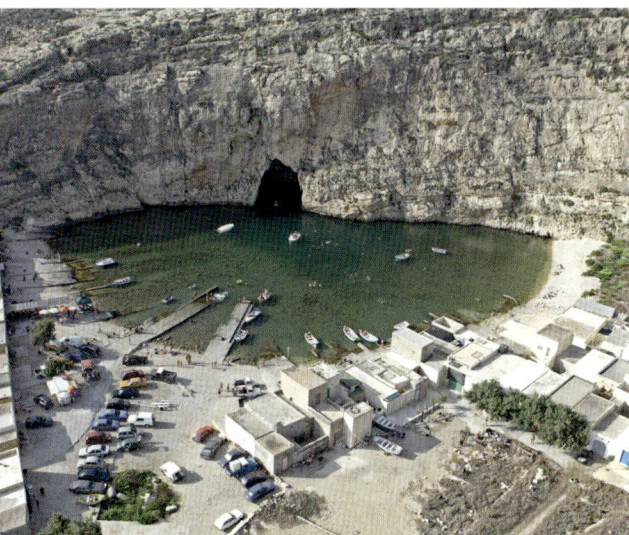

The Inland Sea and Tunnel entrance.

The Inland Sea is a small expanse of shallow water with a maximum depth of 2m linked to the sea by an 80 metre tunnel, inside the seabed drops from 3m at the entrance to 26m at the exit. Both the Inland Sea and the tunnel are used by tourist pleasure boats.

The Azure Reef Created by the collapse of the Azure Window this reef with its pinnacles, huge rocks, gullies and swim throughs, has been designed by nature and just adds to the fantastic variety of diving around the Maltese Islands.

The Blue Hole is a round hole with a depth of 16m where there is a large window which allows you to venture out into the underwater world of Dwejra Point, at the back of the window there is a cave.

> **I strongly suggest that you check out all entry/exit points before you kit up. Please take care when walking these routes especially when it has been raining.**

All these wonders have been created by waves and rough seas over thousands of years, only time and the sea will change these structures. Dwejra point attracts many divers, not only from Gozo but Malta as well. With its normally excellent visibility and a number of unique dive sites, it is no wonder why it is so popular. I have selected just six dive sites for you, but of course you can plan your own dive.

There are many species of fish, types of marine plants and coral to be seen in these areas. Watch out for groupers lying on rocks and under the over-hangs. Don't forget to keep an eye out in the blue, for this is where you are likely to see the larger fish such as dentex and shoals of barracuda.

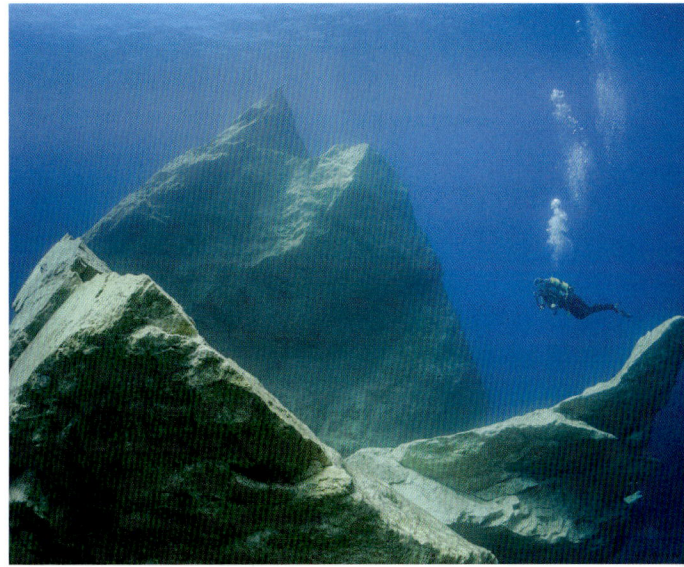

A diver dwarfed by the three Peaks of the Azure Reef.
PHOTO: PER EIDE STUDIO www.pereide.no

Dwejra's fantastic Blue Hole, entry point E2.

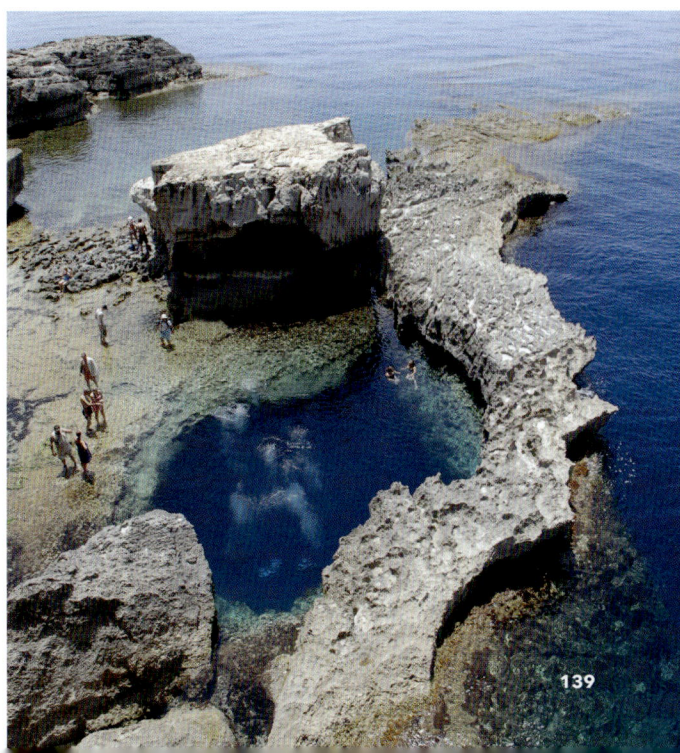

Little Bear to Crocodile Rock — Area 1

To find this entry/exit point E4, is not easy, you first have to navigate your way to a small ledge opposite the rock called Little Bear, which is 220° from the café by the car park. This is not a straight path over the rocks and gullies to E4 and the entry ledge is not visible until you are immediately above it. This is the only place along this coastline that you can enter or exit the water. (See aerial photograph)

This is an excellent dive with a reef which runs from Little Bear to Crocodile Rock and continues to the north point of Dwejra Bay. The average depth on the reef is 8m, with drop-offs from 25m to 36m, depending on your location. Swim away from the cliff face and the depth will quickly increase to 50m plus. During a dive along this ridge, I had a visit from a lone barracuda which came right up alongside me, we made eye contact and within a minute he was gone, I felt I had had a visit from an alien.

THE DIVE — Minimum time - 50 mins

Enter the water at E4, when on the bottom move over to the right-hand side of Little Bear, then drop over the edge of the reef, down to 25m. Face the reef and on your left will be the entrance to Rogers Cave, when you have had a look follow the reef in a south westerly direction, allow around 30 minutes to reach Crocodile Rock. This of course depends on how long you spend at the cave and exploring on route.

Exploring this reef with a torpedo DPV.

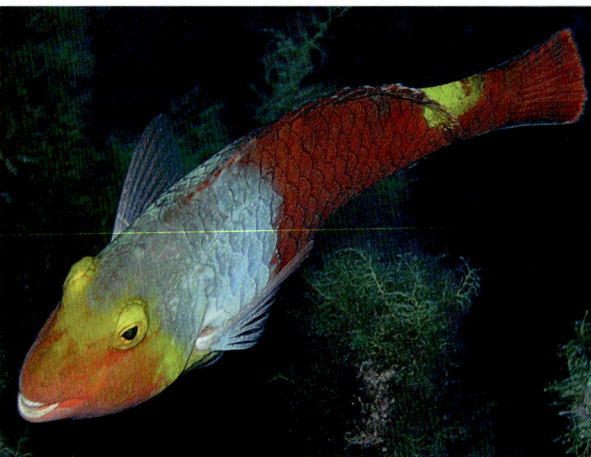

The colourful male parrotfish. PHOTO: VICTOR FABRI

Normally, when you are below Crocodile Rock you will be able to see the reef rising to the surface, another indication that you are below Crocodile Rock is that the line of the reef changes to a southerly direction. When it is time to return ascend to the top of the reef to retrace your steps at a shallower depth along the ridge to Little Bear and your exit point E4, an excellent area for photography. Don't forget to look out into the blue for that elusive alien (barracuda) and other large fish that may pass by.

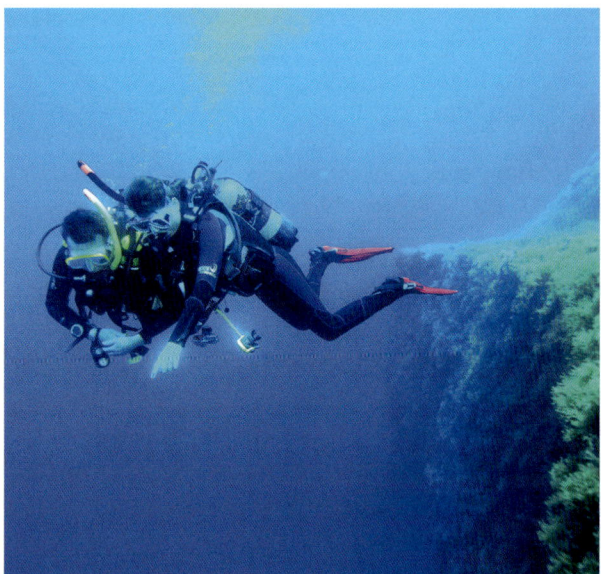

Marine life spotted below the drop-off.

This lone barracuda visits the reef.

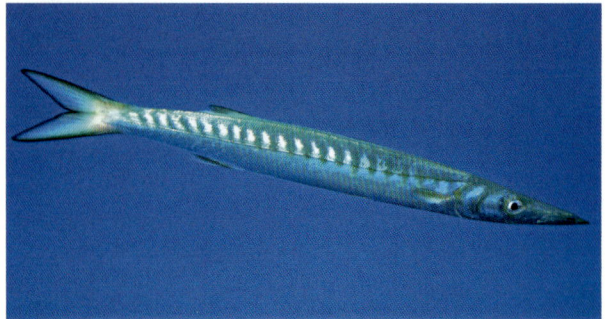

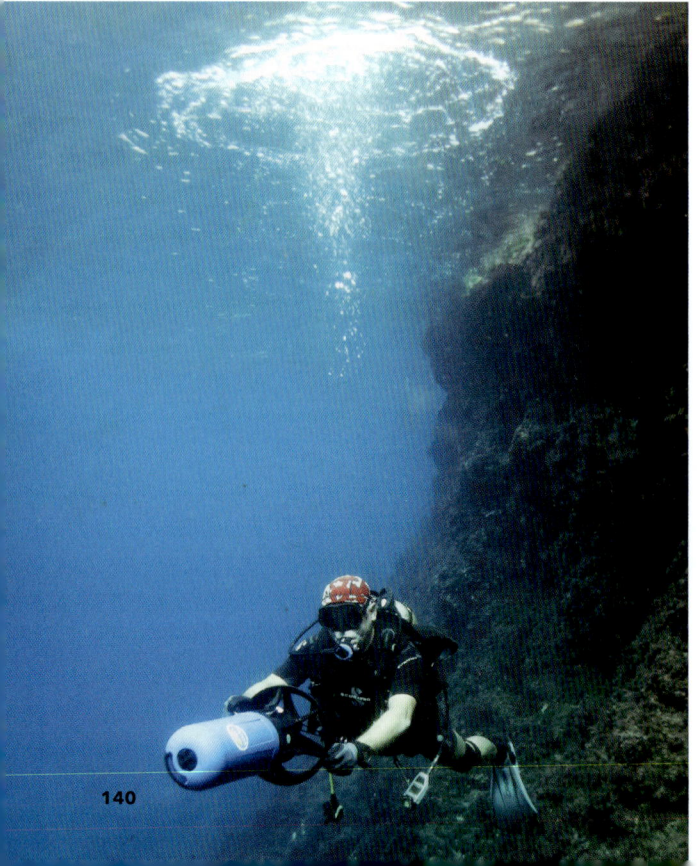

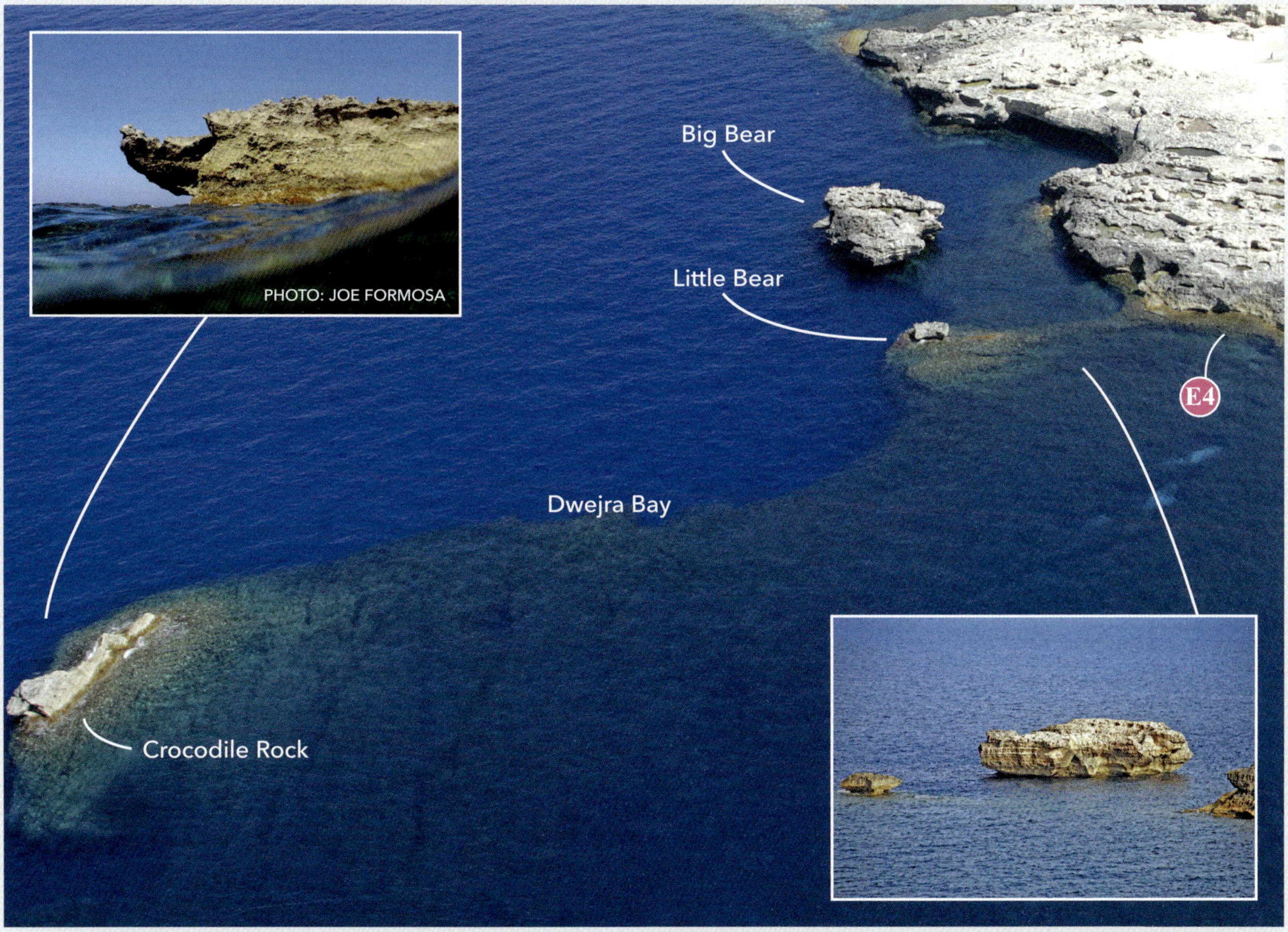

LITTLE BEAR TO CROCODILE ROCK - DWEJRA

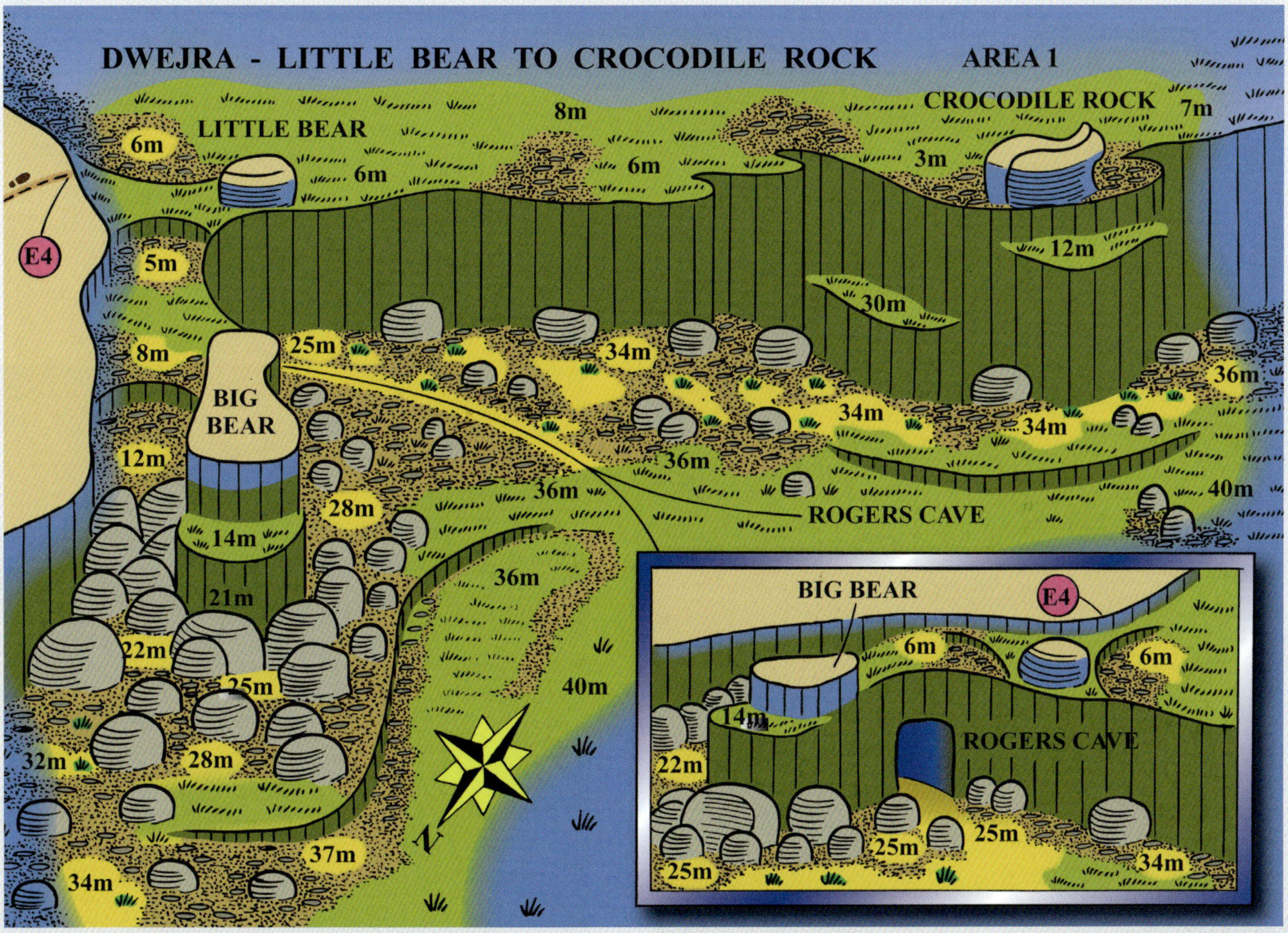

Coral Gardens to Big Bear — Area 2

For this dive site I would use entry/exit point E3, from the main car park head in a westerly direction towards the sea, down the steps and bear right; down more steps into the gully. Bear left, then on your right the route continues over the rocks, this is not easy be careful over the rocks. Once you reach sea level go through a narrow gap between the cliff face and a large boulder, now bear round to your left and E3 will be in front of you. Here you have a nice reef with a drop-off to 30m, away from the reef, like many areas here it slopes away quite quickly to 50m plus. Big Bear is the largest of the two rocks and can be explored all the way round. To the west and south side are the deepest area with a number of large boulders surrounded by areas of sand. On the far side is Rogers Cave. The valley on the inside is shallower with rocks and boulders covering the seabed.

> **Coral Cave has a very large opening and goes back into a secondary cave. I am going to give a warning and make a request! Sadly in 1999 two divers tragically lost their lives within this cave for it is difficult to navigate when the silt has been stirred up. If you are in the entrance of the cave, please take care not to damage the coral.**

Salema fish, top of the chimney Coral Gardens.
PHOTO: LEE JELLYMAN RITUAL DIVE CENTRE

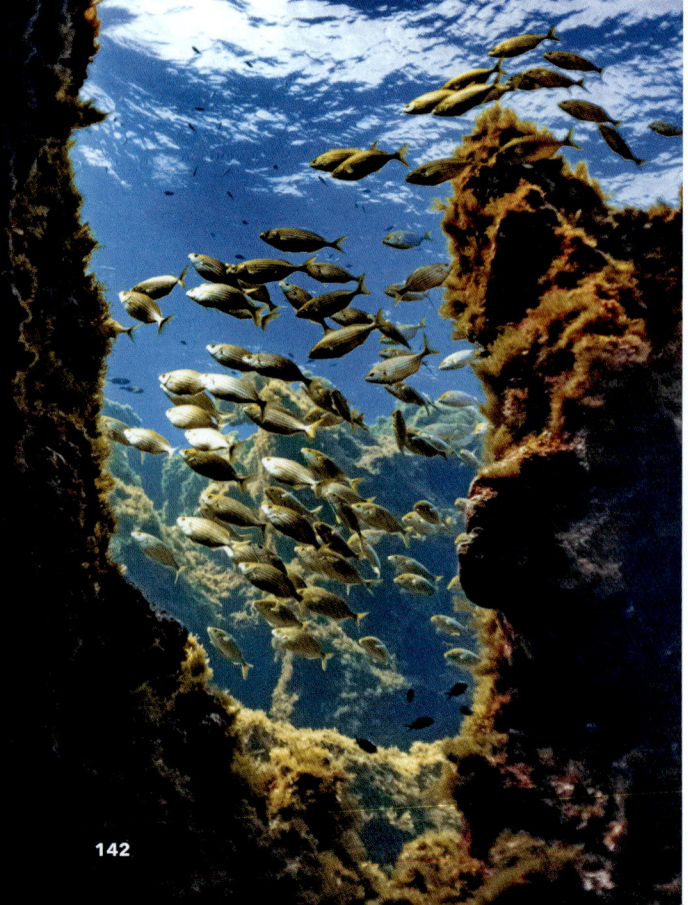

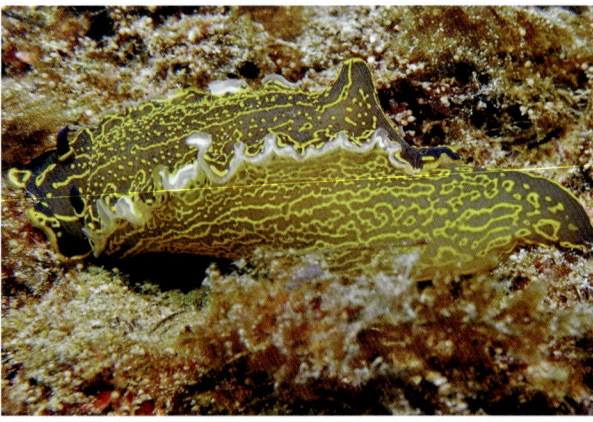

A beautiful yellow nudibranch.
PHOTO: PATRICK SCHEMBRI WALRUS DIVING CLUB

THE DIVE — Minimum time - 45 mins

At E3 the water is very shallow at first, so you have to paddle. Once you have dropped into the water, surface swim out to the middle of the reef where the depth will be around 3m, now swim towards the open sea in a southerly direction and out of the 'U' shaped opening, descend to the seabed at 30m. Turn left and follow the reef you will pass in front of Coral Cave, this is not normally a problem if the visibility is good, otherwise it could be possible to mistakenly enter the cave, as the entrance is very wide. Once past the cave bear to the south and the outside of Big Bear base, over the large rocks down to your selected depth. Now head in an easterly direction up the slope to 25m this is the depth outside Rogers Cave, your dive time could be 35 minutes. Ascend to the ledge at 8m above Rogers Cave, bear left and cross over to the coastline reef, heading in a north-westerly direction at a depth of 9 to 6m, you will pass over the top of Coral Cave. Now look out for the distinct 'U' shape in the top of the reef, at 6m, this is your only route back into Coral Gardens and your exit at E3.

There are many photo opportunities on this reef.
PHOTO: LEE JELLYMAN RITUAL DIVE CENTRE

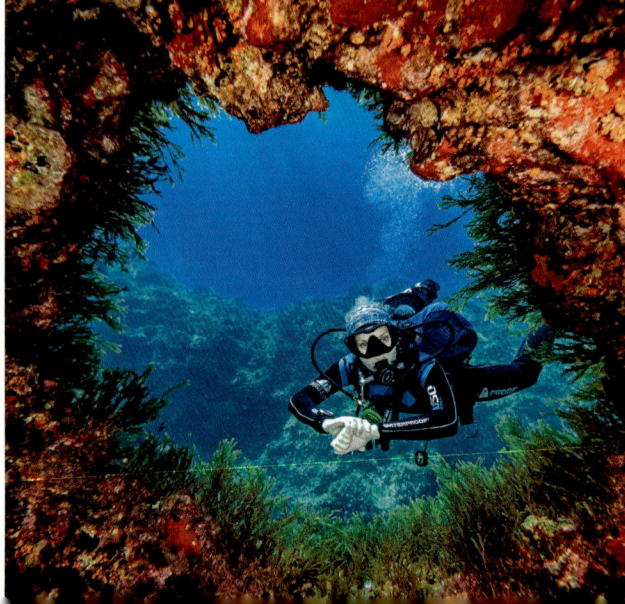

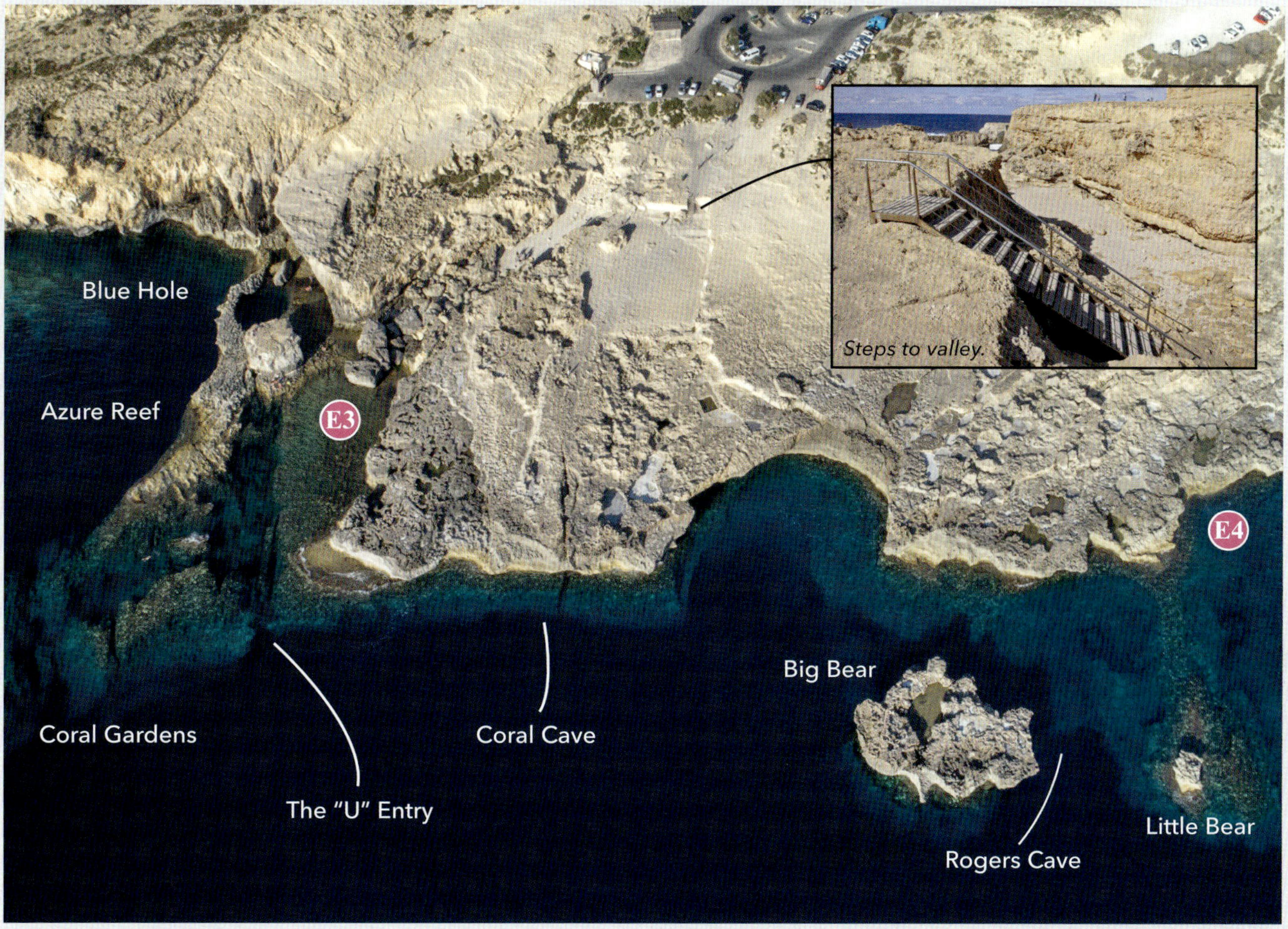
Blue Hole
Azure Reef
E3
Steps to valley.
E4
Big Bear
Coral Gardens
Coral Cave
The "U" Entry
Rogers Cave
Little Bear

PHOTO: PER EIDE STUDIO'S www.pereide.no

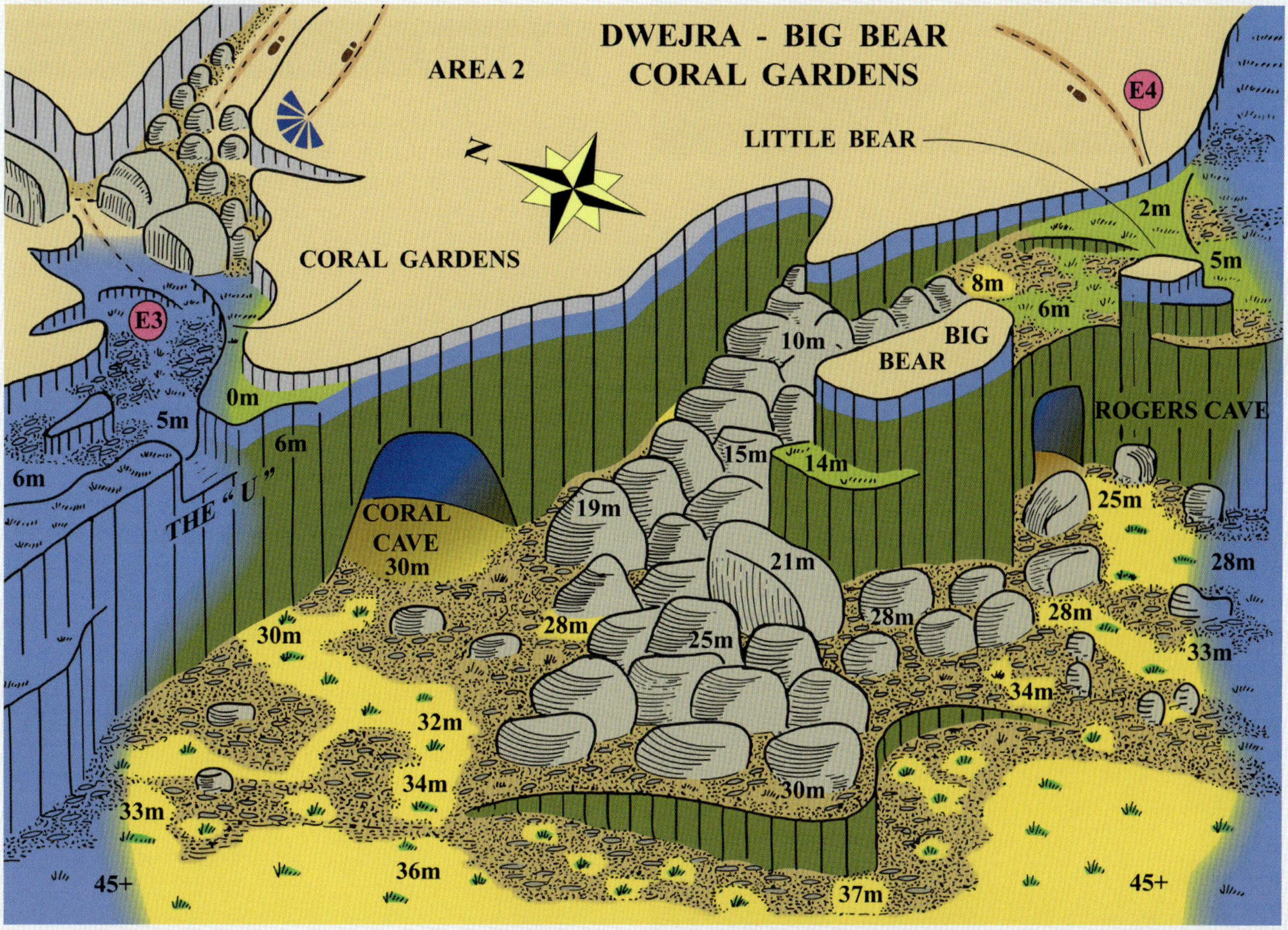
DWEJRA - BIG BEAR
CORAL GARDENS
AREA 2
N
E4
LITTLE BEAR
CORAL GARDENS
E3
BIG
BEAR
ROGERS CAVE
CORAL
CAVE
30m
THE "U"
0m
5m
6m
6m
2m
5m
8m
6m
10m
15m
14m
19m
21m
25m
28m
28m
28m
28m
25m
30m
32m
33m
33m
34m
34m
36m
30m
37m
45+
45+

Blue Hole - Coral Gardens — Area 3

For this dive site I would use entry/exit point E3, from the main car park head in a westerly direction towards the sea, down the steps and bear right; down more steps into the valley. Bear left, then on your right the route continues over the rocks, this is not easy be careful over the rocks. Once you reach sea level go through a narrow gap between the cliff face and a large boulder, now bear round to your left and E3 will be in front of you. Please note you can end this dive at the Blue Hole E2.

Check out the aerial photograph, you will clearly see your entry exit point E3, Coral Gardens, both the 'U' and 'V' openings, the top of the 'crack/chimney and the Blue Hole E2 This dive allows you to explore the outer reef of Coral Gardens, but of course, you can plan your own dive.

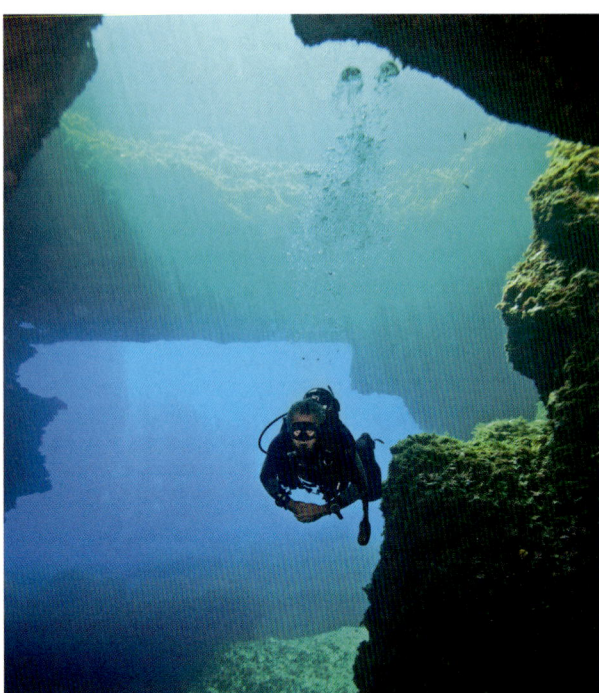

Inside the Blue Hole heading to the cave, and in the background the window to the Azure Reef.

THE DIVE — Minimum time - 50 mins

Once in the water swim away from the shallows and descend towards the open sea, your depth here will be 2m and 6m when you come to the 'U' shaped opening. From this opening the drop off to the seabed is approximately 25m. At this point your minimum time to the Blue Hole is around 15/20 minutes. Once on the seabed, or your chosen depth, turn right and head in a westerly direction keeping the reef on your right, when you reach the end of the reef follow it round, once you have turned the corner you will be heading in an easterly direction., from here it will only take you a very short time to reach the entrance to the 'crack/chimney' here the depth is 27m, now enter this large fissure it will lead you up and into Coral Gardens to a depth of 7m you can end your dive at E3. But if you have the air then bear to your right and follow the gully to the 'V' opening. Your dive time at this point could be 25 minutes depending on your depth and time taken exploring around the headland. Turn right again, keeping the reef on your right-hand side follow it all the way round to the Window and Blue Hole staying at 9/6m this will take you some 20 minutes. Once inside the Blue Hole, whilst completing safety stops if required, admire your surroundings or just diver watch before you exit E2.

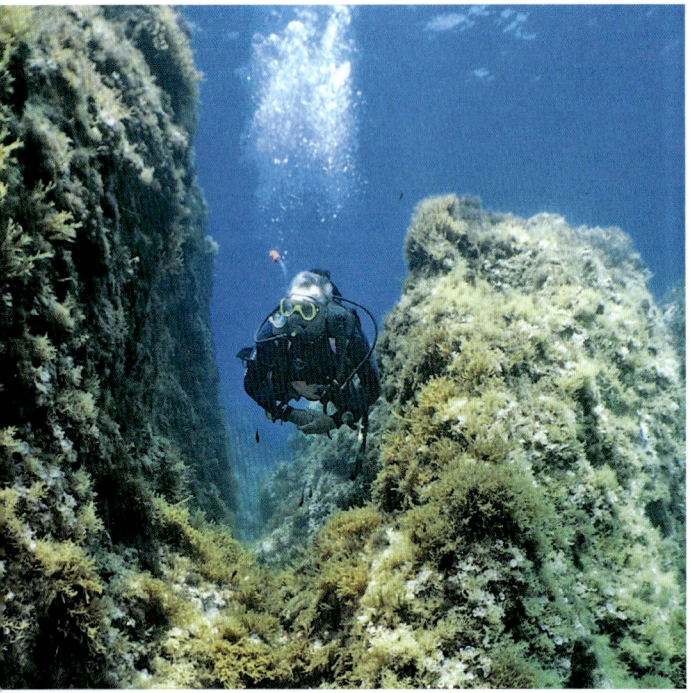

Exiting the "V" opening from Coral Gardens.

The drop-off on the far side of Coral Gardens.

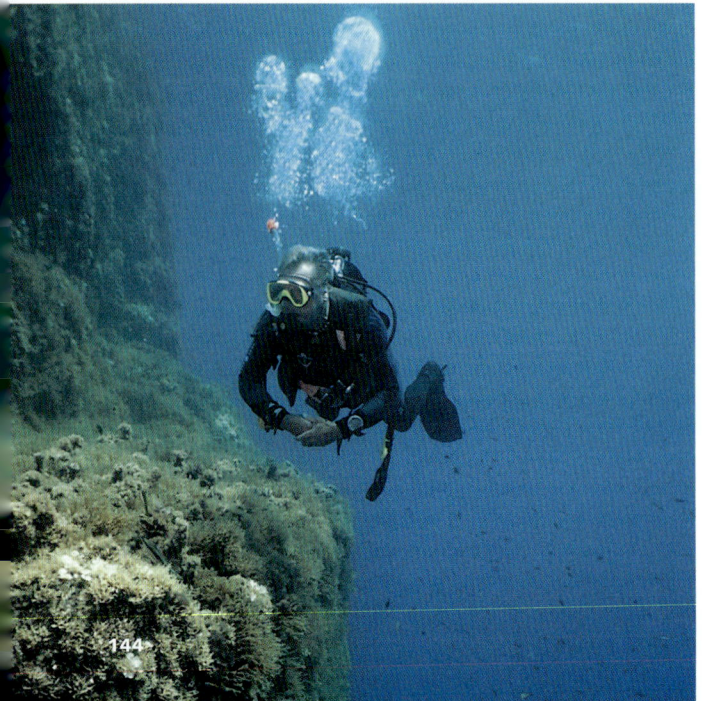

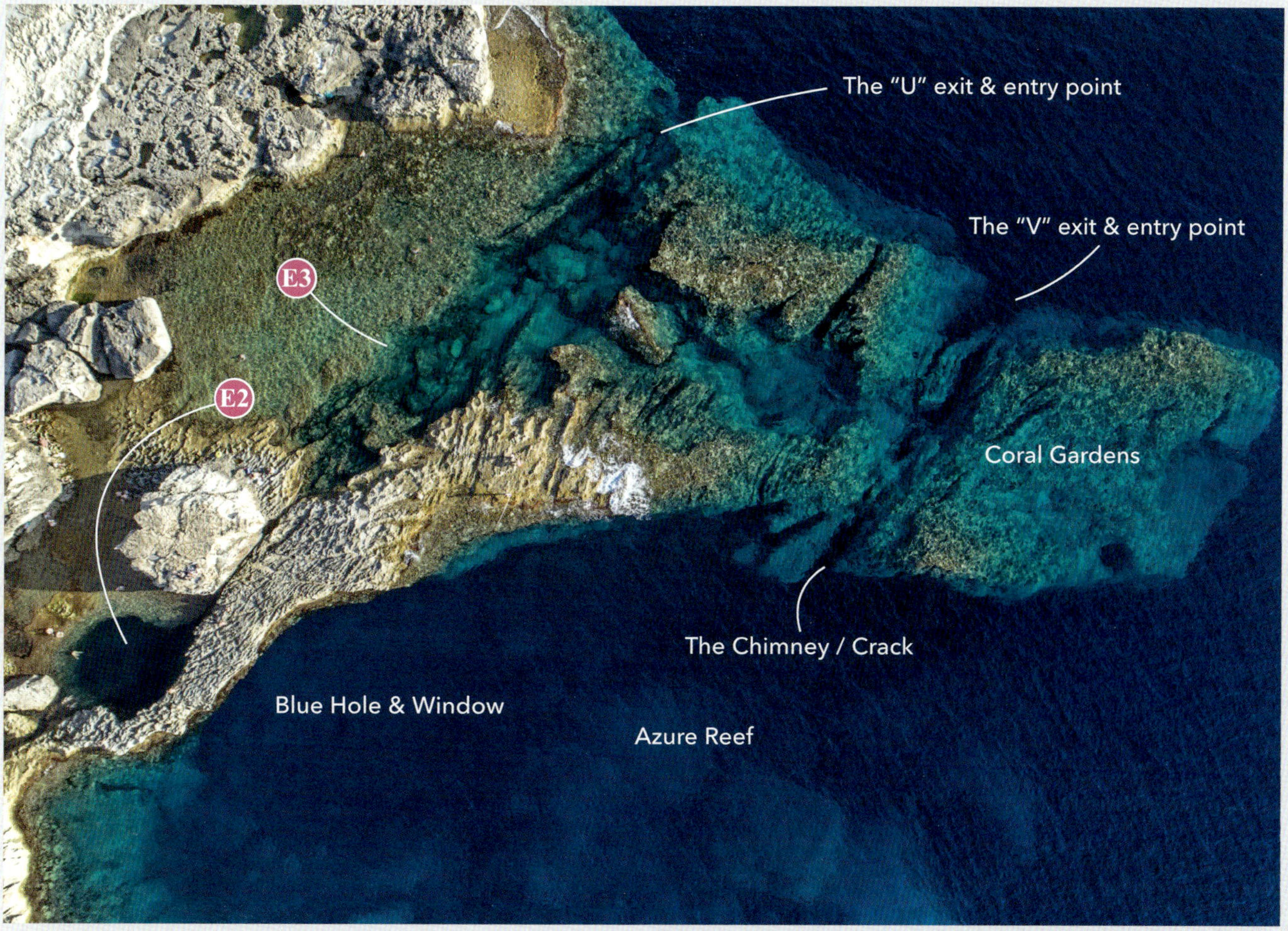

BLUE HOLE & CORAL GARDENS - DWEJRA

Labels on aerial photo:
- The "U" exit & entry point
- The "V" exit & entry point
- Coral Gardens
- The Chimney / Crack
- Blue Hole & Window
- Azure Reef
- E3
- E2

PHOTO: PER EIDE STUDIO'S www.pereide.no

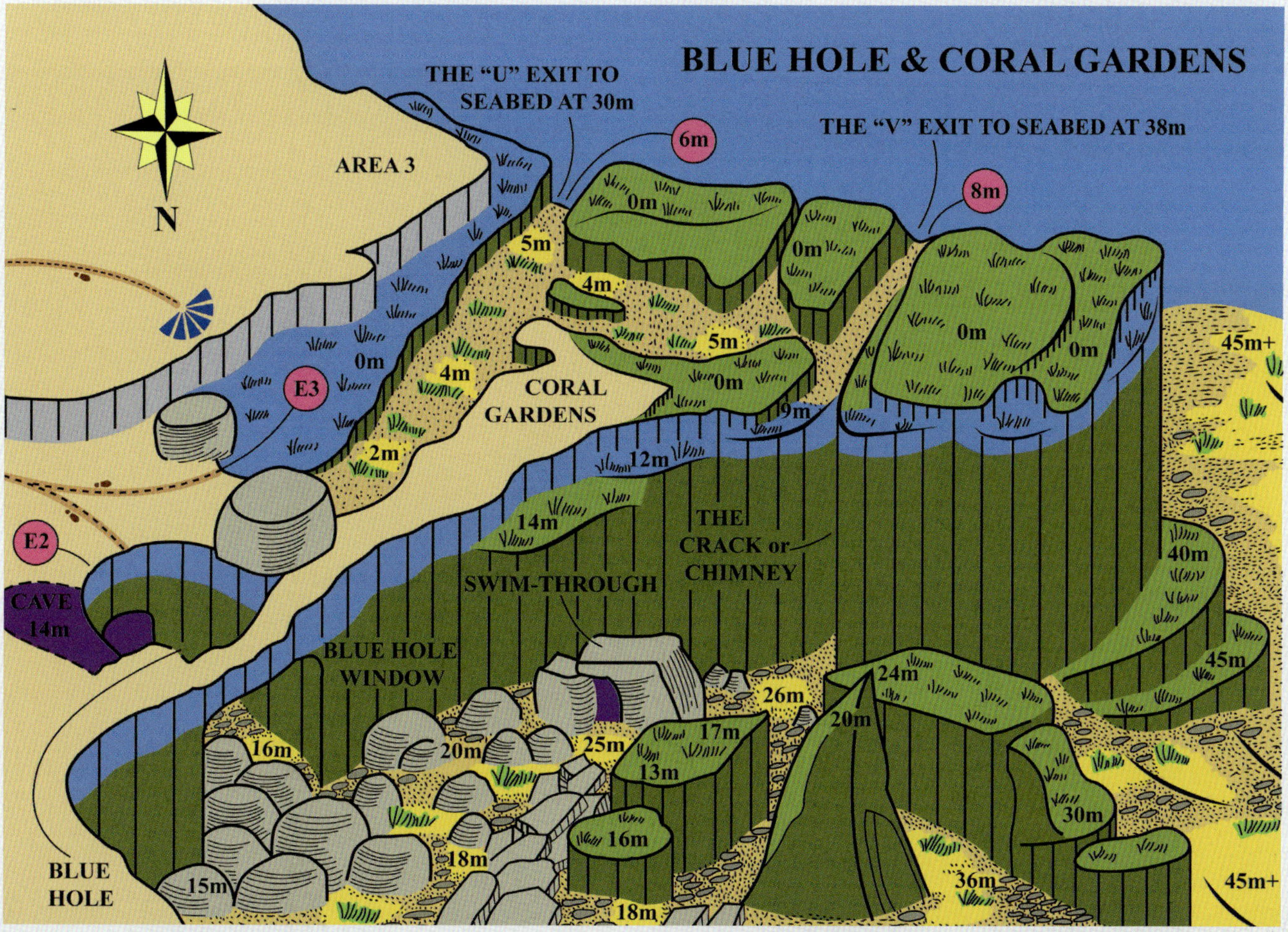

BLUE HOLE & CORAL GARDENS

Map labels:
- AREA 3
- THE "U" EXIT TO SEABED AT 30m
- THE "V" EXIT TO SEABED AT 38m
- CORAL GARDENS
- THE CRACK or CHIMNEY
- SWIM-THROUGH
- BLUE HOLE WINDOW
- BLUE HOLE
- CAVE 14m
- E2, E3

Depths marked: 6m, 8m, 0m, 5m, 4m, 5m, 0m, 9m, 2m, 12m, 14m, 17m, 13m, 16m, 20m, 25m, 26m, 24m, 20m, 30m, 36m, 18m, 16m, 15m, 18m, 40m, 45m, 45m+

BLUE HOLE & CORAL GARDENS - DWEJRA

Azure Reef – Blue Hole — Area 4

For this dive I would use entry/exit point E2, the Blue Hole. Leave the main car park head in a westerly direction towards the sea, down the steps and bear right; down more steps into the valley. Bear left, then on your right the route continues over the rocks, this is not easy be careful over the rocks. Once you reach sea level go through a narrow gap between the cliff face and a large boulder, now bear round to your right and the Blue Hole E3 will be in front of you.

The Blue Hole is very popular with divers, so is the newly formed mountainous Azure Reef, which is quite unique, and at the end of your dive a visit to the cave in the rear of the Blue Hole, a torch will be required.

There are a number of ways you can dive this site I have selected just one and for navigation I will use the reef wall that surrounds the Azure Reef on three sides. An ideal dive site where you could plan your own dive, visiting the peak and large boulder area and the base of the Azure Window.

THE DIVE — Minimum time - 50 mins

While descending the Blue Hole you will pass the top of the window at 7m after passing through the window head in a southwest direction to the swim through at 20m. Now continue to the very large boulder near the entrance to the Crack at 27m, this boulder was the top of the Azure Window, ascend to its top at 24m, dive time now 7/9 minutes. From here take a north westerly bearing this will take you towards the peaks, valleys and the base of the Azure Window. Your dive time now could be 25/30 minutes depending on the time taken to explore the peaks. A compass bearing of 30° will take you to the Azure Windows base, when the base reef comes into view head towards the western end, here there are ledges that step up towards the surface at different depths 30m, 22m, 15m, 8m, the choice is yours. Once here continue round the back of the base, until you reach the coastal reef at 5m, the boulders now below you came from the arch. Now head southeast towards the window of the Blue Hole less than 5 minutes away, your dive time should be 40/45 minutes.

The collapse of the Azure Window has created swim throughs, **care must be taken.**

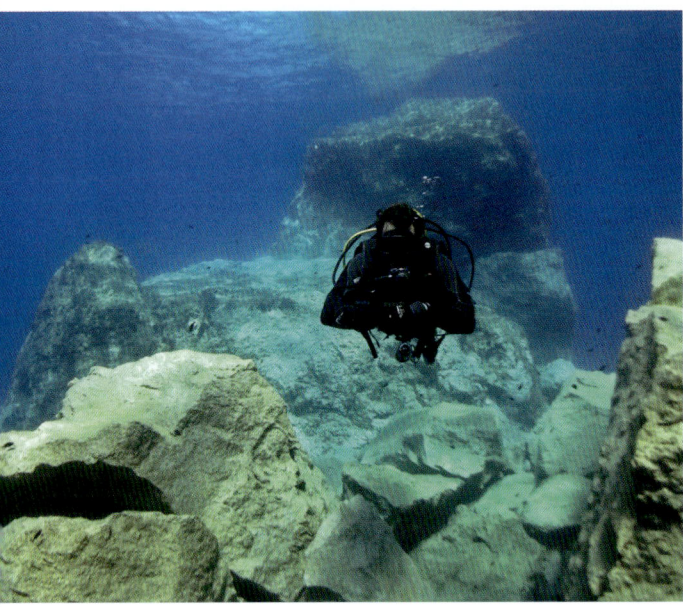

What was the base of the Azure Window.

One of the massive boulders within this reef.

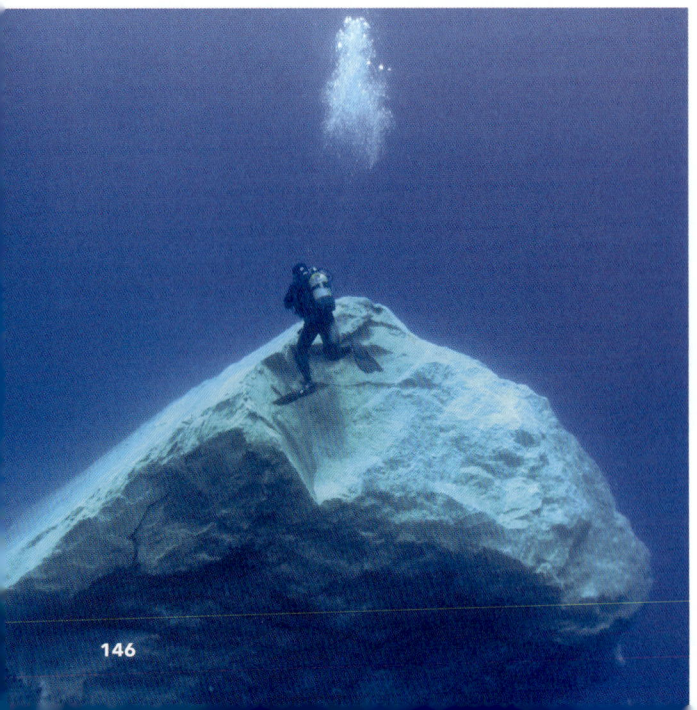

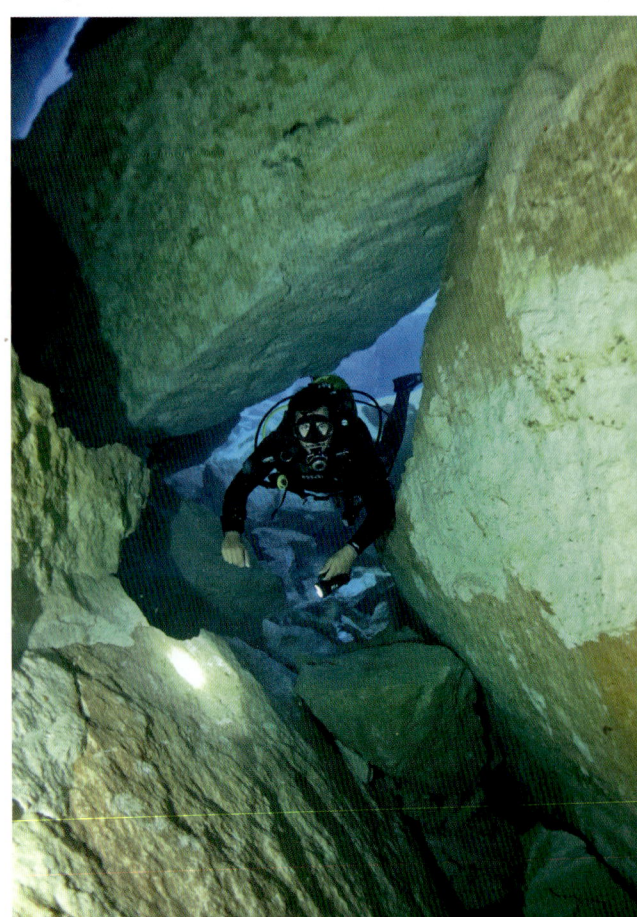

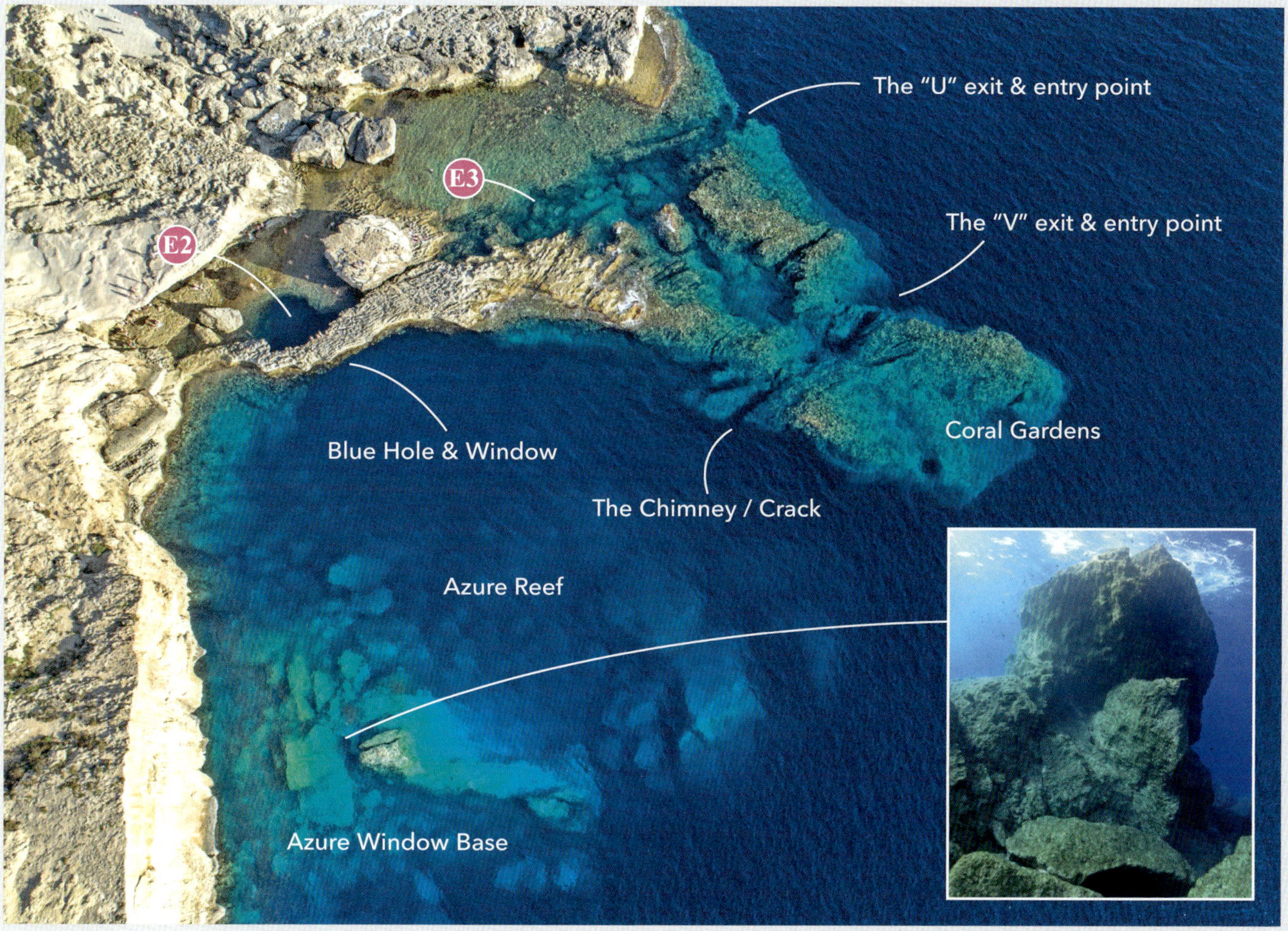
The "U" exit & entry point
E3
E2
The "V" exit & entry point
Blue Hole & Window
Coral Gardens
The Chimney / Crack
Azure Reef
Azure Window Base

PHOTO: PER EIDE STUDIO'S www.pereide.no

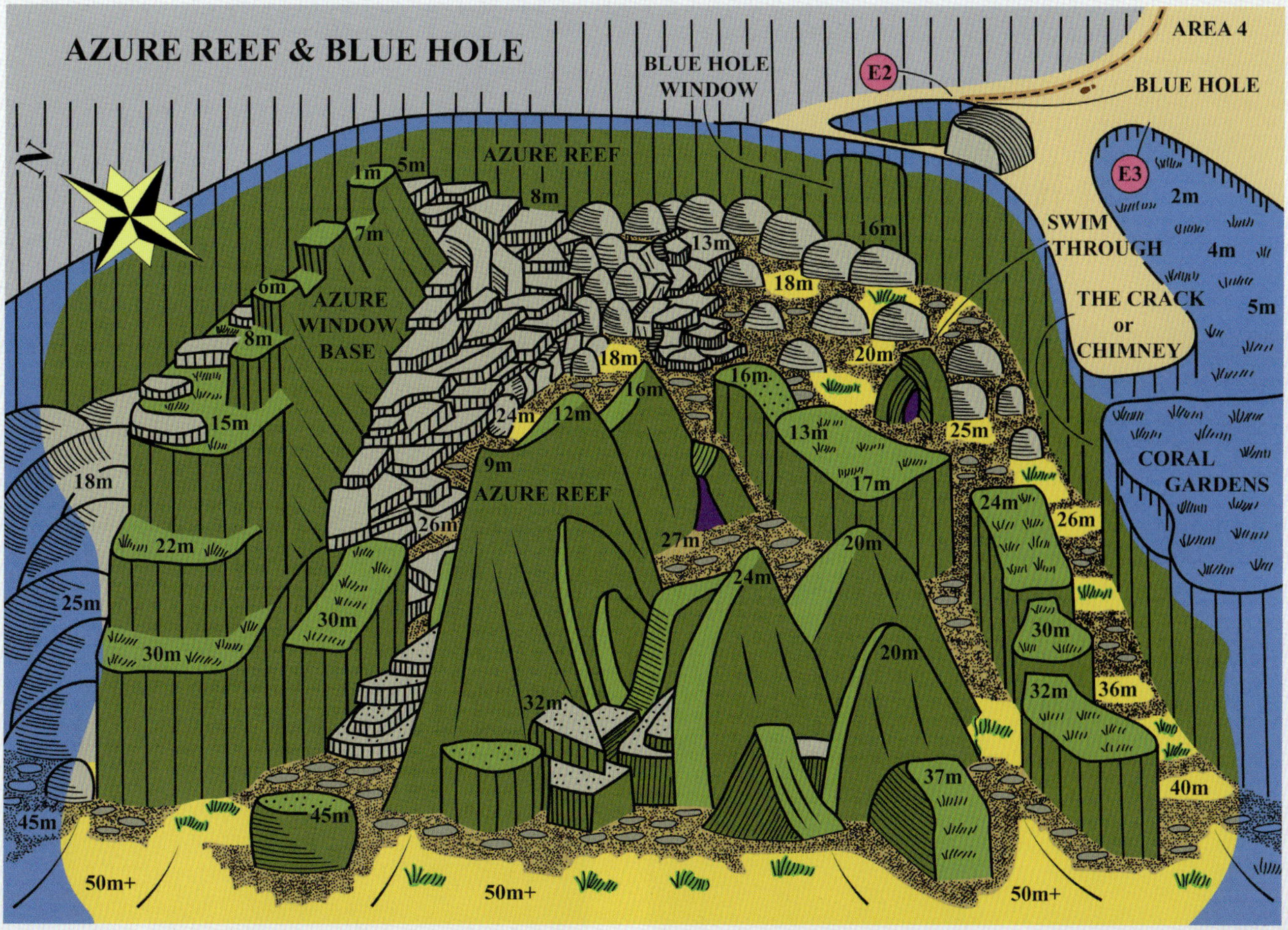
AZURE REEF & BLUE HOLE
BLUE HOLE WINDOW
E2
AREA 4
BLUE HOLE
E3
N
AZURE REEF
1m
5m
8m
7m
6m
8m
AZURE WINDOW BASE
13m
16m
18m
2m
4m
5m
SWIM THROUGH
THE CRACK or CHIMNEY
18m
20m
16m
16m
15m
24m
12m
13m
25m
CORAL GARDENS
18m
9m
AZURE REEF
17m
24m
26m
26m
22m
27m
20m
25m
24m
30m
30m
30m
20m
32m
36m
32m
37m
40m
45m
45m
50m+
50m+
50m+

Inland Sea to Blue Hole — Area 5

> **This dive should only be attempted in calm seas conditions and is only recommended for experienced divers. Beware of the small motor boats carrying tourists in the tunnel, so while in the tunnel it is most important to keep to the sides, if you have to surface.**

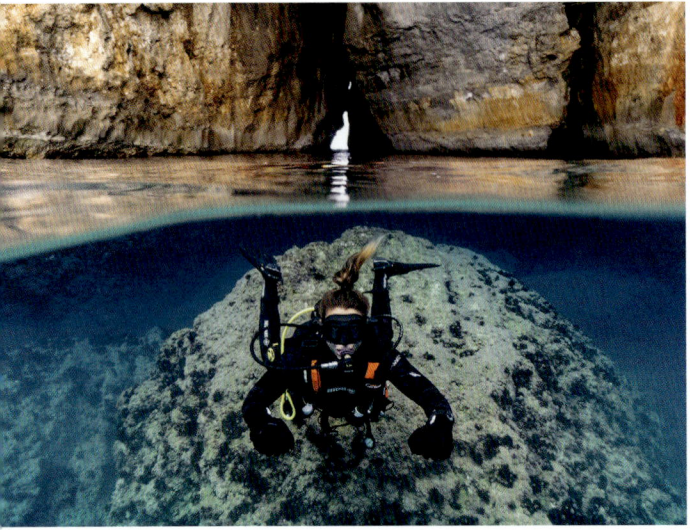

The Inland Sea Tunnel entrance and entry E1.

PHOTO: LEE JELLYMAN RITUAL DIVING CENTRE

This dive plan is from the Inland Sea to the Blue Hole, via the tunnel, a route of approximately 400 metres, a torch, to light up the reef is good idea. There are no exit points along this route, your only help is the pleasure boats if they are running. Once out of the tunnel stay at your required depth and keep to the coastline, there are a number of small ledges at various depths, otherwise the sides drop away to 50m plus.

Inside the 70-metre tunnel, don't forget your torch.

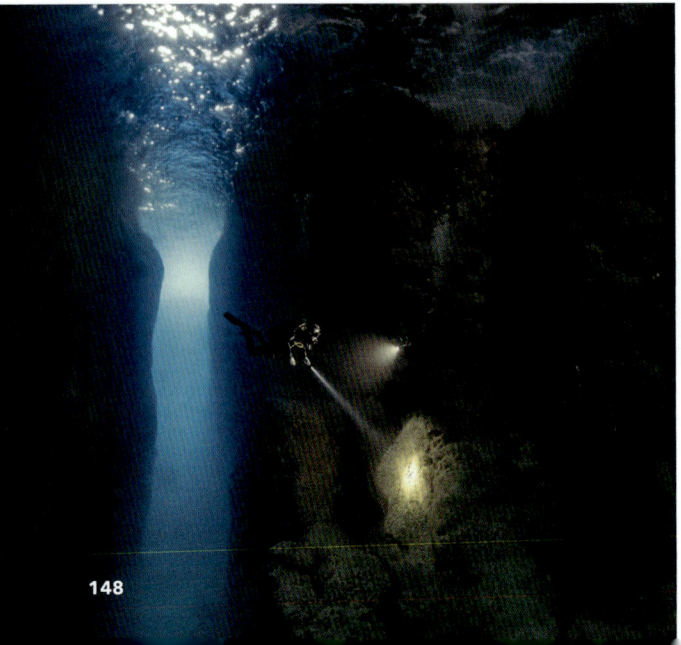

THE DIVE — Minimum time - 50 mins

Your entry point, E1, is by the slipway at the Inland Sea, you then surface swim to the left of the entrance of the tunnel, here your depth is 3m. This will quickly increase to 9m, then to 16m, gradually dropping to 26m at the other end of the tunnel where the bottom is reasonably flat. The length of the tunnel is some 80 metres.

Once out of the tunnel turn left and keep the reef on your left-hand side at all times apart from passing the cove. The first part of the reef will take you in a westerly direction, changing to southerly later.

The following times and depths are where the described pilotage points can be found. 12 minutes 24m a rock wedged in-between a fissure of two rocks. 14 minutes 21m, a rock shaped like a pointing finger. 16 minutes 18m, a triple ledge close together. 20 minutes 18m and halfway with an 18m ledge and two boulders below. After around 22 minutes you will find a cove where the seabed is covered with boulders and you might think that this is leading up to the Azure base, do not enter just cross over to the other side and continue to follow the coastline reef, 26 minutes, 19m and a whitish rock on a ledge. In about 30 minutes, you should have reached the boulders leading up to the Azure base at 5m, from here it is no more than 3 minutes to the window of the Blue Hole and your exit point E2. This is only a guide; you can of course vary your depth and time to suit you and your dive plan.

Just outside the Blue Hole Window.

PHOTOS LEFT & RIGHT: LEE JELLYMAN RITUAL DIVE CENTRE

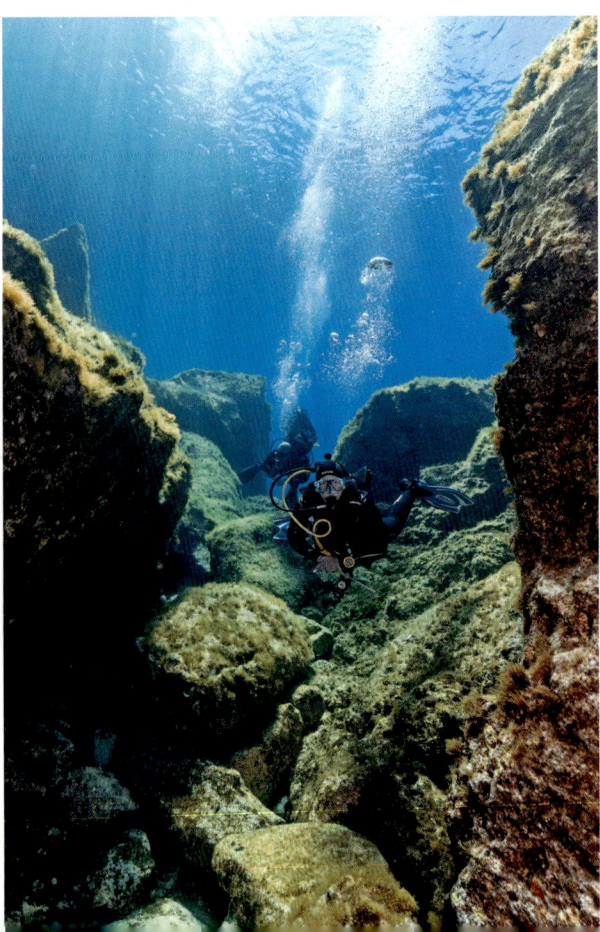

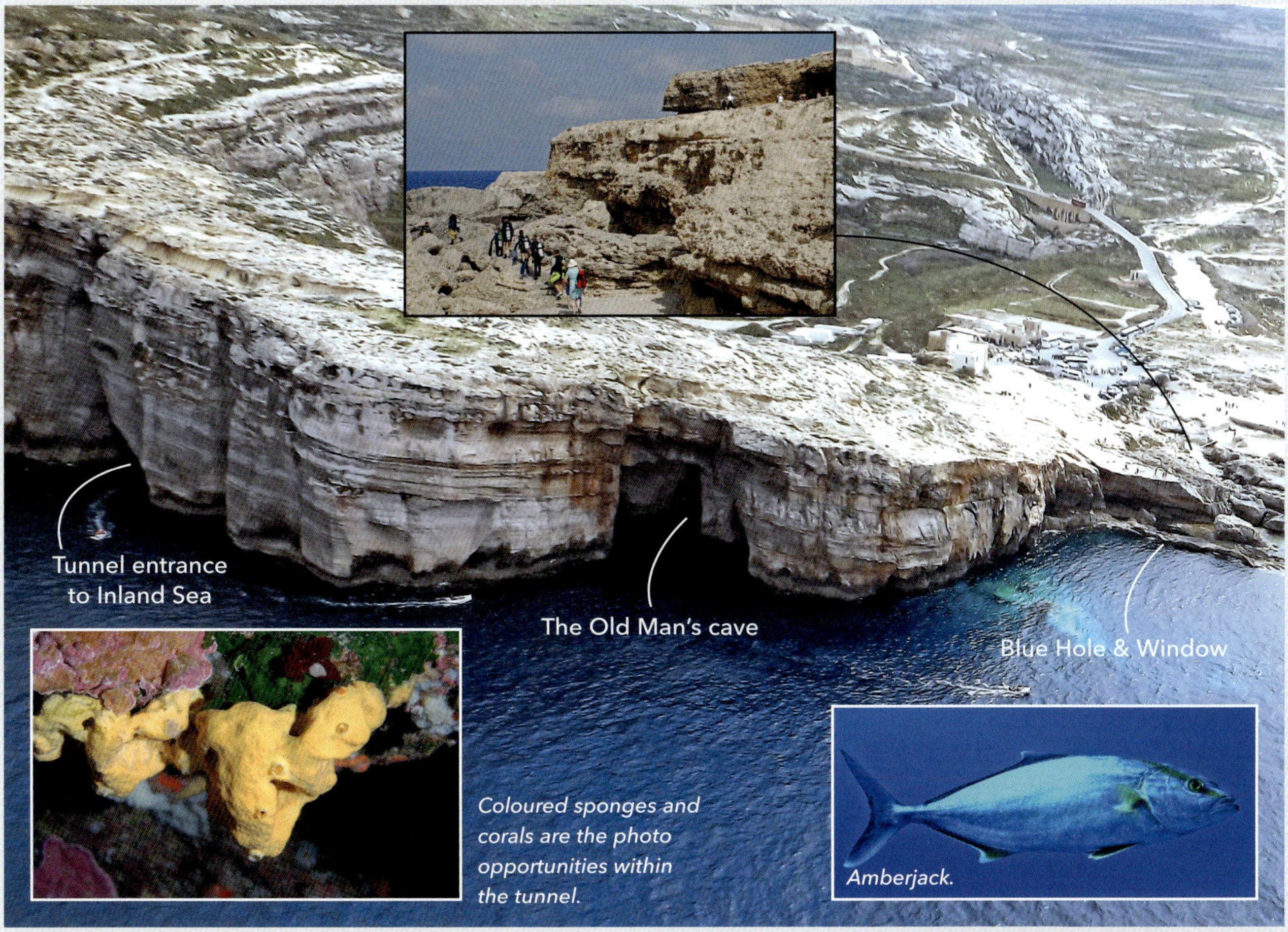

Tunnel entrance
to Inland Sea
The Old Man's cave
Blue Hole & Window
Coloured sponges and corals are the photo opportunities within the tunnel.
Amberjack.

PHOTO: PER EIDE STUDIO'S www.pereide.no

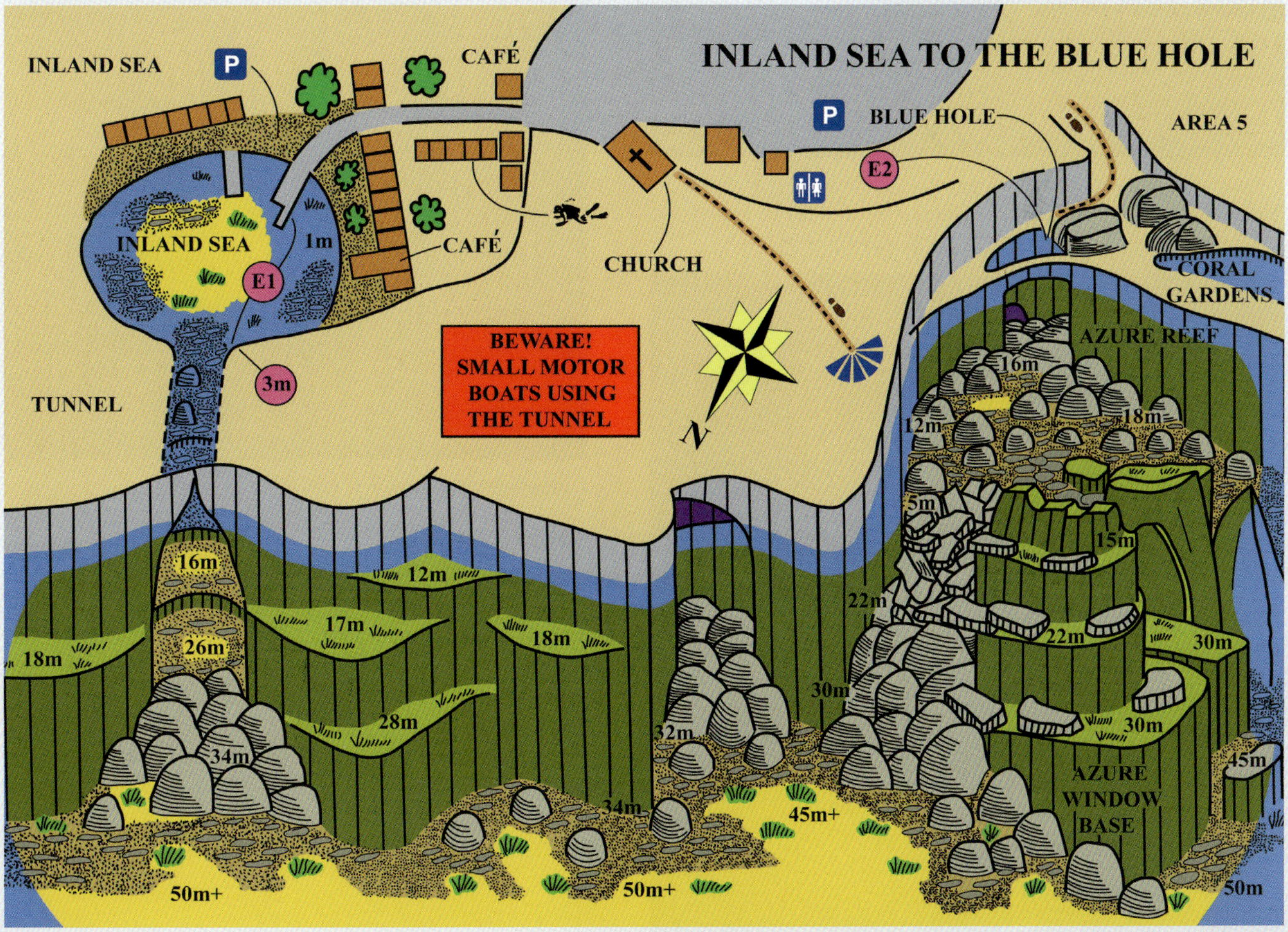

INLAND SEA TO THE BLUE HOLE
INLAND SEA
P
CAFÉ
P
BLUE HOLE
AREA 5
E2
INLAND SEA
1m
E1
CAFÉ
CHURCH
CORAL
GARDENS
AZURE REEF
16m
18m
12m
TUNNEL
3m
BEWARE!
SMALL MOTOR
BOATS USING
THE TUNNEL
N
5m
15m
16m
12m
26m
17m
18m
18m
22m
22m
30m
28m
30m
30m
32m
34m
34m
45m
45m+
AZURE
WINDOW
BASE
50m+
50m+
50m

Inland Sea & Tunnel — Area 6

This unique dive with its 80-metre tunnel with depths from 3m at the entrance to 26m at the exit and is large enough to accommodate a double decker bus with space to spare. Remember the tunnel is the only route to your exit point, the next nearest exit is 400 metres south, and to the north half way round the island. Once out of the tunnel your selected dive plan will determine which way you want to go. I would suggest going right, even though the drop offs are not so dramatic, there is a cave, overhangs and two long ledges at 18m and 10m to explore. Please check outer sea conditions before diving the tunnel.

> **If surfacing in the tunnel it is important to keep close to the sides, due to the boats. Check sea state before diving the tunnel.**

THE DIVE — Minimum time - 40 mins

Your entry point is E1, the same as the previous dive at the entrance your depth is only 3m, so keep to the side until you are safely in deeper water. The tunnel slopes down steeply at first and then levels out to the exit at 26m. Once outside the tunnel, the seabed tumbles down over the boulders to the sand at 50m plus. If you are going to turn right to head for Whale Cave the distance is almost 100 metres and your maximum depth could be 25m, as this is the depth at the bottom of the cave which goes in some 70 metres and rises to a depth inside of 5m.

Please note on your return there is an entrance to a cave/overhang which can be confused with the tunnel, but it is much smaller, so just double check. Hopefully you have brought your torch so you can take your time exploring the tunnel on your way back to your exit.

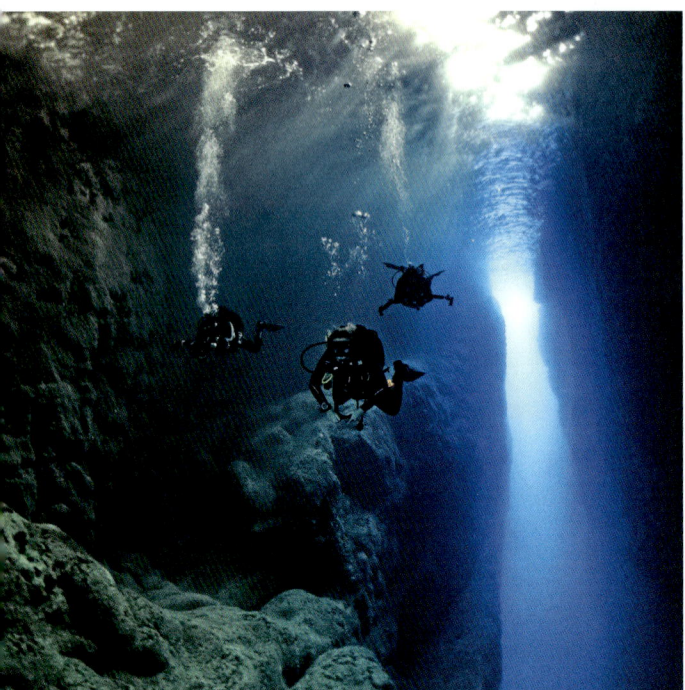

A group of divers returning to the Inland Sea.
PHOTOS: LEE JELLYMAN RITUAL DIVE CENTRE

Excellent opportunity for photos within the tunnel.

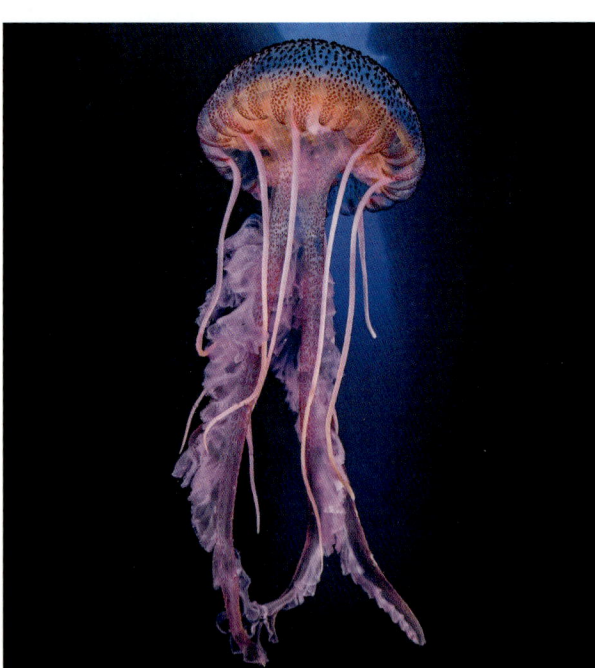

This jellyfish has found its way into the tunnel.
PHOTO: LEE JELLYMAN RITUAL DIVE CENTRE

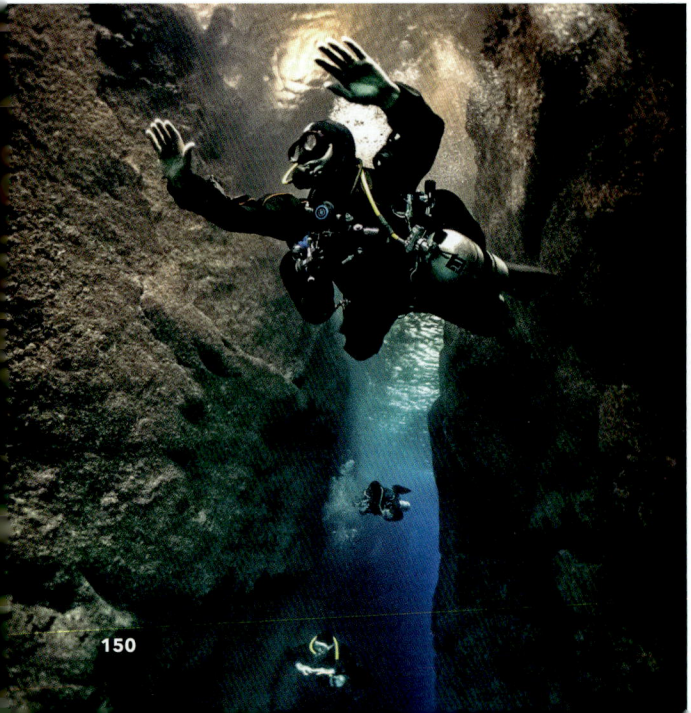

All the normal facilities are here; there is a café at the top car park and another overlooking the Inland Sea, my favourite place here, its reasonably priced and after your dive it nice to sit, rest and fill in your logbook. This area is very popular with the tourists as well as divers, but there is a lot to see and do, so it does not seem to get too crowded. When parking your vehicle by the Inland Sea keep to the area of large pebbles for it has been known that vehicles get stuck where the smaller stones are.

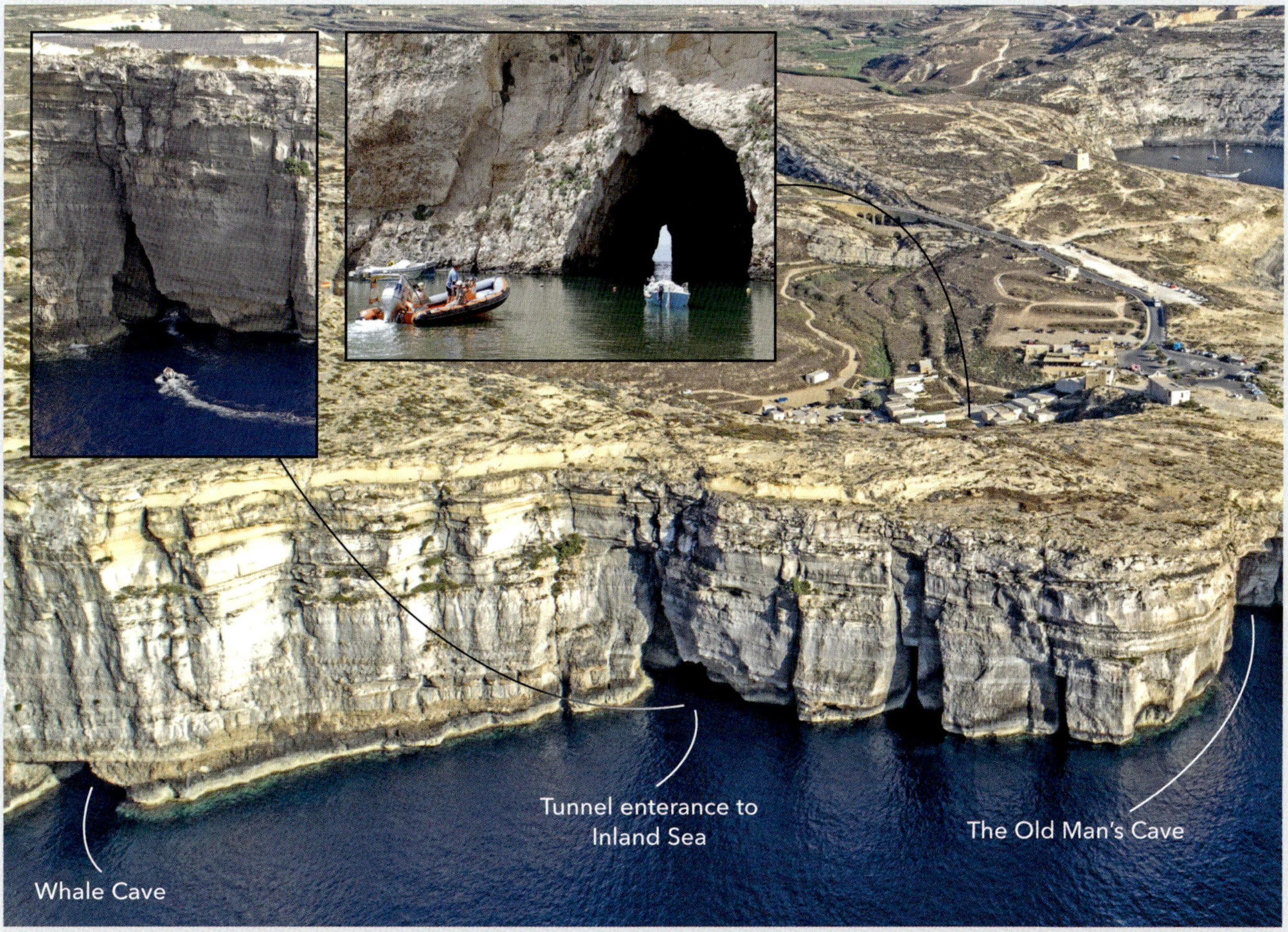

Tunnel enterance to
Inland Sea
The Old Man's Cave
Whale Cave

PHOTO: PER EIDE STUDIO'S www.pereide.no

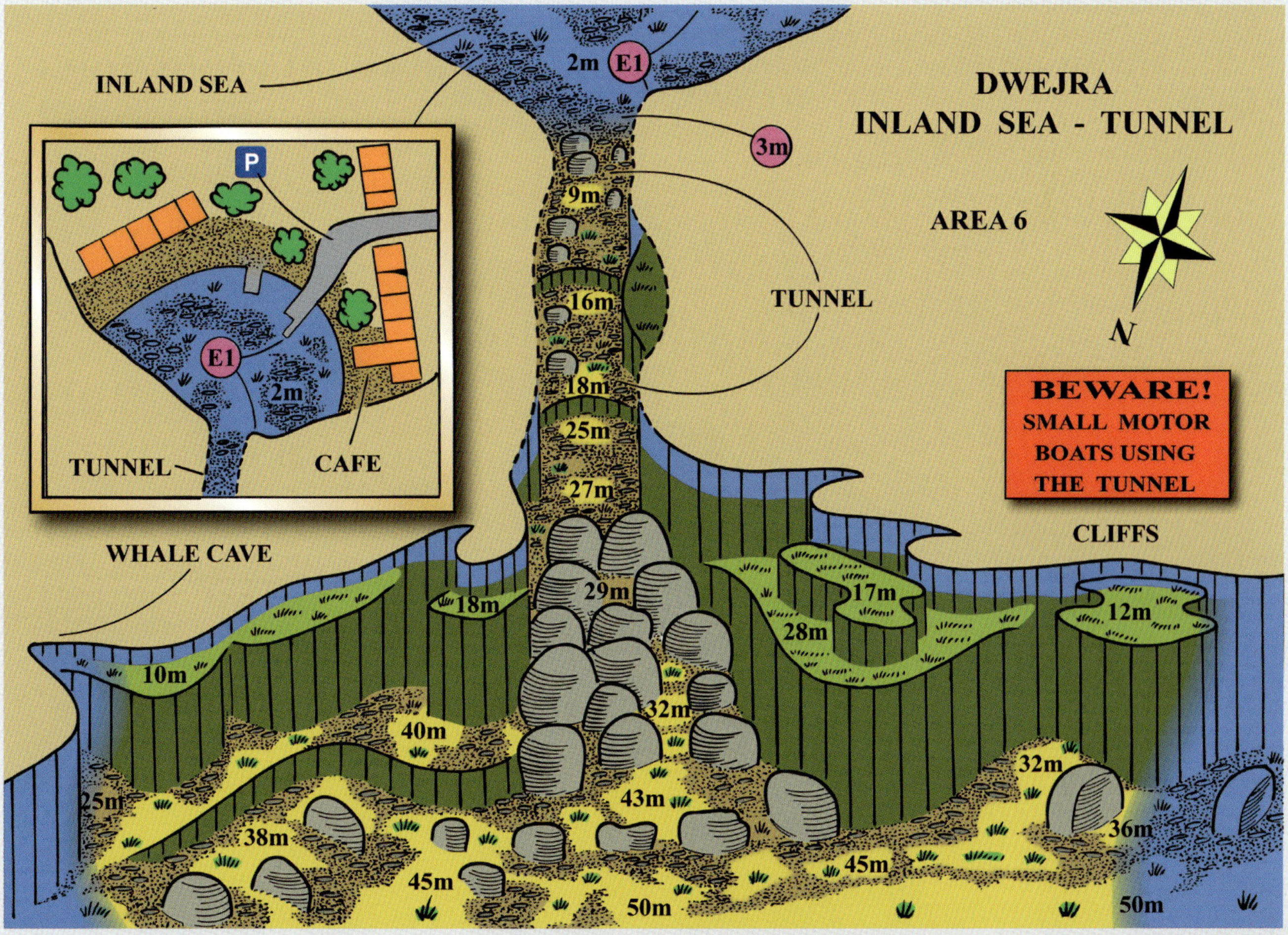
DWEJRA
INLAND SEA - TUNNEL
AREA 6
INLAND SEA
E1
2m
3m
9m
16m
18m
25m
27m
29m
32m
TUNNEL
P
CAFE
BEWARE!
SMALL MOTOR
BOATS USING
THE TUNNEL
CLIFFS
WHALE CAVE
17m
28m
12m
10m
40m
43m
25m
38m
45m
50m
36m
N

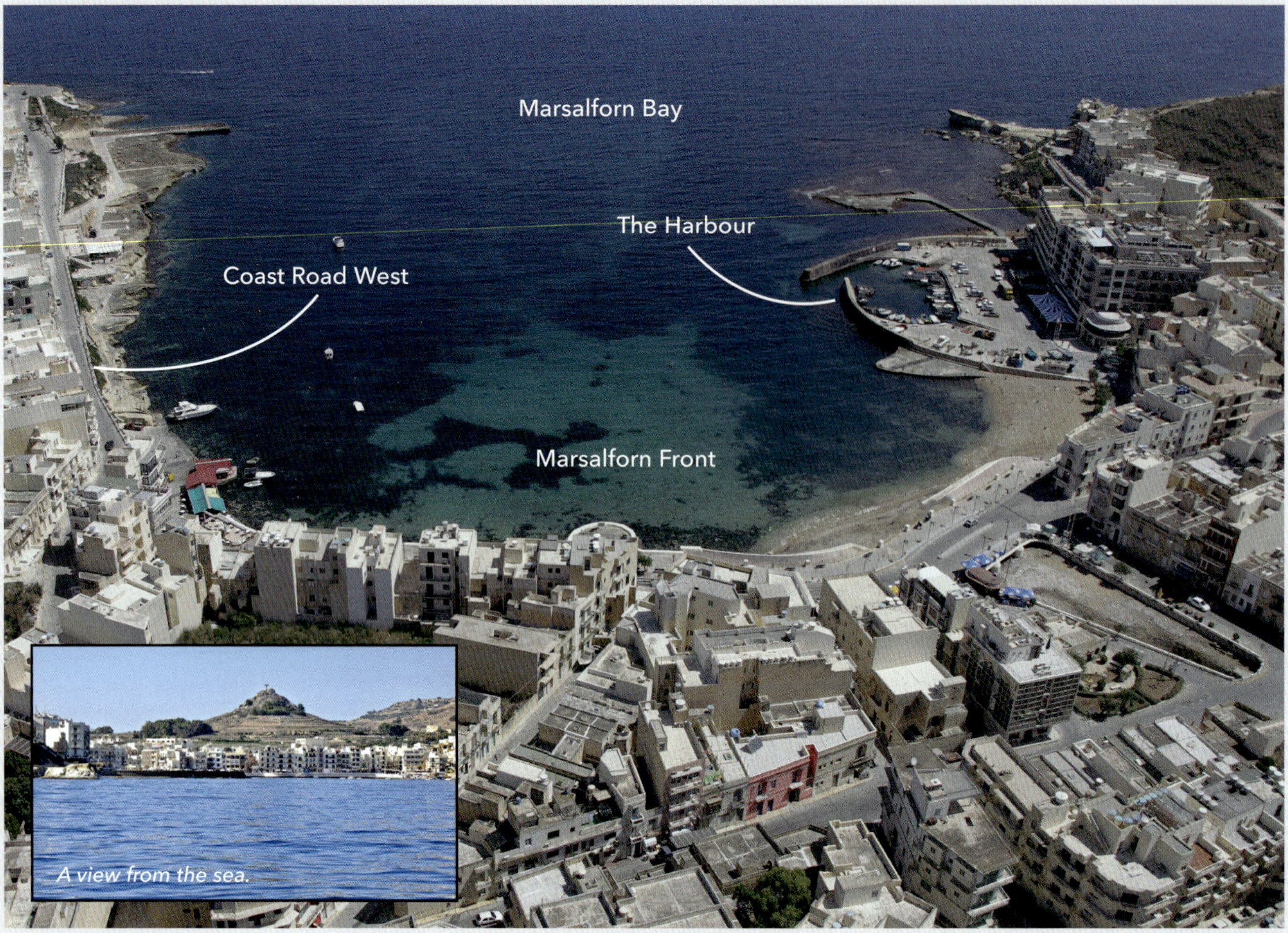

MARSALFORN TO REQQA POINT

Marsalforn Bay
The Harbour
Coast Road West
Marsalforn Front

A view from the sea.

PGL AERIAL PHOTOS

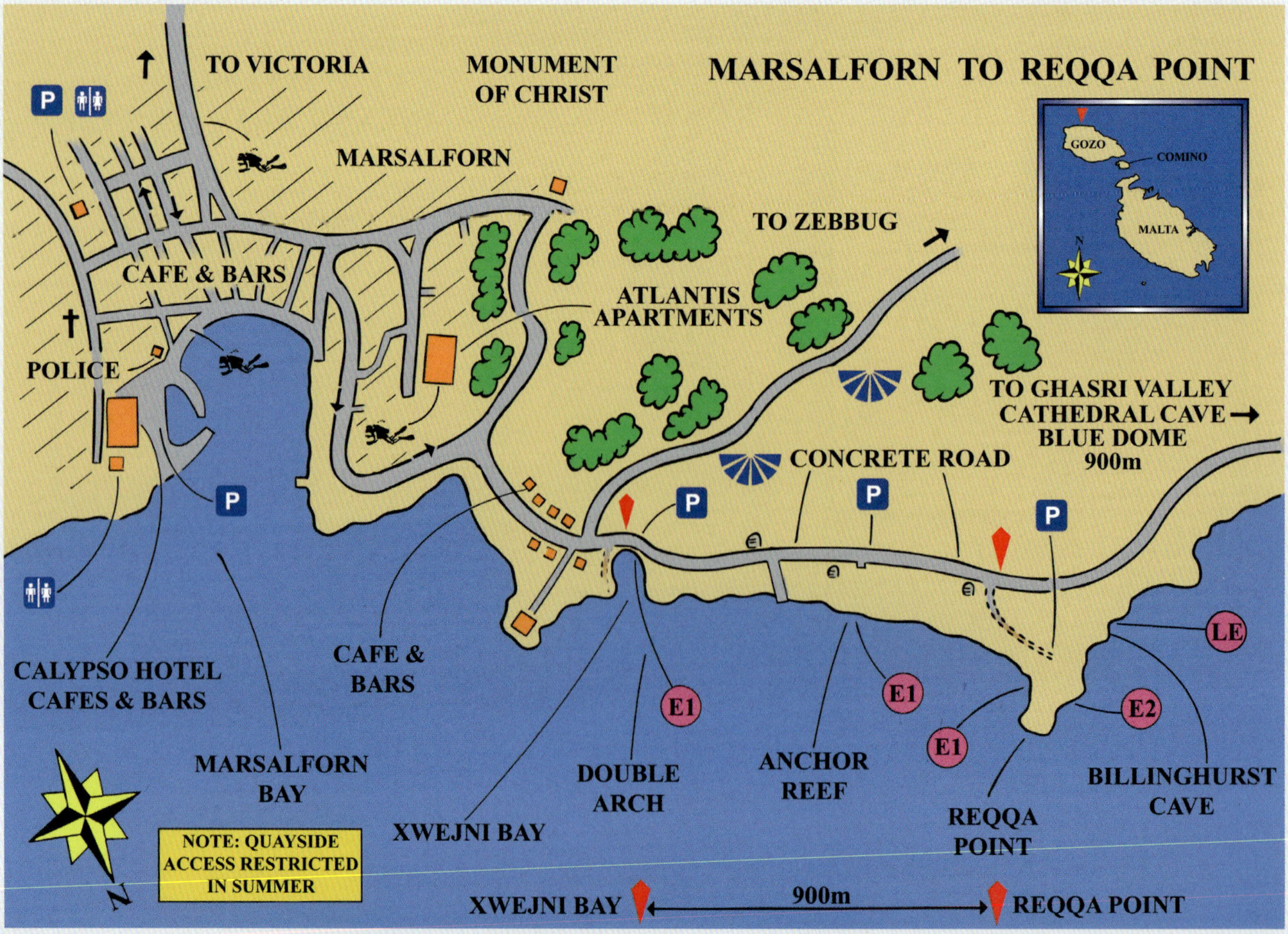

MARSALFORN TO REQQA POINT

TO VICTORIA
MONUMENT OF CHRIST
MARSALFORN
CAFE & BARS
POLICE
TO ZEBBUG
ATLANTIS APARTMENTS
TO GHASRI VALLEY
CATHEDRAL CAVE
BLUE DOME
900m
CONCRETE ROAD

CALYPSO HOTEL
CAFES & BARS
CAFE & BARS
MARSALFORN BAY
DOUBLE ARCH
XWEJNI BAY
ANCHOR REEF
REQQA POINT
BILLINGHURST CAVE

E1 — Double Arch
E1 — Anchor Reef
E1 — Reqqa Point
E2 — Billinghurst Cave
LE

NOTE: QUAYSIDE ACCESS RESTRICTED IN SUMMER

XWEJNI BAY ← 900m → REQQA POINT

GOZO — COMINO — MALTA

Marsalforn - Local Dive Sites

The dive sites, Double Arch, Anchor Reef, Reqqa Point, Billingshurst Cave and Cathedral Cave/ Blue Dome (Ghasri Valley) are on the north coast of Gozo, not far from the resort of Marsalforn. To find these sites head out of Marsalforn in a westerly direction, on the coast road to Xwejni Bay which is 1.8 km. Here the concrete road starts, and your entry point for the Double Arch, see Local Map. **Please do walk over the salt pans it is a cottage industry and they are in use, when open you can purchase packets of sea salt.**

Double Arch

There are a number of dive sites around the world with single arches, but this site with its double arch is quite unique. It is some 200 metres off shore and can take up to 20 minutes to reach and 25 minutes for your return, depending on your speed. An excellent shore dive but you need both good weather conditions and good visibility, and for experienced divers who are skilled in navigation. This dive site can be a boat dive, this means no 200-metre swim, the choice is yours, I have done both, each is a different experience.

If you stay above the Arch and on top of the reef/plateau your maximum depth would be 20m for the more qualified divers there are drop offs and depths of 40m below the arch. The average depth below the arch is 36m, to the west side of the arch which forms a double bridge between the main reef and the plateau. The small reef/plateau has a maximum depth of 17m and is surrounded by depths of 30m plus. Do not miss visiting this area and watch the passing marine life, such as shoals of barracuda coming up from the deep and swimming over the reef descending on the other side. Swimming round the edge this reef will only take you about 5 minutes.

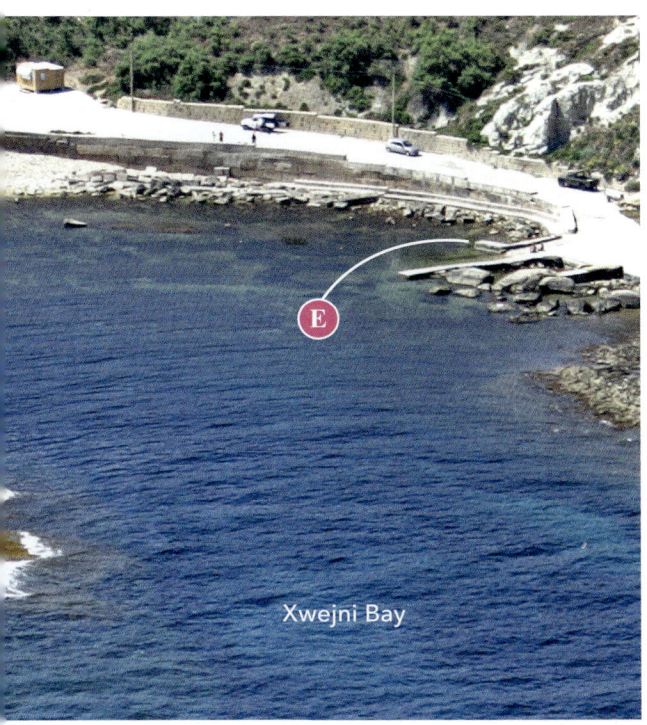
Xwejni Bay

Anchor Reef Entry exit point E1.

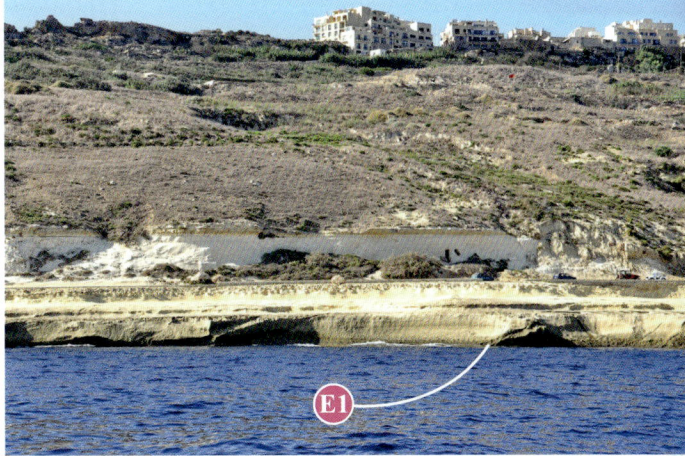

Reqqa Point Entry exit point LE and E1.

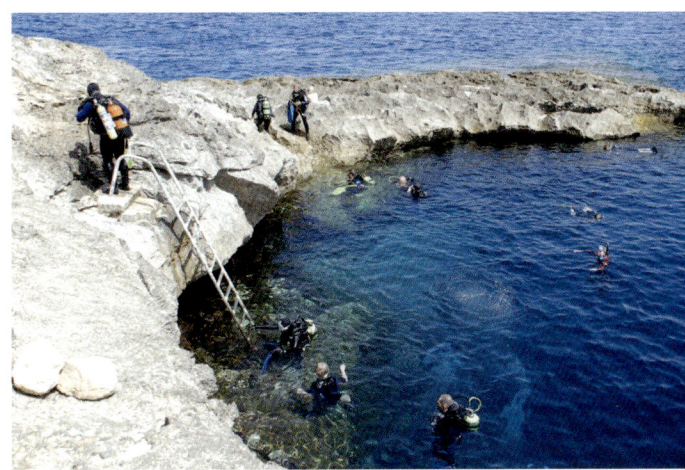

Cathedral Cave Ladder LE entry exit point.

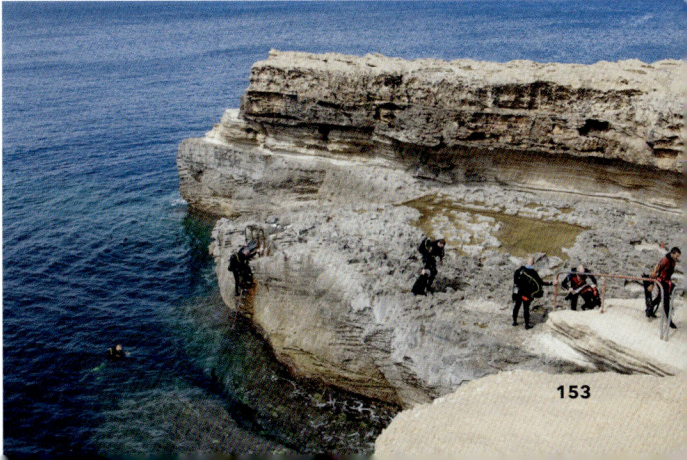

DOUBLE ARCH - MARSALFORN

THE DIVES — Minimum time - 55 mins

Use E1 entry point near the slipway and surface swim just past the point of land on your left, about 8/10 minutes. The depth here will be about 9m, this is where I descend, once under the water take a northerly bearing on the compass and head for the first reef, this will take about 8 minutes, now check for any currents.

Here the sea bed is covered in posidonia grass which slopes gently to the first drop off where the depth is 15m, at this point you should find a double bowl area, on the sand below you at 24m is a broken anchor, maybe from Anchor Reef? From the centre of the two bowls take a northerly compass bearing and cross the deeper area towards the double arch, the approximate distance is 40 meters.

Explore the arches, admire, and maybe take some photographs, then proceed to the top of the arch, here head west onto the plateau and explore this unique area and do not forget the viewing point.

Remember you are at least 25 minutes away from your exit point. When you decide to return take an easterly compass bearing which will take you back to the arch, pass over, and follow the ridge of the reef all the way round until you come back to the double bowl area at 15m, this should take approximately 6/8 minutes. Of course, you can go straight over from the top of the arch to the first reef at 15m compass bearing south. From the Double Bowl continue with a southerly bearing, it will take you about 10/15 minutes to reach Xwejni Bay and your exit point.

This site is often visited by dive boats from Gozo and Malta so it is another option, these boats would normally complete two dives. It also allows you to see the Maltese Islands from a different view point, giving you a great day out.

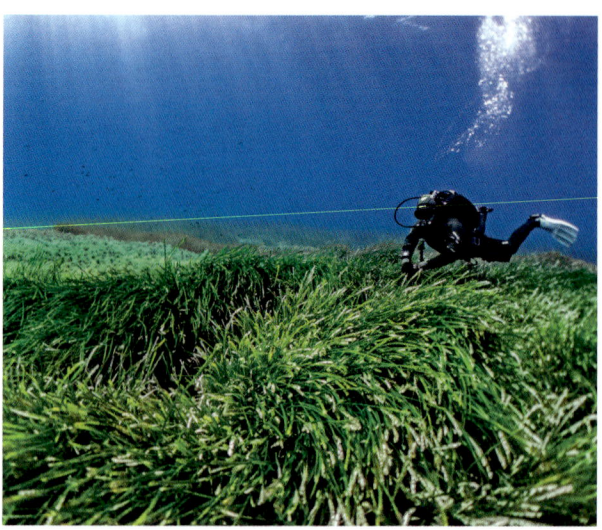

The seabed below at 9m when you first descend.
PHOTO: LEE JELLYMAN RITUAL DIVE CENTRE.

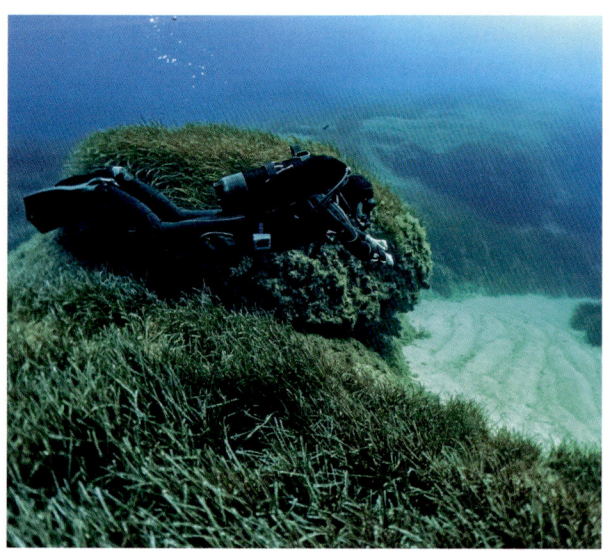

Seabed areas on route to the Double Arch.
PHOTOS: LEE JELLYMAN RITUAL DIVE CENTRE.

Below: Another view of the Double Arch.

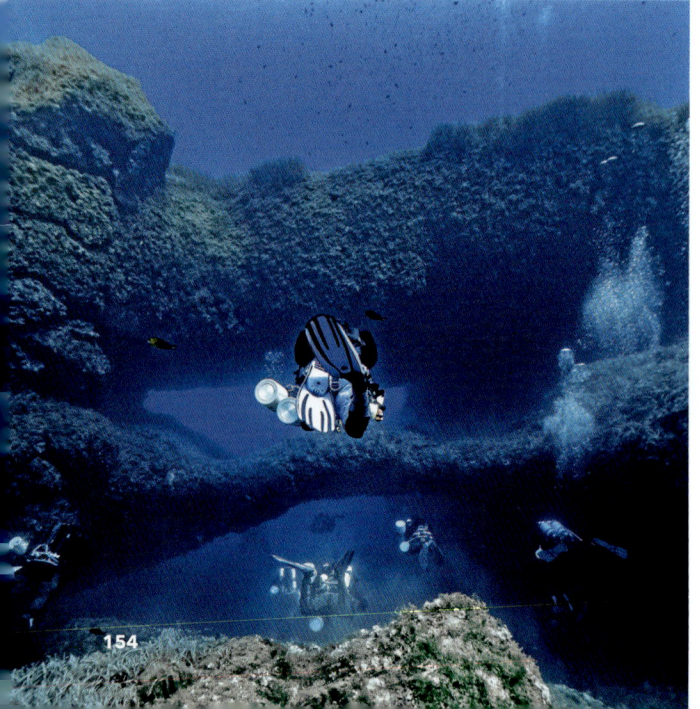

The Double Arch viewed from the open sea.
PHOTO: JON BORG www.jonborg.com

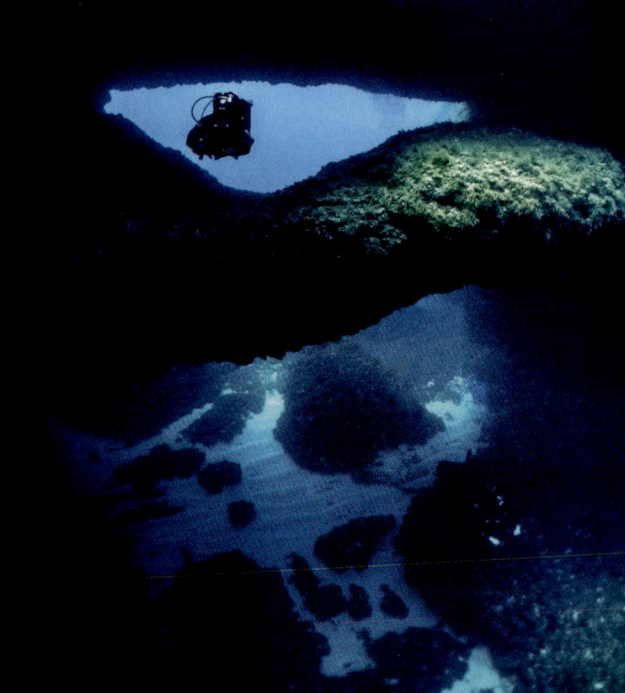

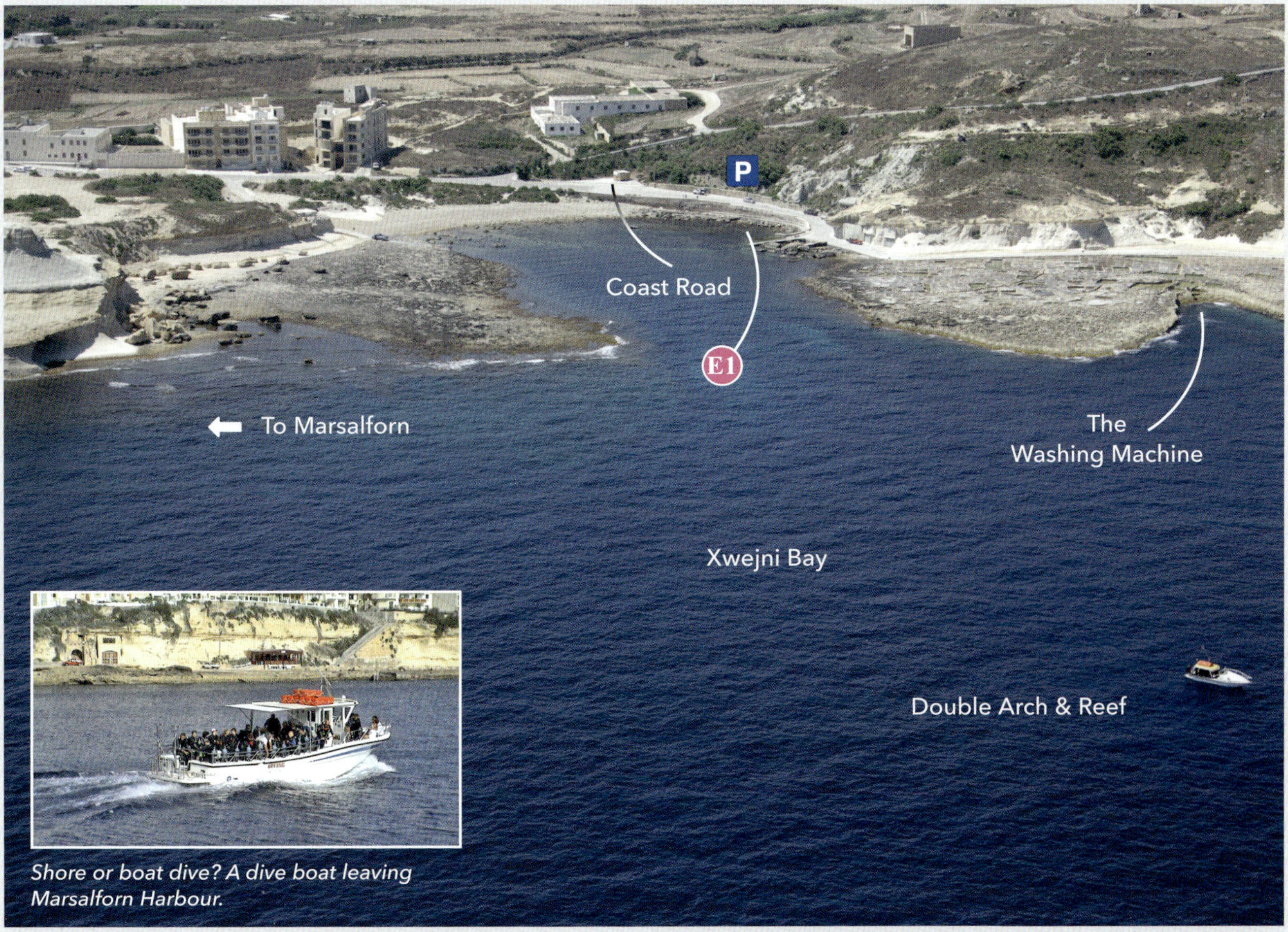

DOUBLE ARCH - MARSALFORN

Coast Road
To Marsalforn
The Washing Machine
Xwejni Bay
Double Arch & Reef

Shore or boat dive? A dive boat leaving Marsalforn Harbour.

PGL AERIAL PHOTOS

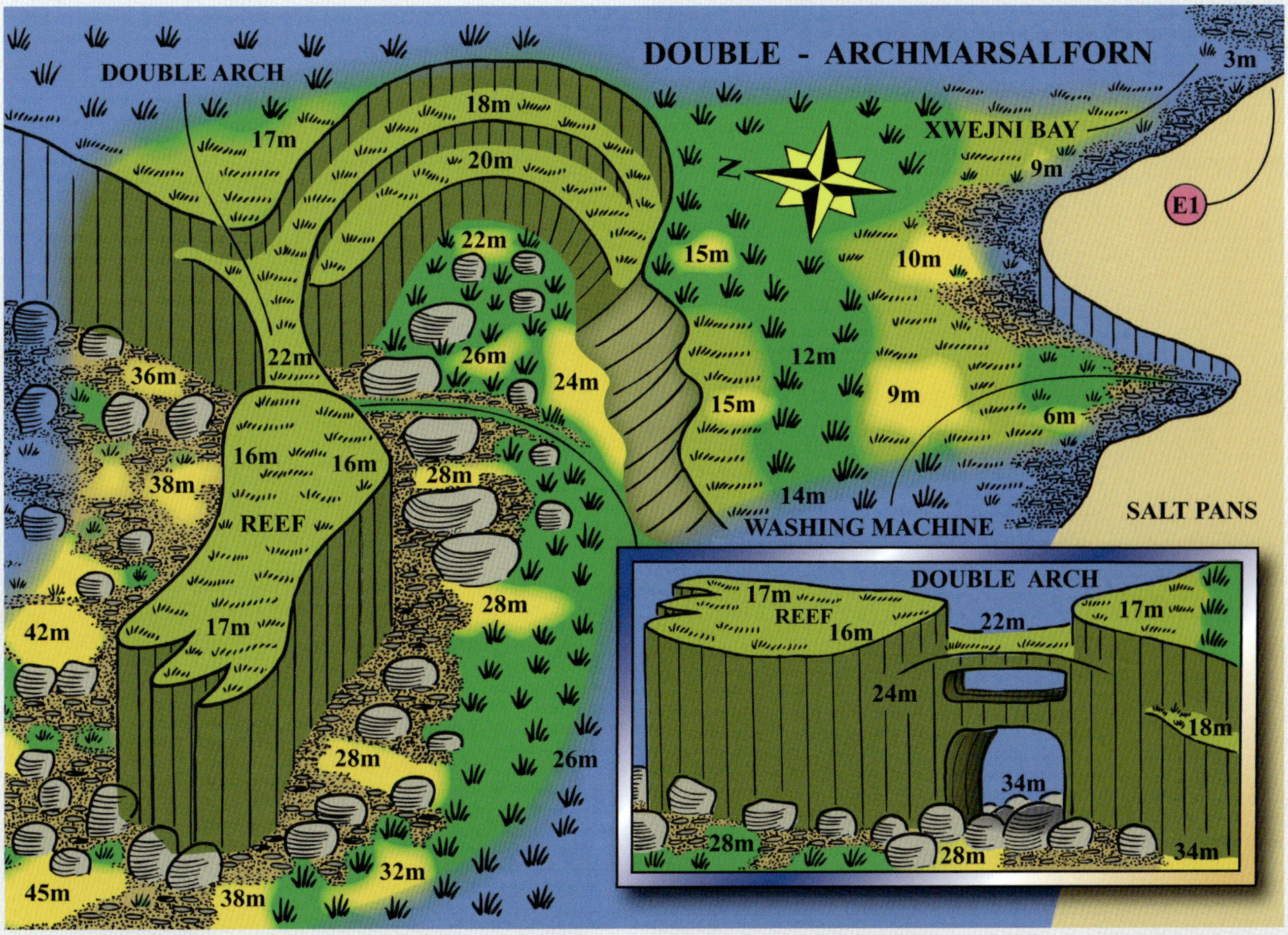

DOUBLE - ARCH MARSALFORN

DOUBLE ARCH
XWEJNI BAY
3m
17m
18m
20m
9m
22m
15m
10m
36m
22m
26m
24m
12m
9m
38m
16m
16m
15m
6m
28m
14m
REEF
WASHING MACHINE
SALT PANS
17m
42m
28m
DOUBLE ARCH
17m
REEF
22m
17m
28m
26m
16m
24m
18m
45m
38m
32m
28m
34m
28m
34m

Anchor Reef - Marsalforn

From Xwejni Bay slipway drive along the concrete road for 500 metres towards Reqqa Point, on the right-hand side a single rock opposite a track leading to a cave dwelling, a further 100 metres on, on the right over the wall is a disused track which leads towards your entry point (see aerial photograph).

Anchor reef has long been the name of this dive site and I have been informed on good authority that there used to be an anchor here. The tales then become a little hazy; one, some visiting divers from a country not too far away, raised the anchor and took it ashore, only to be arrested by the local constabulary, I can only assume that they have been released by now! Or maybe it's the anchor which is in two parts near the Double Arch, originally came from here? Then I was told it was in the Victoria Museum but they were unable to find it, so I am afraid it must still remain a mystery!

This dive is only just a short part of the reef which runs from Reqqa Point in the west, to the Double Arch in the east where the reef has much more dramatic drop offs. The average depth here is 50m plus. Quite often I have seen large groupers just resting on the rocks in this area. Remember you only have one exit point the next closest are some distance away at Xwejni Bay or Reqqa Point.

THE DIVE — Minimum time - 45 mins

Take care when going to entry point E1 and especially down the steps that have by cut out by fishermen. Once in the water descend to around 9m, below you the reef drops away quite sharply, to your left is the start of a 9m ledge, to your right there are a number of ledges ranging from 9m down to 35m, here it's a good idea to ID your exit point. Now descend to your chosen depth, once this is reached head in an easterly direction, after about 12/15 minutes and at a depth of 33m the reef changes from a steep slope to a sheer cliff, continue in the same direction at your chosen depth and around 25/30 minutes into your dive the reef direction will change from a 60° bearing to 120°. Now I suggest you ascend to the top of the reef at 12m and make this your turning point, follow the reef edge in a westerly direction back towards your exit point. Within 50 metres either side of your exit point are two areas of rugged rocks and small boulders to explore, often this area is frequented by large shoals of salema fish which come here to feed. This is an excellent area to complete your safety stops. You can of course plan your own dive.

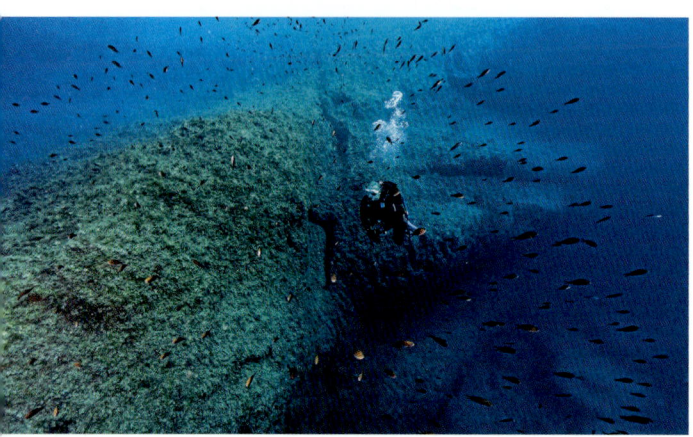

One of the shallow reef ledges along this coast.

PHOTOS: LEE JELLYMAN RITUAL DIVE CENTRE

Along this coastline reefs drop away to 50m plus.

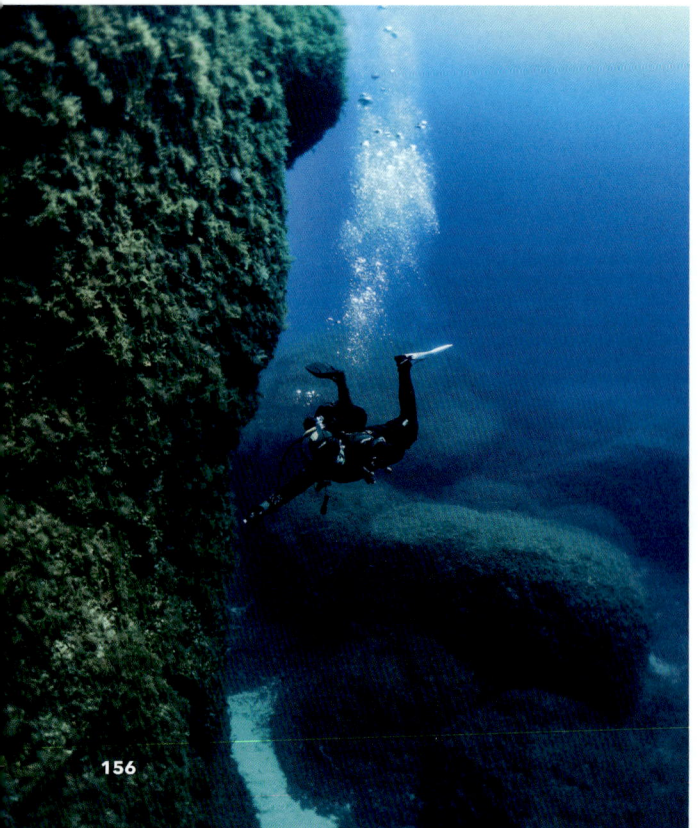

The massive boulders below parts of this reef.

PHOTOS: LEE JELLYMAN RITUAL DIVE CENTRE

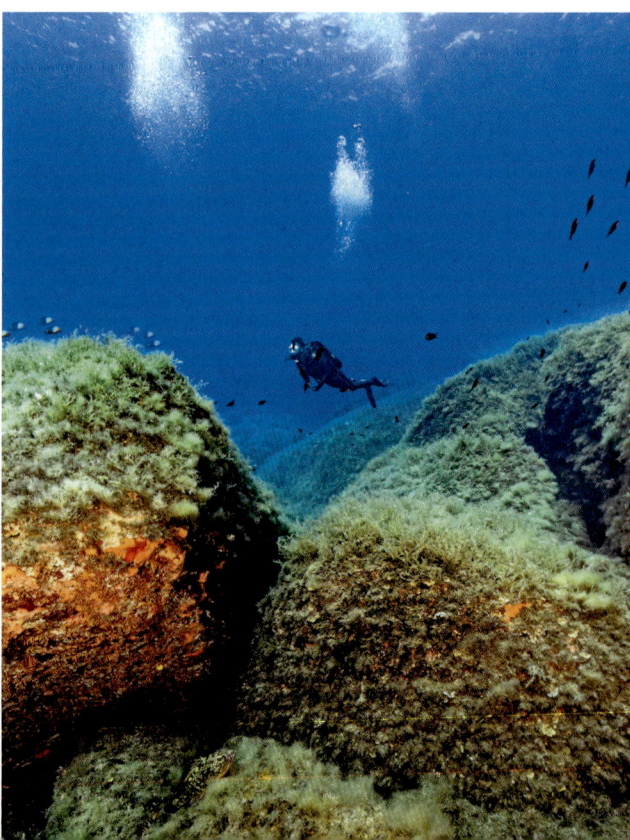

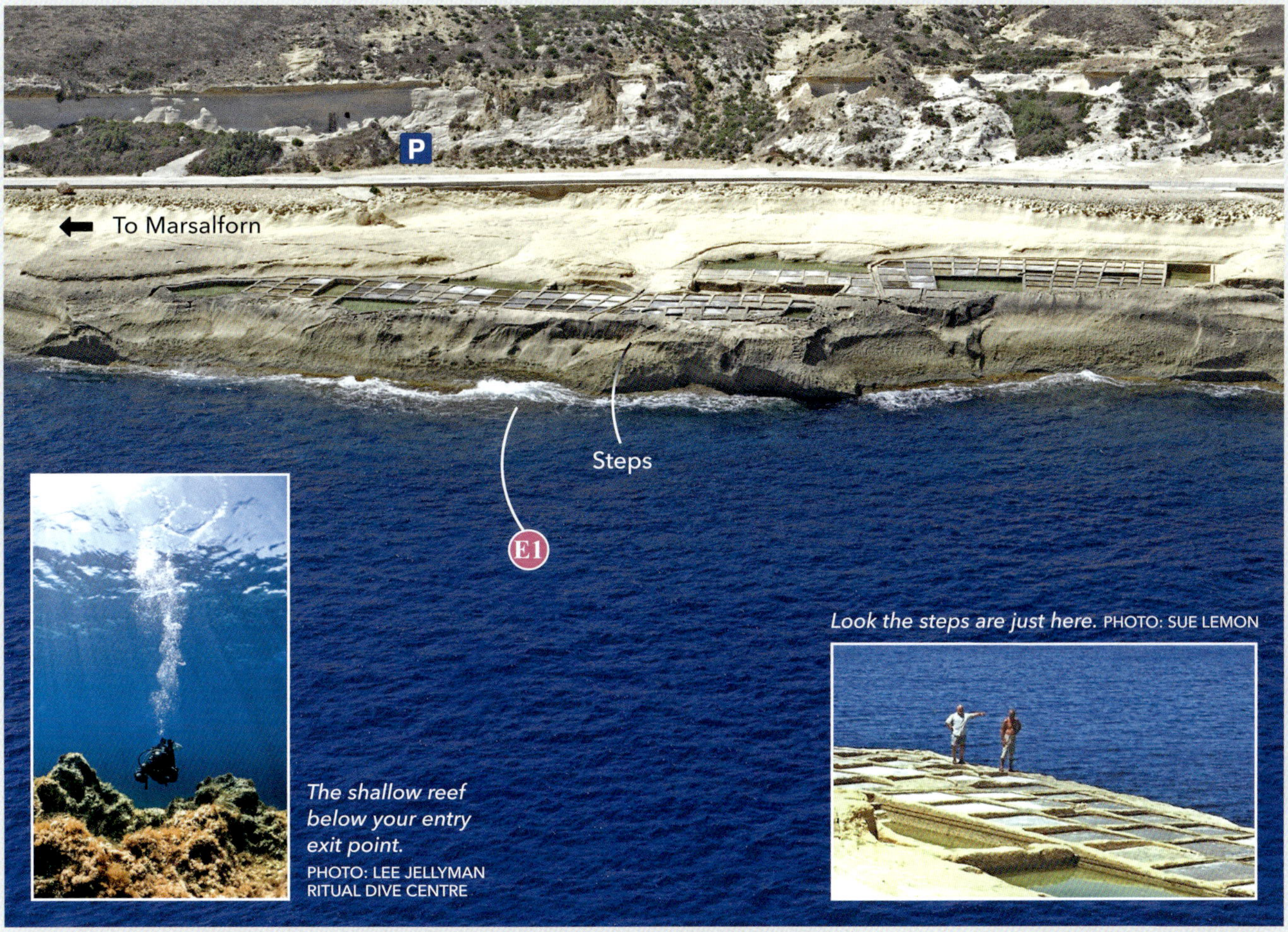

ANCHOR REEF - MARSALFORN

To Marsalforn ←

Steps

E1

The shallow reef below your entry exit point. PHOTO: LEE JELLYMAN RITUAL DIVE CENTRE

Look the steps are just here. PHOTO: SUE LEMON

PGL AERIAL PHOTOS

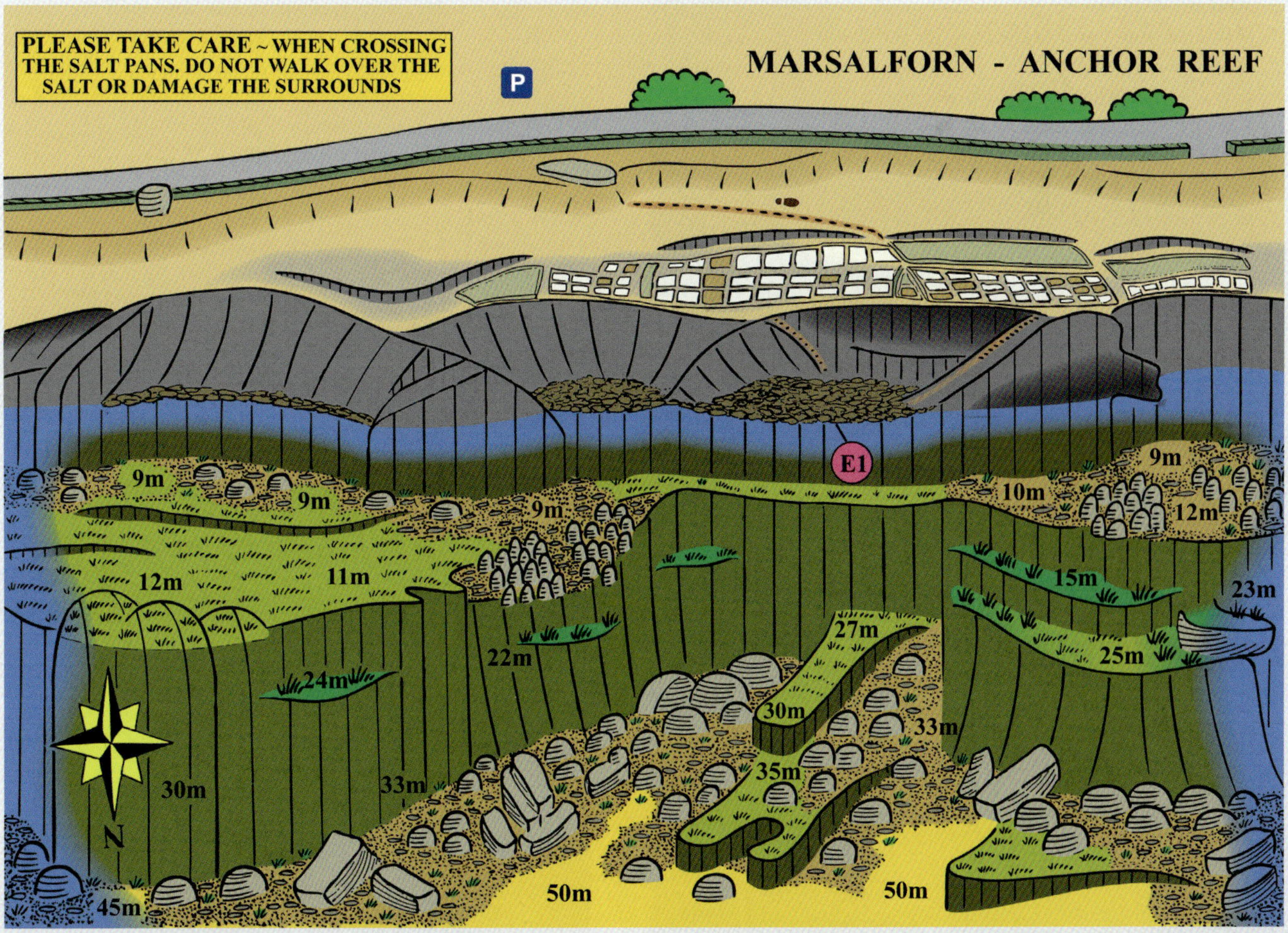

PLEASE TAKE CARE ~ WHEN CROSSING THE SALT PANS. DO NOT WALK OVER THE SALT OR DAMAGE THE SURROUNDS

MARSALFORN - ANCHOR REEF

E1

9m, 9m, 9m, 10m, 9m, 12m, 12m, 11m, 15m, 23m, 24m, 22m, 27m, 25m, 30m, 33m, 33m, 30m, 35m, 45m, 50m, 50m

Reqqa Point - Marsalforn

From Xwejni Bay drive along the road for 900 metres, on your right you will find a track which leads down to your dive site, see aerial photograph. This to me is a very special dive site, with a unique pinnacle at 17m fantastic view point with drop offs to 50m plus. There is also an abundance of marine life, a great place for a photo shoot, all this makes it an excellent dive site, possibly the best in the Maltese Islands, and maybe my favourite.

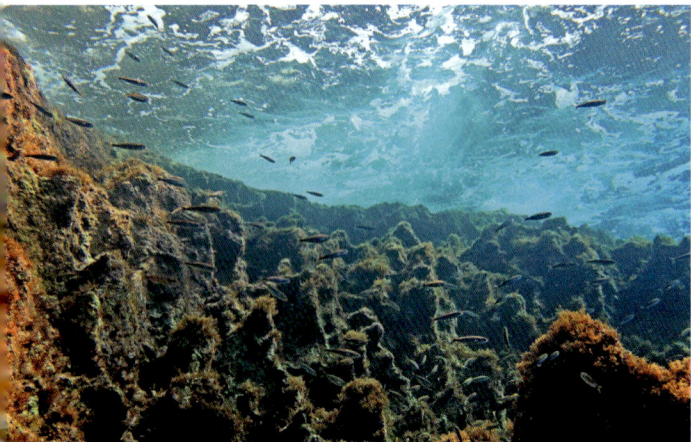

Just below entry exit E2. PHOTO: JOE FORMOSA

There are two entry points, E1, E2 and a ladder LE, is the best option if in place. Take care when walking to them for the ground is very uneven. E1 and E2 are the second options, E2 needs good weather conditions sometimes can be affected by the swell from the north.

The pinnacle cap from the inner reef.

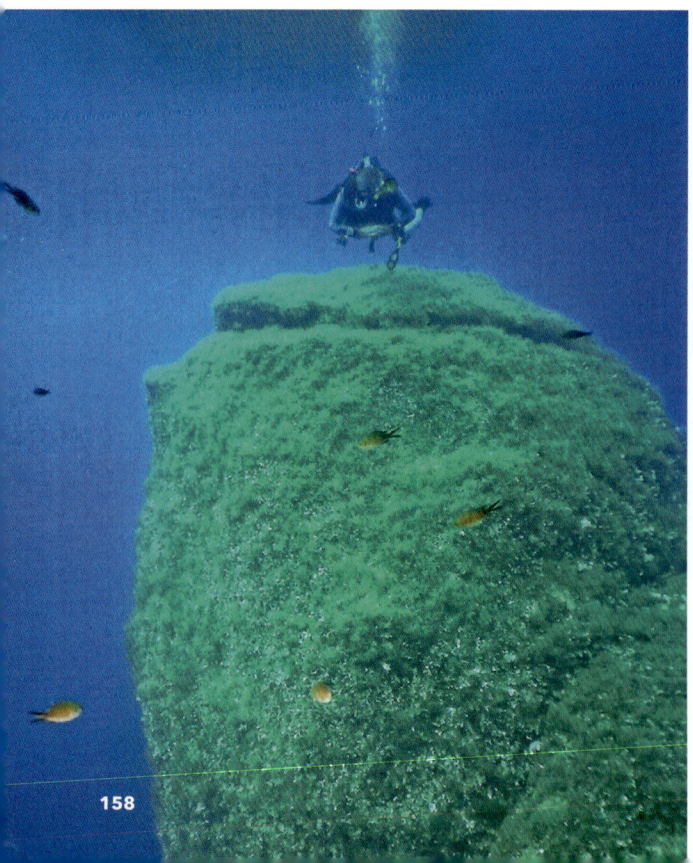

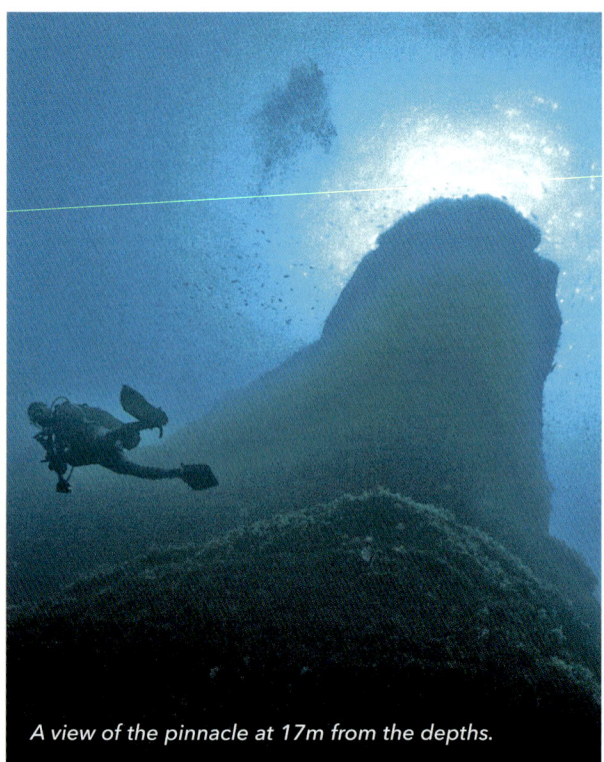

A view of the pinnacle at 17m from the depths.

THE DIVE — Minimum time - 50 mins

Choice 1 using LE or E1, descend to the seabed at 20m you can now follow the wall using it as a guide, all the way round to the pinnacle at your chosen depth, normally it takes about 20 minutes, but this depends on your depth and time while exploring. Below the pinnacle you can reach depths of 45m plus. You should visit the top of the pinnacle at 17m, stop and ponder the spectacular wonders of this reef and the passing marine life.

Divers on the outer reef of Reqqa Point.

PHOTO: LEE JELLYMAN RITUAL DIVE CENTRE

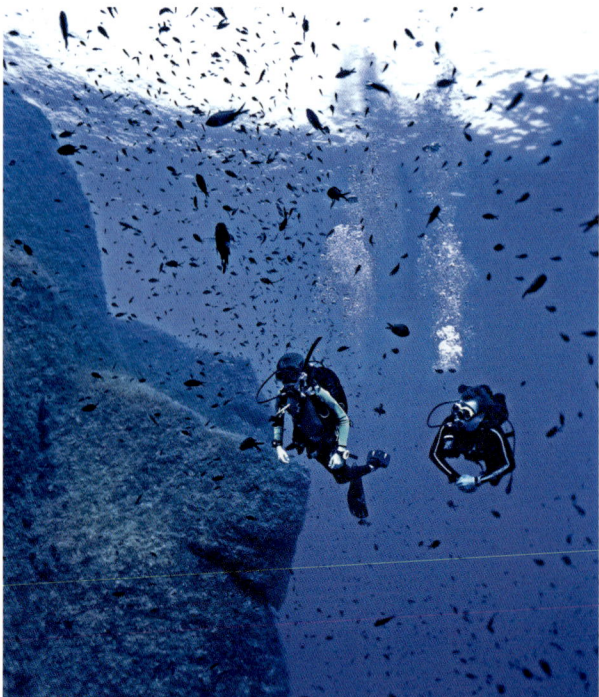

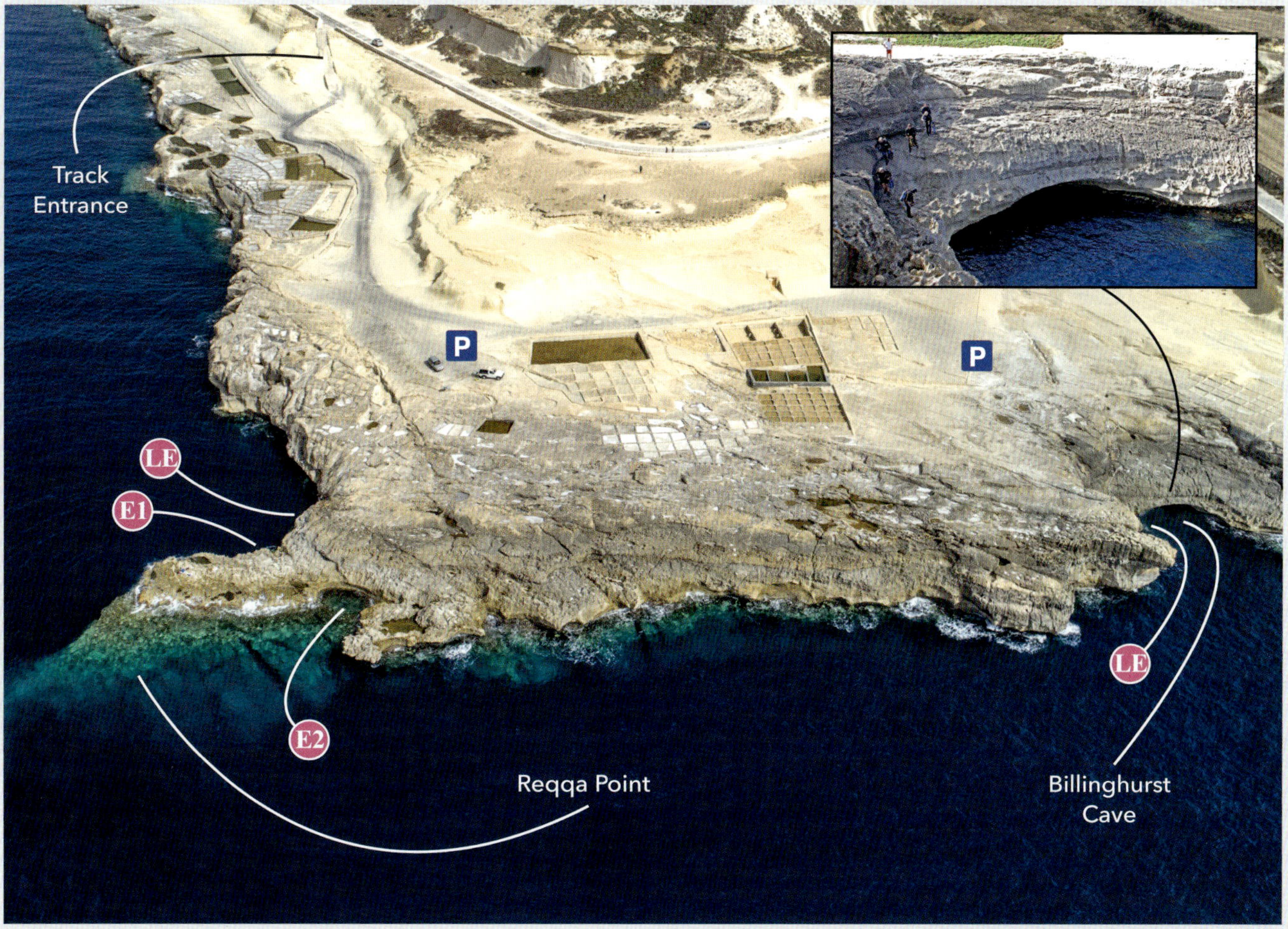

REQQA POINT - BILLINGHURST CAVE - MARSALFORN

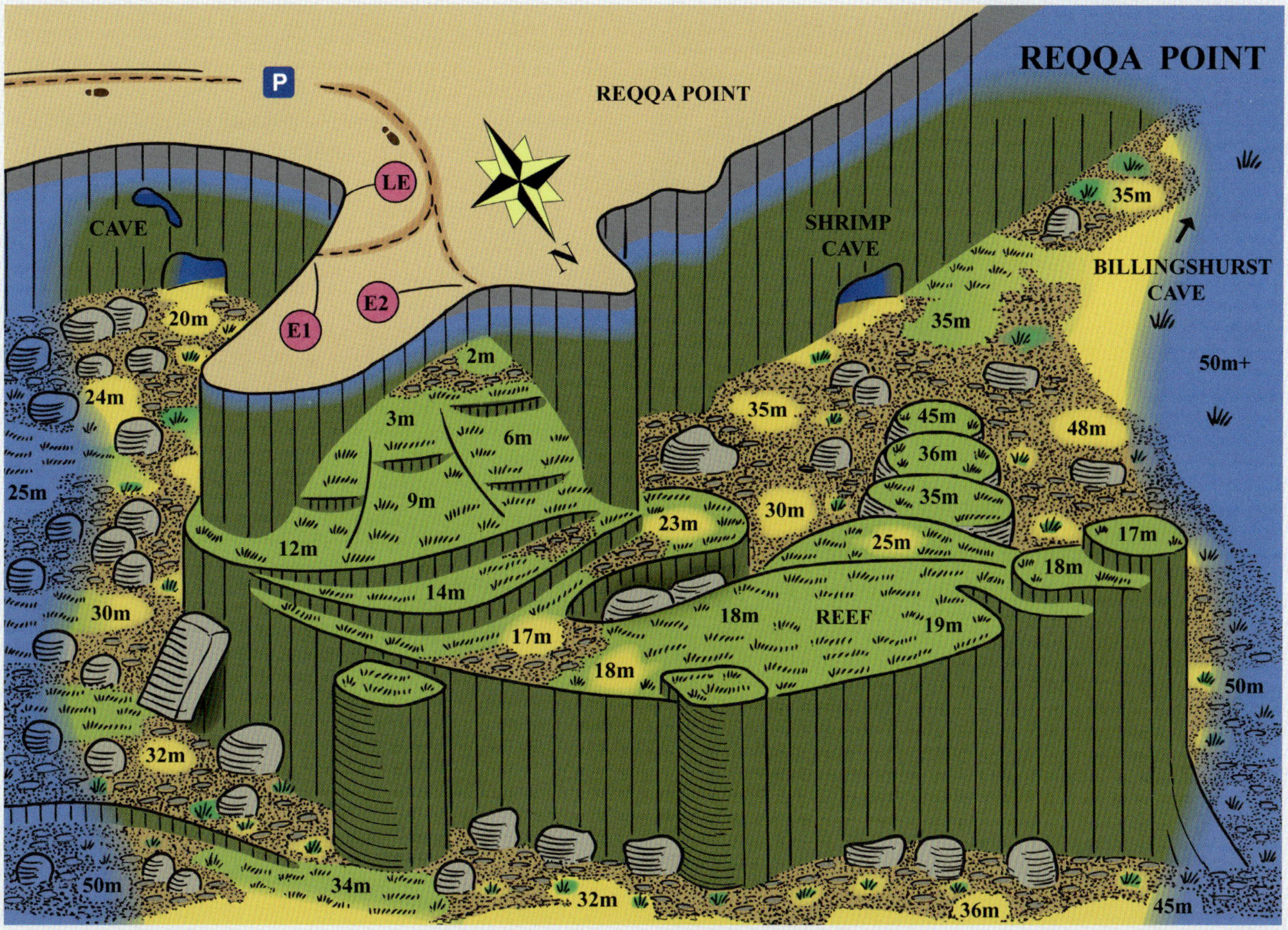

From the pinnacle to exit point LE or E1, follow the edge of the drop off in a south eastly direction, until you reach 12m now follow the wall keeping it on your right all the way round until you are below exit LE and E1. If you have the air and time there are two small caves to the left of your exit point to explore

Choice 2 using entry E2, once in the water surface swim to your left around the little point, then continue for some 20 metres, at this point you can descend to the sea bed at 35m, this gives me a buzz, just slowly freefalling down the rock face. Now swim with the wall on your left for about 20 metres to Shrimp Cave, next head back towards Reqqa Point. When you reach the boulder area use them as stepping stones up to the pinnacle at 17m.

Returning to LE or E1, see first choice.

Returning to E2 take easterly compass bearing and just follow the reef, at 12m head northeast up the steepish slope to your exit point.

Billinghurst Cave

Billinghurst cave is one of the largest in Gozo and named after a branch of the British Sub Aqua Club, also known as the Railway Tunnel.

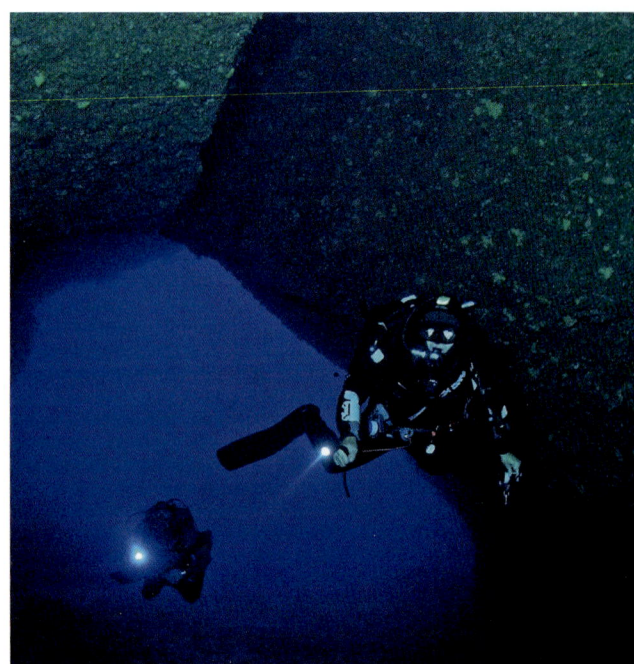

Two divers just inside the cave entrance.

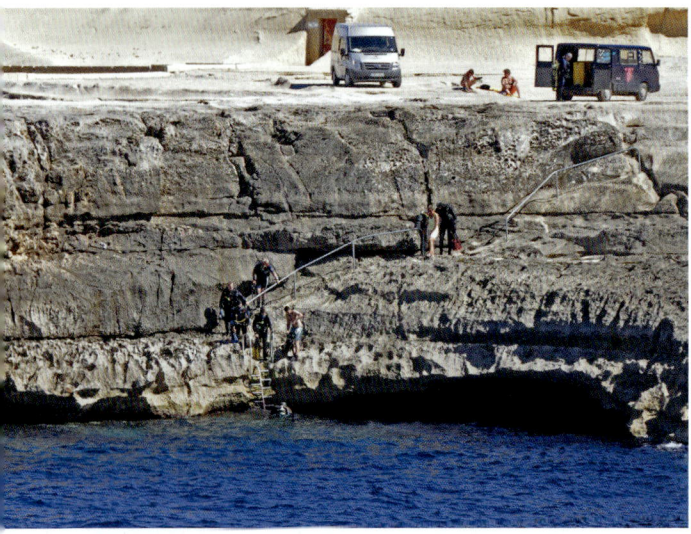

The ladder LE entry exit point for the cave.

Entry is via a ladder LE if in place or a two-metre stride entry by the entrance of the roof of the cave, the depth of the water is 25m. The maximum depth inside the cave is 25m and its width is 20 metres until you reach the boulders it then increases to 40 metres. After 60 metres into the cave the seabed has a gentle incline towards the cavern. At the top of the slope, you can surface inside the chamber which is approximately 20/30 metres in diameter and five meters high. Your exit swim can take up to 14 minutes to reach the cave entrance and your exit point from the water, which is by ladder LE at the side of the cave entrance, alternatively it is just over a 200-metre swim to Reqqa Point E2 if no ladder.

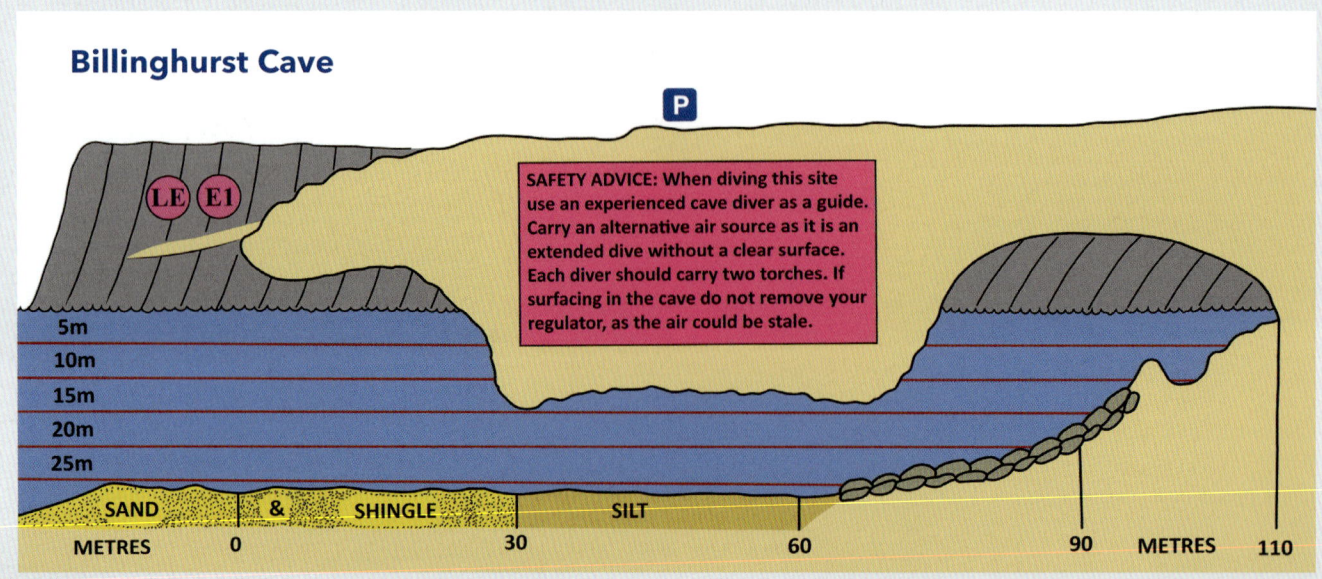

SAFETY ADVICE: When diving this site use an experienced cave diver as a guide. Carry an alternative air source as it is an extended dive without a clear surface. Each diver should carry two torches. If surfacing in the cave do not remove your regulator, as the air could be stale.

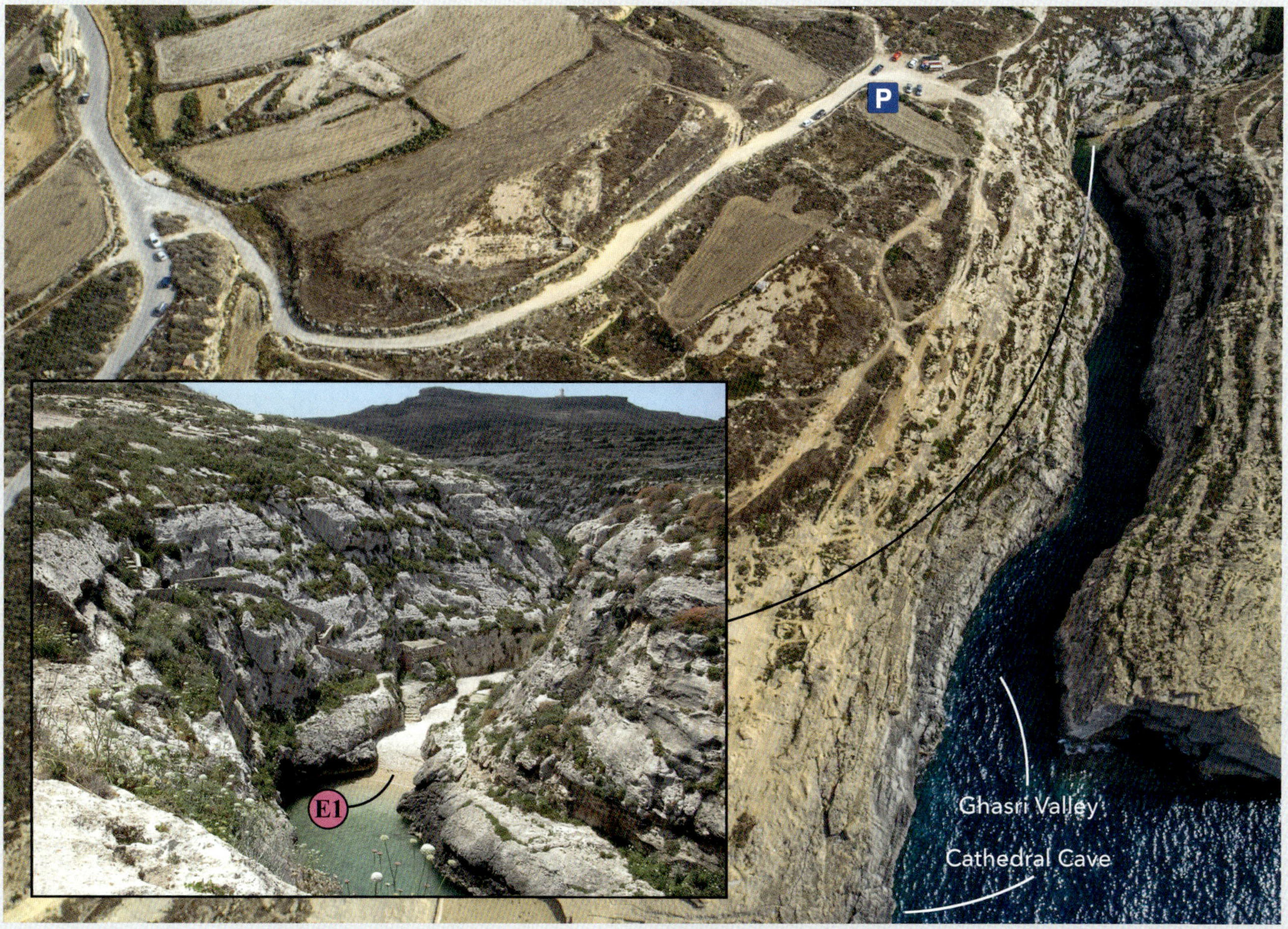

GHASRI VALLEY - MARSALFORN

PHOTO: PER EIDE STUDIO'S www.pereide.no

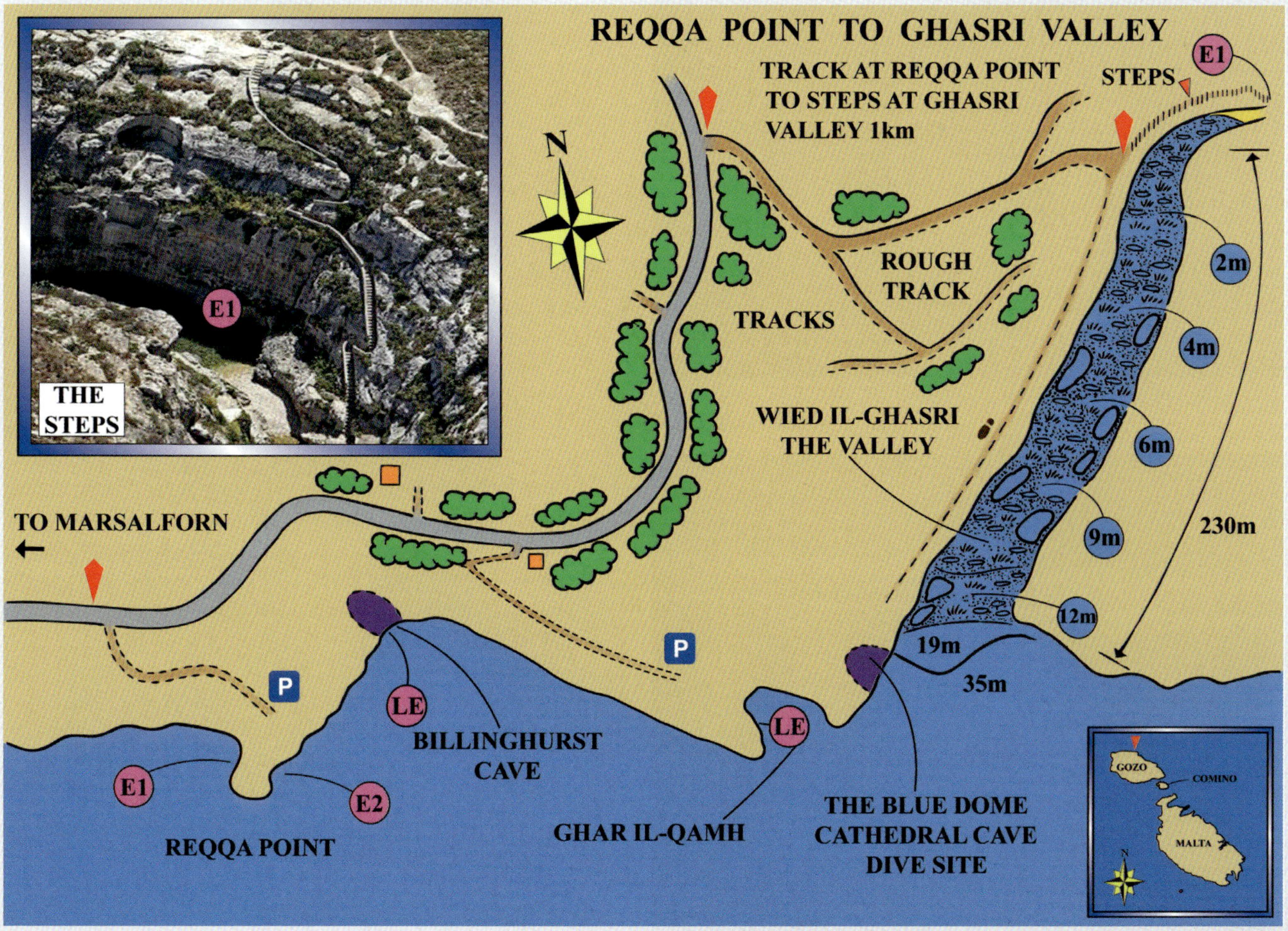

Ghasri Valley
Cathedral Cave

THE STEPS

REQQA POINT TO GHASRI VALLEY

TRACK AT REQQA POINT TO STEPS AT GHASRI VALLEY 1km

STEPS
E1

ROUGH TRACK

TRACKS

WIED IL-GHASRI THE VALLEY

2m
4m
6m
9m
12m
19m
35m

230m

TO MARSALFORN

P

E1
E2

REQQA POINT

LE
BILLINGHURST CAVE

P

LE
GHAR IL-QAMH

THE BLUE DOME CATHEDRAL CAVE DIVE SITE

GOZO COMINO
MALTA

Cathedral Cave - Blue Dome - Ghasri Valley

This dive site is situated on the north coast of Gozo, 3.6km west of the village of Marsalforn. To find this site take the coast road from Marsalforn to Xwejni Bay, now follow local map for the two entry points.

This really is a different type of dive well away from the crowds. There are two entry points for this dive site, one is a ladder entry LE from Ghar il-Qamh. The other entry point with its ninety-nine steps to E1 and the 250-metre narrow gorge with shallow waters to the open sea and the cave, with the magic of the vivid blue colours on the surface in the Dome, has to be seen to be believed. Of course, many divers prefer to reach this dive site by boat.

THE DIVE — Minimum time - 50 mins

Route from Entry E1, once you have negotiated the steps to E1 you will find yourself on a small stony beach, no more than 4 metres wide. Now enjoy a slow surface swim along this narrow gorge for 8/10 minutes, admiring what nature can achieve, just before you exit to the gorge descend. Now you have two choices.

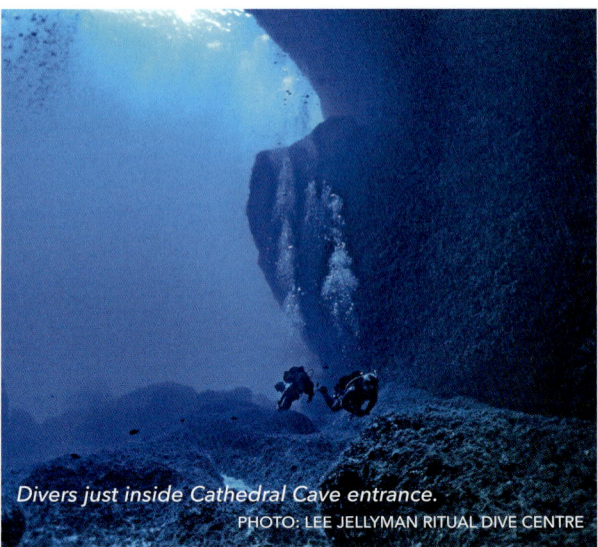
Divers just inside Cathedral Cave entrance.
PHOTO: LEE JELLYMAN RITUAL DIVE CENTRE

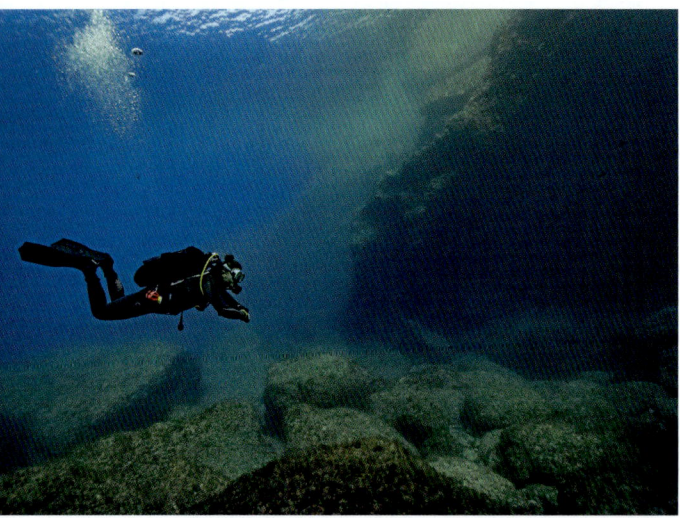
Just outside the cave which is also called The Blue Dome
PHOTO: LEE JELLYMAN RITUAL DIVE CENTRE

Choices 1, head towards the open sea, turn slightly to your left and swim in a northerly direction down to 19m, in front of you, you will see a drop off and to your right the reef will rise to a plateau at 14m, go over the drop off and descend to the sea bed at 33m or your chosen depth.

Once you have explored this area follow the reef around keeping it on your right, up and over the large boulders and slowly into the cave. Your dive time should now be 20/25 minutes here you can complete a safety stop, if you intend to surface within the cave.

Choice 2, once at the end of the gorge descend keeping the underwater wall on your right until you reach the cave entrance at 15m rising to 5m inside. If you do surface in the cave, it will be safe to remove your regulator for there is a crack in the cave above sea level which allows fresh air inside the Dome. With the light penetration from the cave entrance and the light from the crack, turns the surface water inside the dome to a vivid blue, this makes a brilliant photograph even from below the surface.

Route from Entry LE; once in the water swim to the opposite side of the cove, then head northwest along the underwater wall keeping it on your left at all times, exploring this underwater world as you go. When you have rounded the corner, your heading will be south-west this will lead you to the cave entrance.

Return Routes are in reverse depending on your exit point or dive plan. To the ladder exit LE turn right then keeping the wall on your right until you enter the little cove where the ladder is. If your exit point is E1 and the steps, turn left out of the cave and keep the wall on your left. Now enjoy the clear shallow waters of the Ghasri Valley inlet.

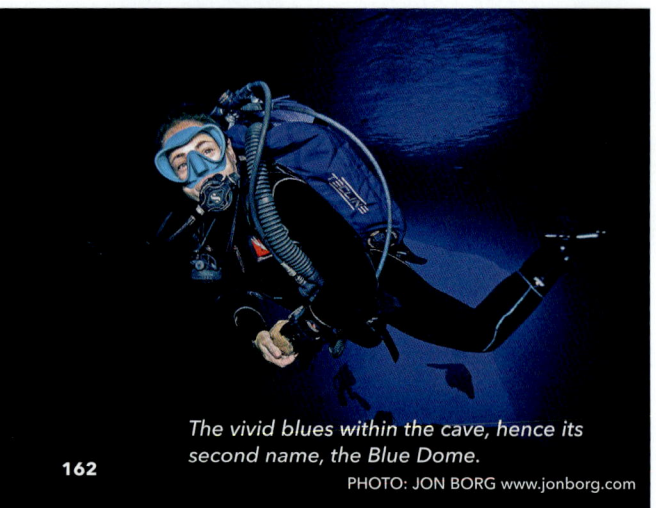
The vivid blues within the cave, hence its second name, the Blue Dome.
PHOTO: JON BORG www.jonborg.com

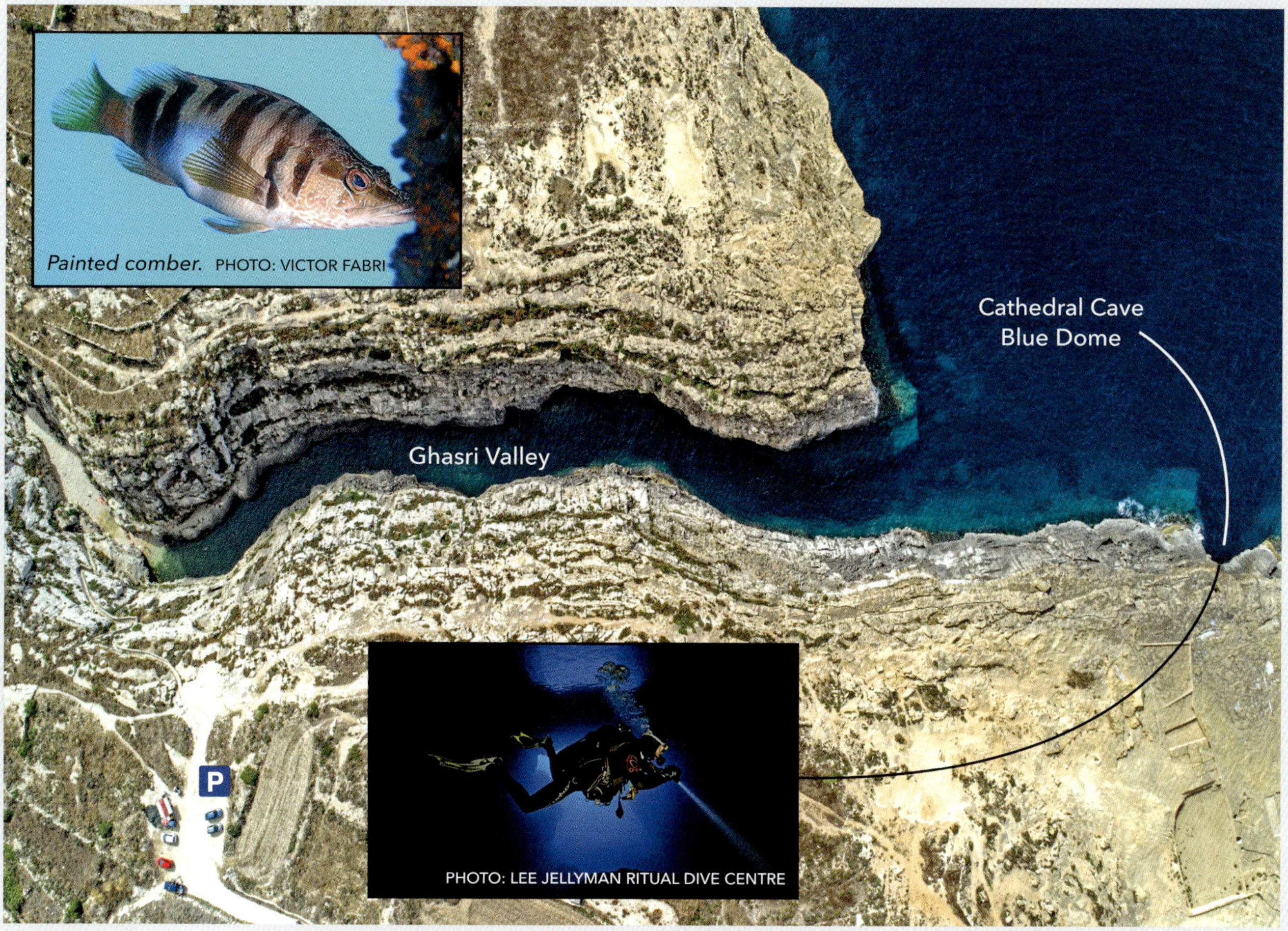

Painted comber. PHOTO: VICTOR FABRI
Cathedral Cave
Blue Dome
Ghasri Valley
P
PHOTO: LEE JELLYMAN RITUAL DIVE CENTRE

PHOTO: PER EIDE STUDIO'S www.pereide.no

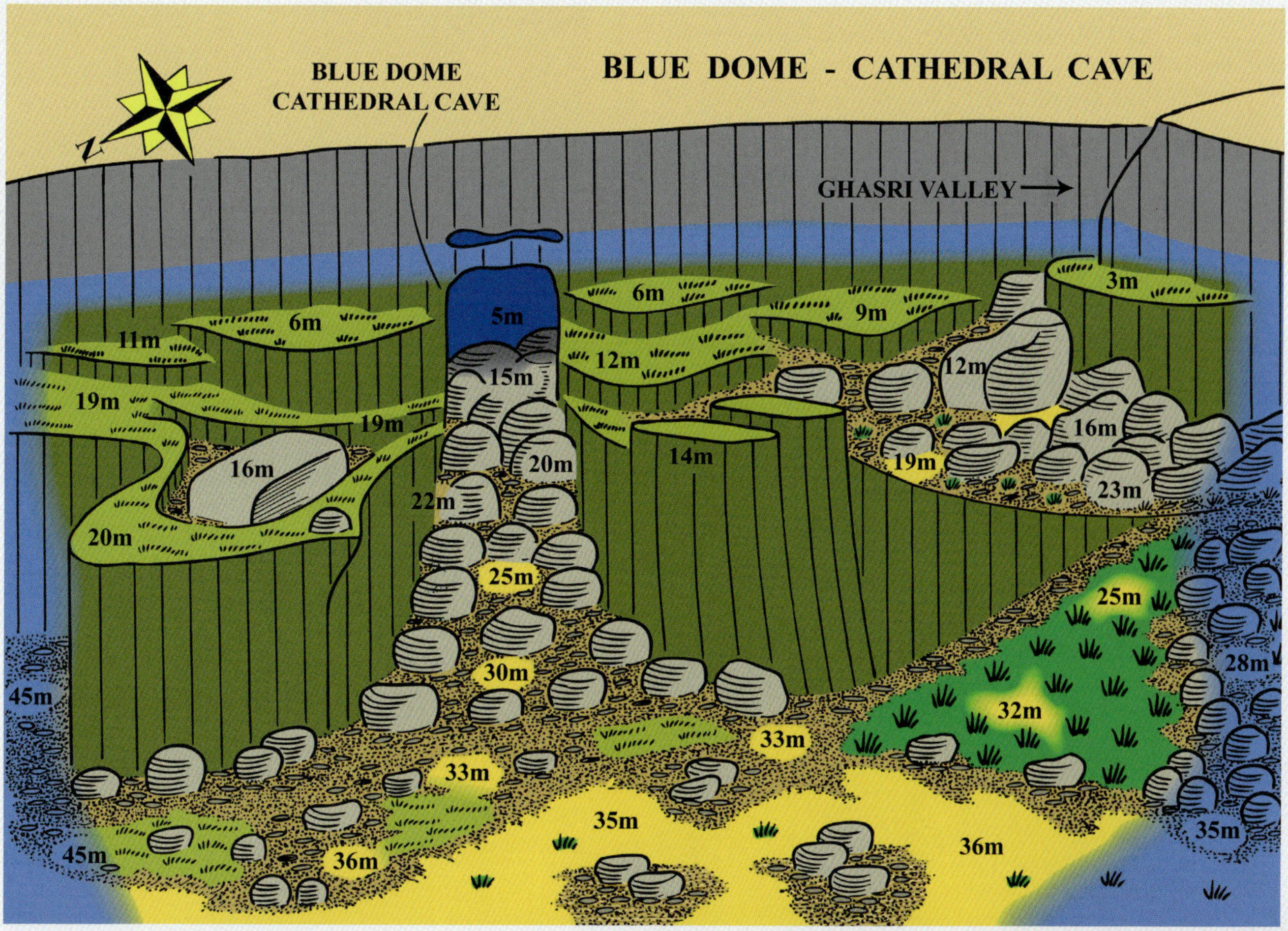
BLUE DOME - CATHEDRAL CAVE
BLUE DOME
CATHEDRAL CAVE
N
GHASRI VALLEY
5m
6m
6m
9m
3m
11m
12m
12m
15m
19m
19m
16m
16m
20m
14m
19m
23m
22m
20m
25m
25m
30m
28m
32m
45m
33m
33m
35m
45m
36m
36m
35m

Malta Boat Diving Sites

01 - The Bristol Beaufighter

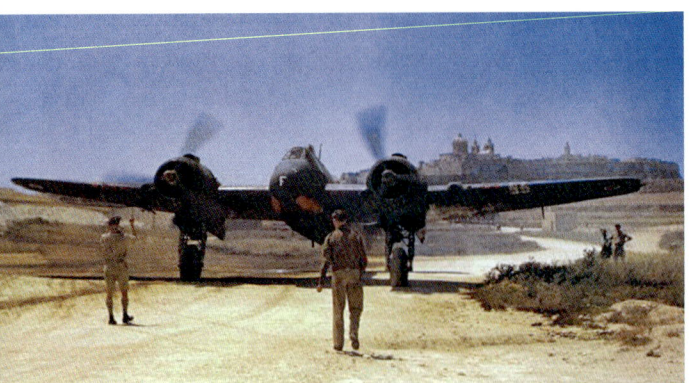

A Beaufighter at Ta'Qali which is now home to the Malta Aviation Museum, in the background the city of Mdina, also known as the Silent City.

PHOTO: FREDRICK GALEA, MALTA AVIATION MUSEUM

The Bristol Beaufighter was built in Filton England, the Mk1 was first taken into service in July 1940. It was a twin-engine strike and torpedo aircraft. It had a wing span of 18 metres and 13 metres in length, armed with bombs, torpedoes and machine guns. Using a gyro angling device and a radio altimeter the Beaufighter could make precision attacks at wave top height with her torpedoes, her long range and able to operate during darkness made her a formidable fighter.

On the 17th March 1943, nine Beaufighters of 272 squadron took off to join up with 39 squadron on a shipping strike off Point Stelo, Sicily. Beaufighter 'N' with her pilot Sgt. Donald Frazee and his observer Sgt. Sandery, started to climb to search for the other aircraft, their speed was around 130 mph when it began to vibrate violently and began to lose height.

Starboard side undercarriage and engine.

PHOTO: SHARON FORDER

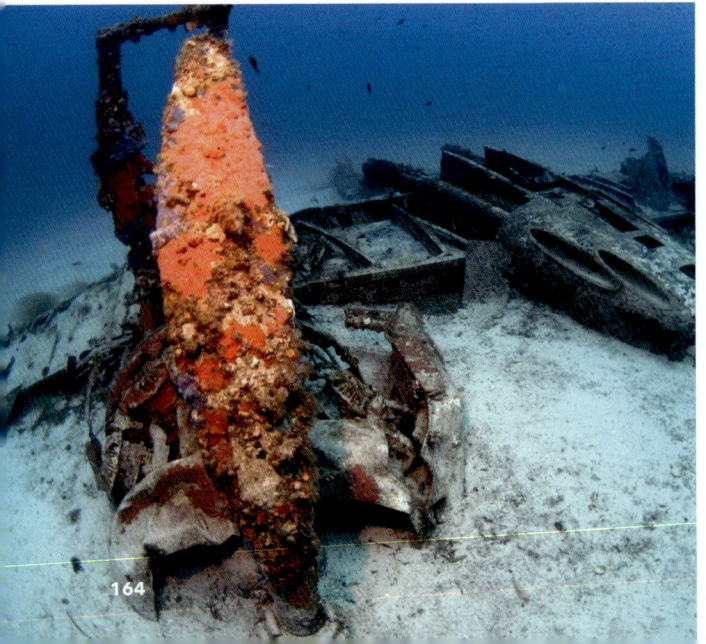

At 600 feet the pilot told his observer they would have to ditch. There was a slight swell and the aircraft hit the water at about 100 mph, they both managed to get out and within seconds the aircraft disappeared beneath the waves. The two men were picked up by a Maltese fishing boat and shortly after that their rescue launch arrived.

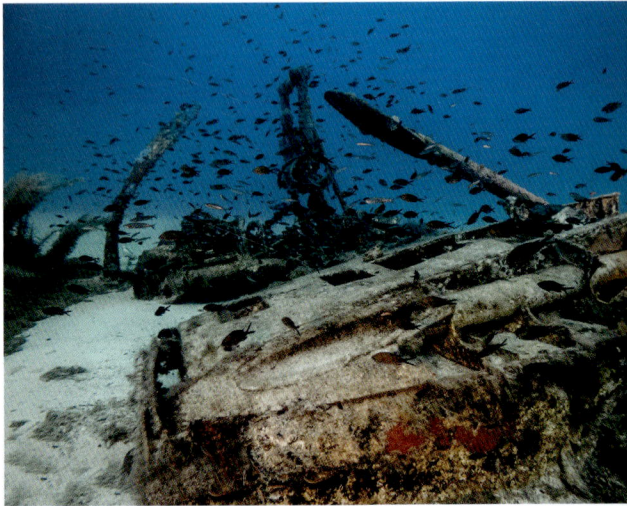

The port side engine with no propeller.

PHOTOS: ARKADIUSZ SREBNIK POLANDDIVINGPHOTOS

Diver above the upturned Beaufighter plane.

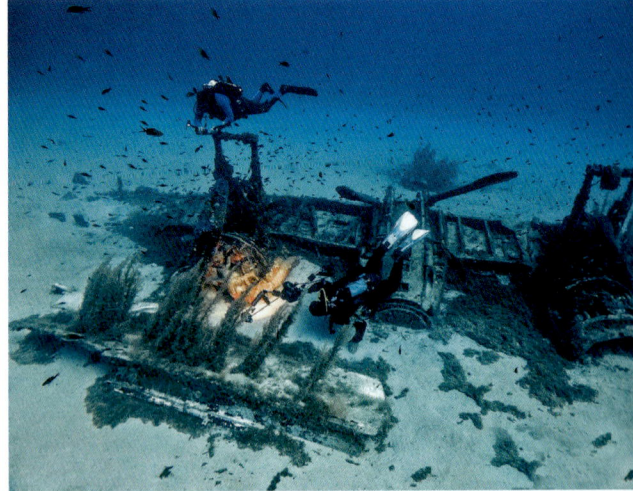

THE DIVE The Beaufighter now lies upside down on a sandy seabed at 38m, which makes her an experienced diver's dive. As you descend you will be able to see what remains of the aircraft, the main fuselage, the wings and undercarriage. This is an excellent dive for the photographer as divers normally stay around the wreckage. Remember that good buoyancy is essential, even touching the sand away from the wreckage will create a cloud which could drift towards the plane to the disappointment of the photographer and the other divers.

02 - HMS *Hellespont*

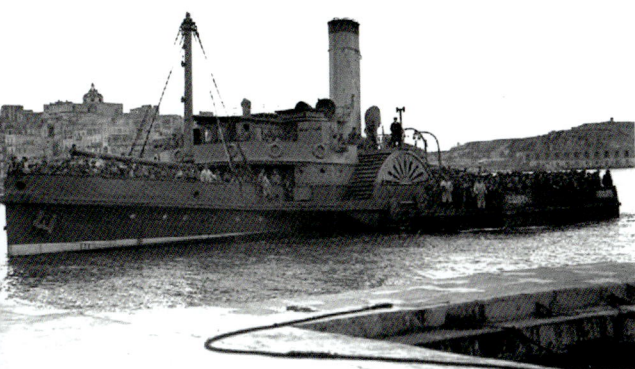

HMS Hellespont in Grand Harbour in 1922.

This deep-sea paddle steamer tug was built by C & W Earls Shipbuilding & Engineering Co. Hull England and launched on the 10th May 1910. Having spent her first working years based at Haulbowline Dockyard, Queenstown, Ireland, she came to Malta in 1922 and for the next twenty years she worked in the seas around the Maltese Islands. On the night of the 6th April 1942 during an air raid she was sunk by German/Italian aircraft, later salvaged, then towed outside Grand Harbour and scuttled three miles off Riscasoli Breakwater lighthouse.

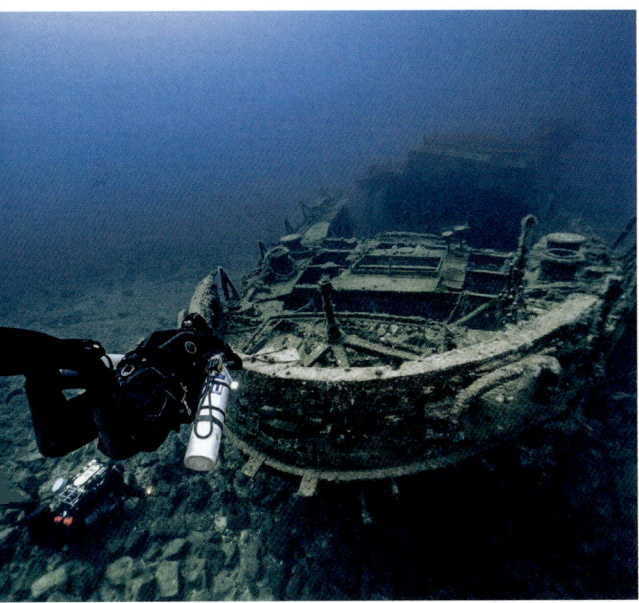

The stern of the HMS Hellespont at 45m.

PHOTO: JON BORG www.jonborg.com

THE DIVE She now lies on a sandy seabed in an upright position at a depth of 45m; the visibility is normally quite good. The metal fittings for the paddles are still in place but the paddles are long gone. An interesting dive with lots to see, including the engine room where the piston rods and boiler are still in place. A great wreck which has remained remarkably intact.

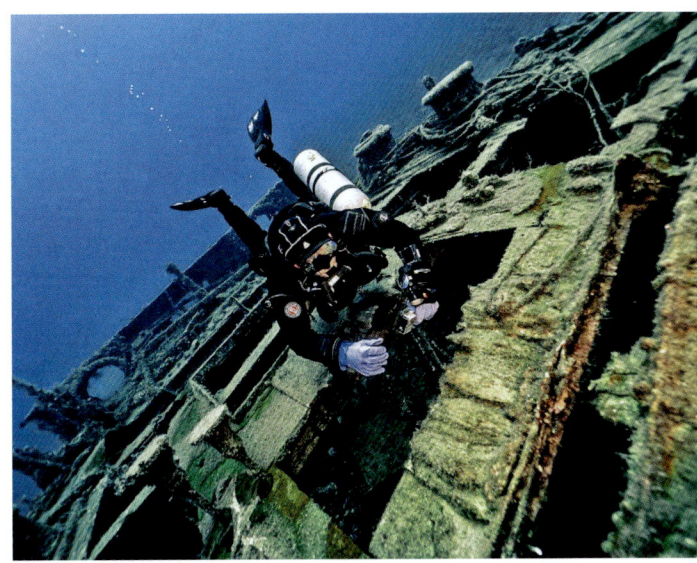

A diver explores the main deck of this wreck.

PHOTO: JON BORG www.jonborg.com

03 - HM *Drifter Eddy*

Built in Aberdeen, Scotland by Alexander Hall Engineering Co Ltd and launched on 6th August 1918. Her first attachment was to a squadron conducting mine clearing duties along the south coast of England at the end of WW1. After the war she was sent to the Mediterranean fleet and based mostly in Malta.

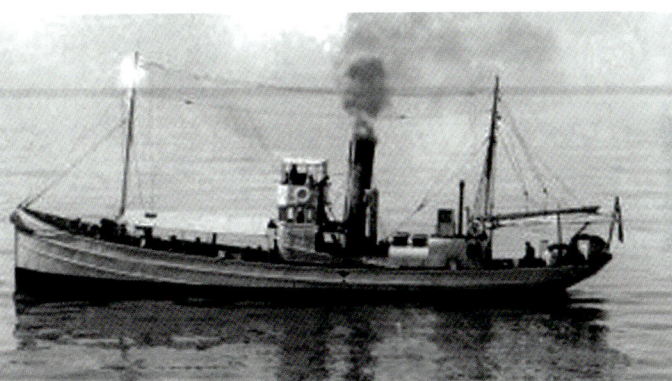

HM Eddy minesweeper, south coast of England.

Below: The bow section HM Drifter Eddy.

PHOTO: GAVIN ANDERSON

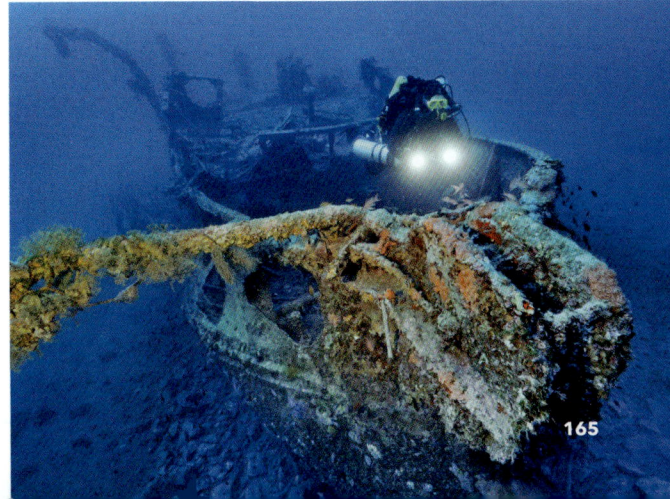

At the outbreak of WW2, the *Eddy* was sent to join the 403rd Minesweeping Group in Malta. She was armed with a three-pounder gun and a Lewis machine gun. Fitted with an anti-magnetic cable around her side at water level as she had a metal hull. Her mine sweeping duties were to clear the approaches to Malta's Harbours. On the 24th May 1942 she left Grand Harbour under cover of darkness to sweep for mines laid by the Italian E boats, whilst on her way back to port the next day at 16-40hrs she struck a mine and sank with a loss of eight crew members, the skipper and ten others survived.

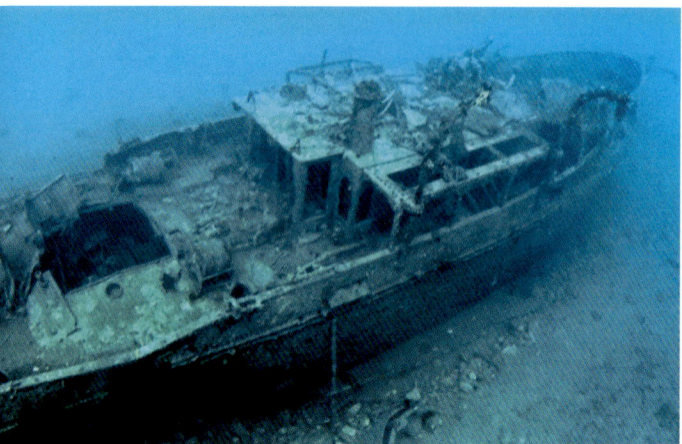

The aft section where the mine damage can be seen.
PHOTO: HUBERT BORG SEA SHELLS DIVE COVE

THE DIVE HM Drifter *Eddy* now lies upright on a sandy seabed approximately 1.3km off St Elmo Point, at a depth of 56m. There is a large hole on the starboard side which was caused by the mine. The main deck and superstructure has collapsed over the years. Beware there is a lot of sediment inside which will quickly reduce visibility, so do not penetrate this wreck.

04 - HMS *Angelo*

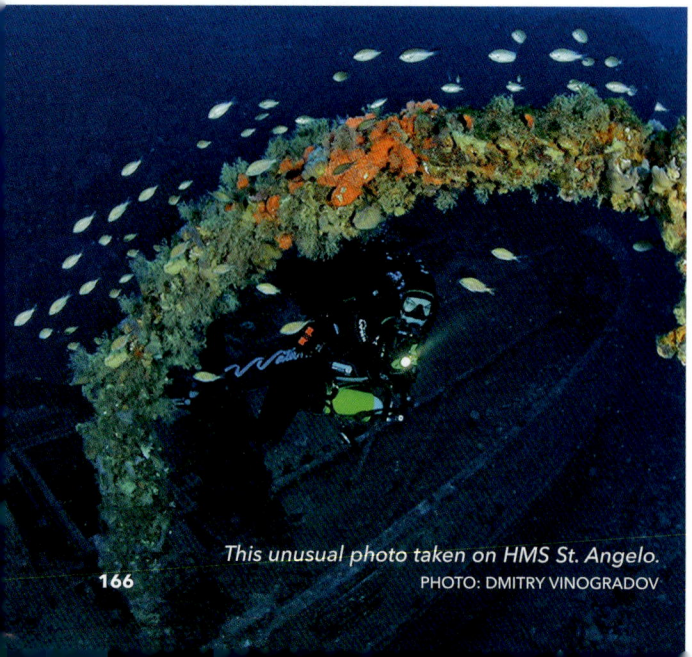

This unusual photo taken on HMS St. Angelo.
PHOTO: DMITRY VINOGRADOV

An auxiliary British tug built by Scott Bowling, originally named HMS *Egmont*, not quite sure when she arrived in Malta. Her duties included, to serve as harbour transport for the Royal Navy Officers carrying personnel from Fort St Angelo to other destinations. During the war she undertook sea rescue duties and later on as a minesweeper.

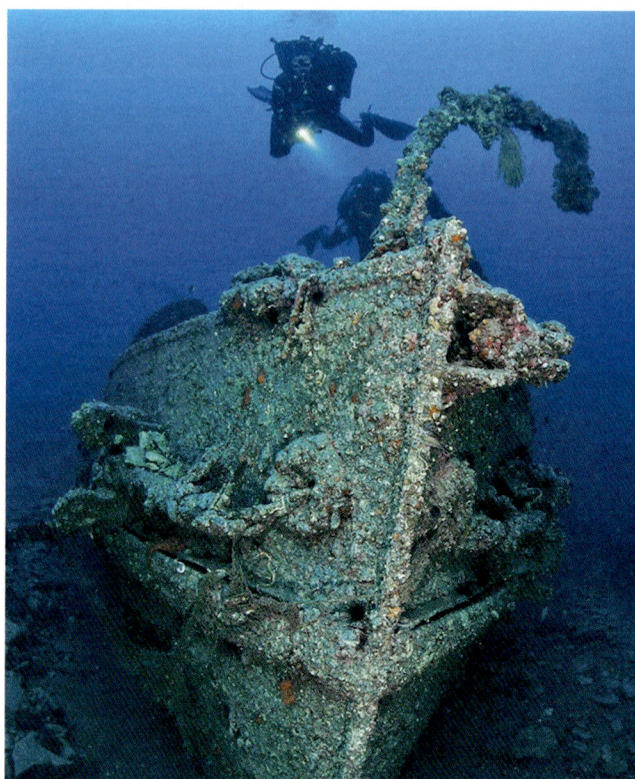

The bows of this British tug just outside Grand Harbour.
PHOTO: DMITRY VINOGRADOV

THE DIVE She was sunk on the 30th May 1942 The bows of this British tug just outside Grand Harbour and now lies upright on a seabed of boulders and sand at a depth of 55m. Permission must be obtained from the Harbour Master before diving this wreck, due to the close proximity of the entrance to Grand Harbour and the shipping lanes. HMS *Angelo* was one of four mine sweepers sunk in this area during May and June 1942.

05 - Bristol Blenheim

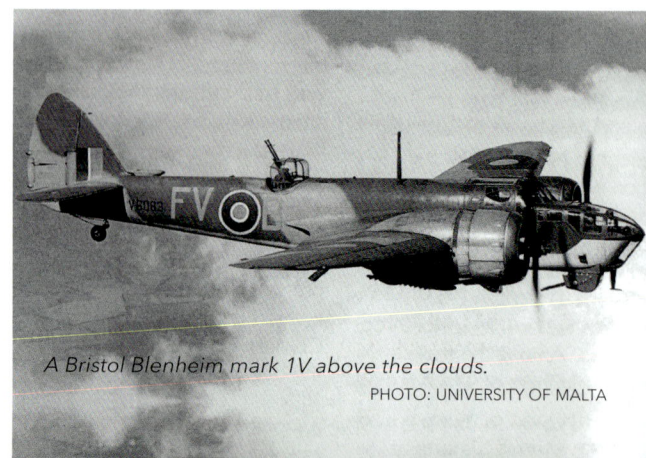

A Bristol Blenheim mark 1V above the clouds.
PHOTO: UNIVERSITY OF MALTA

MALTA BOAT DIVING SITES - BRISTOL BLENHEIM

Nine Blenheim squadrons operated out of Malta during 1941-42. The Bristol Blenheim mark 1V serial No. Z7858 (code M) started service on the 30th August 1941 with the 18th squadron and in October they flew to the Middle East. On 13th December 1941 five Blenheim's took off from Luqa airport Malta. One was the Z7858 with pilot Frank Jury, D.J. Mortimer air gunner and Tom Black navigator. During their flight to their target, they were attacked by a Macchi C200s. Air gunner Sgt Dennis Mortimer was helpless to react as the mid-upper turret with its twin .303 Browning machine guns had jammed. During the attack the port engine was hit causing the propeller to spin off. The Blenheim was left with smoke pouring from the destroyed engine and only about 30 metres above sea level; she was travelling towards Grand Harbour, then turned away and headed south. When a Maltese fishing boat was spotted just off shore, it was decided to ditch nearby.

The Blenheim touched down tail first, despite its battering she remained almost intact and floated allowing the crew to escape, all three were quickly rescued. A Royal Air Force Sea Rescue launch went to the crash site. In his book 'Call – out' Frederick Galea reveals that a launch arrived to find the aircraft still afloat, they attempted to tow it but before this could be achieved, it sank. The other four aircraft returned safely to Malta

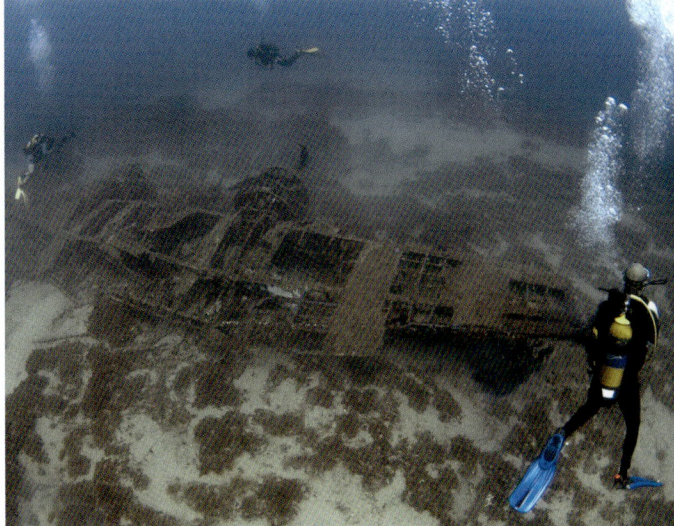

Divers approach the wreck of the Bristol Blenheim.
PHOTOS: SHARON FORDER
The excellent visibility of the wreckage at 42m.

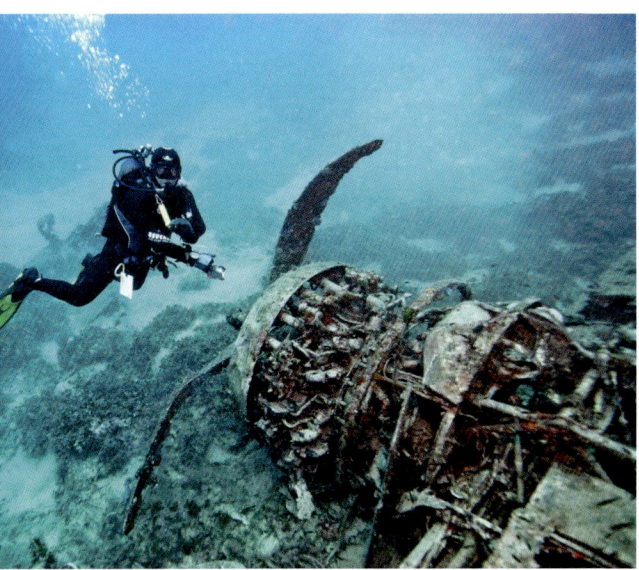

The starboard side engine and the propeller.

A diver enjoys the photographic opportunity.

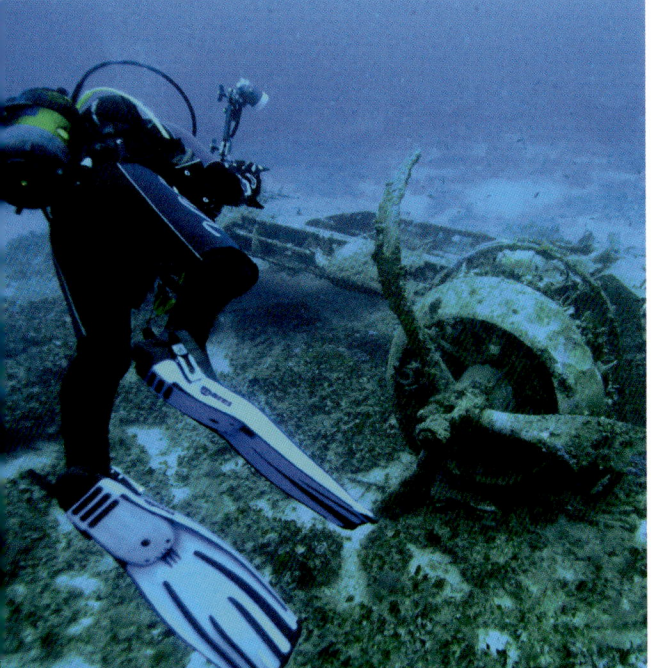

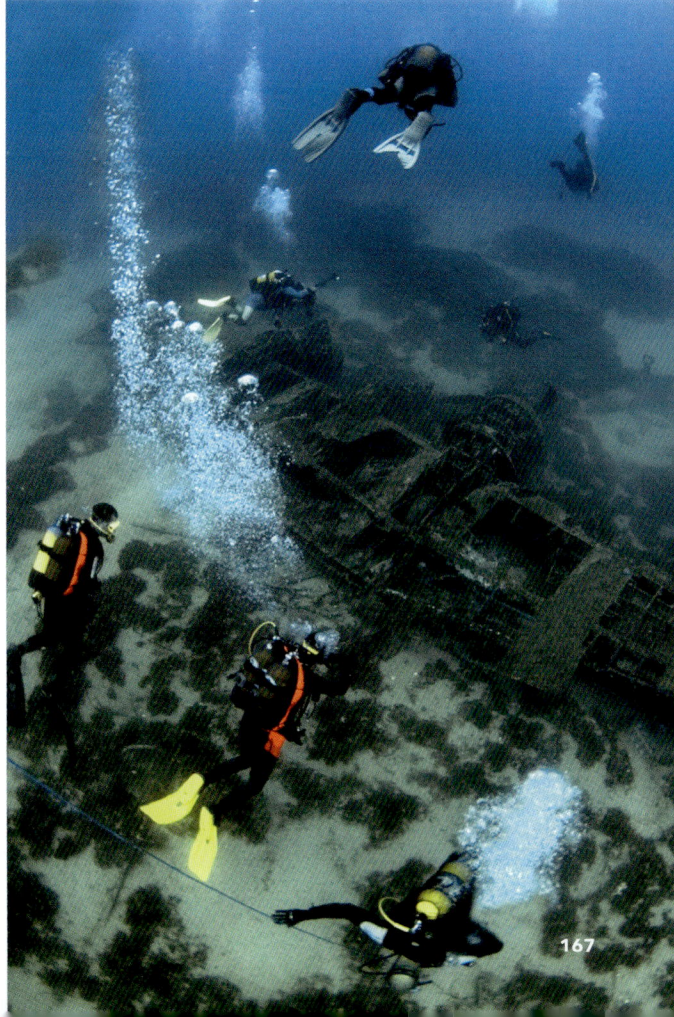

THE DIVE This Blenheim bomber now lies on a sandy seabed surrounded by small reefs at a depth of 42m, less than a kilometre off Xrobb-il Ghagin on the Delimara peninsular in the south of Malta. It is now a highly rated dive and this WW2 aircraft lives up to its reputation. The wings and engines are upright and mostly intact, although the propeller is missing off the portside engine and some of the rear fuselage lays a few metres in front of the wreckage. Very popular with diving photographers, most position their buddies over the starboard side engine. A number of pieces are missing from the aircraft, almost certainly down to early amateur salvage attempts. Only the depth and difficulty in finding this aircraft has stopped further destruction to the Blenheim, so please take care, do not touch and leave it as it is for others to admire.

06 - Filfla Island

Filfla is a small un-inhabited island about 3km south of Ghar Lapsi once used for target practice by the Armed Forces in Malta; it is now a protected nature reserve. This island was made famous as the opening backdrop for the film, The Count of Monte Cristo. A special permit is required to visit or dive this area and is issued by the Malta Maritime Authorities.

THE DIVE In the immediate area close to the island the depths are up to 10m, further away there are drop offs and areas of large boulders to explore, depths vary between 25 and 40m. To the south of the island is Stork Rock which is 6m below the surface, here the seabed then drops away to 60m plus. You have a good chance of seeing large shoals of barracuda large groupers and morays.

A word of warning; do not touch the shell rocket or bombs which litter the seabed they could still be live and dangerous!

This off-shore island is seldom dived and if you wish to do so then pre-plan with your dive centre well in advance.

07 - Ras ir-Raheb

This headland is almost the most westerly point in Malta and is just a part of the magnificent cliffs some as high as 300 feet which dominate this west coast of Malta.

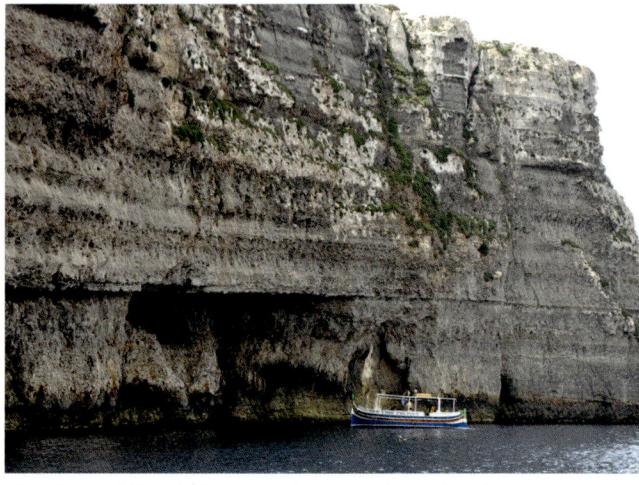

The sheer cliffs which are on this coast line of Malta.

THE DIVE This is a wall dive with caves at varying depths, at 32m on the sand next to the wall is the wreck of the *De Water Joffer*. Not a lot is known about this wreck, there is a hole on the aft starboard side, it is believed to be Dutch.

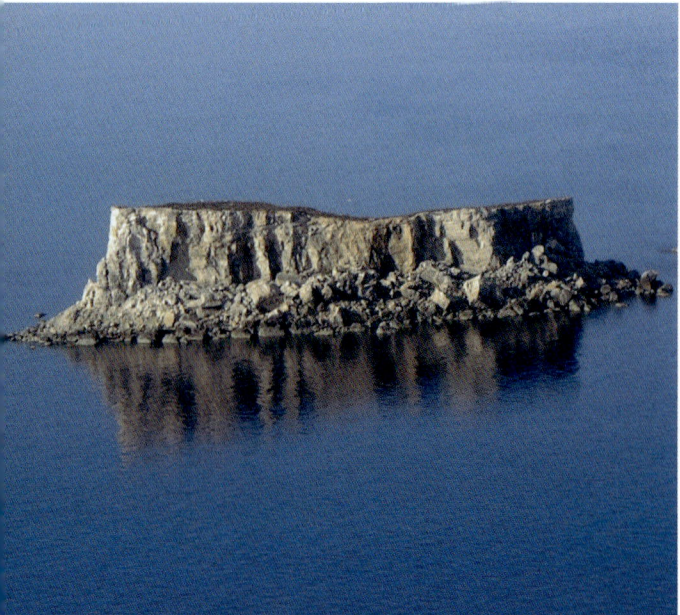

The Island of Filfla. PHOTO: JOE ABDILLA

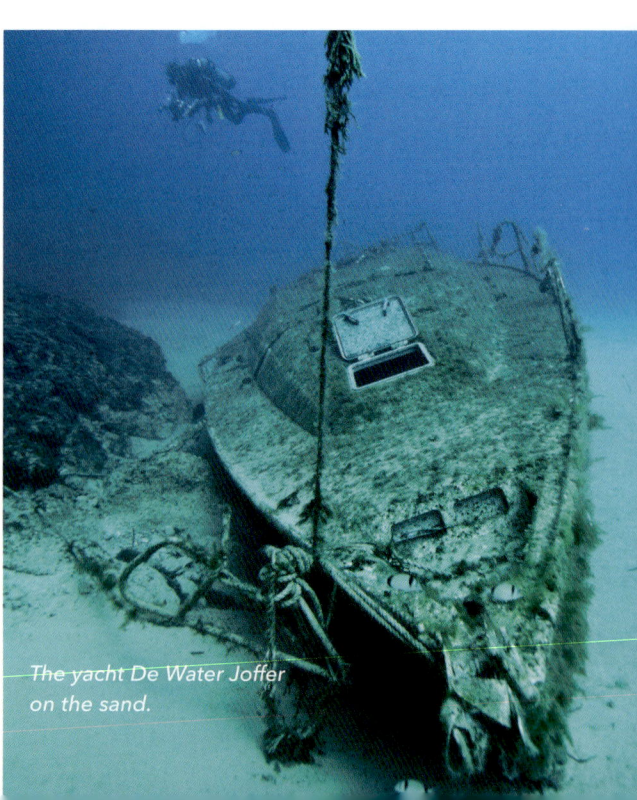

The yacht De Water Joffer on the sand.

08 - *Scotscraig* Barge

The wreck is located at Ic-Cuumnija, 500 metres north of Anchor Bay on the west coast of Malta. This barge was built in 1951, Dundee Scotland, as a ferry from Dundee to Newport across the Firth of Tay, until 1966 when a bridge was built, that's when she came to Malta. She played an important part in building of the Popeye village and the construction of the Anchor Bay jetty.

THE DIVE in 1981 the *Scotscraig* was being towed out to be scuttled in deep water, but on the way she sunk. Now she sits upright on a flat sandy seabed at a depth of 21m almost totally intact. During this dive you will most probably see a number of eels, groupers and octopus and the occasional stingray or tun shell on the sand.

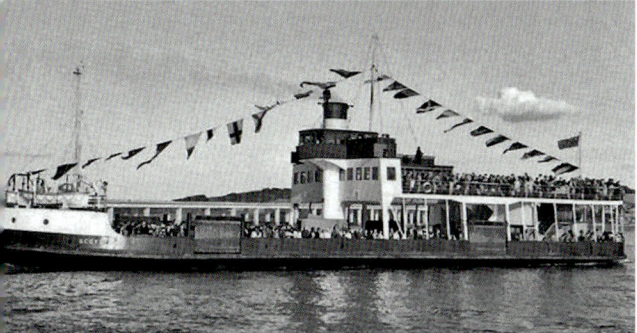
Celebrations of the opening of the bridge.

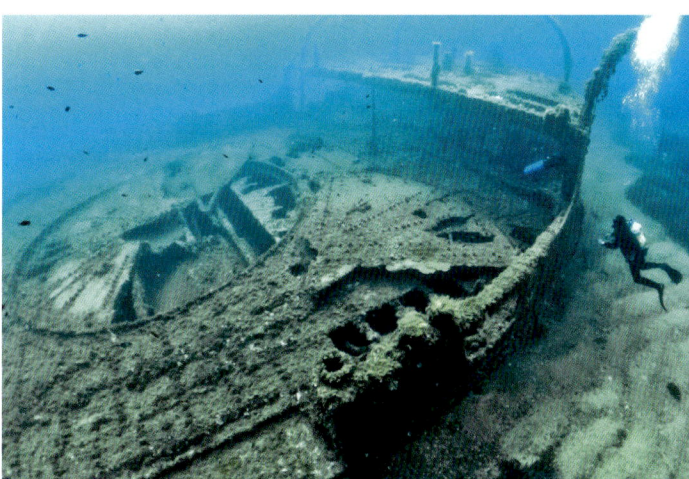
The main deck deck just behind the bows of this barge.
PHOTO: ARKADIUSZ SREBNIK POLANDDIVINGPHOTOS

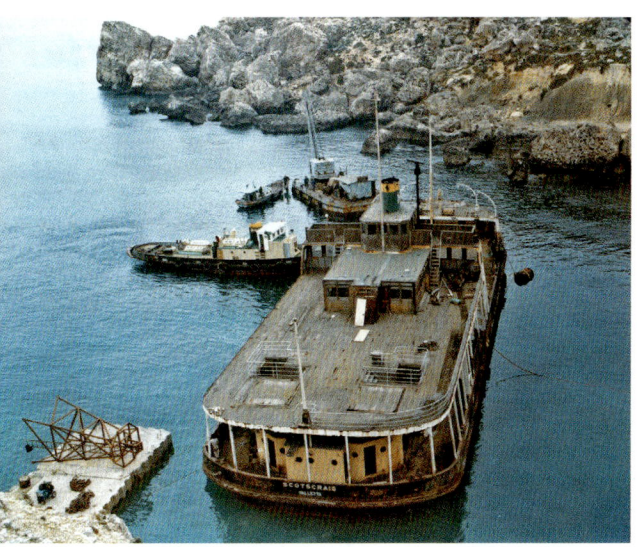
The Scotscraig barge in Anchor Bay.
PHOTOS: WILFRED PIROTTA
She begins to sink before reaching deep water.

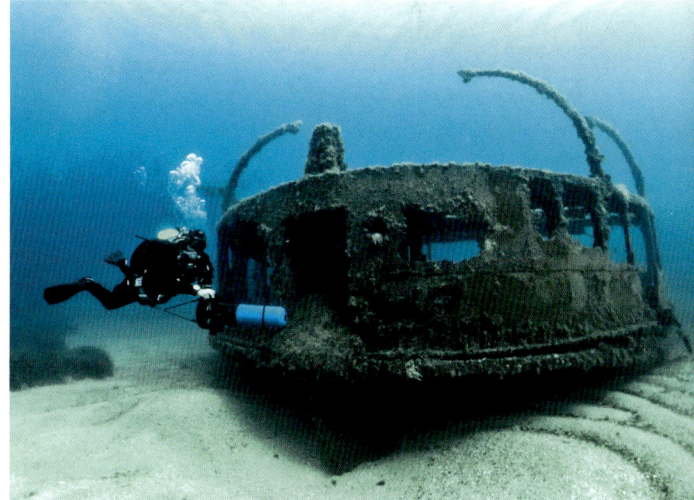
The stern of this barge on the sand at 22m.
PHOTOS: ARKADIUSZ SREBNIK POLANDDIVNGPHOTOS
A diver above the upper structure of the stern.

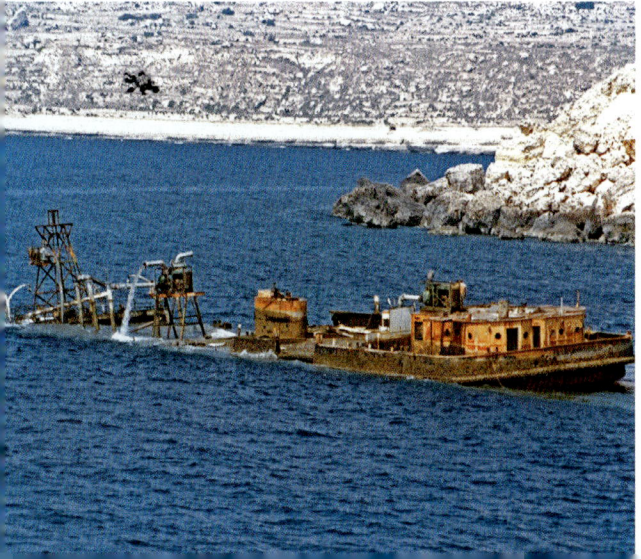

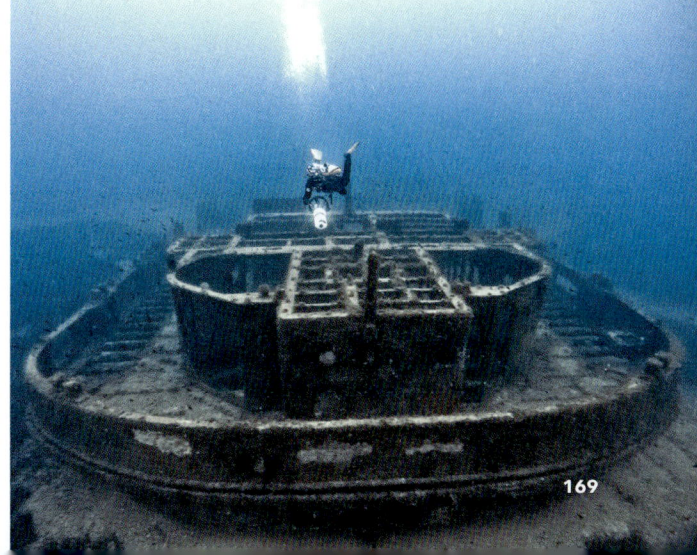

09 - HMS *Stubborn*

HMS *Stubborn* was a 1940 S-Class British submarine launched in November 1942 and commissioned in January 1943. She has a displacement of 990 tons, length 70 metres, beam of 7 metres and a crew of 48. Fuel capacity of 92 tons gave her a range of 6,000 miles, a speed of almost 15 knots on the surface and 9 knots below. She had an armament of 6 forward torpedo tubes and one rear tube, a 3-inch gun and a 20mm Oerlikon gun.

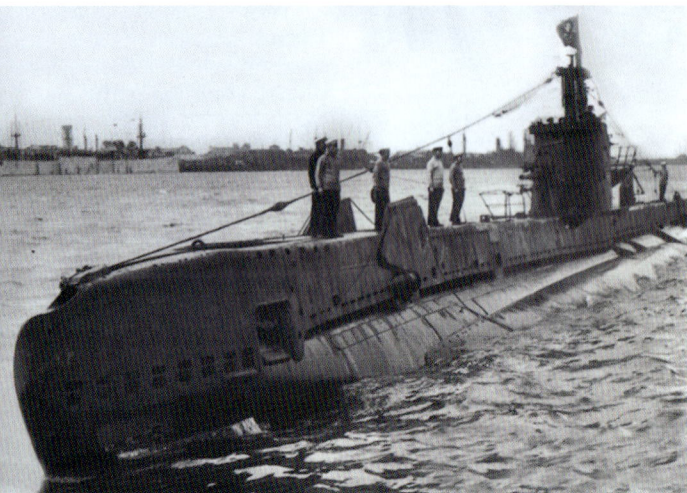

HMS Stubborn leaving harbour.
PHOTO: RN SUBMARINE MUSEUM GOSPORT

During the early part of 1943 she operated out of Lerwick on the Shetland Islands, patrolling the Norwegian Sea. During the summer she headed south patrolling around the Scilly Isles. In September of that year, she was back in the Norwegian Sea, during her operations she was involved in towing and supporting the X crafts which attacked the battle ship *Tirpitz*.

In the late evening in February 1944 HMS *Stubborn* sighted an enemy convoy of 7 ships, she attacked firing, 6 torpedoes and two hits were claimed; then 34 depth charges were dropped by the enemy before she left the area. HMS *Stubborn* returned the next day and sighted another enemy convoy of 5 ships; she attacked firing 6 torpedoes with two hits claimed. They retaliated by dropping 36 depth charges and she was damaged, they surfaced, then quickly blowing all her main ballast, she sunk to 500 feet. She really did have a guardian angel watching over her, for a further 16 depth charges were dropped while she was on the seabed. They decided to wait until darkness before attempting to surface, after many unsuccessful attempts, she was able to surface. It took seven days to reach Lerwick, escorted by 4 destroyers, a Norwegian Patrol boat, a Beaufighter air escort. During these days sometimes being towed and other times under her own steam, she made it.

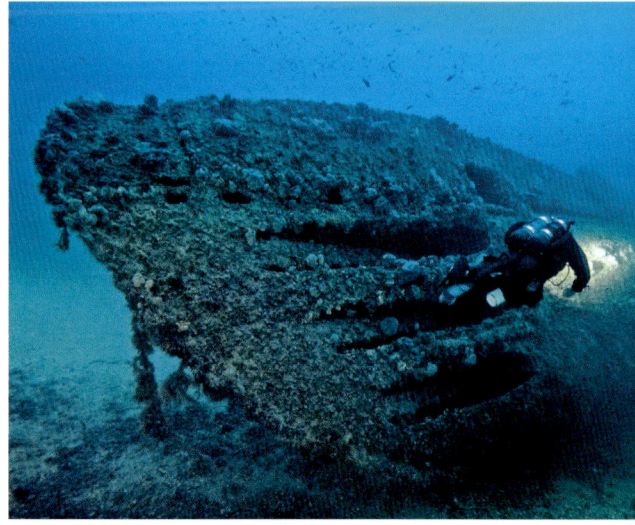

The bow showing her three portside torpedo tubes.
PHOTO: ARKADIUSZ SREBNIK POLANDDIVINGPHOTOS

HMS Stubborn which lies at a depth of 57m.
PHOTO: JP BRESSER - DIVE DEEP BLUE

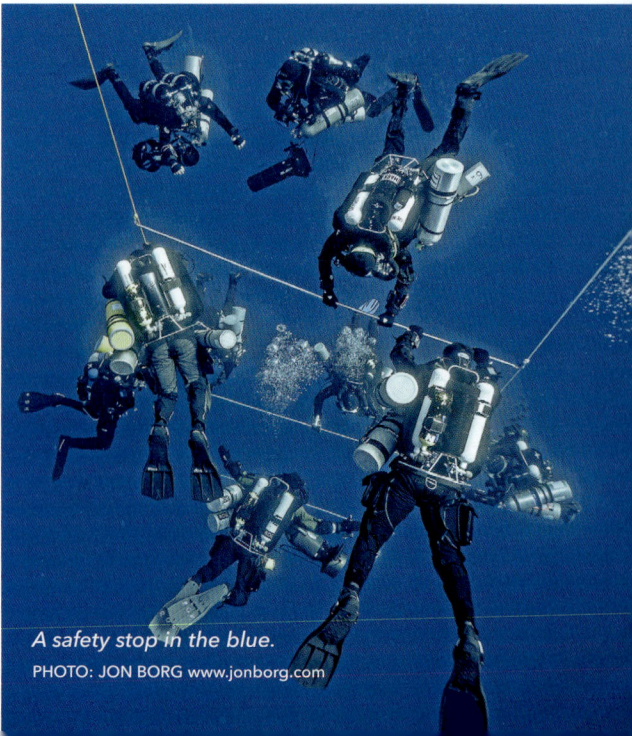

A safety stop in the blue.
PHOTO: JON BORG www.jonborg.com

MALTA BOAT DIVING SITES - HMS *STUBBORN*

After a refit in Devonport, she returned to Holylock and on the 18th March 1945 she left for Freemantle Australia, via Gibraltar, Malta, Port Said, Suez, Aden, Ceylon and arriving in Freemantle on the 1st June, she then saw action in the Pacific. HMS *Stubborn* recorded the deepest dive made during the war by a British submarine, reaching 540 feet. She endured one of the worst attacks of the war and suffered the loss of her complete tail fin which held the aft hydroplanes and rudder. This loss was not caused by depth charges, but from hitting the seabed at 540 feet. During the return voyage from Australia, it became evident that the hull aft had suffered more distortion than was originally thought. HMS *Stubborn* was one of the few British submarines that had art work painted on her conning tower during the war, it was a mule's head.

She was sunk on the 30th April 1946, as an Asdic target two miles off Qawra Point on the north coast of Malta.

THE DIVE This excellent dive to a depth of 57m is for experienced divers only. Descending the shot line through the crystal blue waters and when the HMS *Stubborn* comes into view you will see that she sits almost upright on a sandy seabed. This wreck is remarkably well preserved with its conning tower, torpedo tubes and propellers, there are two open hatches, but please do not enter. For the photographer, even at this depth, normally the visibility will allow you to take some decent shots.

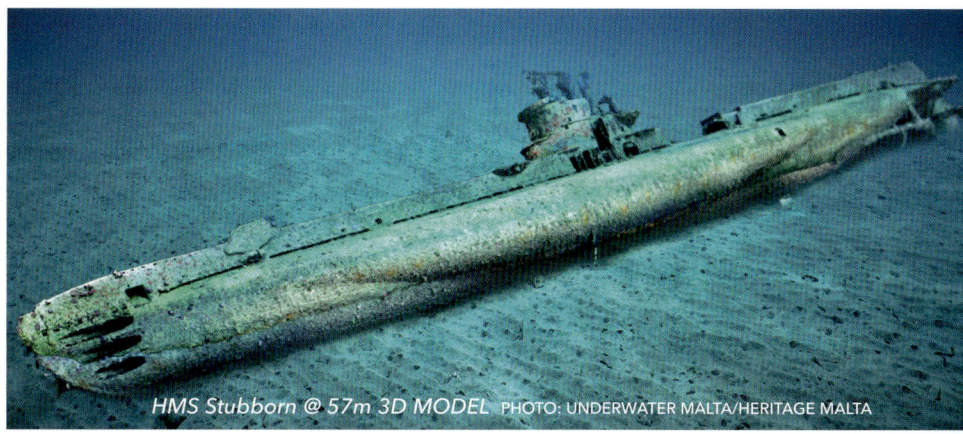
HMS Stubborn @ 57m 3D MODEL PHOTO: UNDERWATER MALTA/HERITAGE MALTA

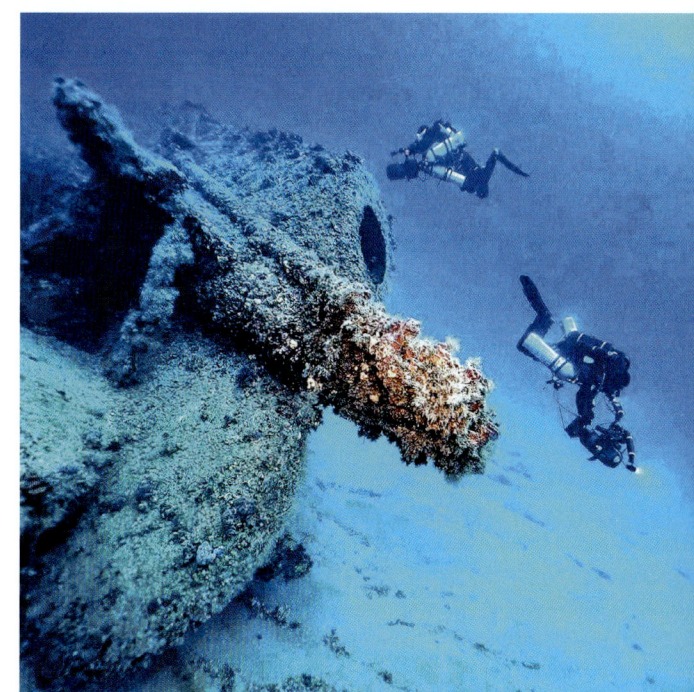
The bow section of HMS Stubborn.
PHOTO: JON BORG www.jonborg.com

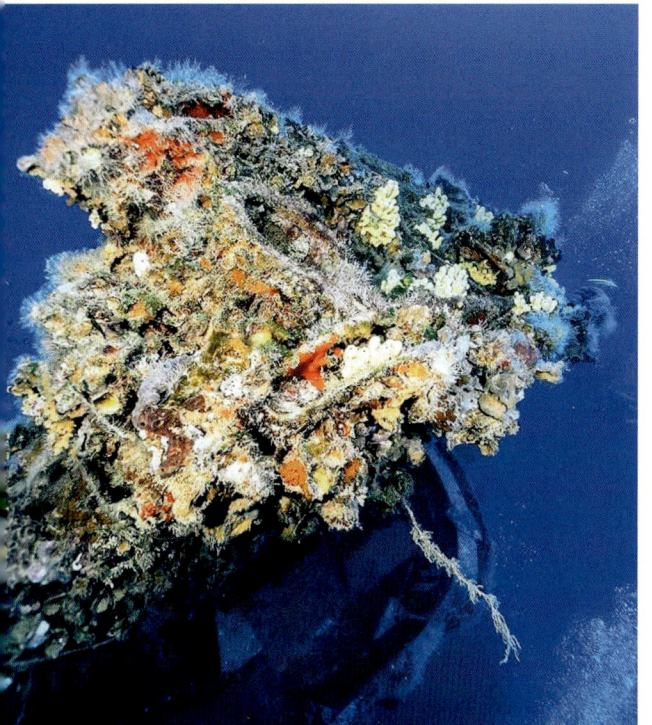
The marine growth on top of the conning tower.
PHOTO: JON BORG www.jonborg.com

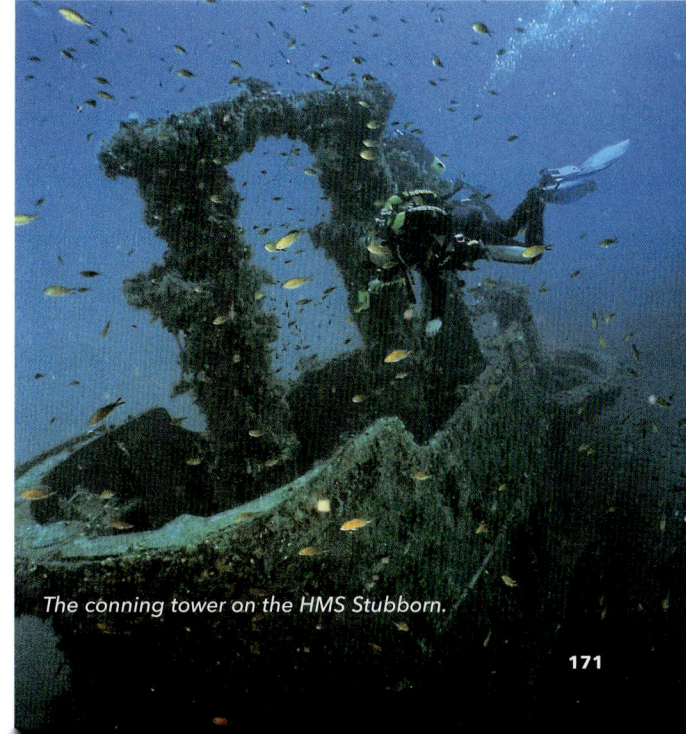
The conning tower on the HMS Stubborn.

MALTA BOAT DIVING SITES

10 - The *Imperial Eagle*

Built in 1938 by J. Crown and Sons Ltd in Sunderland England, weighing 257 gross tonnes with a length of 45 metres. Named *New Royal Lady*, originally requisitioned by the Royal Navy for transport duties, and then transferred to port defense duties. In 1947 she was sold to John Hall, Kirkcaldy for service on the Firth of Forth and re-named *Royal Lady*. Later that year she was sold to the General Steam Navigation Co. Ltd, London, for Thames dock cruises and re-named *Crested Eagle*.

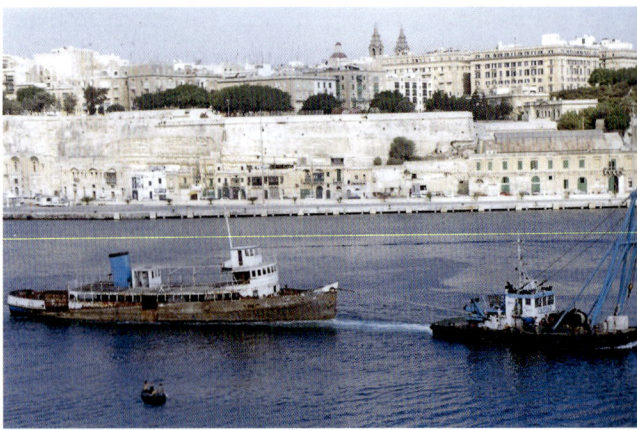

Imperial Eagle leaving Grand Harbour under tow.
PHOTO: CHARLIE SCICLUNA

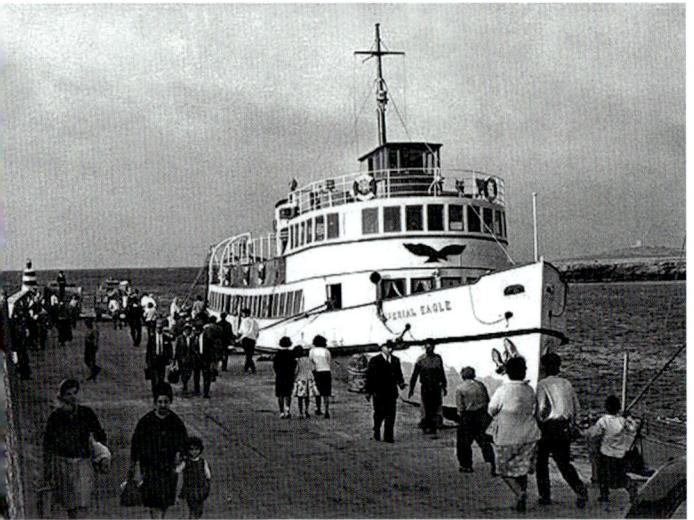

Passengers embark the Imperial Eagle at Marfa Quay, Malta.
PHOTO: ALEX DUNCAN - ISLE OF WIGHT

In 1957 she was purchased by Magro Bros. Malta, after modification to carry 70 passengers and 10 cars, she was re-named *Imperial Eagle* and carried out ferry services between Malta, Marfa Quay and Mgarr harbour in Gozo until the mid-1970's after which time she was used for storage in Grand Harbour.

A group of divers at the bow of this wreck.
PHOTO: ARKADIUSZ SREBNIK POLANDDIVINGPHOTOS

THE DIVE After laying half submerged next to the old cattle sheds in Grand Harbour for a number of years she was refloated, made environmentally safe. She was scuttled some 500 metres off Qawra Point at the end of the reef on the 19th July 1999 and has come to rest in an upright position at an approximate depth of 38m. An ideal extended range dive with the added extra attraction of a photo session with the Statue of Christ, which is only a short distance away.

The forward deck and bows of the Imperial Eagle.
PHOTO: ARKADIUSZ SREBNIK POLANDDIVINGPHOTOS

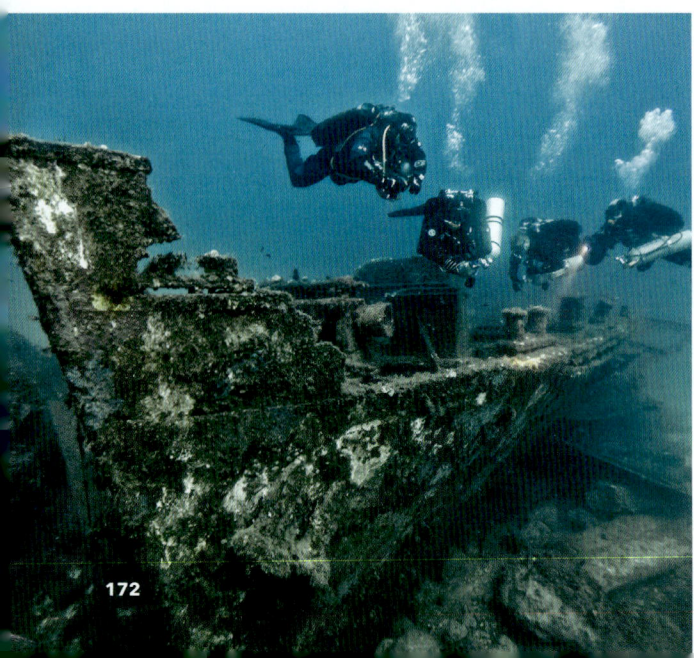

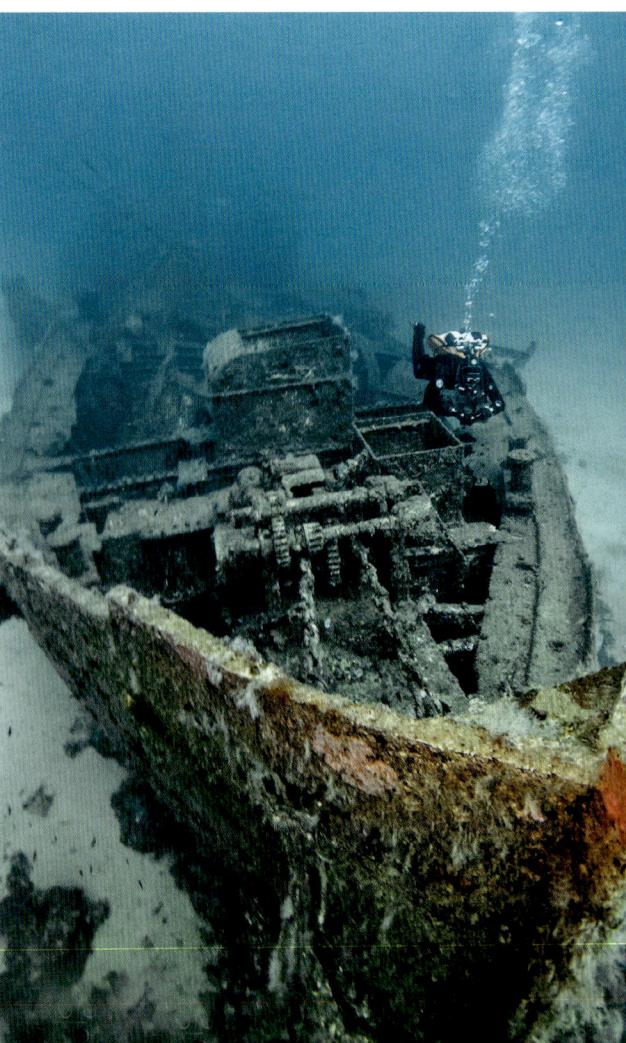

MALTA BOAT DIVING SITES - MV *IMPERIAL EAGLE*

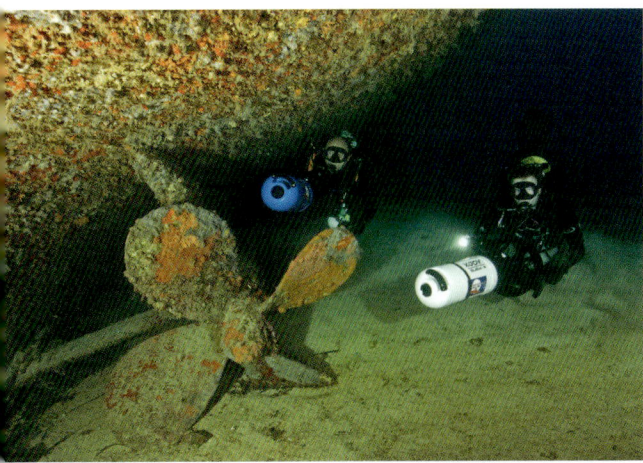

PHOTO: MAX VALLI ORANGE SHARK

Using a DPV is a great way to explore a wreck.

PHOTO: JON BORG www.jonborg.com

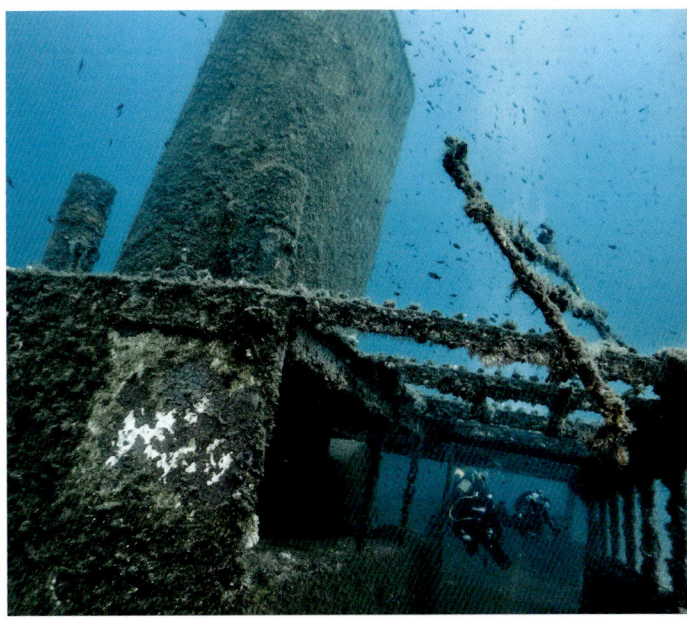

The forward deck and bows of the Imperial Eagle.

PHOTO: ARKADIUSZ SREBNIK POLANDDIVINGPHOTOS

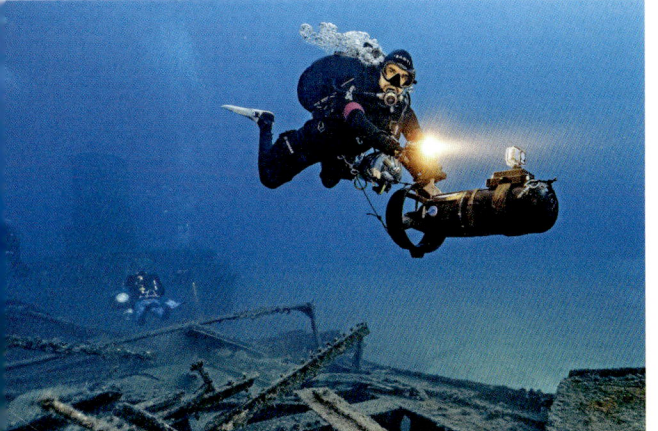

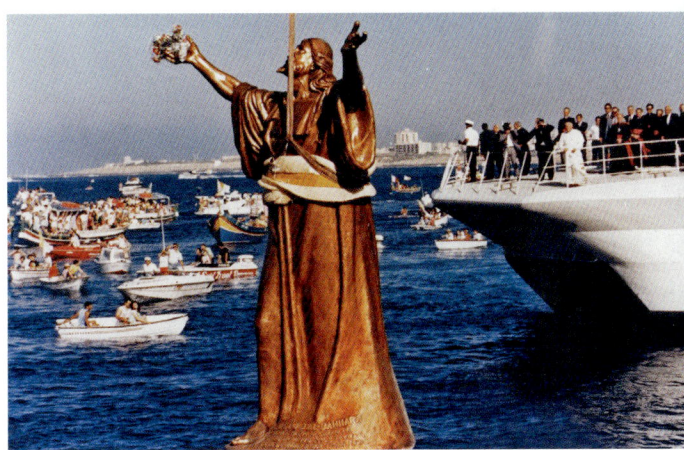

Bottom left: A view of the stern deck and midships.
Bottom right: The Statue of Christ not far from the wreck.

PHOTOS: ARKADIUSZ SREBNIK POLANDDIVINGPHOTOS

Pope John Paul observes the lowering of the statue of Christ off St Pauls Island May 1990, later moved to a new site off Qawra Pont.

PHOTO: WILFRED PIROTTA

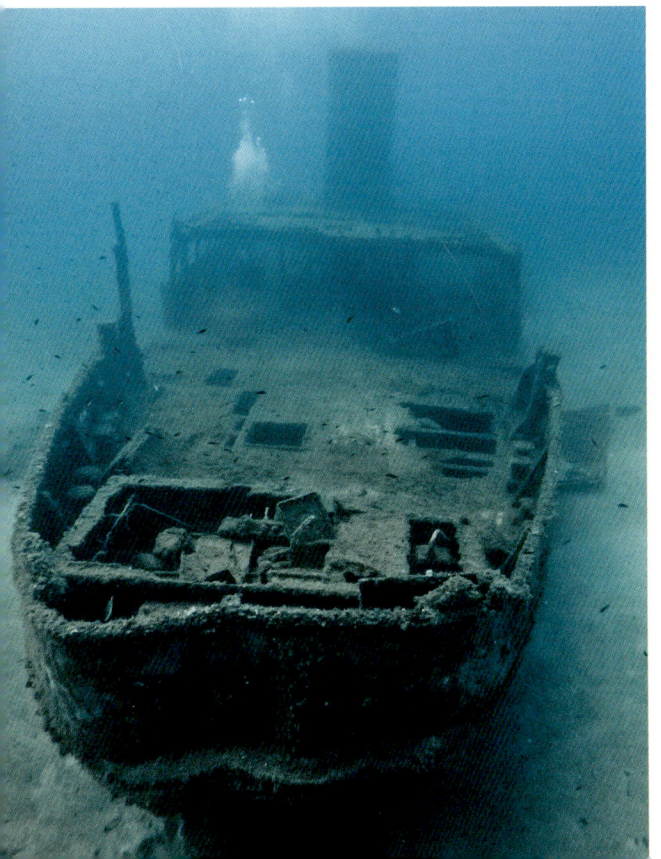

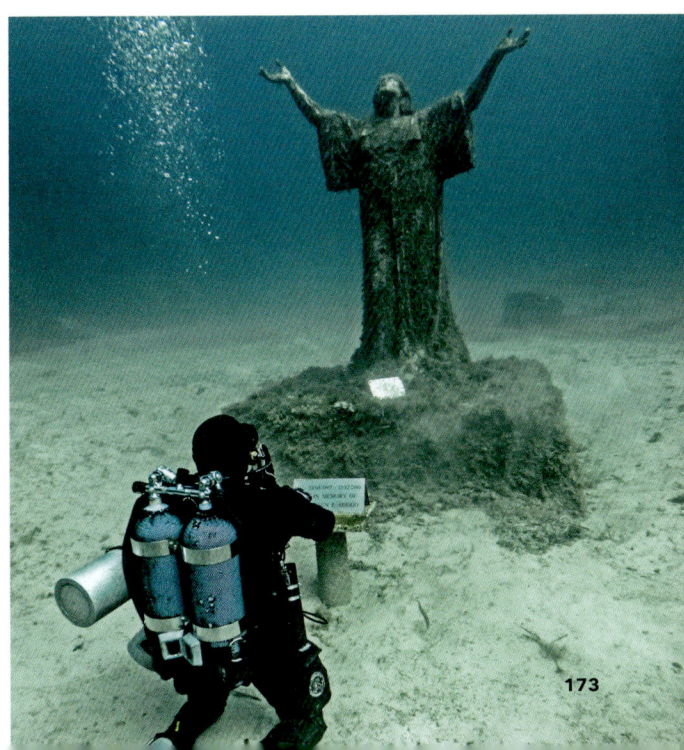

173

Gozo Boat Diving Sites

Around the shores of Gozo there are many hundreds of boat dives to list them all would almost be impossible, I have chosen a few of the most popular ones, bearing in mind that some of these dives can be done from the shore. Gozo has so much to offer the scuba diver with dramatic reefs, never ending drop-offs, caves of all sizes, arches, tunnels, blue holes, windows and wrecks all with marine life to match, the diving is just brilliant.

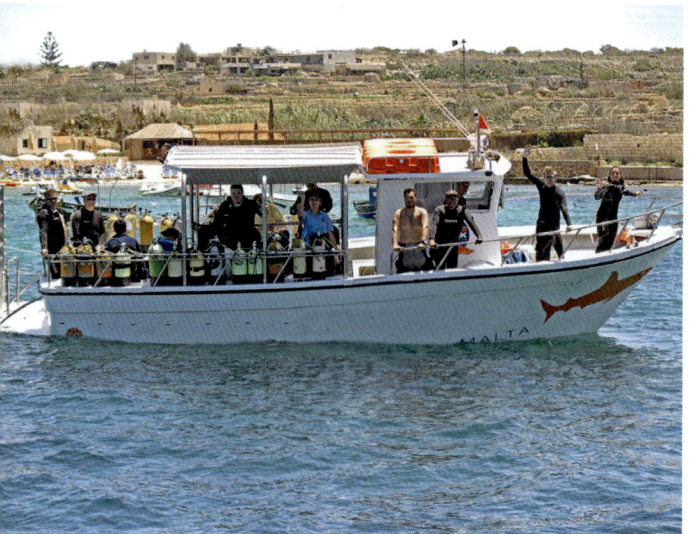

A dive boat leaves Malta for a trip to the Gozo dive sites.

01 - MV *Hephaestus*

Built in Linkoping, Sweden in 1965, she is a steel-built tanker with a tonnage of 595, registered in Lome Togo. 62 metres long and a beam of 8 metres. It had one 6-cylinder 4 stroke diesel engine, with a single shaft and propellor, giving her a speed of 11 knots.

Divers visit this latest artificial reef / diver attraction.
PHOTO: ARKADIUSZ SREBNIK POLANDDIVINGPHOTO

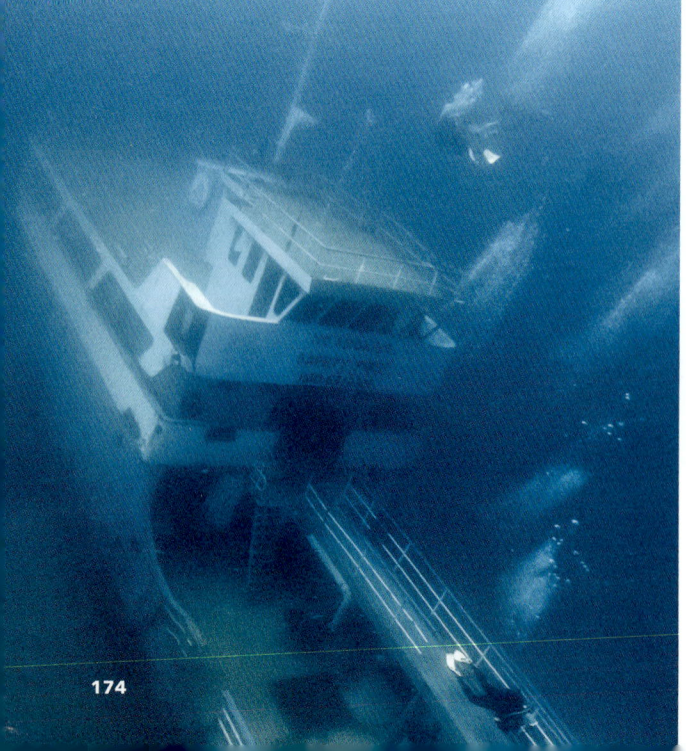

She was a bunkering oil tanker had a mixed crew, with a captain from Bangladesh. Her first years at sea had been uneventful as she went about her work, up until when she arrived off the coast of Malta, late in 2017. The vessel had been at sea for about four months and was anchored 3 miles off Qawra Point, while there was a dispute relating to payment of the crew's wages. During a severe storm on the morning of the 10th February 2018 the ship began to drag its anchor. the crew attempted to sail the ship into sheltered waters, unfortunately the ship was washed ashore on the north side of Qawra Point. Thankfully, her tanks were empty, only a minor leak of fuel was reported and all the crew were rescued safely.

Six months later and after temporary repairs she was pulled off the rocks and towed to Marsa shipyard, the severely damaged ship was too costly to repair so would have to be sold for scrap.

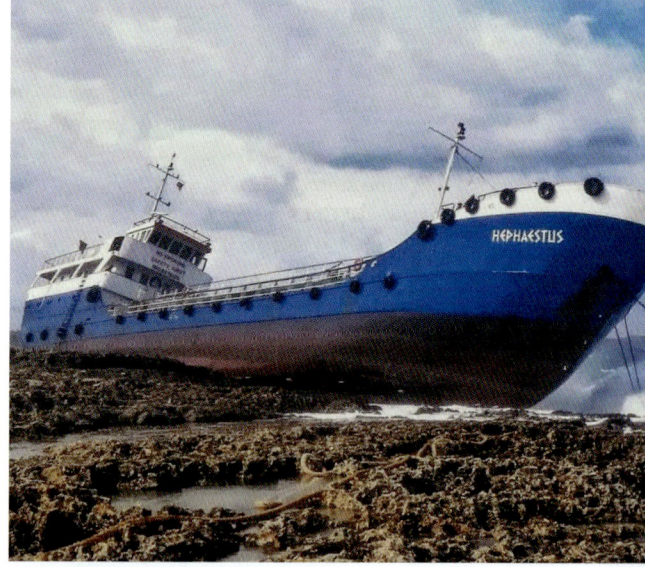

MV Hephaestus grounded at Qawra Point Malta.
PHOTOS: MALTA TOURISM AUTHORITY
MV Hephaestus off Xatt L-Ahmar before the sinking.

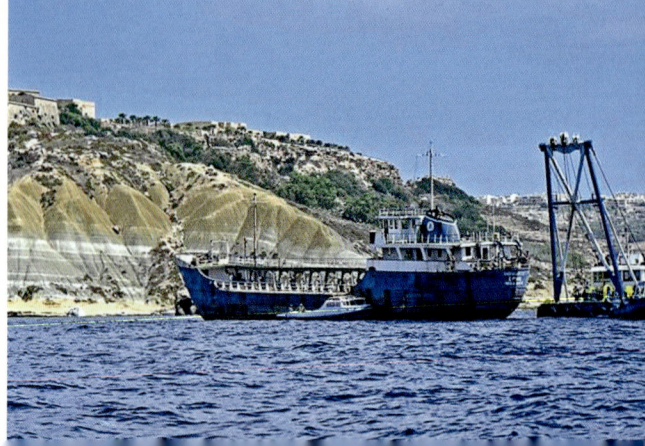

By 2019 working together the Malta Tourism Authority, Professional Diving Schools Association and the Ministry for Gozo made plans to have the ship cleaned and made environmentally safe and then to be sunk off Xatt l-Ahmar as a diver attraction. The MV Hephaestus was scuttled 29th August 2022 and now sits upright on a sandy seabed at 46m.

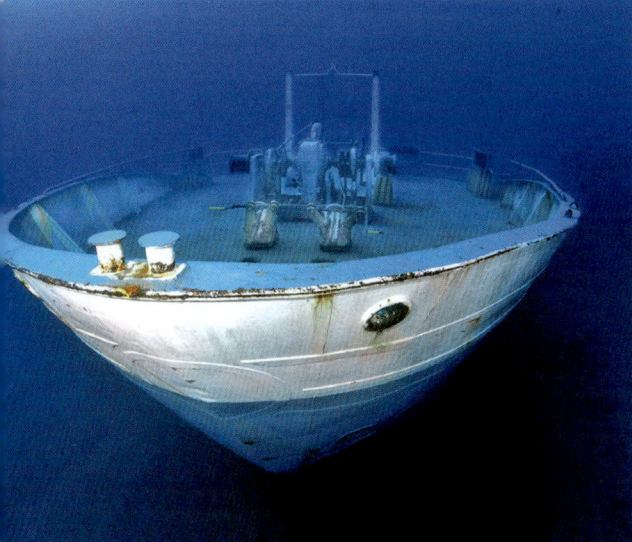

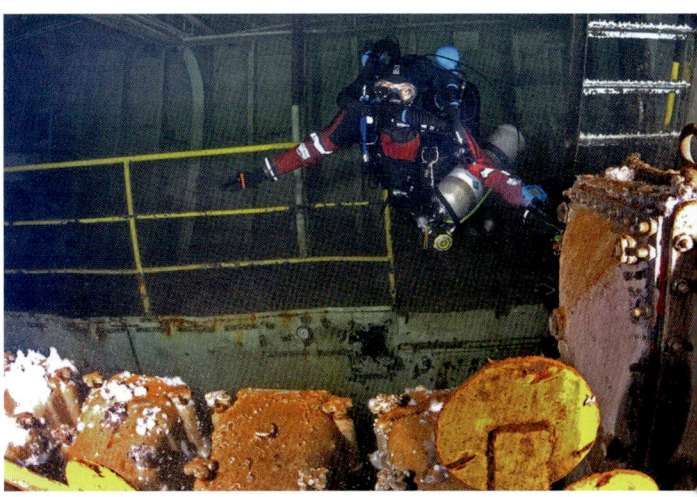

Top right: The MV Hephaestus's engine room.
Top left: An underwater view of the bow of this ship at 34m.
PHOTOS: GRAHAM OWEN MALTAQUA
Below: Marine growth has started to grow on this hatch.

THE DIVE The wreck is now sitting on a slightly sloping sandy seabed some 200 meters from the shore line. Depths to the seabed are, the bow 45m, the stern 42m, average deck depth 37m top of the bridge 33m. You can penetrate inside the wreck including the engine room with the correct procedures being carried out. It will take time for the marine vegetation to take over bare metal areas, but slowly it will happen. That's after other early arrivals of marine life take up residence on this new found home.

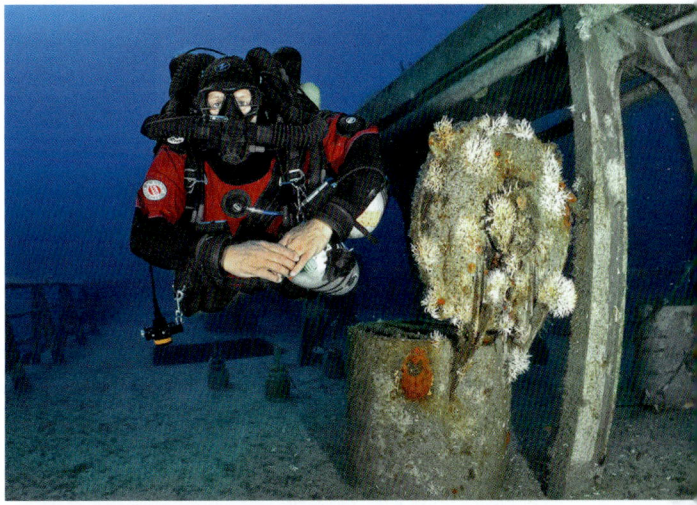

Bottom right: The bow and upper deck at a depth of 33m.
PHOTOS: ARKADIUSZ SREBNIK POLANDDIVINGPHOTO
Bottom left: The stern resting on a sandy seabed at 45m.

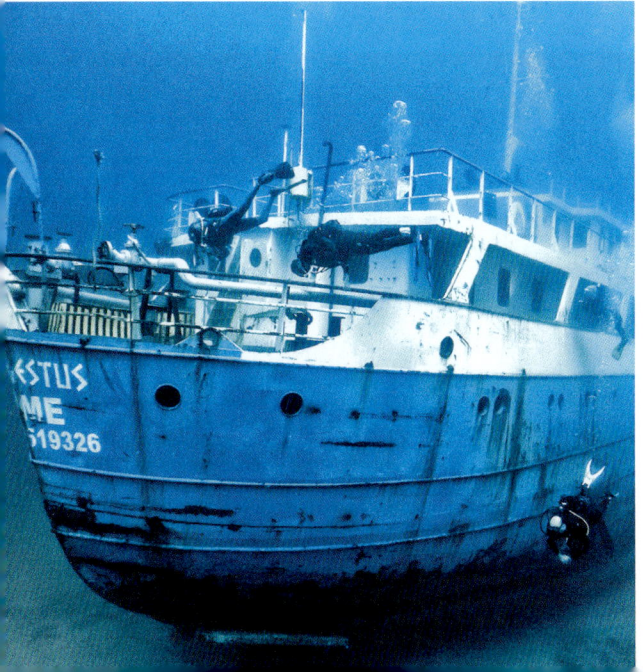

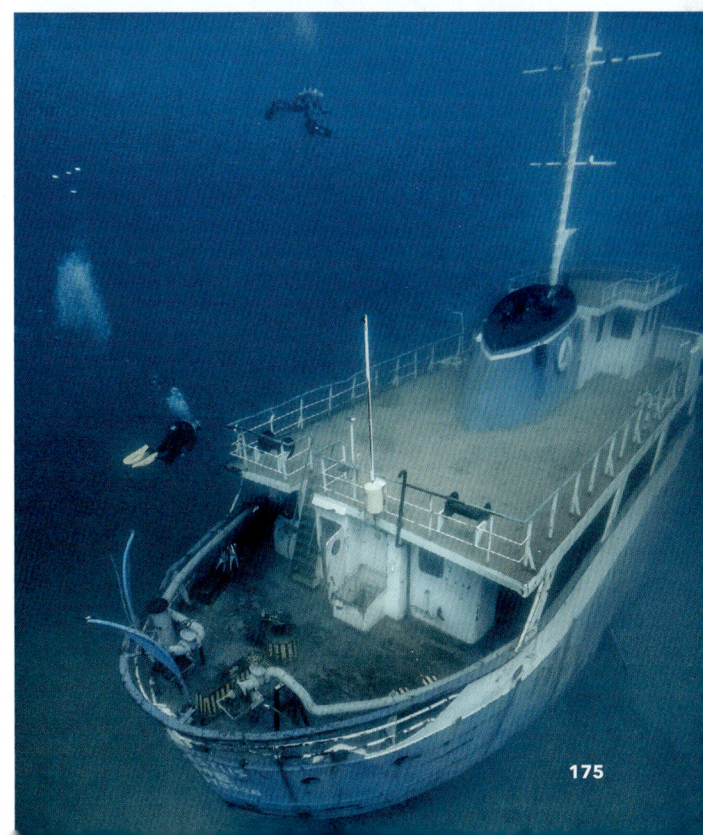

02 - Fesse Rock

This rock is situated some 400 metres off the entrance to Mgarr ix-Xini on the south coast of Gozo. The top of rock rises almost 15 metres out of the sea; below the sides quicky drop down to almost 50m plus.

THE DIVE I think the dive plan is up to you, the most impressive drop offs are on the eastern side. Around the base are areas of large boulders surrounded by the sandy seabed. The sides of the column are littered with cracks, small and large fissures, these areas are all covered in soft and hard corals and many tube worms. Fire worms, starfish, coloured nudibranch and of course octopuses are just some of the marine life which have made this reef their home. Looking out into the blue on the southwest side you may see passing shoals of barracuda, dentex and amberjacks. A great dive site, and for those non divers there is always snorkelling.

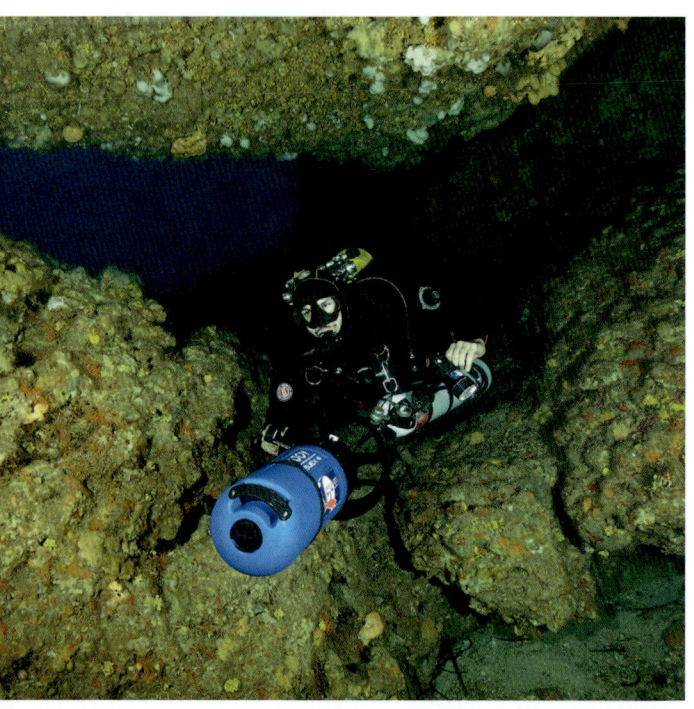

These DPV's are now available to hire at many dive centres.
PHOTO: MAX VALLI ORANGE SHARK DIVE CENTRE

03 - Dawra Tas-Sanap & Cave

This dive site is the first sheltered inlet to the southeast of Xlendi Bay and has an underwater landscape suitable for all divers, there is a shallow reef, where the boat will normally anchor.

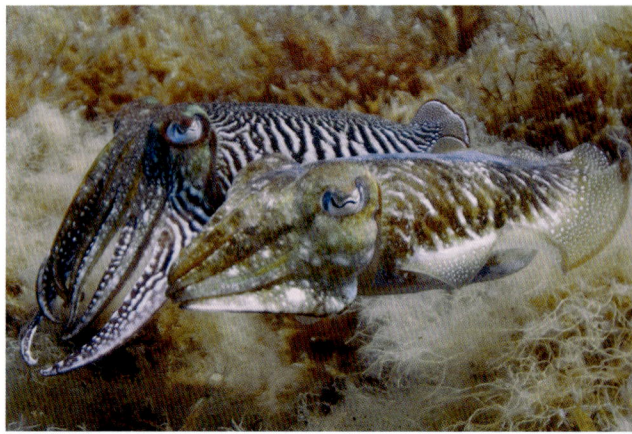

Cuttlefish changing their colours, makes a fantastic photo.

THE DIVE To start head in a south-westerly direction to find the ledges, drop offs, massive boulders, an arch and nearby the large semi-circular cavern at 18m. Further along in the cliff face is a cave/tunnel 15 metres wide, continue just round the corner where there is a second entrance at 11m this could also be your turning point. Below this area there are large boulders and depths of 50m plus. Here the walls rise almost vertically to the surface, they have been carved out by the sea over thousands of years. Dentex roam this area so keep an eye open in the blue.

After you have reached your selected depth return to 15m and enjoy the wonderful sight of the big arch in the sunlight and the large shoals of salema fish moving across the reef. Now you can return to the shallow reef for your safety stops and the boat. This is a great dive with much to explore.

The fried egg jellyfish, large shoals arrive during summer.
PHOTO: JANEZ KRANJC ORANGE SHARK DIVE CENTRE

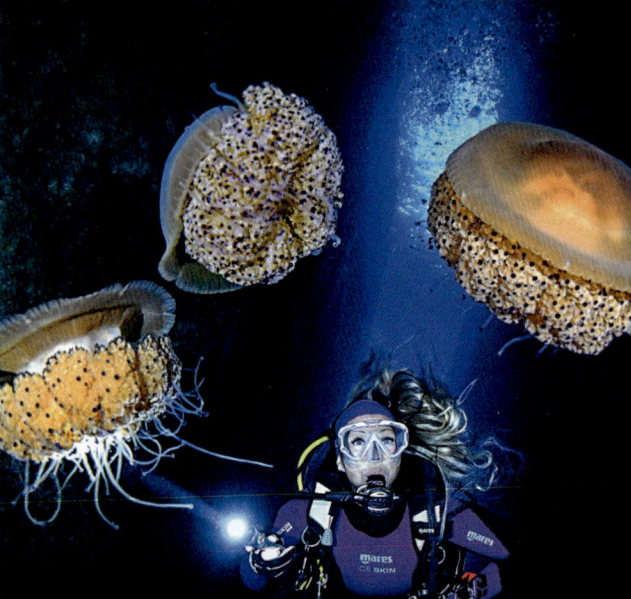

04 – Zurzieb Cavern & Reef

Another great boat dive on the south coast, just a short distance west of Xlendi Bay, the boat will anchor above a 6m little ledge.

THE DIVE The main area of this dive site is shaped like an upside-down triangle, with an inner route, with a maximum depth of 18m. This route includes gullies, arches at shallower depths, below 10m there is an area of large boulders ending at the point with a single very large boulder, the top of which has a depth of 18m, the seabed below is 35m. The outer route first heads east, before heading west, it is longer and deeper and includes gullies, arches, then the tunnel at 16-18m. Moving south towards our maximum depth at 35m, below the very large single boulder at the point. Now to shallow waters and the cave/cavern to the west of the ledge area.

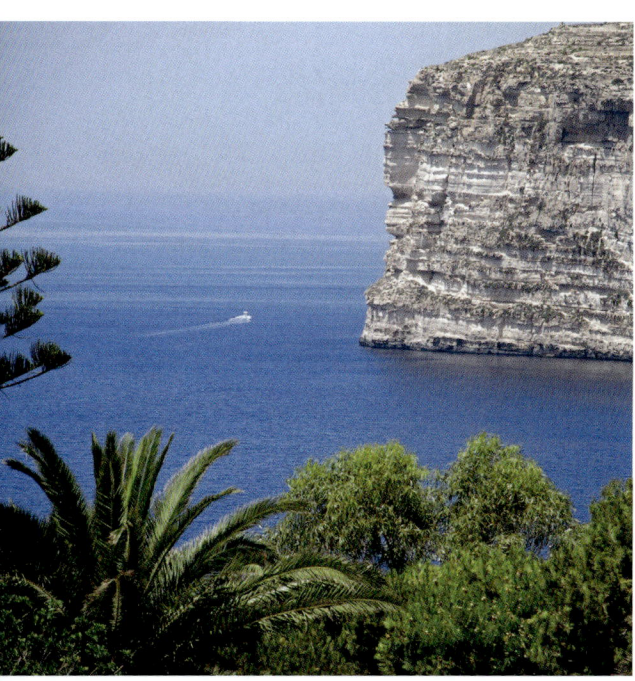

A view of the cliffs to the west of Xlendi Bay

A photo shoot by these colourful underwater reefs.
PHOTO: JANEZ KRANJC ORANGE SHARK DIVE CENTRE

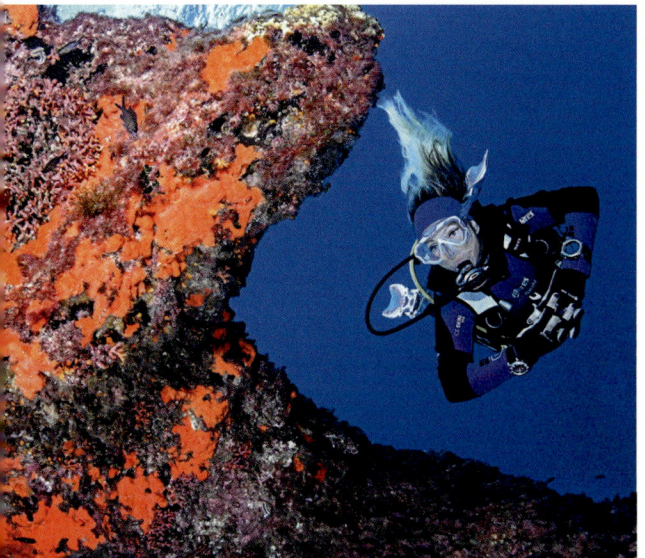

05 - Fungus Rock - Dwejra

This large limestone rock dominates Dwejra Bay, originally named 'The Generals Rock' famous for the rare shrub like fungus known as general's root, whose red juice was treasured for its medicinal properties. Used by the Knights of St John against dysentery, bleeding, impotence and other healing properties. The bay behind Fungus Rock is often used by yachts for stop-overs whilst travelling around the islands. The 'Qawra Tower' which overlooks the bay is occasionally open for visiting tourists.

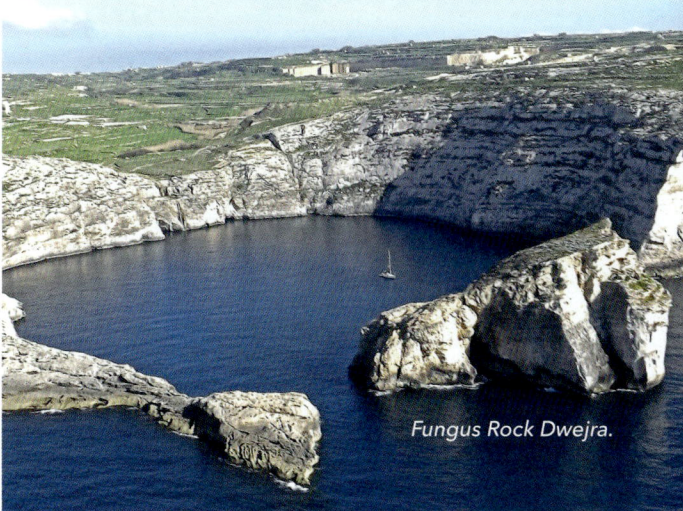

Fungus Rock Dwejra.

THE DIVE Below the surface on the outer side of this fascinating rock wall drops vertically to a depth of 50m plus where you will find the area covered in large boulders, this is the best area to explore they provide excellent habitat for large groupers. From the north-eastern corner of the rock as you begin your slow ascent you will find that the underwater features become more interesting, as ledges and gullies present themselves for closer inspection.

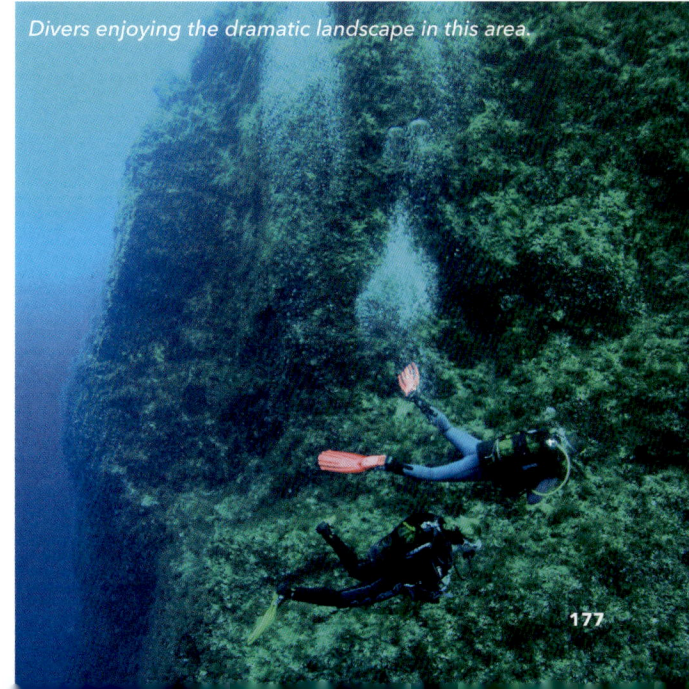

Divers enjoying the dramatic landscape in this area.

GOZO BOAT DIVING SITES

06 - San Dimitri Point

San Dimitri Point is the most westerly point of Gozo; here the impressive cliffs rise out of the shimmering blue waters to a height of 80 metres. While admiring the beauty of this area you will realise that the boat is your only exit. Below where the boat will anchor is a shallow plateau with an average depth of 6m, great area for safety stops if required.

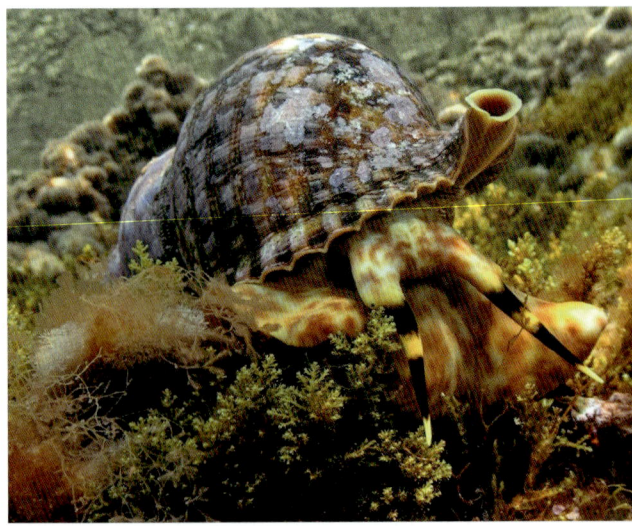
A night dive reward, a colourful trumpet triton shell.
PHOTOS: VERONICA BUSUTTIL

In the clear blue waters, amberjacks on a feeding frenzy.

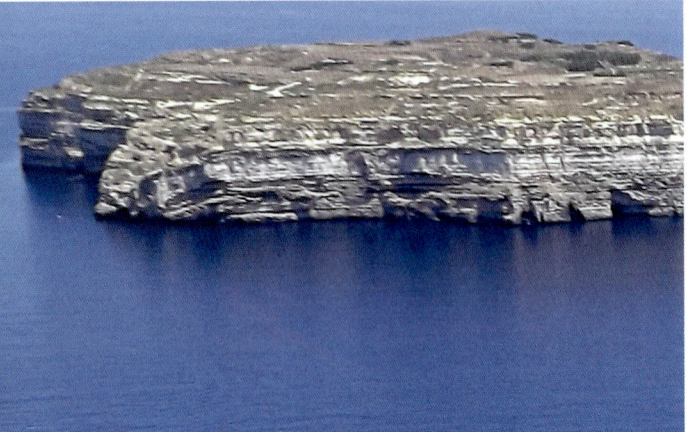
The cliffs of San Dimitri Point, during calm waters.

THE DIVE This area is well known for its fantastic visibility, that means, clear deep blue waters, alive with shoals of spectacular fish such as barracuda, dentex and tuna passing by. The first part of the drop off is more of a steep slope leading down to house sized boulders with vertical walls; here you might spot groupers resting on the algae covered ledges. A dive with a difference! This surely is one of Gozo's best boat dive sites.

A shoal of barracuda which are often seen in this area.
PHOTO: VERONICA BUSUTTIL

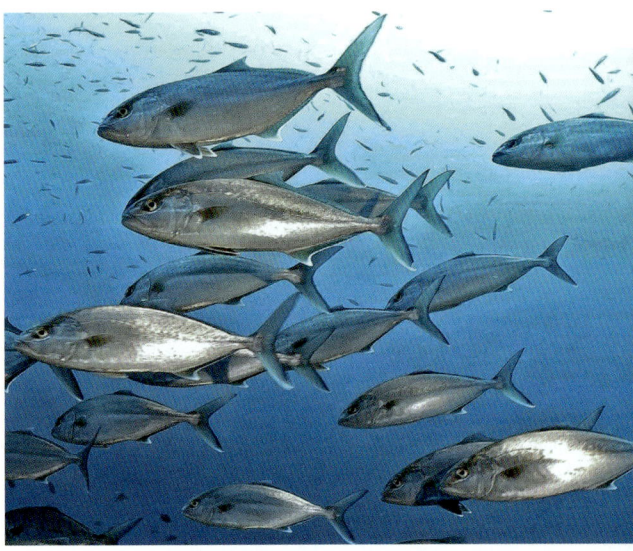

Divers with excellent visibility, explore the San Dimitri reef.

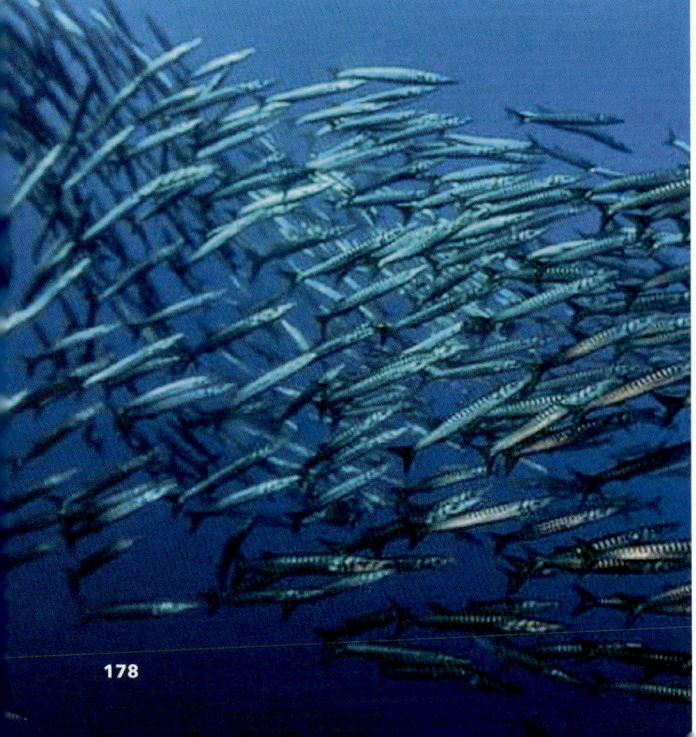

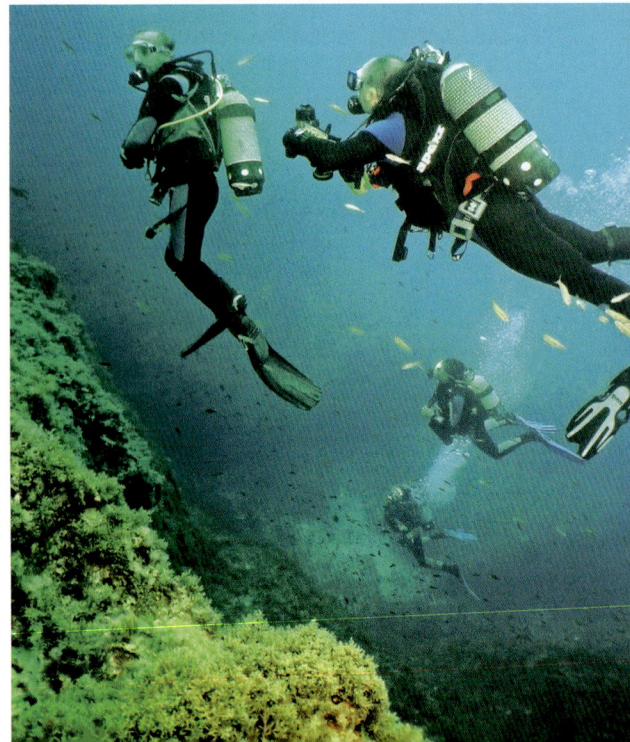

The Legend of San Dimitri

The legend of San Dimitri Point is that there was an old widow who lived with her son near to the chapel of San Dimitri. When Turkish invaders came and captured her son, taking him away to become a slave, she ran to the chapel praying to San Dimitri to return her son to her. The painting in the chapel came alive, and San Dimitri on his white horse rode out of the picture to follow the Turkish ships, rescuing the boy and returning him to his mother. Then San Dimitri vanished back into the painting. As a thanksgiving the mother and son promised to light an oil lamp under the painting every day until they died. However, one day a big tremor shook the surrounding cliff side; the earth subsided and the chapel sunk to the bottom of the sea. The area has a reputation for abundant fish life, because they are attracted to the lamp of San Dimitri, which still shines to this very day! Research for this legend kindly carried out by Marthese Matusiak.

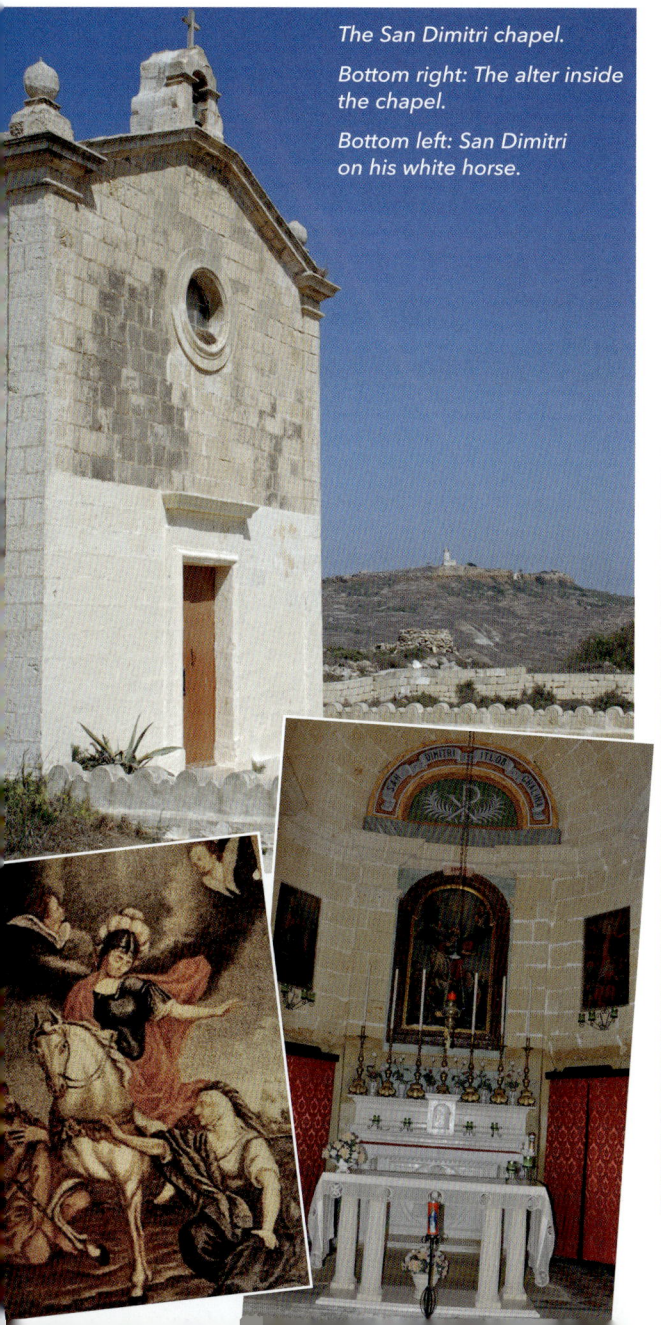

The San Dimitri chapel.

Bottom right: The alter inside the chapel.

Bottom left: San Dimitri on his white horse.

07 - Ta'Camma - Gudja Cave

This dive site is on the north coast of Gozo is quite unique for it has five caves, three of which including Gudja Cave rise to above sea level. Of course, the dive brief will be given before you enter the water on which caves will be on your dive plan.

THE DIVE Cave 1 Gudja Cave is on the western side of the plateau near where the boat will anchor, the top part drops to 8m below the surface, the lower part starts at 15m down to the seabed at 30m, you can swim from one part to another, but you will need a torch. Now you will have to travel east for 20 metres to cave 2, height 15m seabed 28m, another 26 metres will take you to cave 3, height 15 metres seabed 33m, further on for another 20 metres will take you to cave 4, this cave is much larger 30 metres wide and from the seabed at 30m rises above the surface. Cave 5 is further on to the east and is the largest of them all, from the seabed at 33m rising high above the surface. Your dive plan may not include all five caves.

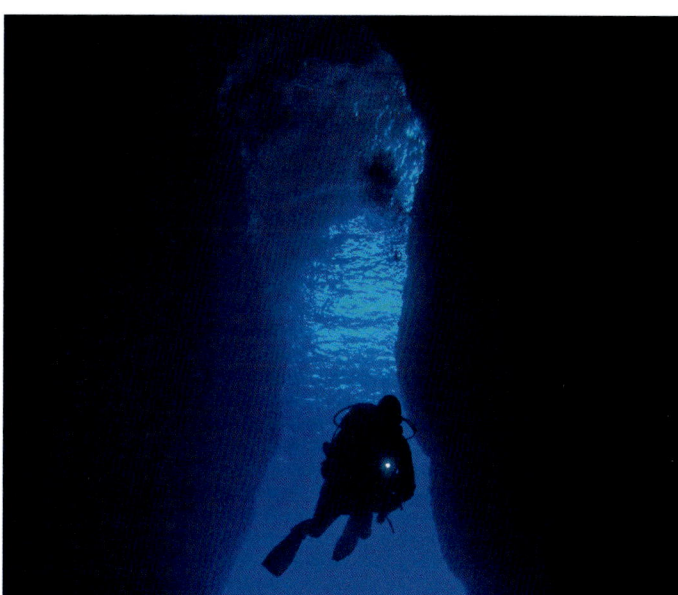

One of the many caves /caverns along this coastline.
PHOTOS TOP: SHARON FORDER BOTTOM: IAN FORDER

This nudibranch sometimes called a Spanish Dancer.

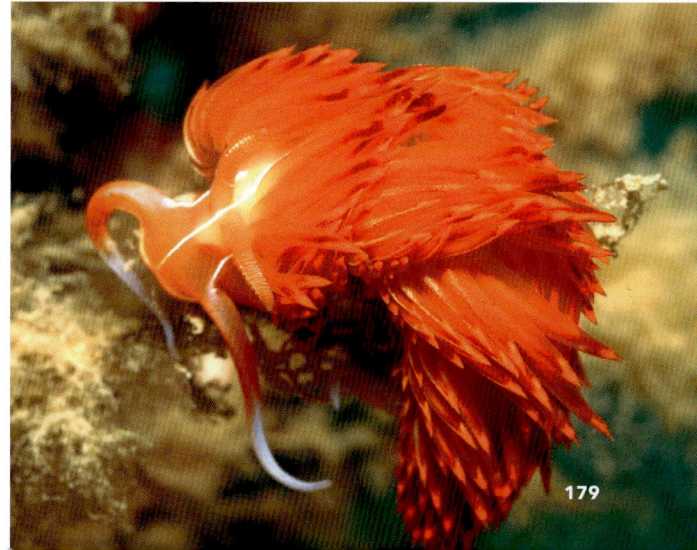

08 - Wied il-Meilah The Valley of Salt

This is another dive site on Gozo's north coast and is just over one mile from the village of Gharb and not far from Ghasri Valley. The mayor and the local council were able to spend 800,000 euros on this beauty spot, the valley and local area were in a very poor state, the work was completed in 2003 and 2011 and is now one of 21 European Destination of Excellence EDEN winners, it now attracts many visitors each year. You can almost reach the waters edge but the site cannot be dived from the shore.

THE DIVE The boat will anchor near the arch over a 12m plateau from here you can complete the whole tour, heading down to your maximum depth of 30m before turning east when you reach the boulders, explore, then head southeast up to your chosen depth, on your way you may see Vera's bike, a father pushed this bike over the cliff to stop his son from riding it, so the story goes.

Now head west along the reef wall before turning left into the area of two caverns when you leave do not miss the swim through. Massive boulders are now in front of you, their top depth averages around 14m, ascend the reef wall to complete your safety stops before returning to the boat.

It's a must to take your camera and torch on this dive which will give you many opportunities to use them.

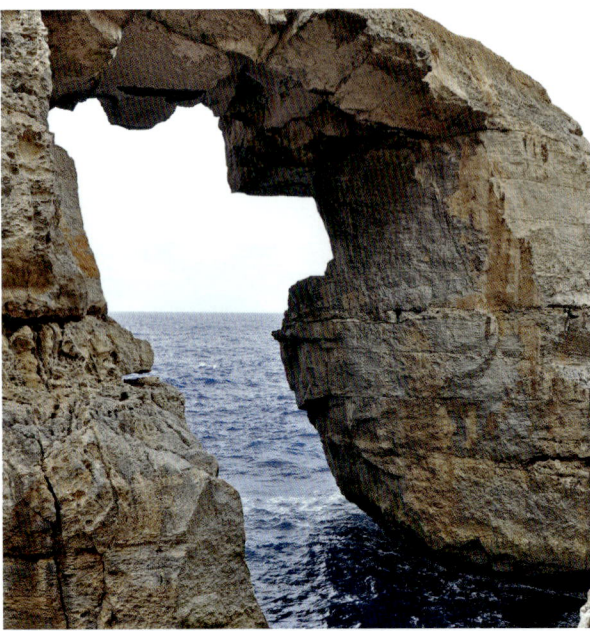

At the end of this picturesque valley is the arch.

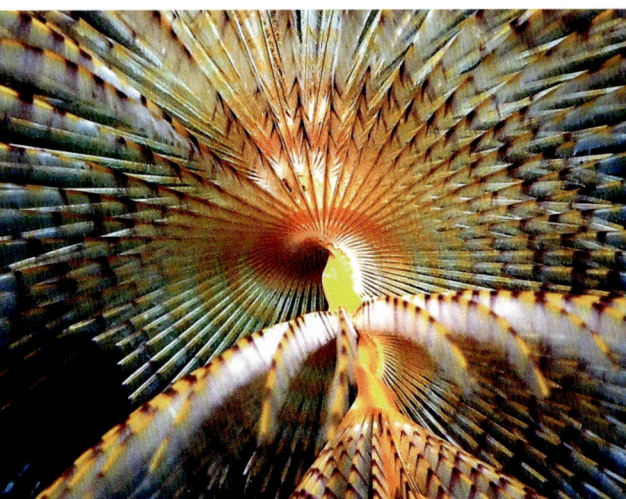

The amazing colours of this tube worms.
PHOTO: PATRICK SCHEMBRI WALRUS DIVING CLUB

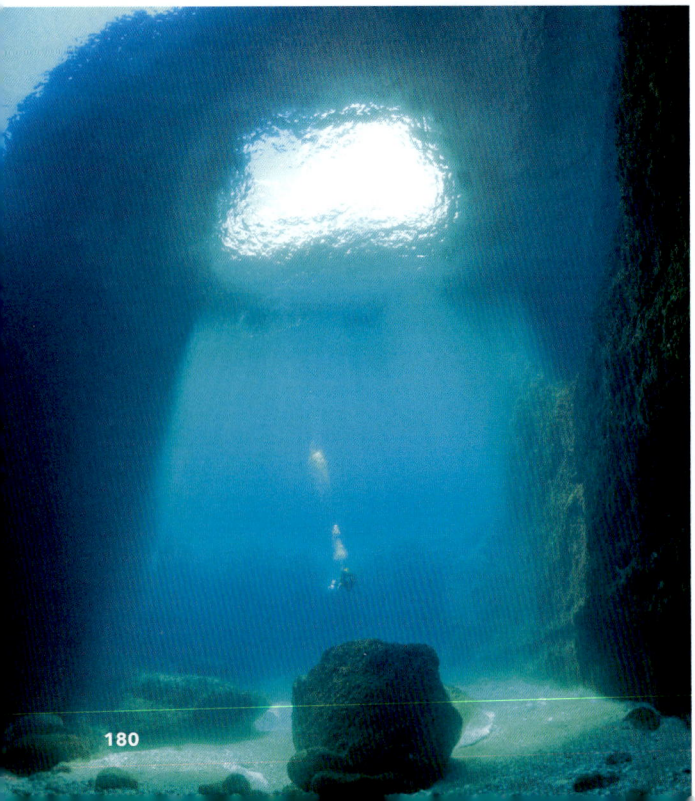

A diver's view of the arch from below the surface.
PHOTO: PER EIDE STUDIO'S   www.pereide.no

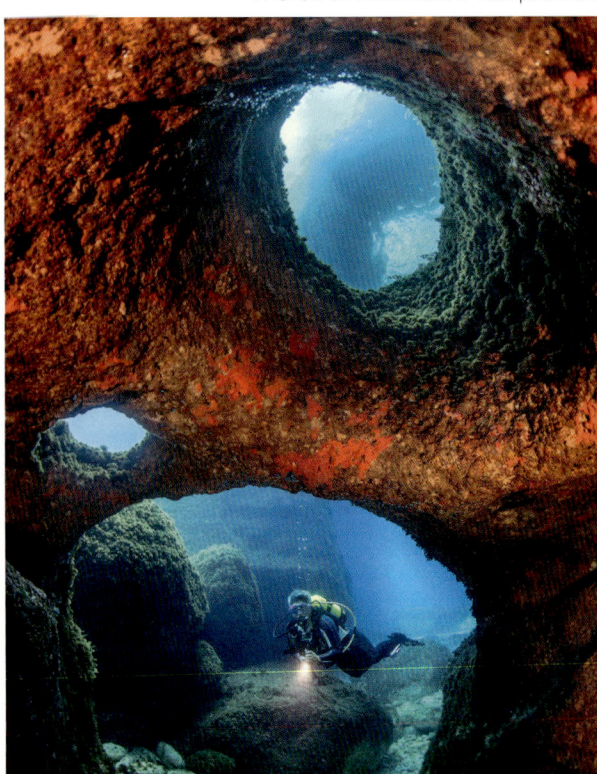

Fantastic photo opportunity! you could call it Swiss Cheese.
PHOTO: PER EIDE STUDIO'S   www.pereide.no

09 - Calypso Tunnel / Cave

Just a short distance to the west, from the seaside resort of Marsalforn, is the lovely Xwejni Bay. The landmark here is the large lump of sandstone on the eastern side of the bay which has been shaped over the years by the wind and sea. The reef wall where the dive site is located is a continuation of the same reef wall that leads to the Double Arch 100 metres away, Anchor Reef and then on to Reqqa Point.

Top right: Many groupers live and hide on these colourful reefs. PHOTOS: IAN FORDER
Below: A shrimp cleans the mouth of this moray.

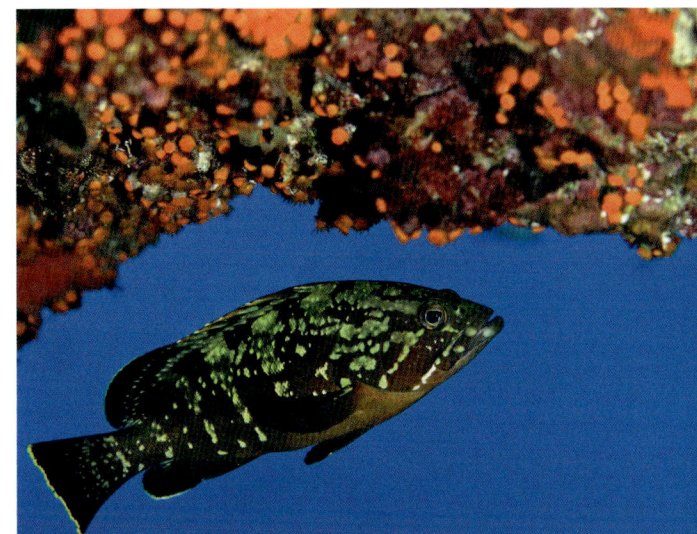

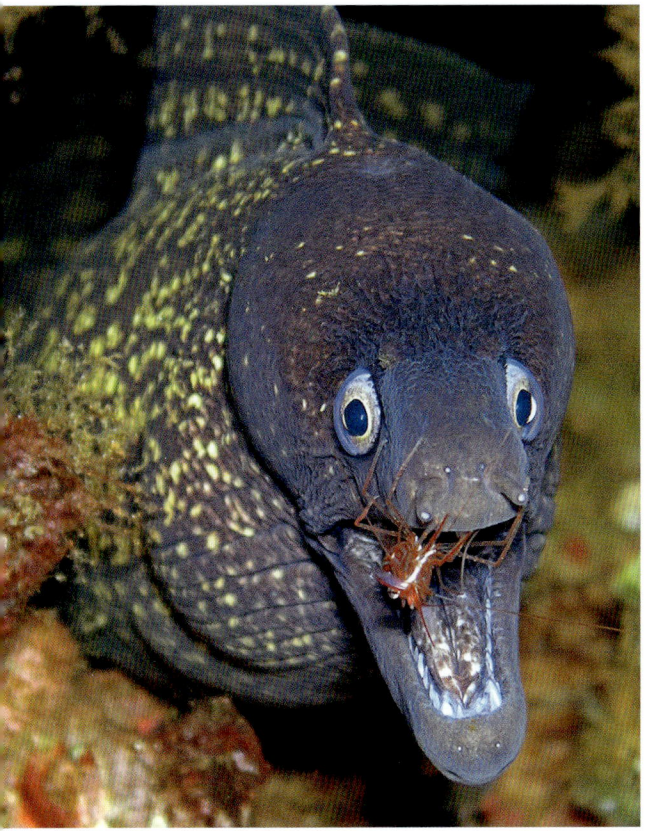

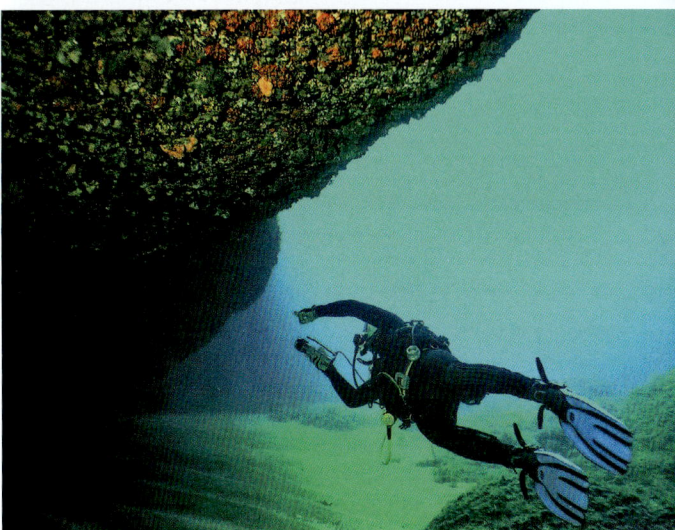

Leaving the Calypso cave via the mouth.

The face of the Calypso Cave, divers at the mouth and at the top the two eyes.

THE DIVE The first part of your dive is a small valley with boulders, grass and sand, depth 25m, which is surrounded by meadows of posidonia grass depth 16m. This sunken area was originally the back of a very large cave, the ceiling collapsed thousands of years ago leaving only a small arch. At its northern end is the Calypso Cave/Tunnel which leads to the open sea, depth here on the sand is 35m. As you leave the tunnel turn around and take a look back, you will see the resemblance to a face, the mouth, which you have just passed through and high up the two eyes at 21m. Once outside your dive plan will continue east or west along this outer reef. When returning to the boat you have two choices, return through the spectacular reef to the small valley, or just go upon to the posidonia meadows and head south back to the boat. You can shore dive this site if sea conditions are perfect, but the boat is the best option.

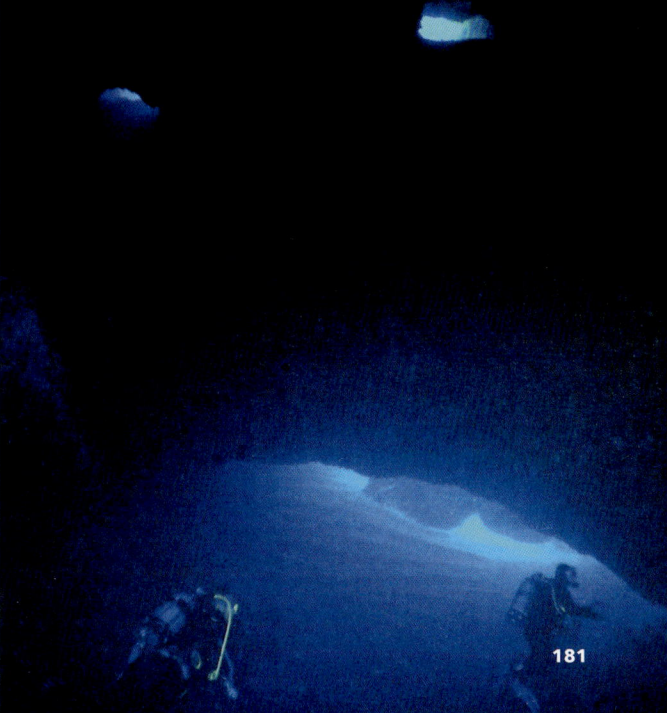

COMINO BOAT DIVING SITES

01 - Lantern Point

Named Lantern Point, due to the small light on its end, often called Lighthouse Point, possibly the most popular dive on Comino, and with good reason.

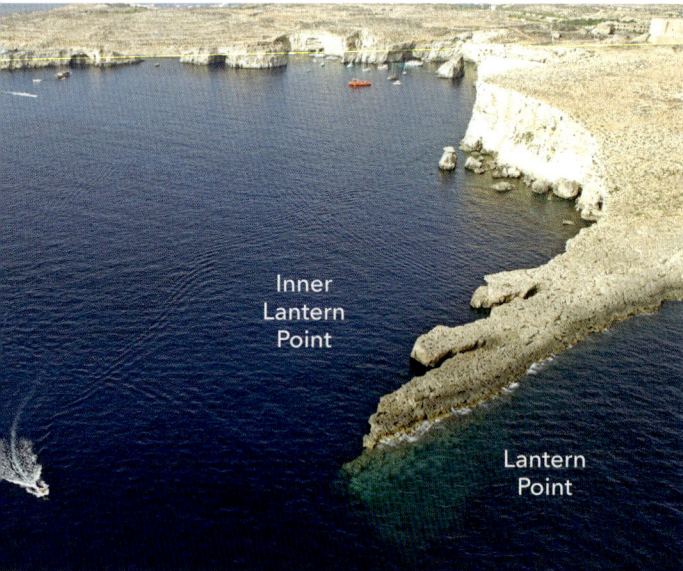

Lantern Point, this finger of land jutting out into the sea.

The underwater topography here is simply stunning, and includes tunnels, caves and swim-throughs, a sheer wall, massive boulders, and a maximum depth of 50m, ideally take a torch. The boat will usually anchor to the south of the point, quite close to the Lantern which gives the point its name. Below the boat is a plateau with an average depth of 8m, just the place to end your dive and safety stops

A diver ascending from the chimney to the plateau on the south side of Lantern Point.

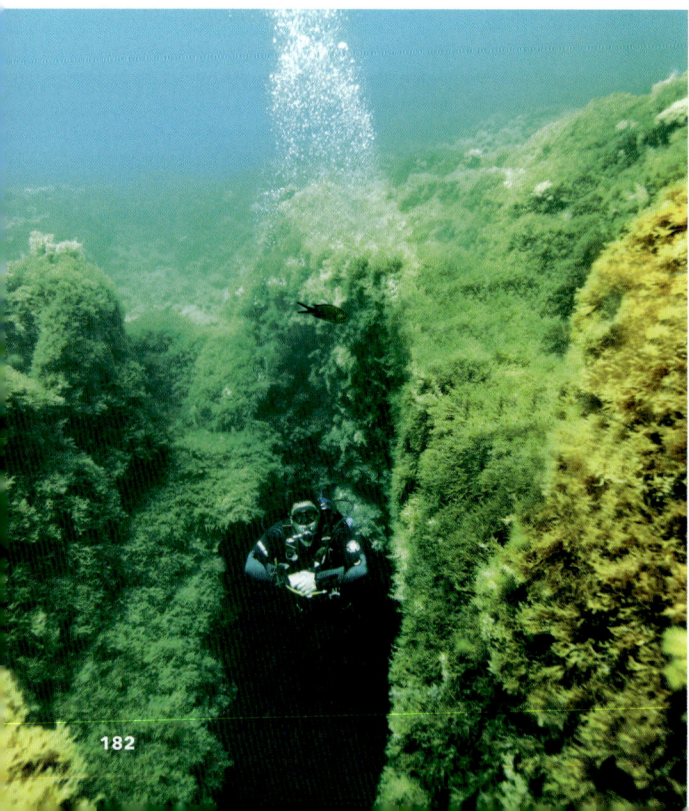

THE DIVE The chimney is normally the start of the dive, close to the Lantern at a depth of 4m the entrance is large enough for divers to enter one at a time and exits at 18m and is relatively straight. Your torch will illuminate the corals, fans and sponges which decorate the walls. On exiting the tunnel, you will find yourself in a gully leading down to 25m, with the sheer wall of the headland to your right.

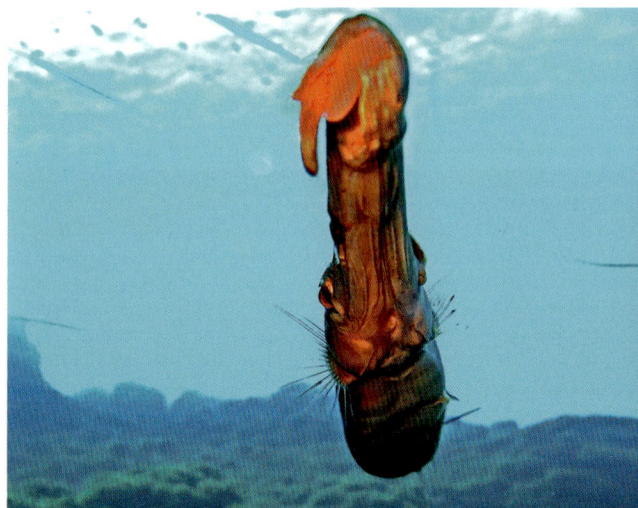

This squid would not normally be found close to shore.
PHOTO: JOE FORMOSA

Continue straight ahead towards a huge boulder known as "The Mushroom" at 28m. It is possible to swim under this massive rock using a series of swim-throughs for a complete circuit of the central pillar that gives the boulder its name. Take your time and light up your surroundings for an array of beautiful sponges, corals, fans, and occasionally lobsters or huge urchins. Now head south for the plateau and reef wall, which would now be on your left, depth 25m, to your right are large boulders, surrounded by sandy areas sloping away to 50m plus.

Almost at the exit of the chimney at 18m.

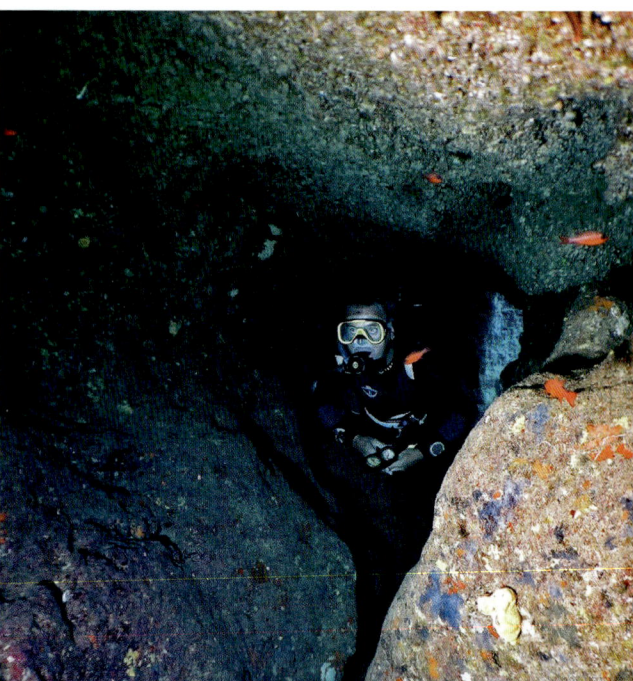

Look out for large groupers resting on the rocks, continue down to 35m where there is a U-shaped cave near the headland. On reaching the headland ascend to the top of the reef at 20m, look out in the blue for a chance to see larger fish such as dentex and amberjacks. Follow the reef with the drop off on the left, keeping your depth at 18m, once you reach the gulley at the start of the wall you can either, return through the chimney to the plateau or ascend the reef wall. Once on the plateau take your time to explore this area, you will normally find octopus and other marine life, also you will see bubbles being released from the chimney through the porous limestone rock forming a curtain, which is good for an unusual photograph.

Here an overhang starts to form above the surface, and within the plateau you will find two large well shaped holes carved out of the limestone by wave action over the centuries. You can see the rounded stones responsible lying at the bottom of the holes. Moving further on you will reach a shallow cave on your right, with an entrance at 5m. Within the cave there is an air space above you, and it is possible to continue along the wall in a U-shape until you exit at only 2m deep. Before you go too far, look behind you at the cave entrance and the overhanging rock framing a dazzling blue window. A great photo opportunity, if you can dive this site in the afternoon you will benefit from natural sunlight on the wall.

02 - Inner Lantern Point

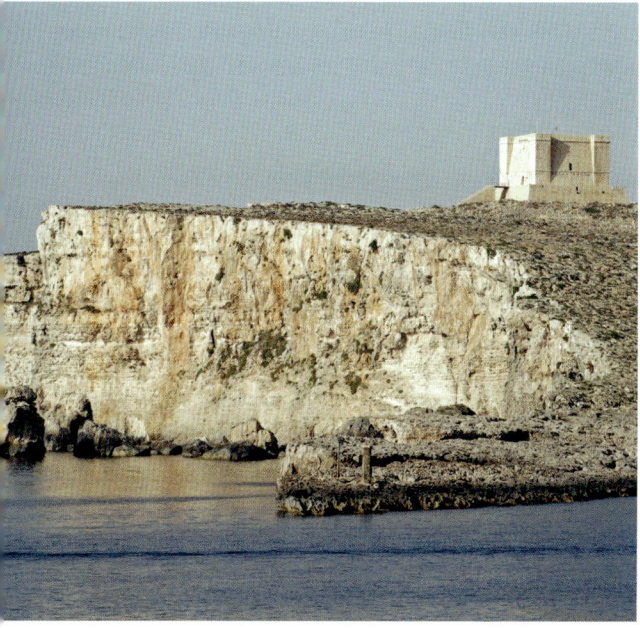

Comino Tower Fort, and the cliffs by Lantern Point.

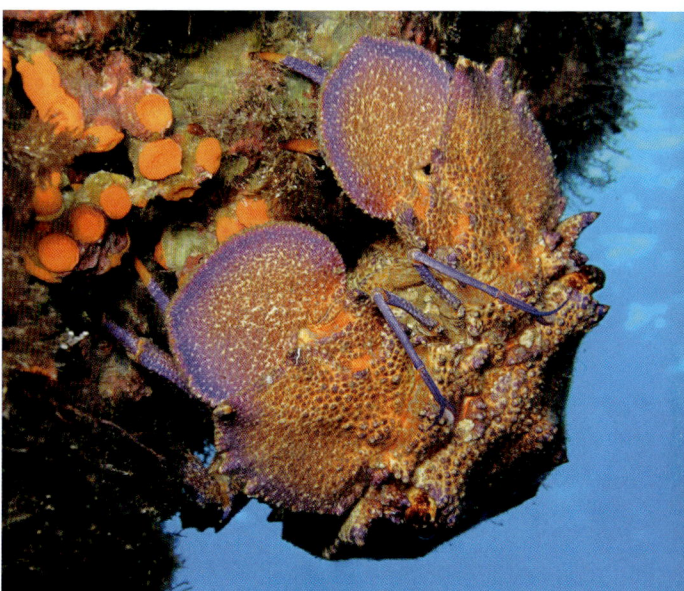

Slipper lobster hanging up-side down.   PHOTO: JOE FORMOSA

Underwater landscape, reef, boulders, grass and sand.
PHOTO: LEE JELLYMAN RITUAL DIVE CENTRE

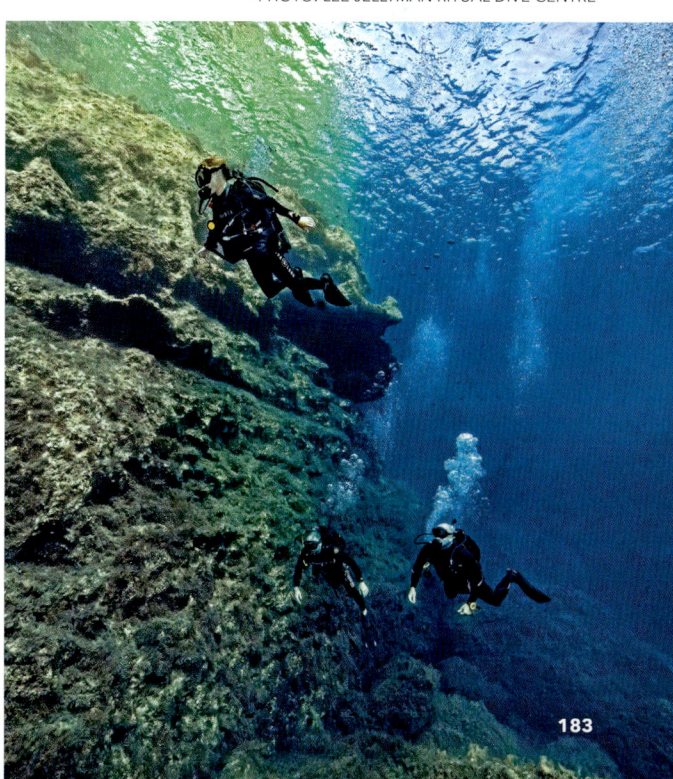

This site is on the inner side of the thin peninsula of rock at Lantern Point. Depths here range from 30m to less than 5m and it is suitable for all levels of diver. The underwater landscape is almost as beautiful as Lantern Point, but no tunnel.

THE DIVE Here you have a sheer wall, a shallow cave, with many large boulders lying against each other, giving several swim-throughs. There are two large inlets which can be seen on the aerial photograph: these are great to explore when sea conditions are right. The wall itself is covered in colourful growth, including sponges of all colours. Look out for the marine life that you might see, octopus, painted combers, ornate and cuckoo wrasses. Beyond the boulders the seabed slopes down to a sandy area around 30m. On this side you will find some of the tallest boulders, their tops only 12m below the surface. Towards the end of your dive, swim with the wall on your right until you reach a little plateau 6m deep.

COMINO BOAT DIVING SITES

03 - Crystal Lagoon

This shallow, popular dive site is suitable for all levels of diver with depths ranging from 5m to 16m, and is just a short distance from the famous Blue Lagoon. The seabed is a mixture of sea grass, small boulders and dazzling sandy patches; this area is a nursery for young fish and is great for taking photos. Your boat will normally tie up at the little jetty in the lagoon next to the tunnel entrance, allowing non divers to embark, snorkel, or swim.

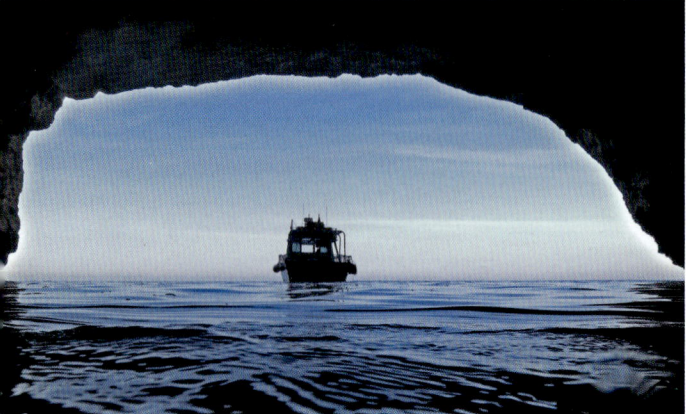

A view from the tunnel. PHOTO: JOE FORMOSA

THE DIVE — Maximum depth 16m

The dive starts at the entrance of this 60 metre tunnel, depth 5m, with vertical walls and a seabed of rocks and gravel, large enough for small boats to pass through, **please take care when while diving the tunnel**. While passing through check the walls for nudibranch.

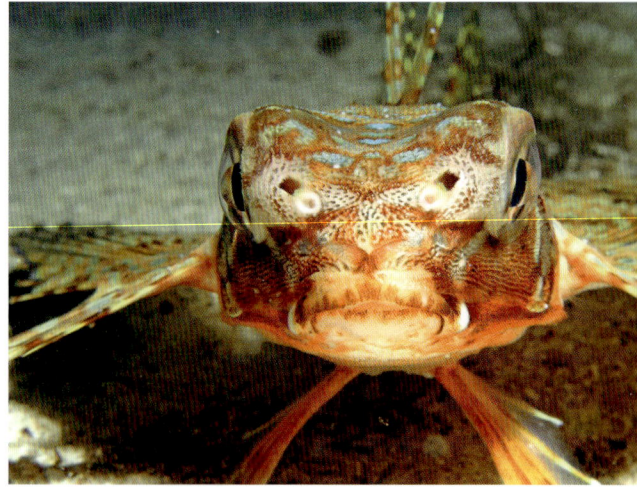

Flying gurnard resting on the sand.

Once out of the tunnel at 8m, turn right to where you can find a false tunnel, explore, next on to a rocky overhang, which gives the appearance of a rhino's head; the walls and ceiling are covered in marine growth this will attract nudibranchs.

Out over the sand is a pinnacle which rises up above the surface, it is known as Mushroom Rock, it is over 10 metres tall, this area is the octopus garden, look for clues, empties shells they have discarded, and there may be a painted comber outside their hiding place.

Now continue to the arch where you may find lobsters and cuttlefish. To return to the lagoon you can use the tunnel or go round the headland where the seabed is made up of small boulders, sea grass and sandy patches, 10m. Here there are usually flying gurnards picking their way across the sand. Try not to spook them and you may be rewarded with a wonderful display of their iridescent blue wings.

04 - *P31* Patrol Boat

The Armed Forces of Malta Maritime Squadron decommissioned the *P31* Kondor class offshore vessel in the latter months of 2004, ending her thirteen-year chapter in Malta's history.

P31 in Grand Harbour. PHOTO: JOSEPH TONNA AFM

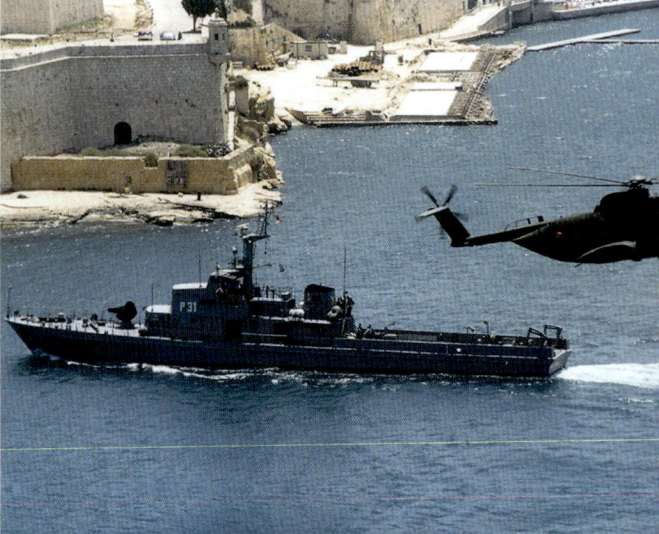

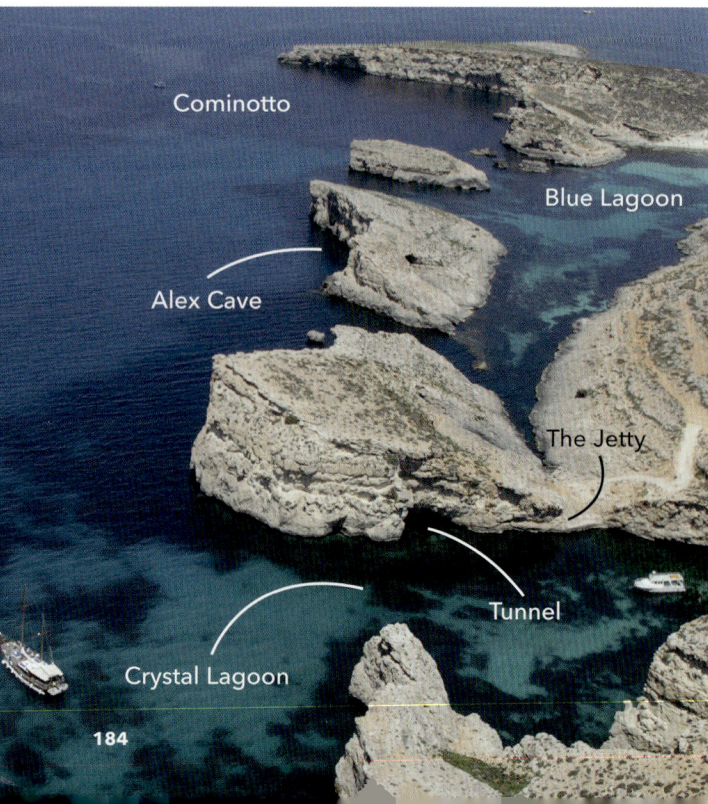

COMINO BOAT DIVING SITES - P31 PATROL BOAT

The *P31* began her life in former East Germany, she is a Kondor class boat designed and built in East Germany in the 1960's. Like her sister ship the *P29*, she is 52 meters in length, with a width of 7 metres and weighs 360 tons and was primarily a mine sweeper. In August 1992 the *P31* and the *P30* left Germany undertaking a three-week long journey to Malta, for two days they battled through force 9 winds, before entering calmer seas off Dover their next port of call was Brest, home of the French Navy's Atlantic fleet.

Whilst crossing the Bay of Biscay they encountered thick fog and the *P31* developed a fault with her radar and the *P30* guided her along to the port of Vigo in Spain. They entered the Straits of Gibraltar and into the Mediterranean, finally the ships arrived in Malta where they were greeted by the crew's family, friends and the Armed Forces of Malta's top brass.

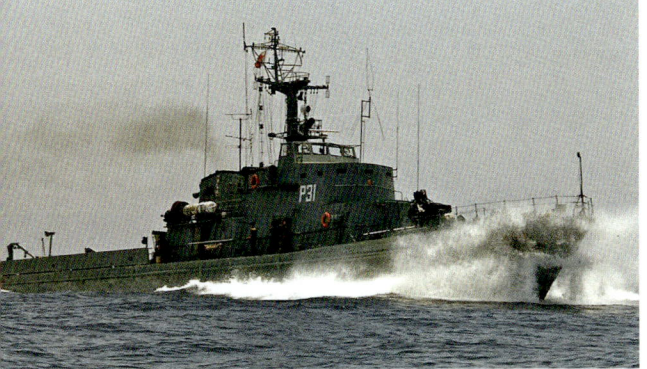

The P31 patrolling the coast of the Maltese Islands.
PHOTO: ARMED FORCES MALTA

After being made environmentally safe for her new surroundings, the *P31* patrol boat was scuttled as a diver attraction on the 25th August 2009 off the island of Comino. She now lies on the seabed, at 22m, with a slight list to the portside, surrounded by a sandy seabed and areas of sea grass, midway between Lantern Point and the small island of Cominotto.

Watched by many, she sinks to her final resting place.
PHOTO: DAVID P. ATTARD ARMED FORCES MALTA

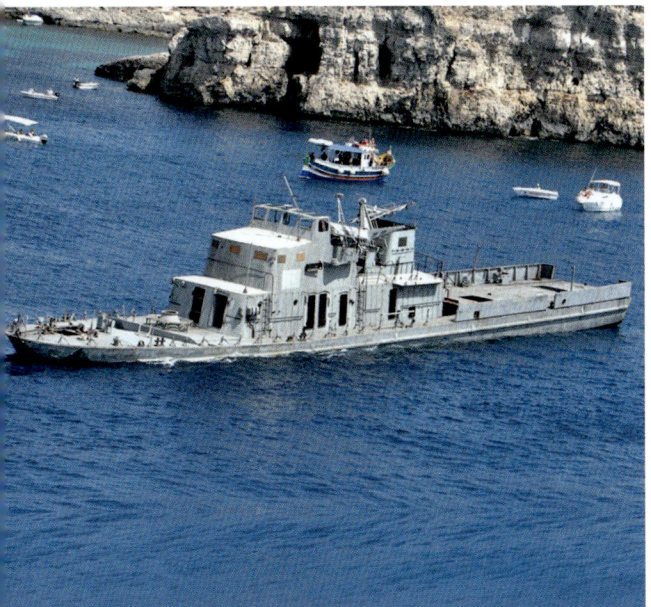

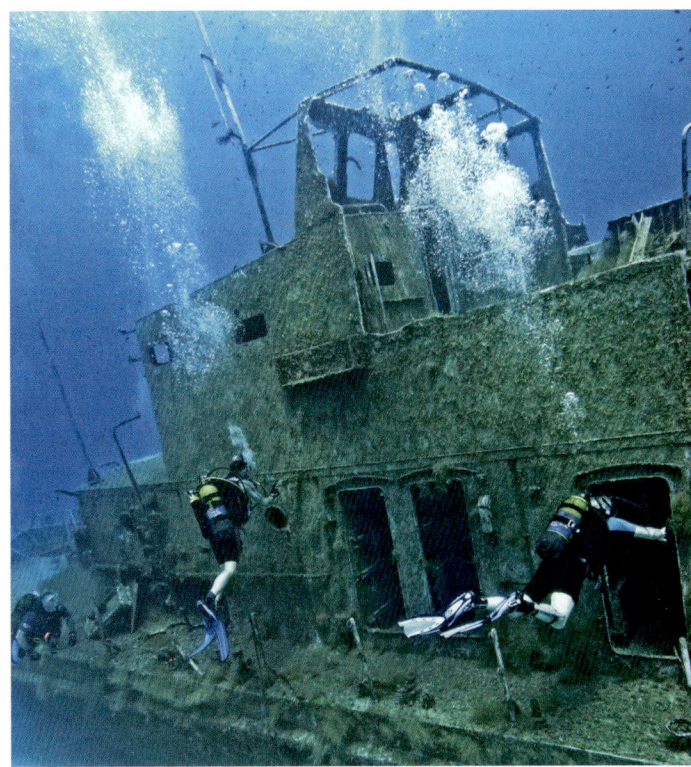

Divers enjoying the fantastic visibility on this wreck.

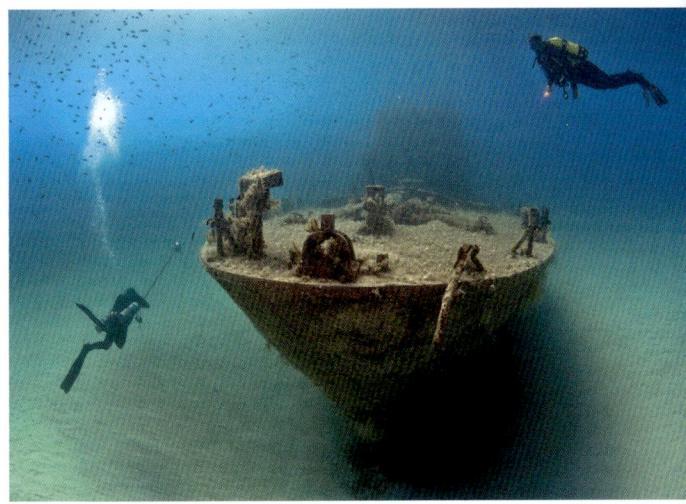

The bow of this interesting shallow wreck.
PHOTO: PER EIDE STUDIO'S www.pereide.no

Divers on the port side and upper structure of the P31.

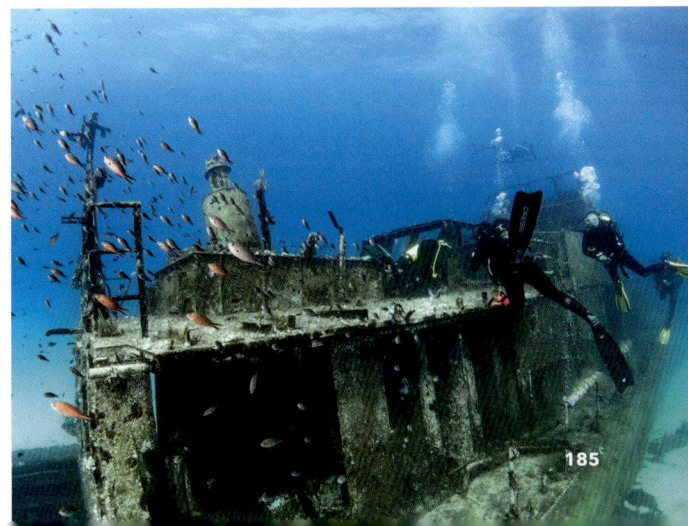

COMINO BOAT DIVING SITES - *P31* PATROL BOAT

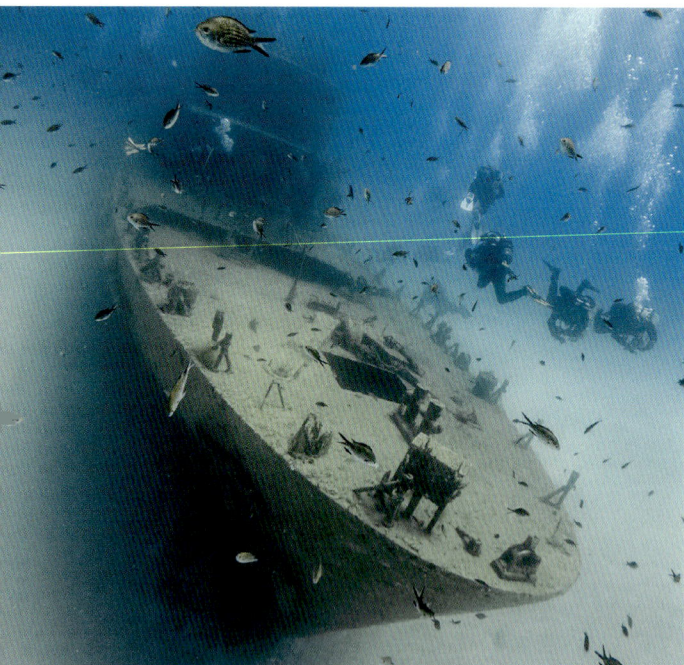

Most divers are able to explore this wreck at 22m.
PHOTO: ARKADIUSZ SREBNIK POLANDDIVINGPHOTO
The bridge and fore deck of the P31 Patrol Boat.

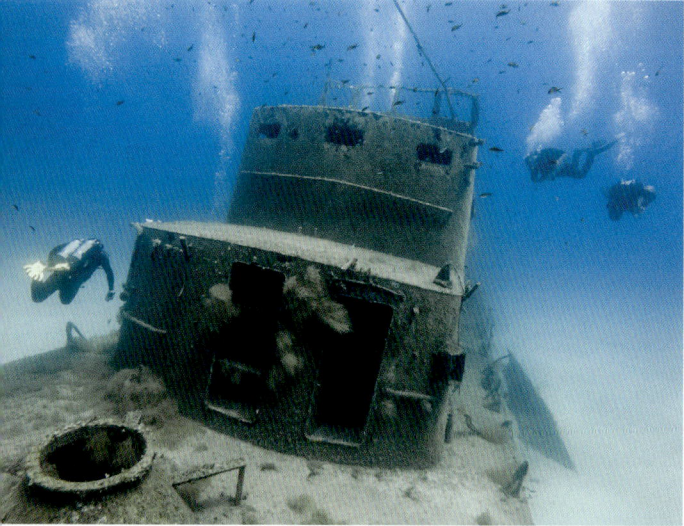

A cuttlefish, who seems to be trying to hide.

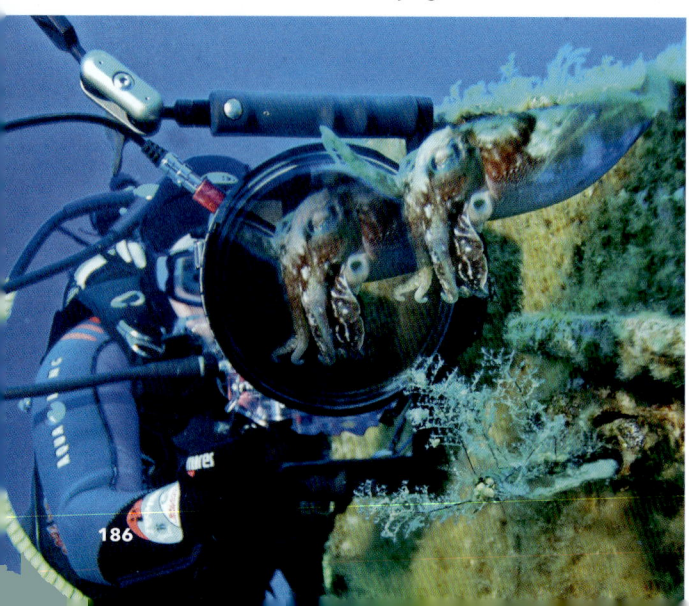

THE DIVE — Maximum depth 22m

After you have entered the water and before you descend, check out the wreck as often it can be seen from the surface. With the *P31* being at a shallower depth than the *Rozi* or the *P29*, some of the upper structure walls and chimney have been damaged by winter storms, even though she faces in a westerly direction. Protected from north and easterly storms by Comino and the north eastern coastline of Malta.

As you travel over the sand along the side towards the bow her number A126 now covered over by marine growth was used as a photo opportunity. When you reach the bow, move away a little and look up at it, rising up towards to the surface some five metres high. You can also see that she has a slight list to port.

Moving on to the deck you will find a depth of approximately 16m, at this point you may wish to penetrate the wreck. Although light penetrates into many parts of the interior of the ship, for other areas you will need a torch This can be done through the bow deck hatch; doors in the main structure, and the two rear holds. On the port side, below where the mast was and just in front of the missing chimney, you can enter the wheel house and central area but you have to exit through the same door.

The *P31* was made as safe as possible for divers to enter this wreck, so the hazards are minimal, please use your penetration procedures, depending on your experience or at least for the first time you have a dive guide. **This wreck has been under the water for over fourteen years**. So, when entering take care. Look out for cuttlefish around this wreck and into the blue for amberjacks and other large marine life.

Diver carefully explores the inside of this wreck.
PHOTO: LEE JELLYMAN RITUAL DIVE CENTRE

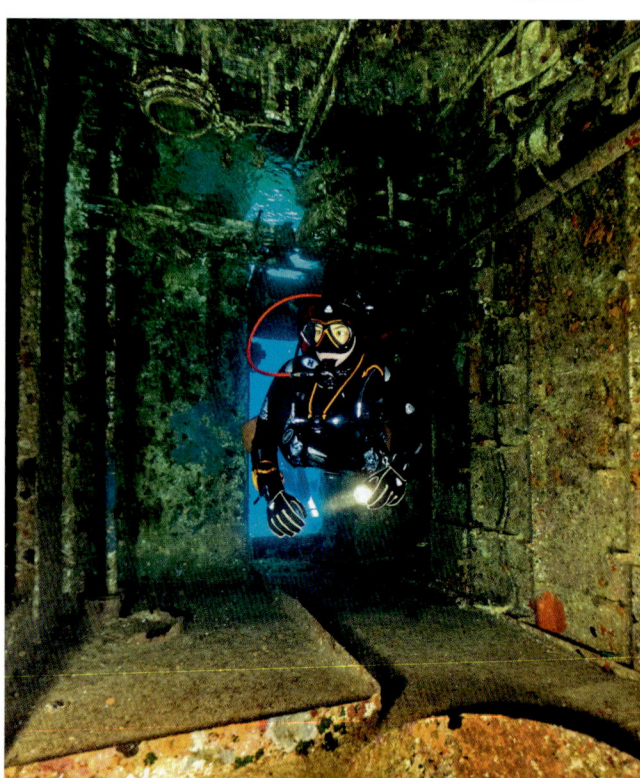

The stern is quite open, here there are two openings to the holds, a small one to the rear and a much larger one just behind the upper structure. Moving along the side of the upper structure towards the bow, you will pass the bridge, the mast was removed due to the fact that it was too close to the surface and could have been a hazard to shipping. At first it was laid along the top of the upper structure, during a storm it became unstable, so for safety reasons it was totally removed. Entering the bow deck the first thing you will see something which looks like a round seat, this was the mounting for the 14.5mm AAMG anti-aircraft machine gun, in front of this is the forward hatch. The railings around the bow deck and other areas shows the growth of marine life. Moving up and on to the bridge, here the depth is 12m. If you are not using a shot line you will need to deploy your delayed surface marker buoy, due to possible boat traffic.

Fish possibly to be found here are flying gurnards, saddle bream, parrot fish, cuttlefish, dusky groupers, amberjacks and many other varieties of marine life.

05 - Alex's Cave

Alex's Cave is in the largest islet and not far from Comino's Blue Lagoon, this large, friendly, underwater cave, which has a high chamber with an opening allowing fresh air to enter. At the rear there is another smaller entrance called the Rabbit Hole, this dive is suitable for all levels of qualifications.

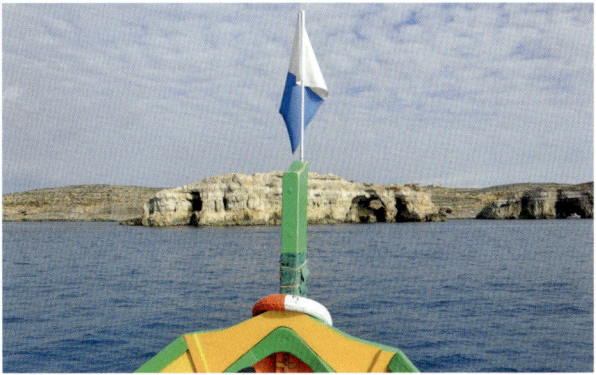

Straight ahead is the islet where Alex's Cave is found.

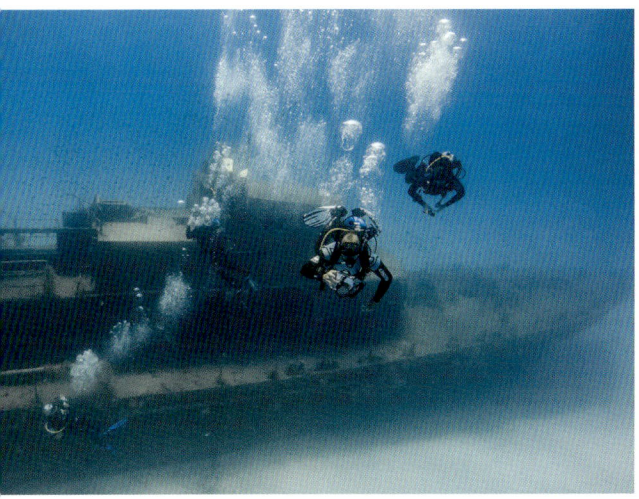

Divers leaving this wreck and heading for the boat.
PHOTOS: ARKADIUSZ SREBNIK POLANDDIVINGPHOTO
The bow and the bridge of the P31 on the sand at 22m.

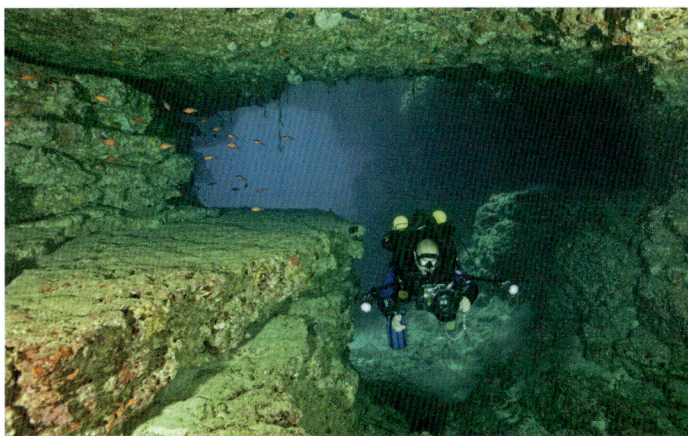

ABOVE PHOTO: MAX VELLA ORANGE SHARK DIVE CENTRE
Divers enter the main and larger entrance of the cave.
BELOW PHOTO: LEE JELLYMAN RITUAL DIVE CENTRE

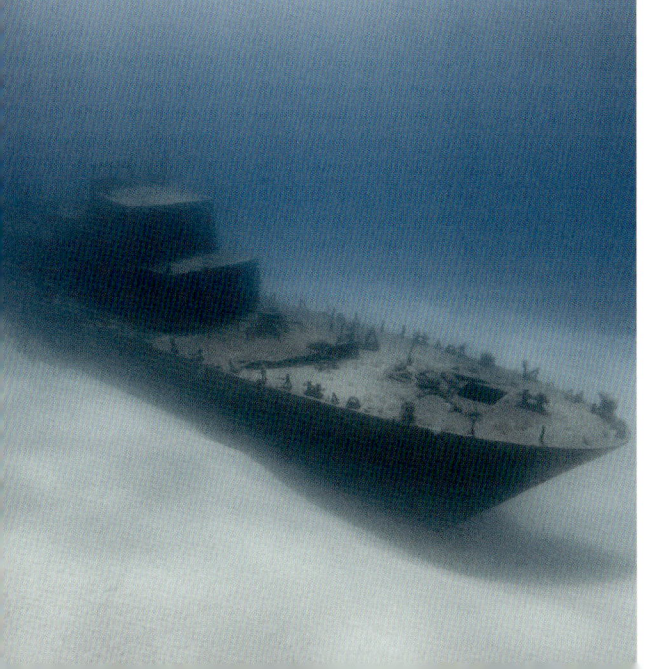

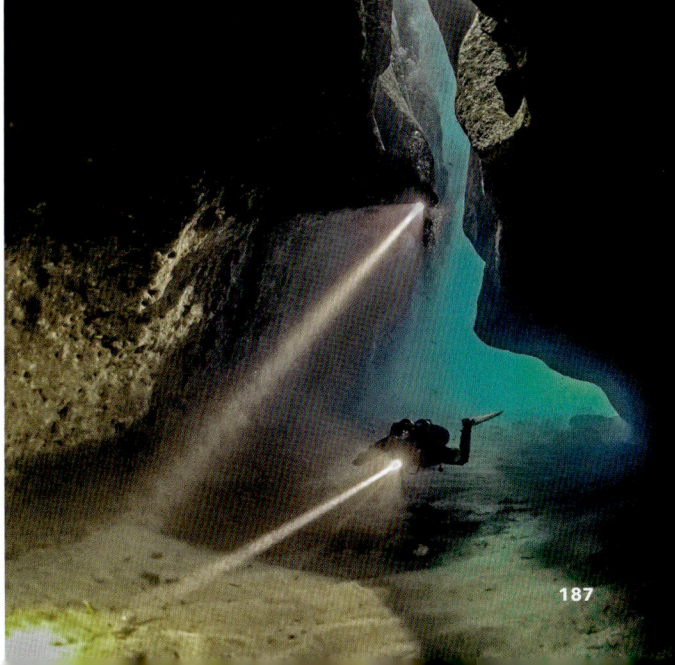

COMINO BOAT DIVING SITES

THE DIVE — Maximum depth 16m

Your boat will normally anchor near the entrance to the cave, depth 16m. The cave, which has an average depth of 8m and is some 40 metres long, so you will need a torch. The dive boat brief will cover the cave and your location.

While diving you may hear and see small boats near the entrance of the cave where the depth is 14m.

The entrance to Alex's Cave is 8 metres wide, sort of hidden by boulders which litter the area outside. The cave is well lit due to a crack in the roof, until you reach a slight left-hand bend where it becomes almost completely dark. Use your torch explore the side walls and ceiling of this wonderful underwater cave and chamber. It is easy to navigate, as most of the time you can see the light of the entrance. This makes Alex's Cave a great first cave dive, the floor of the cave is fine sand, so good buoyancy control is important. The walls and ceiling are inhabited by shrimps, and there is also a resident conger eel called Alex. When you reach the dead end, depth 10m, ascend and you will find a chamber above sea-level with room enough for half a dozen divers. There is a crack in the roof which allows a little sunlight to come through, also fresh air to enter the chamber. When you descend turn off your torch and enjoy the intense blue arch which is your exit from the cave.

When you leave the entrance turn left and follow the reef wall around keeping it on your left over the grass and rocky area past the small arch, the swim-through of The Rabbits Hole will be on your left, it takes about 5 mins. On your way back to the boat and if you have the time and air maybe a visit to Mushroom Rock, its on your left about half way back.

06 - Anchor Reef - Cominotto

The dive site is located of the southwest coast of this small island, diving here is just as dramatic as on Comino, with tunnels, overhangs, swim-throughs and an anchor with depths of 45m plus. Normally the boat would anchor on the west side of Cominotto, a short distance north of the point, depth below the boat 10-12m, your dive will start here.

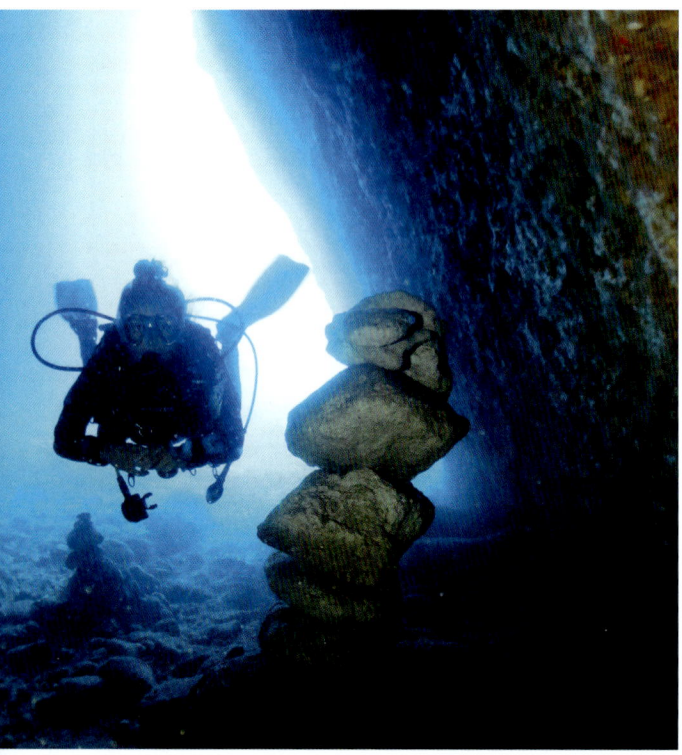

Built by divers, these finely balanced columns of stone.

The Rabbit Hole swim through at the back of this islet.
PHOTO: LEE JELLYMAN RITUAL DIVE CENTRE

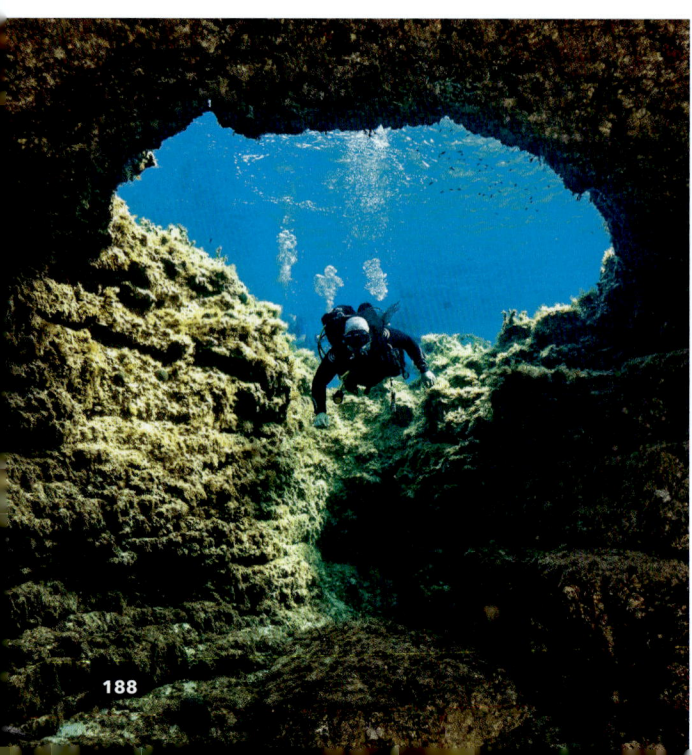

Many similar drop-offs on the reef around Cominotto.

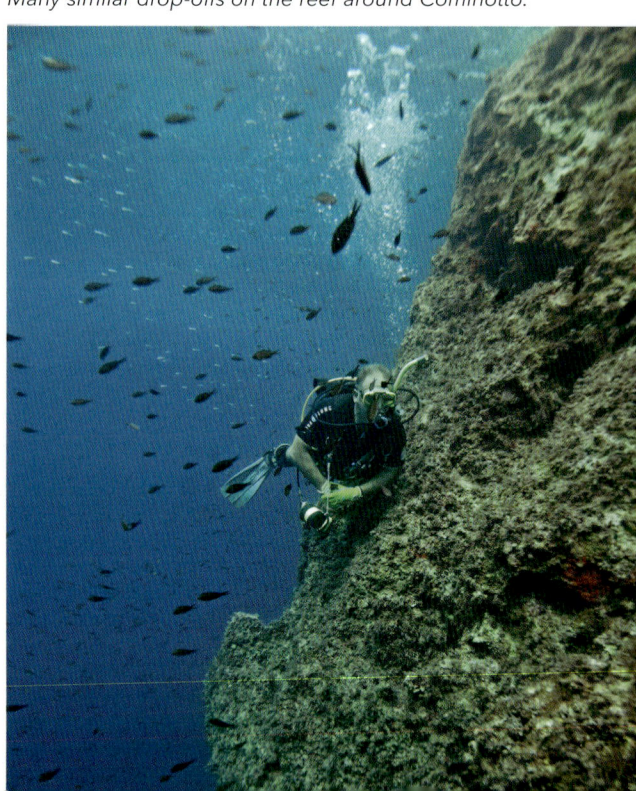

THE DIVE This dive usually starts by the large V-shaped cut-out in the cliffs. Here the cliffs drop away underwater giving a wall all the way to Cominotto's southern point; depths are between 15m and 25m, with lots of interesting overhangs and ledges. Take a torch to explore two swim throughs and you will find lots of colourful marine growth and marine life such as tube worms, hermit crabs, octopus, just to name a few.

For the more experienced divers there is a drop off for a deep and exciting wall dive, with depths up to 50m plus. At 35m is a relic from Malta's maritime history a large WW2 anchor, completely encrusted in corals and sponges, which gives this dive it's name.

07 - Santa Marija Reef

Located on the north coast of Comino, close to the Comino Caves, depths very from 12 to 25m, suitable for all grades of divers. Within this area there are tunnels, overhangs and swim-throughs. Parts of this dive will cover areas of the Comino Cave dive, as the boat will anchor just outside of these caves above a sandy area in 10m.

THE DIVE — Maximum depth 20m

There are numerous gullies, caverns, swim-throughs to explore and take that special photo, especially with the wide-angle lens. The large swim through to the north has a large colony of red anemones in its roof, schools of salema fish that feed on the algae, red mullet, saddle bream, painted combers and cuttlefish are just some of the marine life to look out for.

Part of this excellent underwater landscape.
PHOTO: LEE JELLYMAN RITUAL DIVE CENTRE

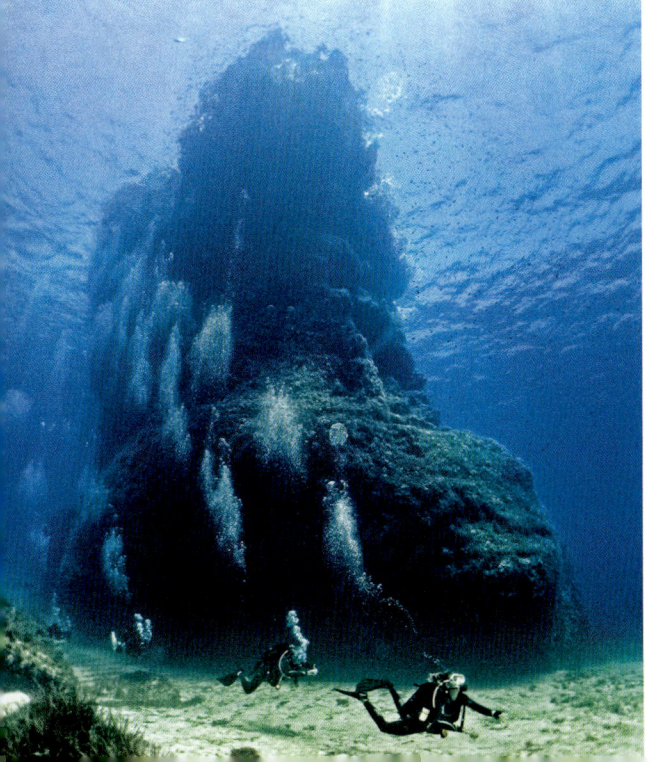

08 - Comino / Santa Marija Caves

Almost the perfect dive? situated on the rugged north coast of Comino often referred to as the Comino Caves. With its large interconnecting cave in which you can surface. A number of smaller caves/caverns and a large arch, all of which you can explore. At the end of your dive below the boat, meet the saddle bream in a feeding frenzy, this is very popular with most divers, it is a fantastic feeling when in very close contact with so many fish.

Your dive boat will anchor in the little bay; a short distance from the Comino Cave, from here you will be able to see some of the caves from the boat. as their entrances rise above the surface. Below the boat the gentle undulating seabed is made up of sand, posidonia (sea grass) and some small boulders, with a depth of 10m.

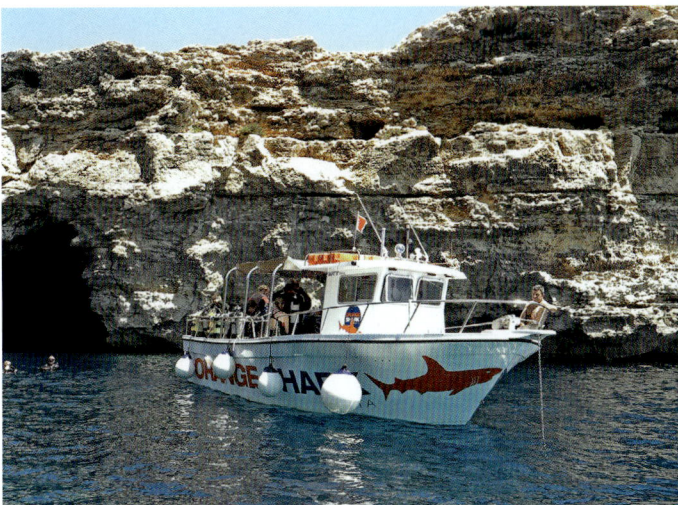

The boat is anchored a short distance from the caves.
PHOTO: MAX VALLI ORANGE SHARK DIVE CENTRE

PHOTO: LEE JELLYMAN RITUAL DIVE CENTRE
Zorro's swim-through, the mark from the sword "Z".

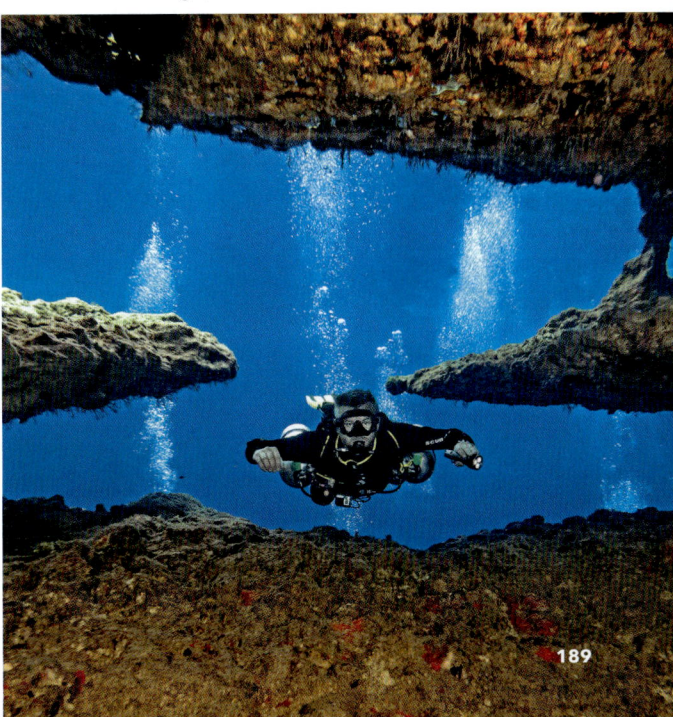

THE DIVE Normally the dive will start at the entrance of the cave at 10m, which extends all the way through the headland; there are at least two routes through it. Once in the cave bear round to the right, the floor slopes upwards making the height of the tunnel lower, this gives way to a wide-open area with a brilliant azure blue of your large exit ahead.

When leaving the cave go left; and you will see the wonderful swim-through in the shape of a Z, almost as if Zorro carved it with his sword. This is a fantastic photo opportunity, normally the camera person would be on the inner side and the model on the outside. After the photo shoot explore the outer area with its swim-throughs and overhangs with large horizontal crevices filled with corals, sponges, tube worms and nudibranchs.

On your return of course you can go round the cliff wall back into the bay where the boat is anchored, but most divers return through the cave. If you keep to the right about half way you will see sunrays coming from a hole in the roof where you can surface. Do not be surprised to see tourists who have climbed down into the cave from above.

Continue to the cave exit, once outside there are further caves and a large arch to explore. Below the boat there is an area of sand where you could feed the fish, or, if you have a camera, take some exceptional photographs. I have been diving this site for over 36 years and each time it still gives me a buzz to see this event. The photographic opportunity with the light blue of the sea and hundreds of silver fish on a sandy seabed is too good to miss. Whether you feed the fish, take photographs or just watch this spectacular show I cannot see how you will not be impressed.

The best way to do this, is for one person to start feeding, the fish will surround that person, then others can move in and feed by hand or take photos.

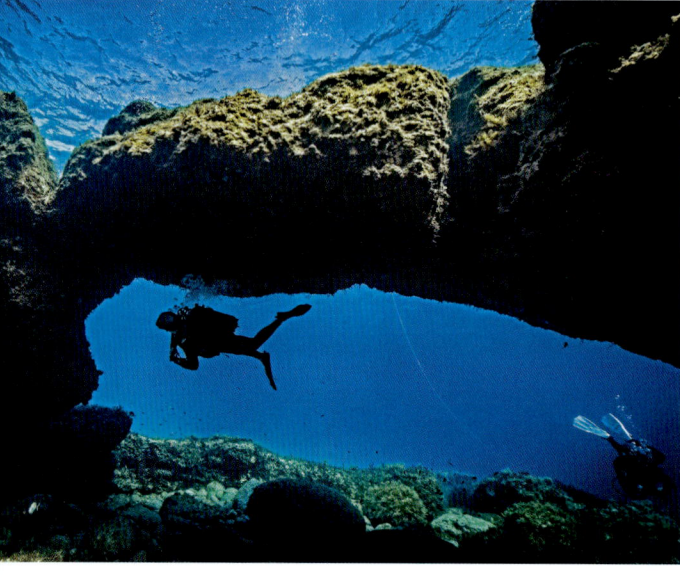

The arch not far from the main cave/tunnel entrance.
PHOTO: LEE JELLYMAN RITUAL DIVE CENTRE

It's a great feeling to be surrounded by saddle bream.

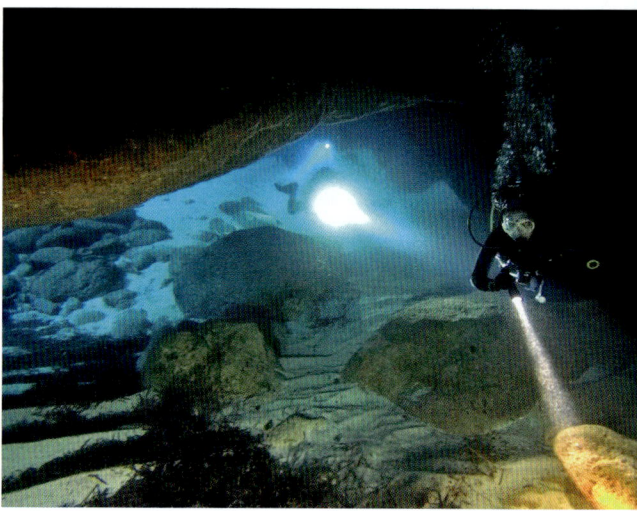

Inside the Santa Marija cave system.
PHOTO: SERGEY MARKOV DIVE SYSTEMS DIVE CENTRE

PHOTO: MAX VALLI - ORANGE SHARK DIVE CENTRE
The far side exit of the Santa Marija cave.

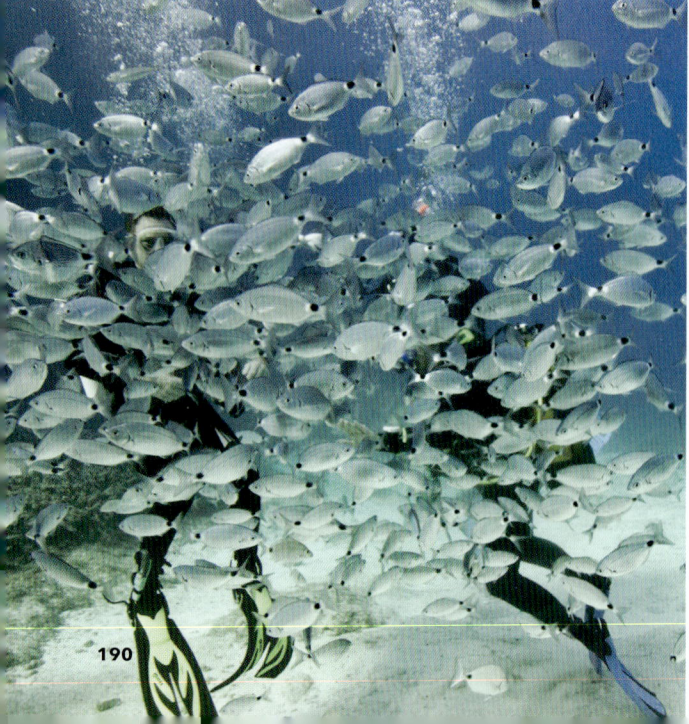

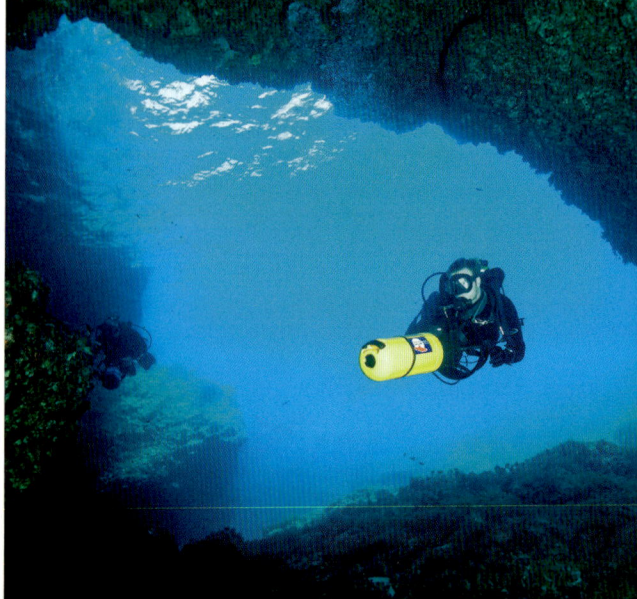

COMINO BOAT DIVING SITES - SANTA MARIJA CAVES & REEF

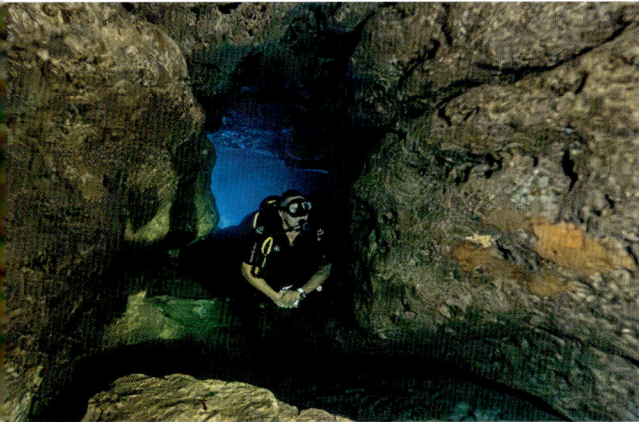

The middle section of The Santa Marija main cave.
PHOTOS: LEE JELLYMAN RITUAL DIVE CENTRE
Within the cave, light from where you can surface.

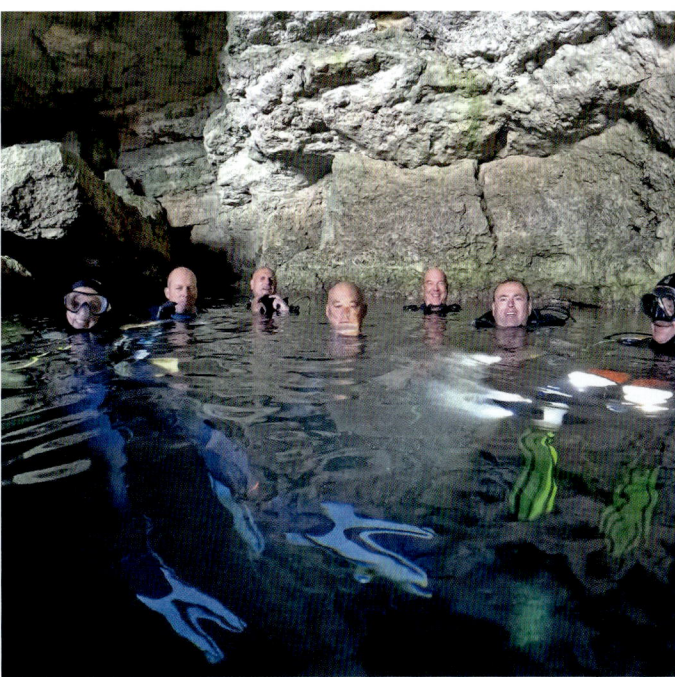

Happy divers have surfaced in this fantastic chamber.
PHOTO: SERGEY MARKOV DIVE SYSTEMS DIVE CENTRE

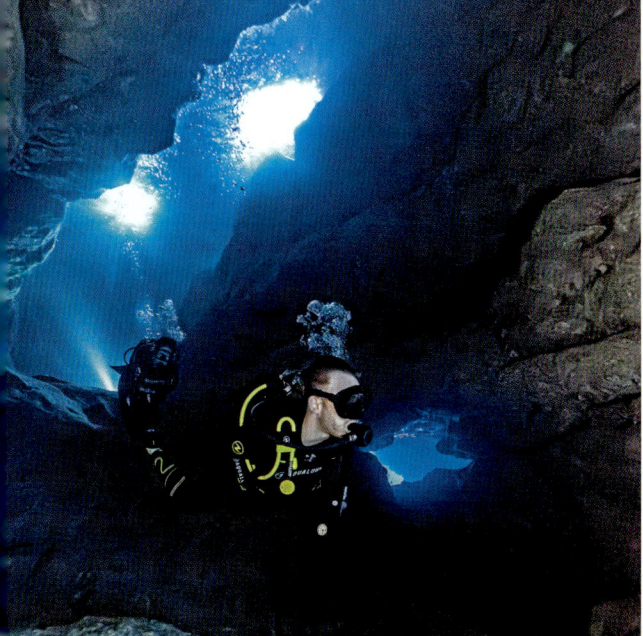

09 - Comino / Blue Lagoon

Comino is a very small island with a land area of 2.5 square km, located between the islands of Malta and Gozo. Normally there are no more than ten residents, including a priest and a policeman living on Comino. During the late spring, summer and early autumn the Blue Lagoon is very popular with locals and their boats, day tripper boats will arrive with tourists, anchor in the lagoon for lunch and a swim. Boat taxis will operate through the day, from Cirkewwa, Malta, Mgarr, Gozo, to the Blue Lagoon. There is a hotel on Comino which only opens in the summer.

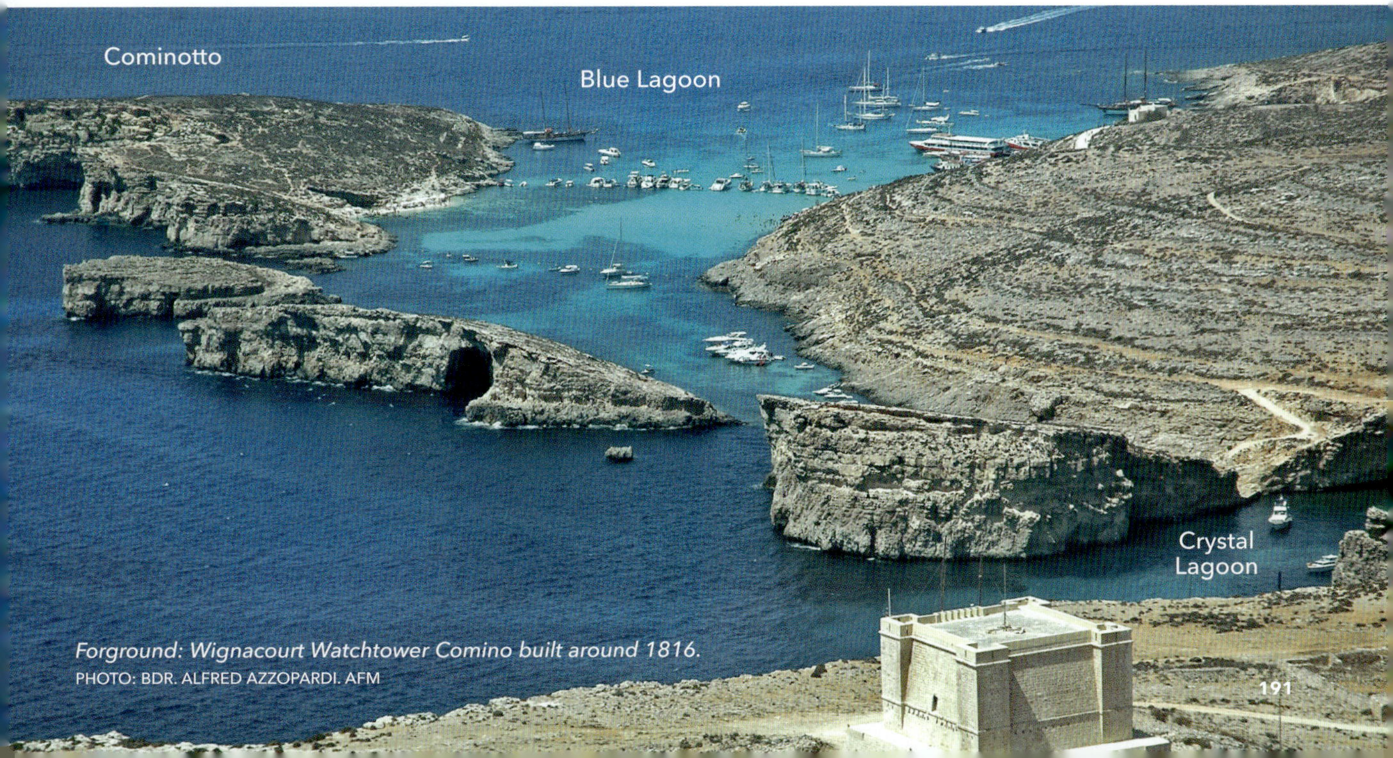

Foreground: Wignacourt Watchtower Comino built around 1816.
PHOTO: BDR. ALFRED AZZOPARDI. AFM

TECHNICAL DIVING SITES

01 - SS *Le Polynesien* War Grave

SS *Le Polynesien* was built in France and launched in April 1890. With a length of 152 metres, a beam of 15 metres, a gross tonnage of 6659. Powered by 12 coal fed-boilers, which generated 7500 hp, allowing her four-bladed propeller to give her a top speed of 17.5 knots, easily recognised by her two large black funnels.

She was designed as a luxury cruise liner to carry 252 passengers between France, Australia and the French Colonies via the Suez Canal. She began service in 1891 sailing to Australia until the outbreak of WW1 in July 1914, when she was requisitioned by the French government, then armed and used as a troop carrier.

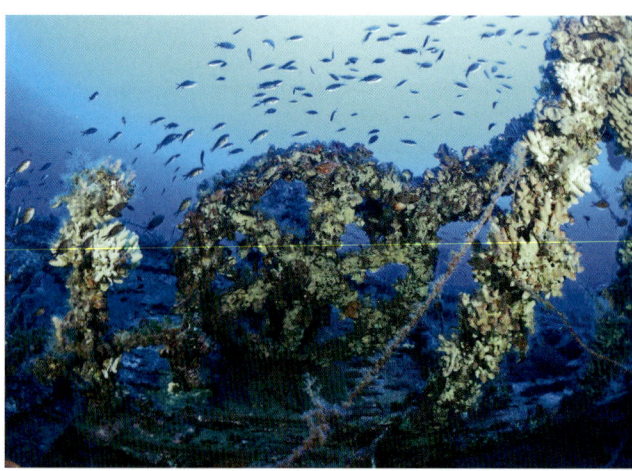

Marine growth on this upper wheel. PHOTO: CATHY DE LARA

Just before the end of the war, on route from Tunisia to Thessaloniki in Greece, with Serbian troops and cadets of the Royal Serbian Army. The French steamer was torpedoed on the 10th August 1918. by the German submarine *UC-22*, only 2 miles off Malta. She was hit on the port side near the engine room and sank within half an hour. Eleven crew and six passengers died, the survivors were taken to Malta and recuperated at Cottonera Hospital.

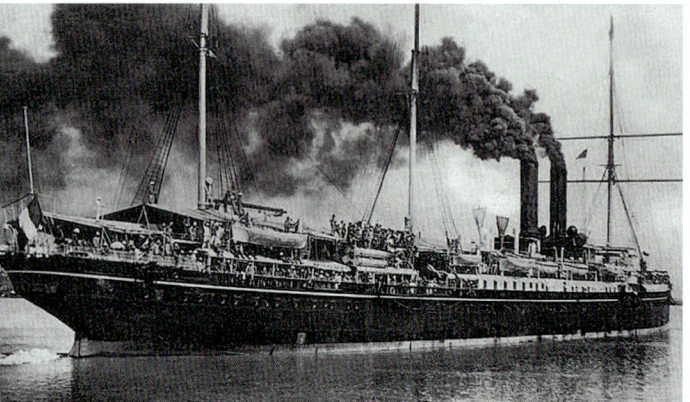

SS Le Polynesien as a troop carrier in 1914.

A diver above the stern gun on this magnificent wreck.
PHOTO: JON BORG www.jonborg.com

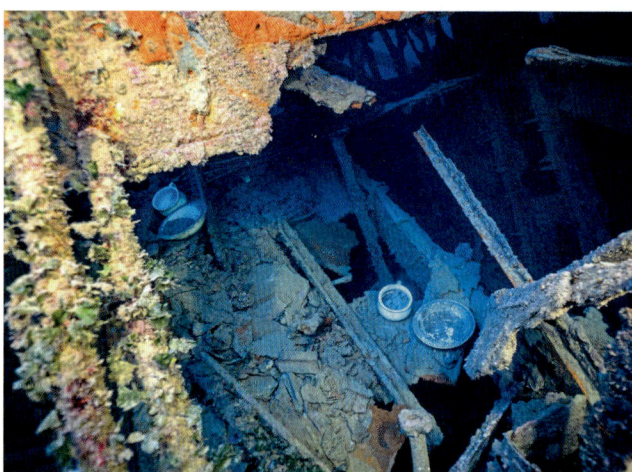

Ceramics can still be seen PLEASE DO NOT TOUCH.
PHOTOS: DAVE GRATION HERITAGE MALTA
One of the twelve boilers that this ship had.

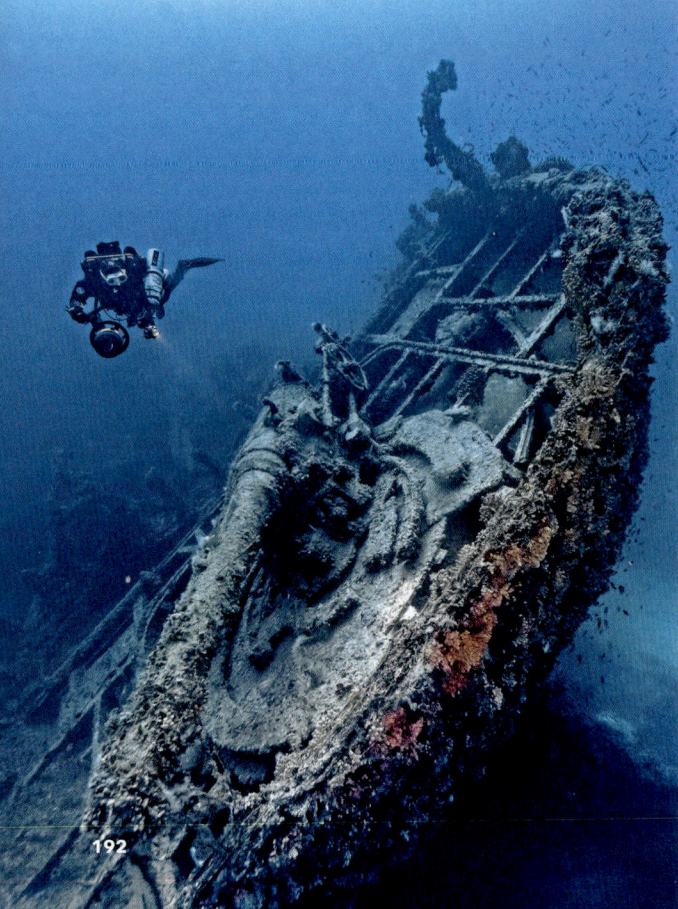

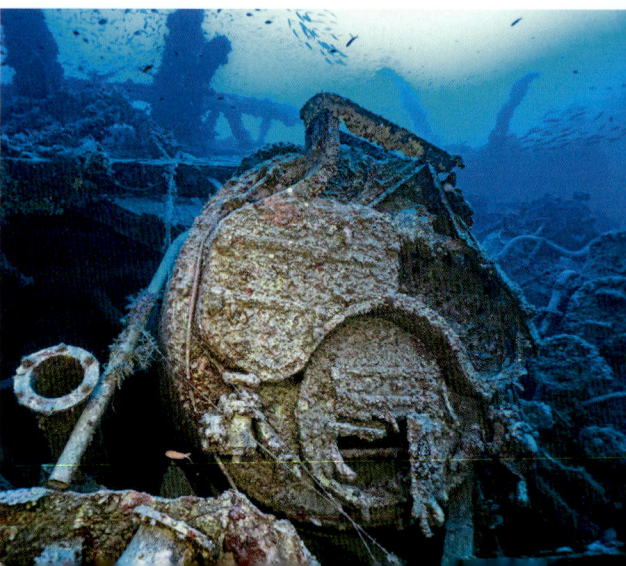

TECHNICAL DIVING SITES - SS *LE POLYNESIEN*

Nick-named the 'plate' ship due to the many ceramic artefacts which remain on this wreck, unfortunately many of these have been taken over the years, including chandeliers from the first-class dining areas.

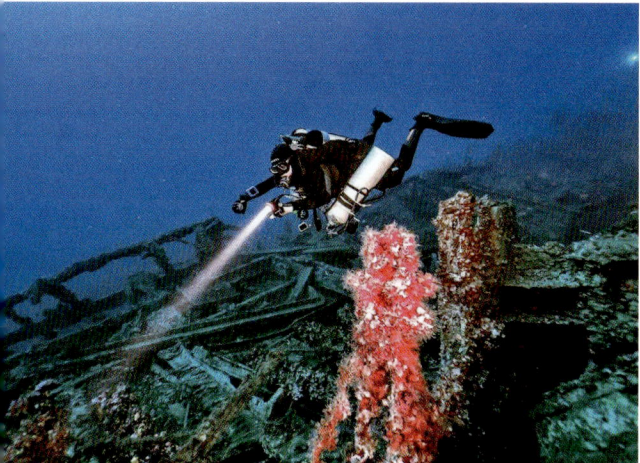

The colourful encrusted parts on the upper structure of this wreck at 50m. PHOTO: JON BORG www.jonborg.com

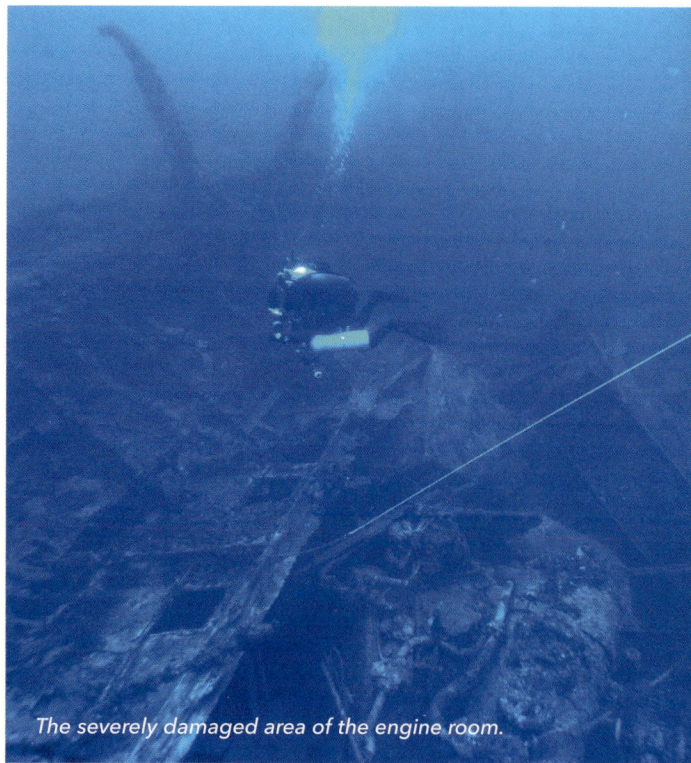

The severely damaged area of the engine room.

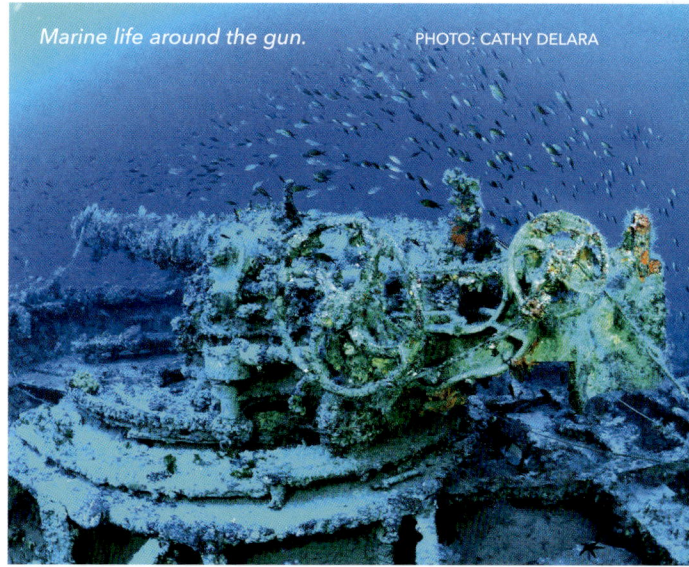

Marine life around the gun. PHOTO: CATHY DELARA

THE DIVE The *SS Le Polynesien* is now lying about 2 miles from Marsaskala on a sandy seabed at 65m, almost intact, on her port side, the highest point of the wreck is 50m. There is so much to see and many areas to explore and needs multiple dives. The engine room is severely damaged, but the large engine block and several boilers are visible, it was here the torpedo hit.

Visit the knife edge bow that rises majestically from the seabed, the two large anchors are still stowed on either side. There are two encrusted deck guns which can be found, one at the bow and the larger one at the stern, maybe the most photographed areas on the wreck. A further 10m below the stern gun, you can see the four bladed propeller and rudder. The wreck acts as a safe haven for large shoals of fish, when predators such as barracuda and tuna are around. There can be strong currents in this area. Quotes by experienced divers: "One of the most spectacular shipwrecks in the world". "Excellent wreck, could spend a month diving this one".

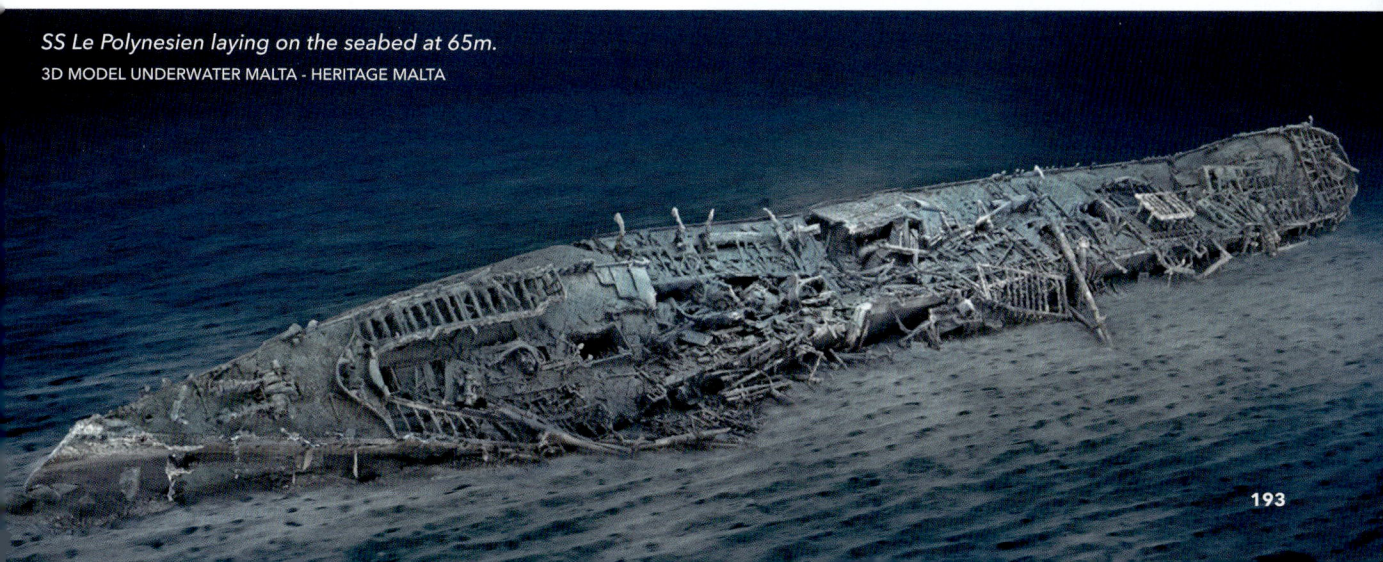

SS Le Polynesien laying on the seabed at 65m.
3D MODEL UNDERWATER MALTA - HERITAGE MALTA

TECHNICAL DIVING SITES

02 - HMS *Nasturtium*

When WW1 broke out, the Admiralty had a problem with not having enough ships for mine-sweeping operations. So, they embarked on a rapid program to increase the number of smaller anti-submarine ships. HMS *Nasturtium* was one of 36 Arabis Flower class ships intended for these duties in European waters. Built by A. McMillan & Sons, Ltd., Dumbarton, Scotland, and laid down on the 1st July 1915 with a yard number of 464.

HMS *Nasturtium* was based in Malta, on the 23rd March 1916, the liner SS *Minneapolis* with a displacement of 13,543 tons was torpedoed and sank northeast of Malta with the loss of 12 lives. HMS *Nasturtium* was one of the ships involved in the rescue operations of 177 persons.

On the 27th April she entered the same minefield that had sunk HMS *Russell* earlier that day, it is now known that these mines were laid by the *U73*. About 7.45pm she struck a mine on her starboard side, close to the foremost funnel, the explosion killed 7 of the crew. Her boiler rooms began to flood but she did not sink straight away, by now most of the crew left the ship. HMS *Sheldrake* started to tow her, but it was very difficult due to her list, a heavy swell and darkness. Assistance was given by HMS *Wallflower* and HMY *Aegusa*, the latter also hit a mine and sank during the rescue operations.

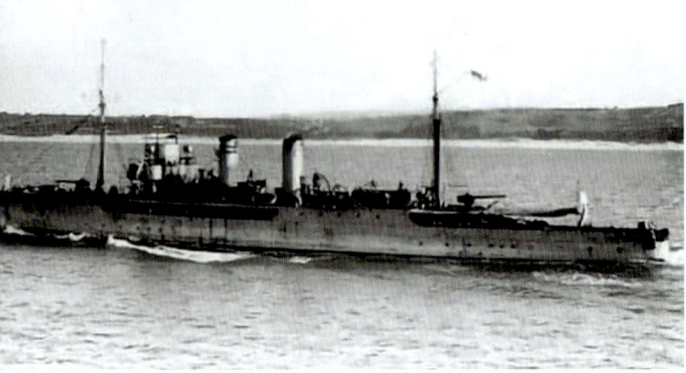

HMS Nasturtium an Aribis Flower class ship.
PHOTO: UNIVERSITY OF MALTA

Launched, 21st December 1915 she had a displacement of 1250 tons, overall length of 81.6 metres, a beam of 8.2 metres. She was driven by two coal fired cylindrical boilers supplying steam to a 4-cylinder triple expansion engine connected to a single propeller shaft, giving her a speed of 15 knots and a range of 2,300 miles. With an armament of 2 X 4-inch guns, fore and aft, 2 X 3-pounders, and anti-aircraft guns and a crew of 79.

The stern gun, see the topside photo or 3D Model
PHOTO: STEVEN GALICIA www.galicia.be

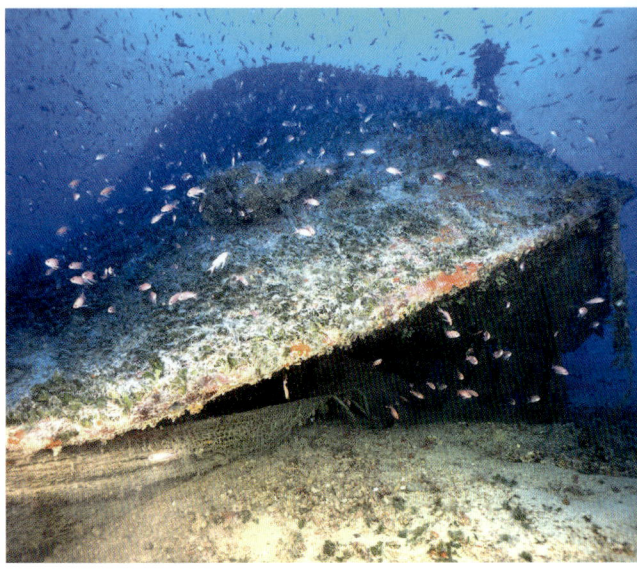

The bows of this minesweeper laying on her port side.
PHOTOS: DAVE GRATION HERITAGE MALTA

The large anchor on the bow now covered in coral.

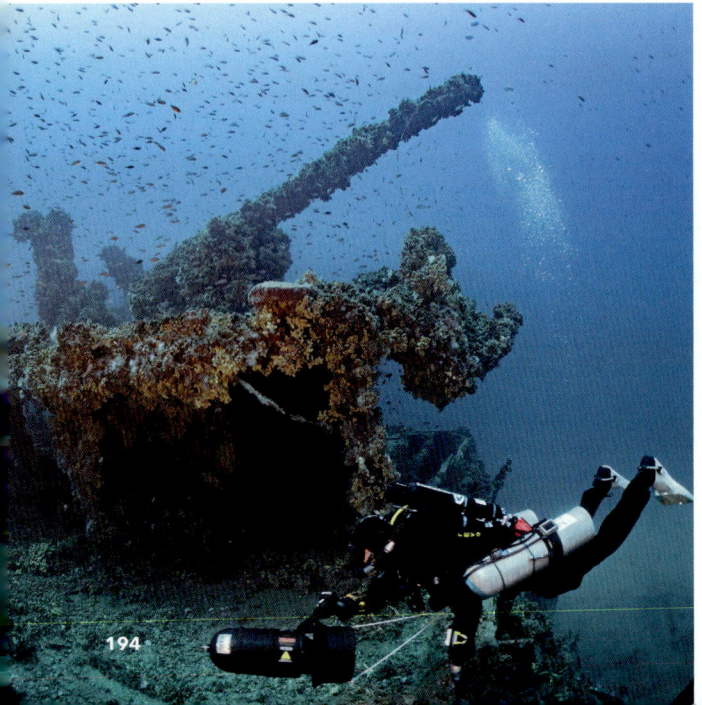

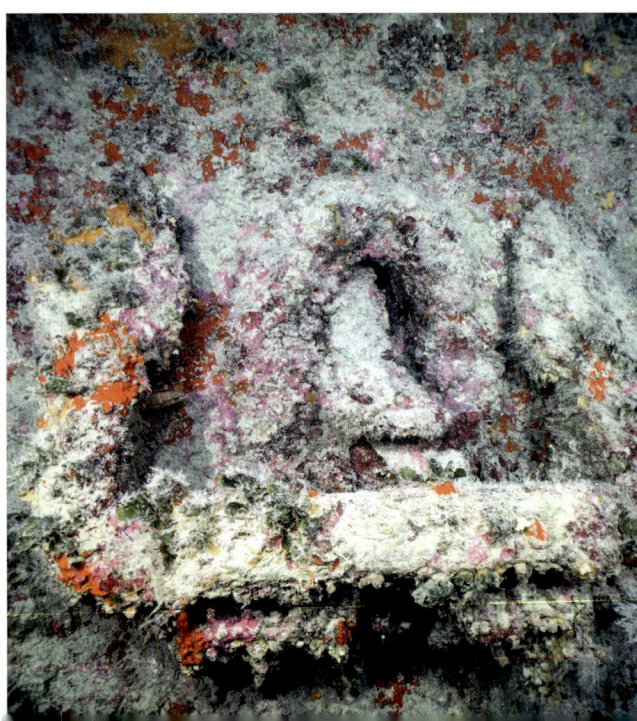

TECHNICAL DIVING SITES - HMS NASTURTIUM

In the early hours of Friday, the 28th April, the captain and crew who had remained on the ship till the last moment, abandoned the ship as her list had increased. Then she rolled gently over on her port side with both masts well submerged; there she lay for a short time until she reared her bow in the air and slowly sank.

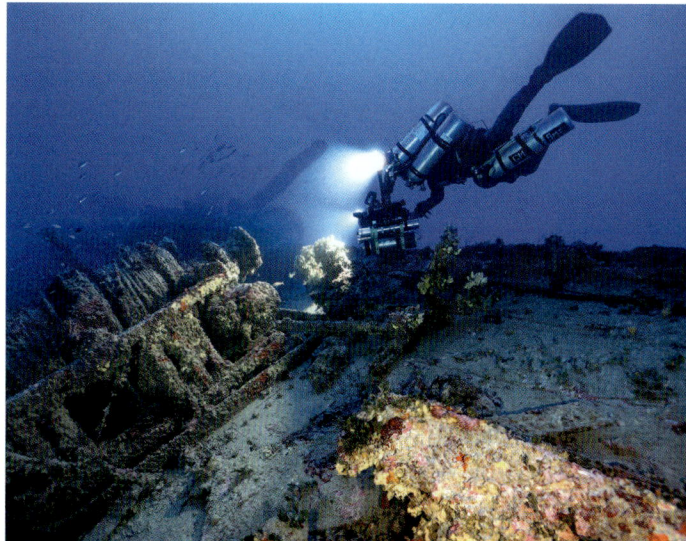

The large winches on the main forward deck.
PHOTO: JOHN WOOD HERITAGE MALTA

Exploring this wreck for that special photograph.

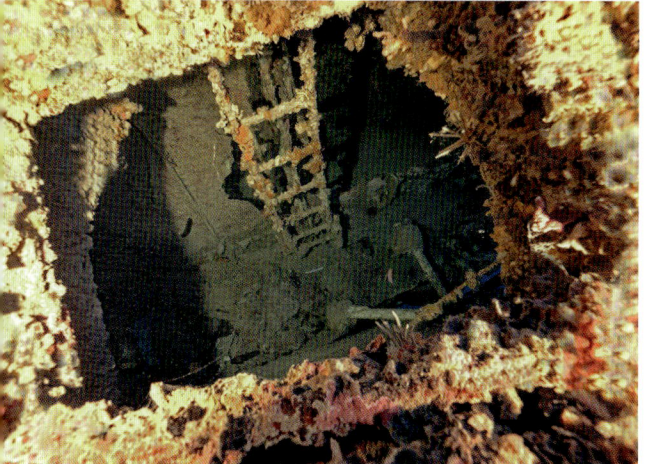

A deck hatch and ladder. PLEASE DO NOT ENTER!
PHOTO: JOHN WOOD HERITAGE MALTA

THE DIVE This excellent wreck of the HMS *Nasturtium* now lies approximately 10 miles from St Elmo's light Valletta, at a depth of 67m on a flat sandy seabed. The bow lays almost parallel with the sand, but the remainder of the ship is listing to one side, the bow and the stern guns can easily be found, also the winches on the main deck. Look for the ammunition on the port side laying on the sand. Visibility is normally 30 metres and the currents here are listed as medium, strong and variable. The marine life is really amazing, with shoals of barracuda, and many other varieties of fish life. Quotes from experienced divers "This wreck is amazing" "Coral growth is fantastic" "Items belonging to the ship are still there"

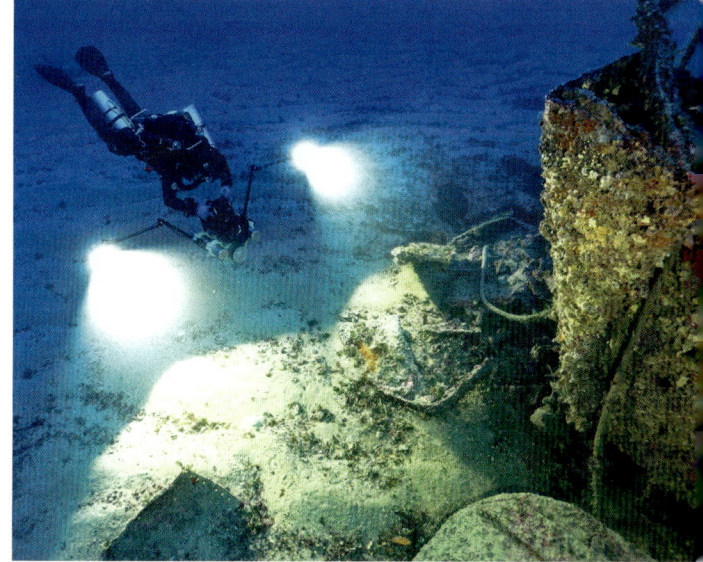

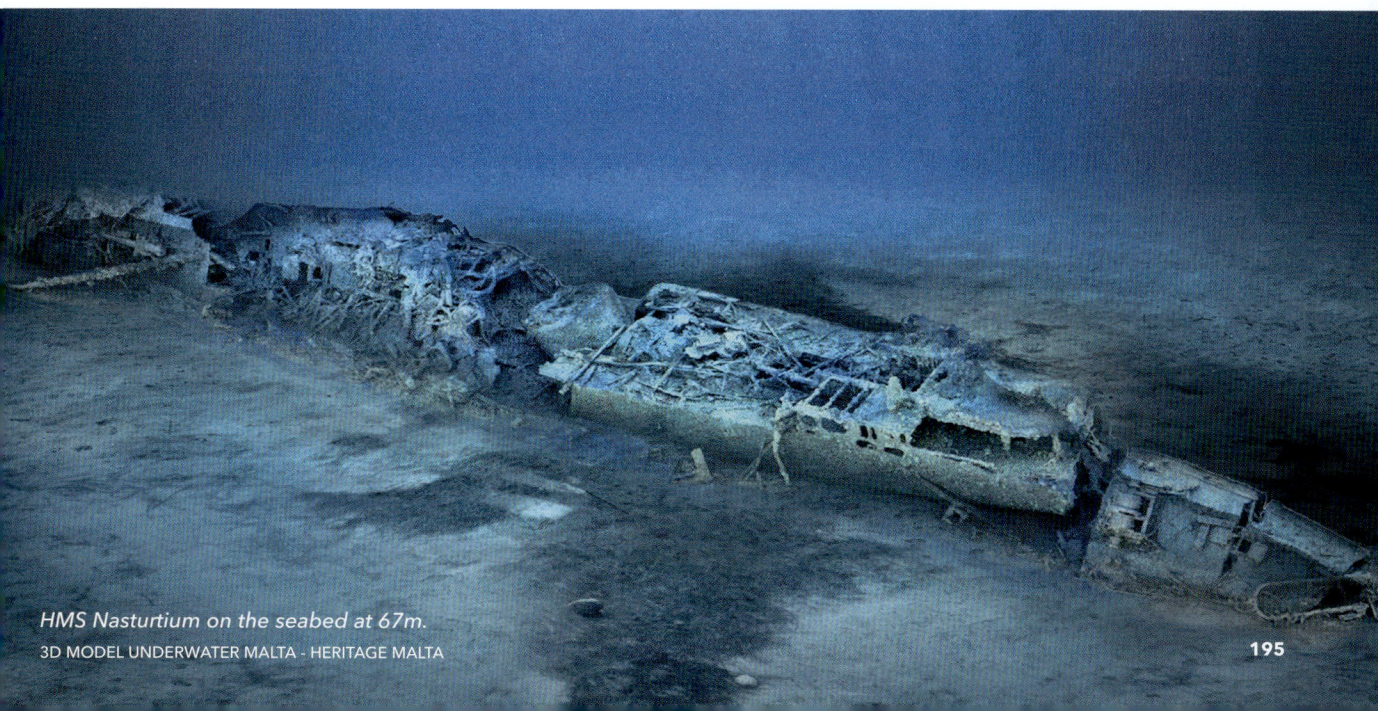

HMS Nasturtium on the seabed at 67m.
3D MODEL UNDERWATER MALTA - HERITAGE MALTA

TECHNICAL DIVING SITES

03 - HMS *Southwold* L10 War Grave

HMS *Southwold* was a Hunts Class Destroyer built in East Cowes England in 1941 job number J6274, a total of 86 ships of this class were built for the Royal Navy. She was 86 metres in length and a beam of 9.5 metres, with a tonnage of 1050, a top speed of 27 knots and a range of up to 4,000 miles Her armament consisted of 3 turrets with 4-inch guns, one at the bow and two aft, anti-aircraft guns and submarine depth charges. She had a crew of 168 Officers and men.

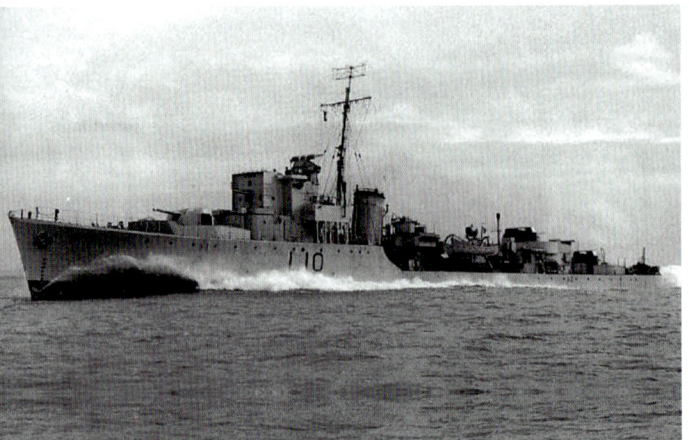

HMS Southwold L10, a Hunt-class destroyer.
PHOTO: UNIVERSITY OF MALTA

HMS *Southwold* was launched on the 25th May 1941 and commissioned in October the same year. She went to Scapa Flow for her sea trials, before joining the Mediterranean Fleet. In January 1942 she joined the 5th Destroyer Flotilla in the Mediterranean for convoy duties, anti-submarine patrols and transporting troops and supplies to Tobruk and Alexandria.

The forward gun turret of this Hunt-class destroyer.
PHOTO: JON BORG www.jonborg.com

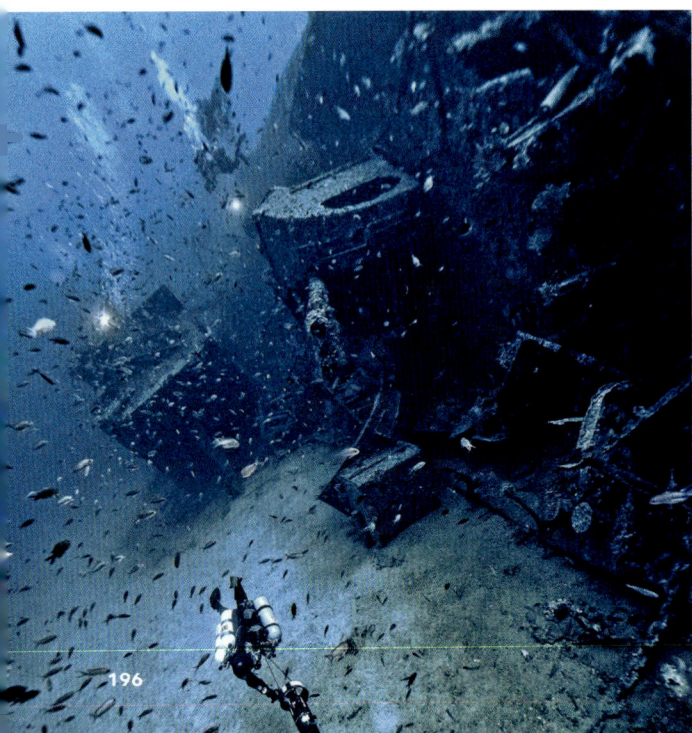

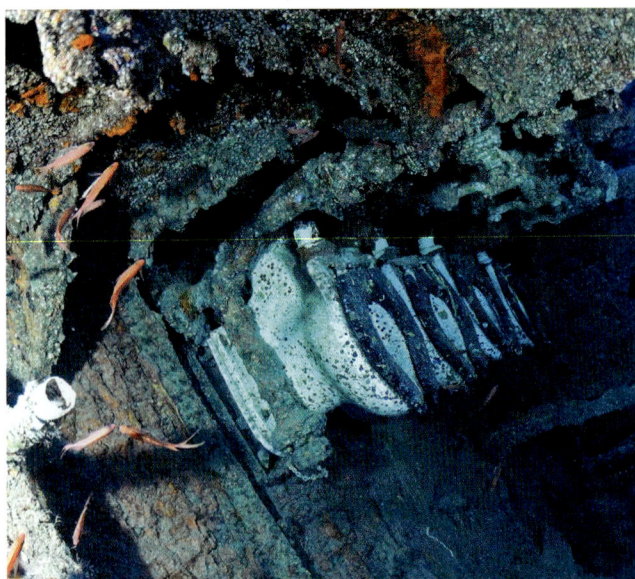

These toilets are out of order. PHOTO: CATHY DE LARA

On the 20th March she was carrying out anti-submarine patrols with other destroyers to make a safe passage way for the Malta relief convoy MW10. The next day, she joined this convoy and took part in the Second Battle of Sirte. They were outnumbered and outgunned, so a smoke screen was laid, preventing the Italians from taking proper range. They dashed in and out of the smoke screen firing damaging salvoes. The engagement was broken off that morning, but the Italian squadron approached again in the afternoon. Again, it was the smoke screen that was giving the destroyers, including HMS *Southwold* a chance to get close to the enemy, on one attack they hit the Italian battleship *Littorio* and the cruiser *Giovanni delle Bande* with torpedoes.

The Italian fleet withdrew and German planes took over the attacks to prevent the convoy reaching Malta. When the convoy was 20 miles from Malta, the Germans sank the *Clan Campbell* but by now the convoy was within reach of fighter protection from Malta.

A diver hovers over the forward gun turret with its 4" gun barrels. PHOTO: STEVEN GALICIA www.galicia.be

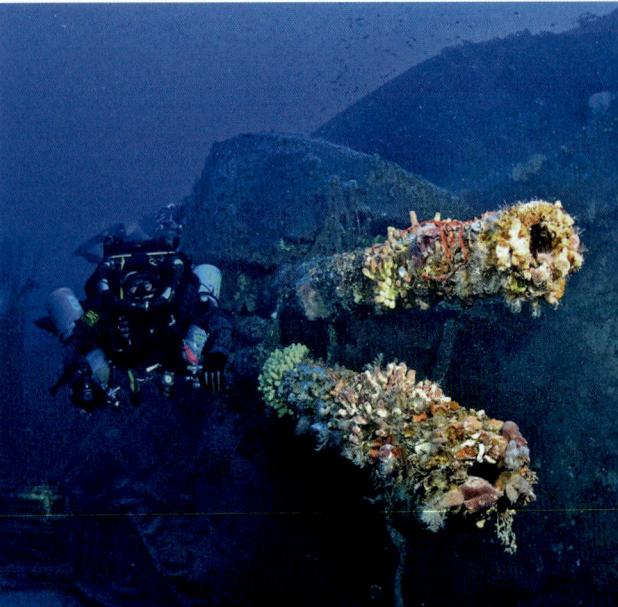

TECHNICAL DIVING SITES - HMS SOUTHWOLD

On the 23rd March 1942 one of the merchant ships, the *Breconshire* in this convoy was hit by enemy bombs a few miles off Zonqor Point, Malta. Under deteriorating weather conditions, the crew managed to drop her anchors. HMS *Southwold* and HMS *Beaufort* left the convoy to render assistance to the merchant ship *Breconshire*.

The next day, 24th March *Breconshire* was dragging her anchors on the sandy bottom and she started to drift helplessly towards shore. HMS *Southwold* was ordered to give her a tow, but while trying to pass a line to the disabled ship a mine exploded under her engine room.

One officer and four ratings lost their lives, she sustained major structural damage and the engine room flooded while electrical supplies failed. While she was being towed by the tugboat *Ancient*, the ship's hull plating, abreast of the engine room, split right up to the upper deck on both sides and she began to sink. HMS *Dulverton* rescued the survivors.

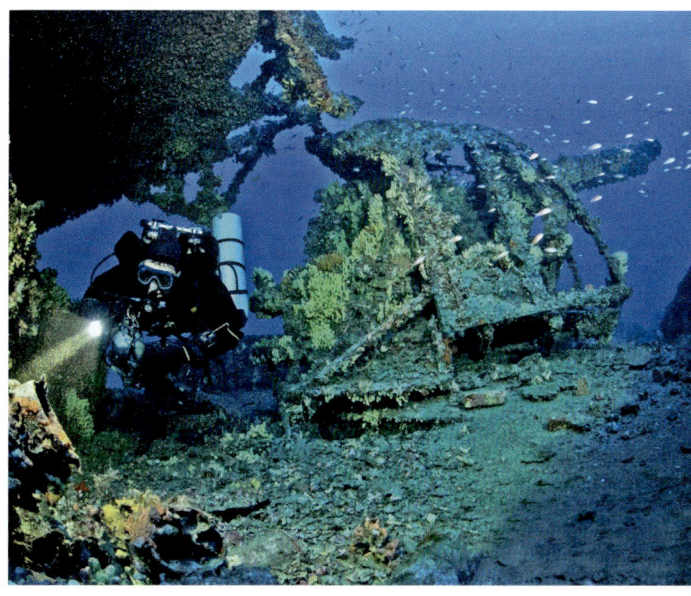

One of the turret guns which are still visable today.

PHOTOS: STEVEN GALICIA www.galicia.be

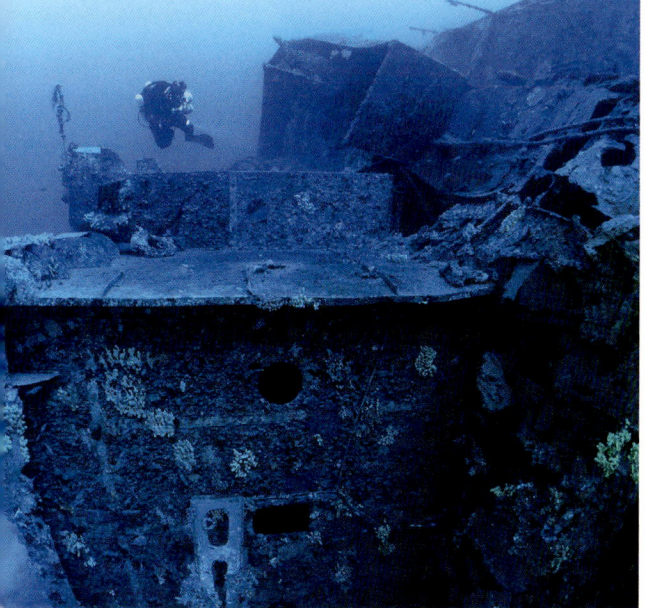

The bridge laying on the sand. PHOTO: CATHY DE LARA

Coral growing on the bows of this popular wreck.

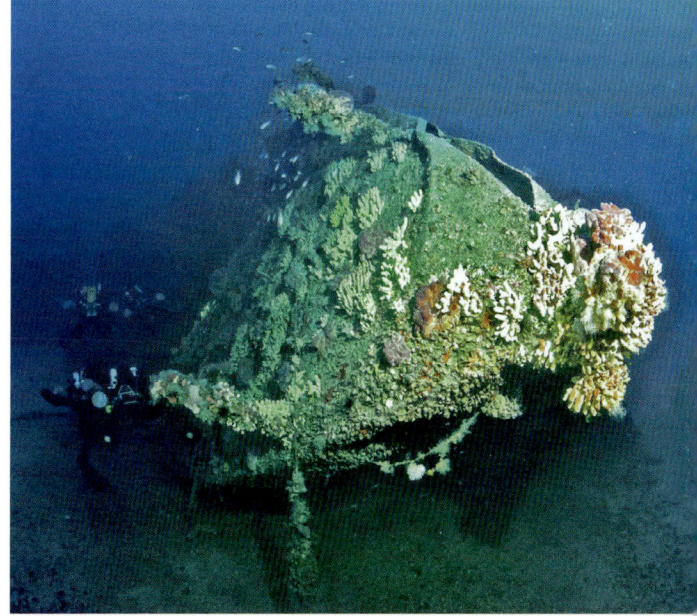

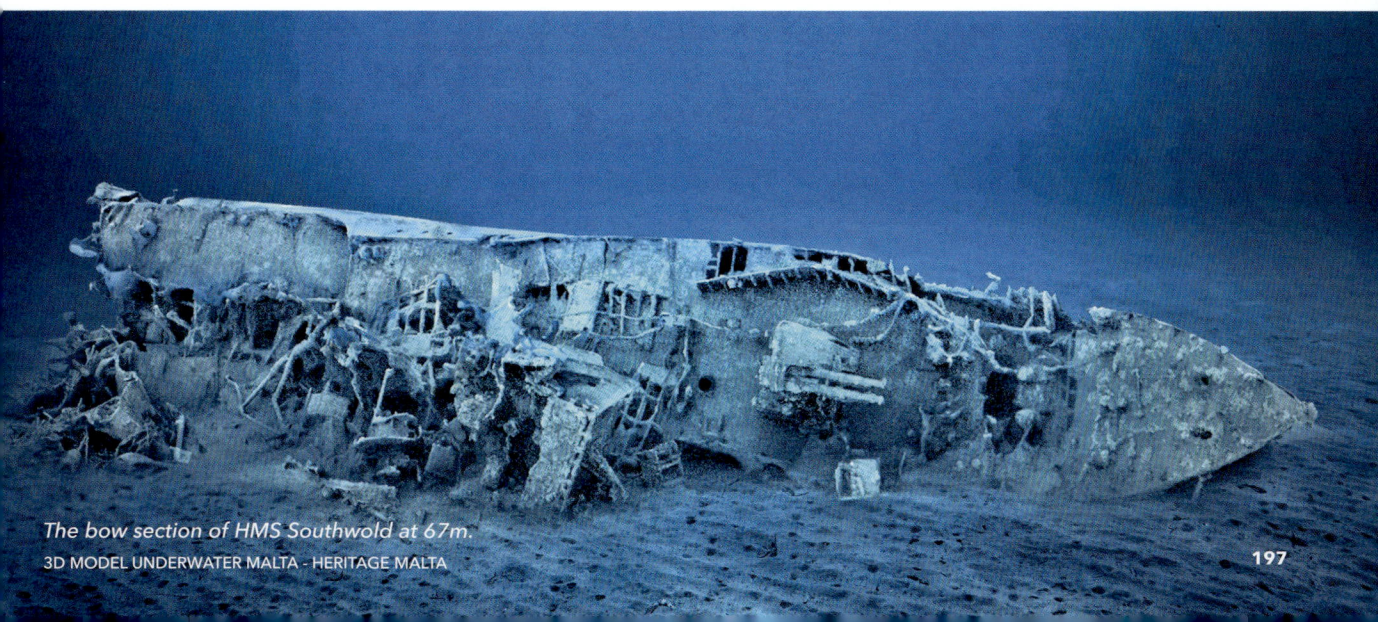

The bow section of HMS Southwold at 67m.
3D MODEL UNDERWATER MALTA - HERITAGE MALTA

TECHNICAL DIVING SITES - HMS SOUTHWOLD

THE DIVE HMS *Southwold* now lies on a sandy, shingle sea bed with small rocky areas at a depth of 67m, less than 2 miles northeast of Marsascala and 3 miles from Valletta's Grand Harbour, the seas in this area are well known for the unpredictable strong currents, these waters should be checked before you dive.

On the bottom in two parts, the bow section which is the largest part of the wreckage, is just over 40 metres in length. Laying on her starboard side, most parts of the wreckage rise up almost 10m towards the surface. Her forward 4-inch guns are still in position, the turret and barrels are now covered in marine life and coral. The ships bridge and control room lay out on the sand still attached to the forward deck, now check out the wash room and the angle of the toilets, out of order, there are many other areas to explore on this wreck.

Quotes; by experienced divers: *"Excellent dive" "This wreck is a gem and maybe one the best technical dives in Maltese waters".*

The upright stern and propeller of HMS Southwold L10.
PHOTO: STEVEN GALICIA www.galicia.be

The stern section lies upright some 300 meters away at a depth of 74m, this section of the wreck is some 30 meters long. Like the bow section there are many areas to explore including one of the rear 4 inch gun and the turning mechanism of the second rear guns.

Both sections of this wreck are alive with marine life and covered by hard and soft corals, often fantastic visibility for photo-shoots.

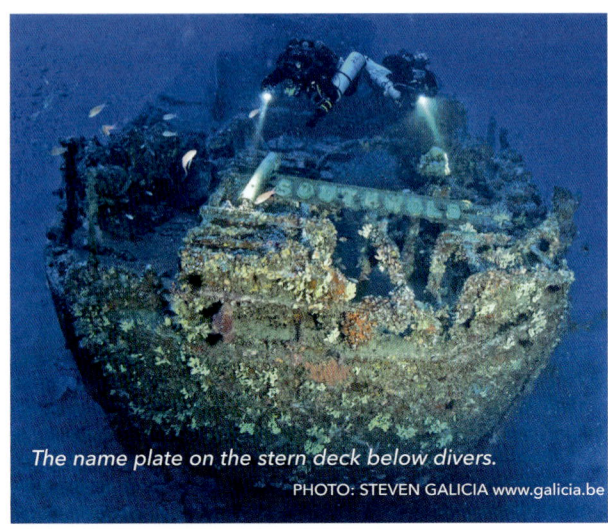

The name plate on the stern deck below divers.
PHOTO: STEVEN GALICIA www.galicia.be

Below: HMS Southwold L10 a Hunts-class destroyer.
PHOTO: ROYAL NAVAL MUSEUM PORTMOUTH

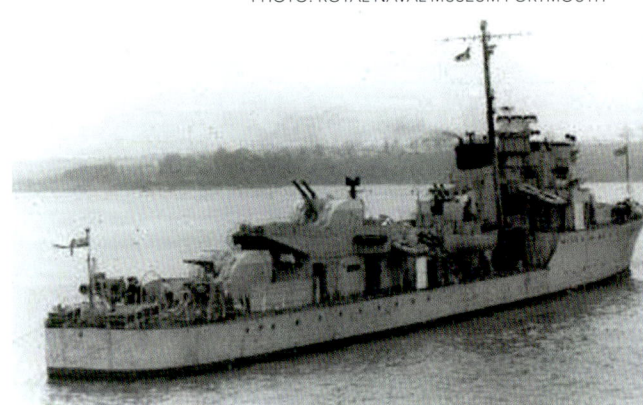

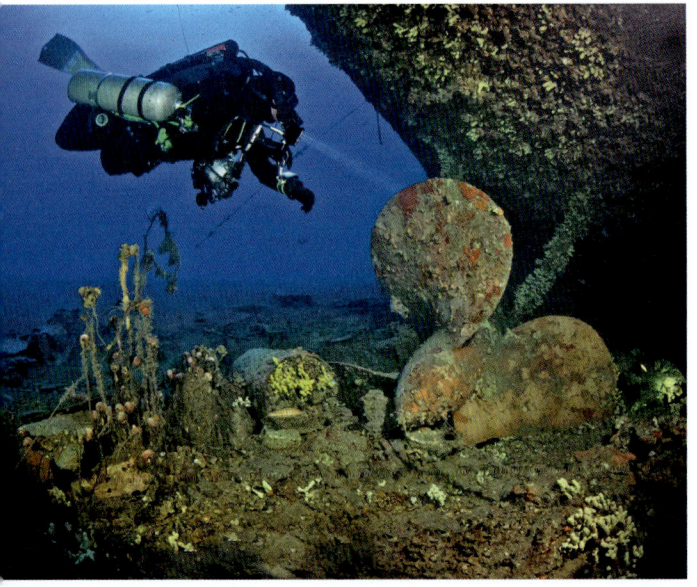

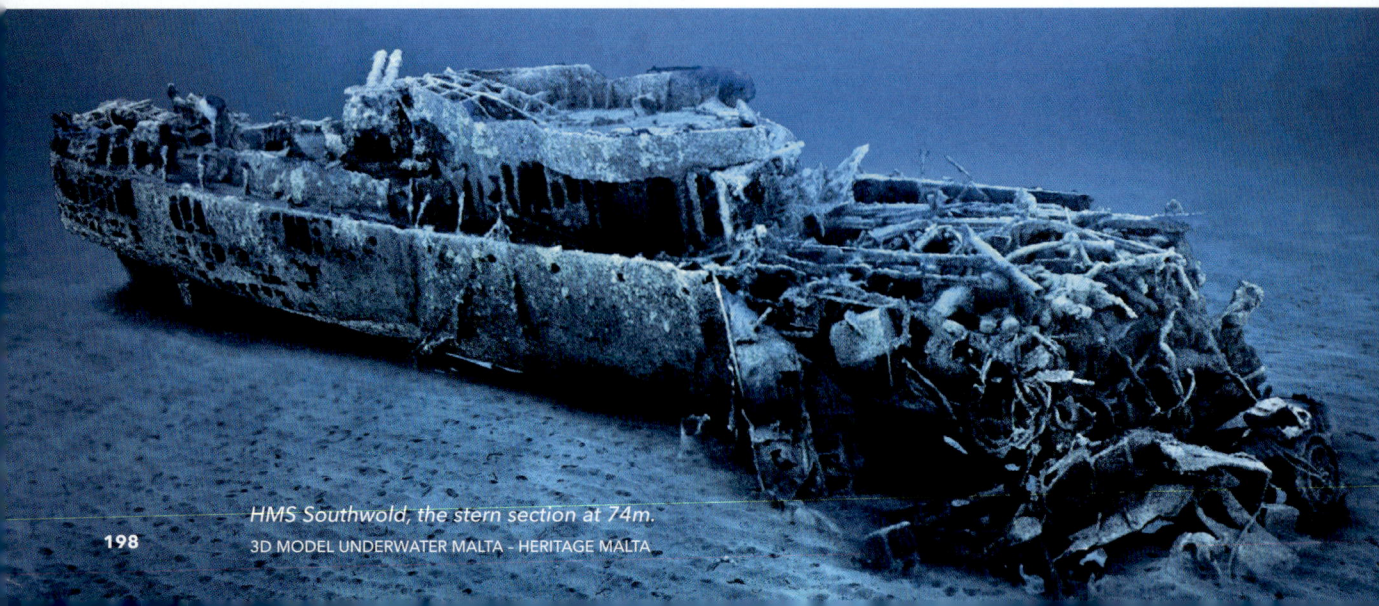

HMS Southwold, the stern section at 74m.
3D MODEL UNDERWATER MALTA - HERITAGE MALTA

04 - B24 Liberator War Grave

The B24 Liberator was an American heavy bomber, designed and built by Consolidated Aircraft Corporation in San Diego, USA, it was the world's most produced multi-engine plane, 18,000 were built during WW2. Used extensively in all branches of the American Armed Forces as well as some Allied Forces, even serving as a transport aircraft for Sir Winston Churchill.

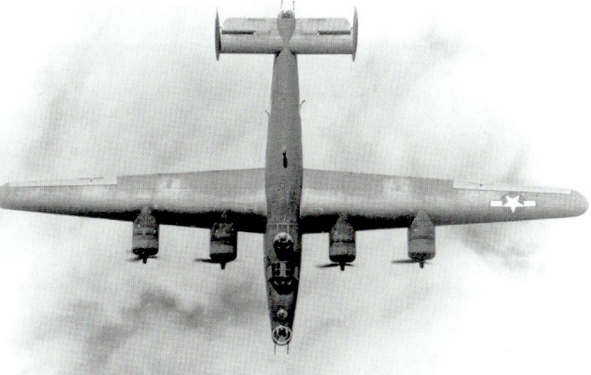

B24 Liberator an American WW2 bomber.
PHOTO: U.S. AIR FORCE - UNIVERSITY OF MALTA

Many of the bombing missions in WW2 which were carried out over western and southern European countries, were carried out by the B24 Liberators. This also included most of the heavy bombing that was part of the Italian, Sicily Campaign between 1942-1943, early in May 1943 the port of Reggio in southern Italy, was the target, being only eight miles across the sea from Sicily, this city was subjected to a series of heavy bombing raids. During one raid on the 6th May 1943, two waves of B24 Liberators, totaling fifty aircraft and flying from North Africa, dropped a record 110 tons of bombs over the city, mainly targeting the harbour.

Divers descend to the B24 Liberator laying on the flat silty sandy sea bed at 58m.
PHOTO: STEVEN GALICIA www.galicia.be

During one of these raids this B24 aircraft developed engine trouble and was hit by anti-aircraft fire over the city, and after dropping its bomb load, the crew decided to fly to Malta, which was often used as a safe haven for damaged aircraft returning to North Africa from Italy and Sicily.

They attempted to reach Malta, but the aircraft lost power as it approached the island, forcing the plane and her crew of 10 to ditch in the sea. The wheels of the aircraft were down when it hit the sea, flipping the plane over, and after floating for a few minutes, she sunk, the tail section first followed by the wings and nose. One member of the crew remained unaccounted for, whilst the other nine survived and were rescued by the Royal Air Force rescue boat.

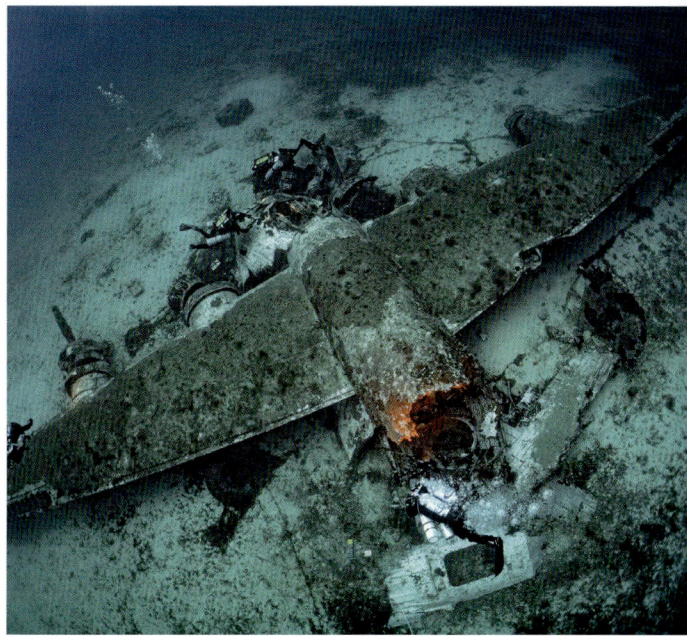

Exploring this aircraft in excellent visibility.
PHOTOS: STEVEN GALICIA www.galicia.be
A diver above the badly damaged cockpit.

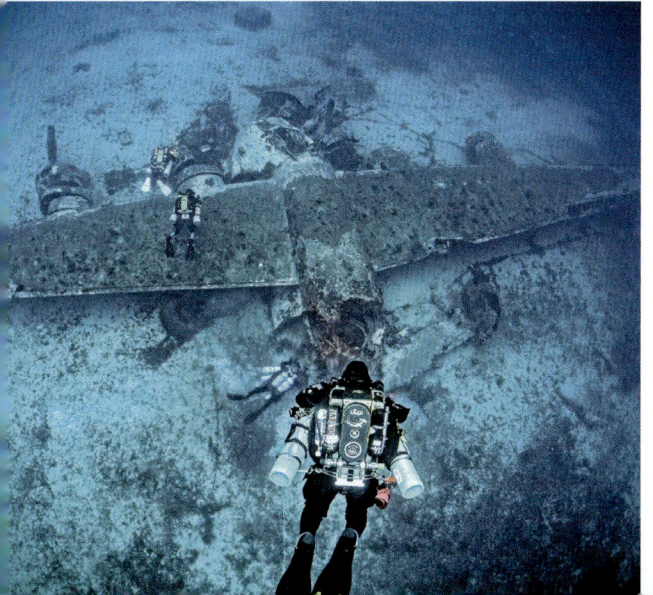

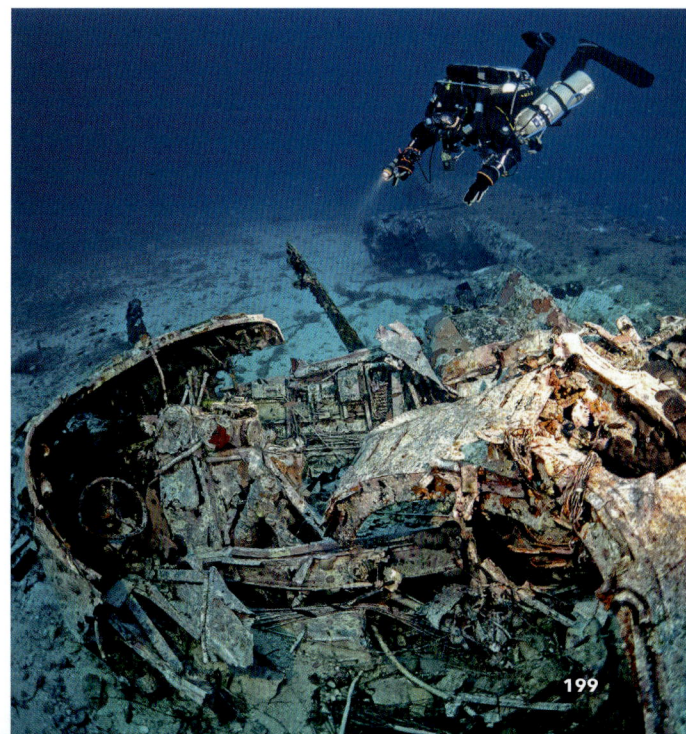

TECHNICAL DIVING SITES - B24 LIBERATOR

The University of Malta Maritime Archaeology team started looking in 2015 for this B24 Liberator aircraft that crashed landed in the sea off Malta in 1943. This aircraft was located early in 2016, using a side-scan sonar. It was unusual to have a USAAF bomber in Maltese waters as they never flew out of Malta's airfields.

The wreckage of the B24 Liberator was first dived in 2018, but it was not until June 2023 when the Maritime Archaeology Team in collaboration with the DPAA, that all the remains of the missing airman Sgt. Irving R. Newman aged 22 years, were found and carefully removed to the surface by this diving team.

THE DIVE The B24 Liberator now lies approximately 1.6km south-west of Marsaxlokk at a depth of 58m on a silty, sandy seabed, most of the wreckage is intact, projecting prominently from the seabed, with visible damage to the nose and tail sections. The starboard outboard engine is still attached to the wings, whilst the other three are detached at varying degrees. The entire wing structure of the aircraft is almost intact, whilst the nose of the aircraft is destroyed and the cockpit is torn open, the tail section of the aircraft lies collapsed under the main fuselage.

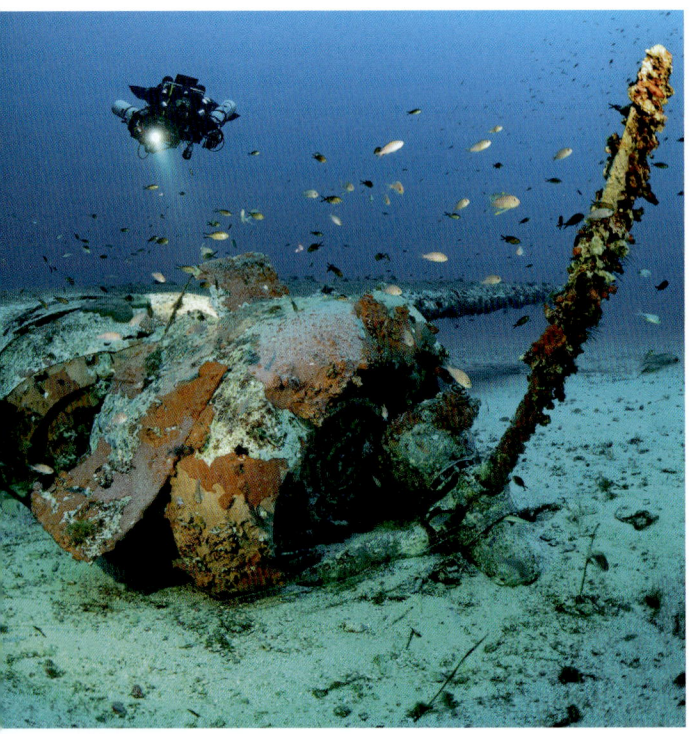

The far port engine and propeller on the sand.
PHOTO: STEVEN GALICIA www.galicia.be

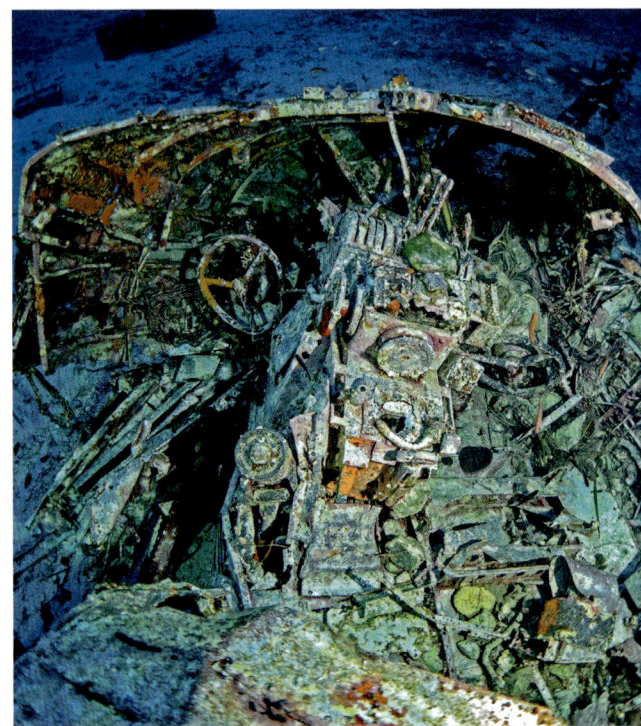

An inside view of the badly damaged cockpit.
PHOTO: STEVEN GALICIA www.galicia.be

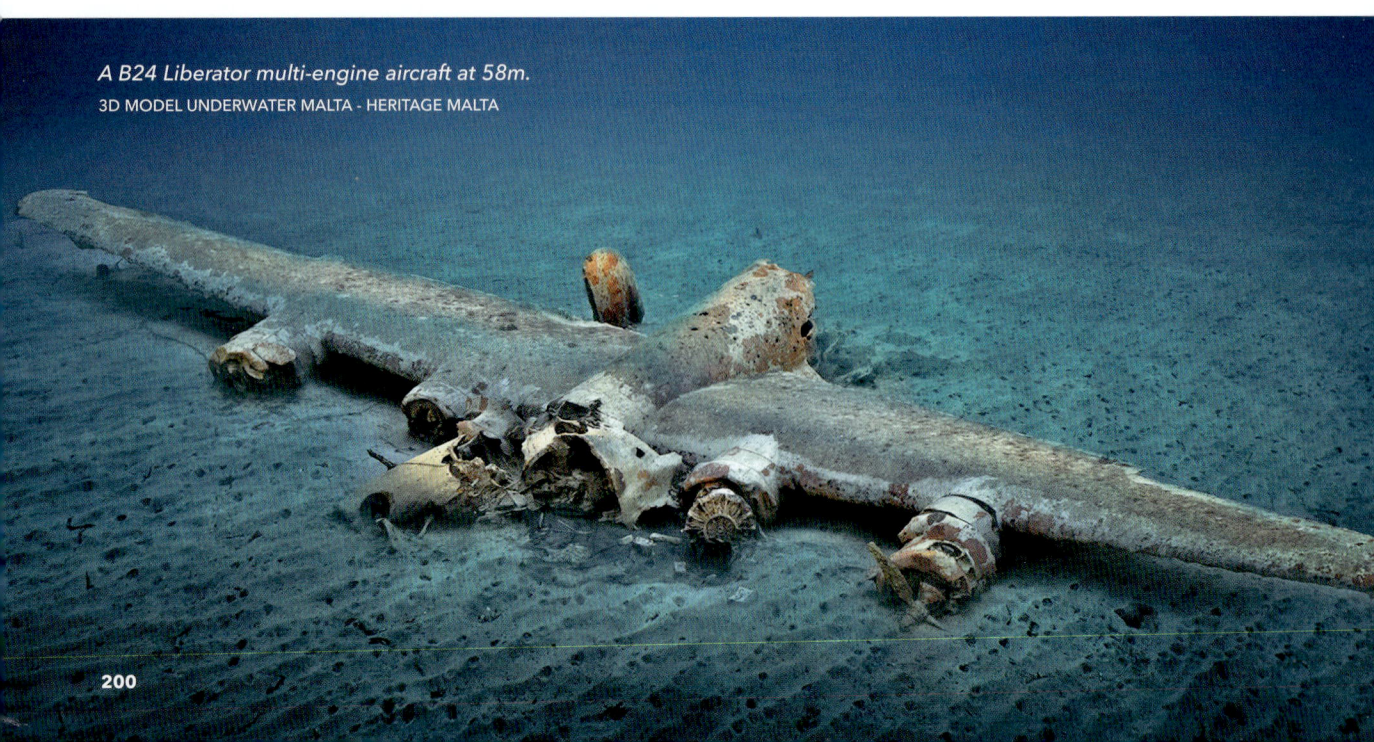

A B24 Liberator multi-engine aircraft at 58m.
3D MODEL UNDERWATER MALTA - HERITAGE MALTA

05 - Junkers Ju88 Aircraft

The Ju88 was a German twin engine multirole combat aircraft which entered service on the very same day Germany invaded Poland. It was 15 metres in length, with a 20-metre wingspan, with a top speed of 316 mph. Built by Junker Aircraft Motor Works. Designed to operate day or night, carry both bombs or torpedoes and offer low level ground support. There was a crew of three, pilot, an observer and a radio operator/rear gunner.

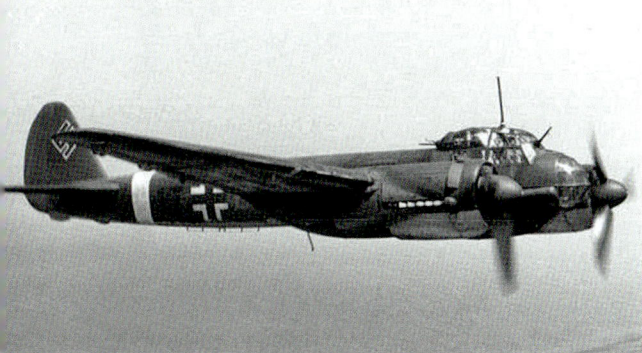

The Ju88 was a versatile twin-engine fighter aircraft.
PHOTO: UNIVERSITY OF MALTA

The Maltese Islands played a critical role during WW2 and at this time was a British Colony. Throughout the conflict it was the only Allied base in the Mediterranean Sea between Gibraltar and Alexandria in Egypt, it became a military and naval fortress. In 1940 the North African campaign increased its strategic importance and Malta became a prime target for the Axis Luftwaffe based on Sicily only sixty miles away.

The Axis attempted to destroy Malta and starve its people by attacking ports, cities and the Allied convoys transporting supplies to the island. This became known as the Second Siege of Malta which took place between 1940 and 1943.

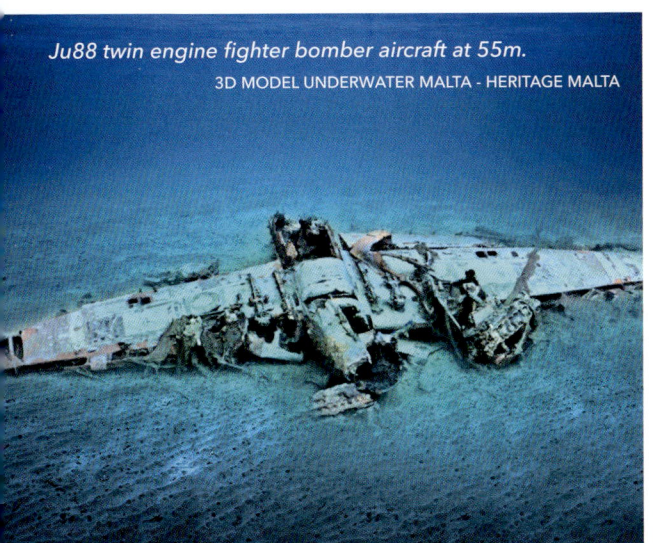

Ju88 twin engine fighter bomber aircraft at 55m.
3D MODEL UNDERWATER MALTA - HERITAGE MALTA

In 1943 the Luftwaffe increased their activity and launched wave after wave of air raids. It was during one of these raids that the Ju88 was shot down after being hit by flak or during a dogfight in the blue skies high above the Maltese Islands. It now lies on the sea bed at 55m a short distance off the east coast of Malta. Throughout the campaign, many ships and planes on both sides were destroyed however, by this stage the Allies had built up their own indomitable defence system. Malta was now the base for 35 squadrons consisting of over 600 modern fighters and bombers, which led to eventually ending WW2 in victory for the Allies.

At the end of the war King George VI awarded the Maltese Islands and its people the George Cross.

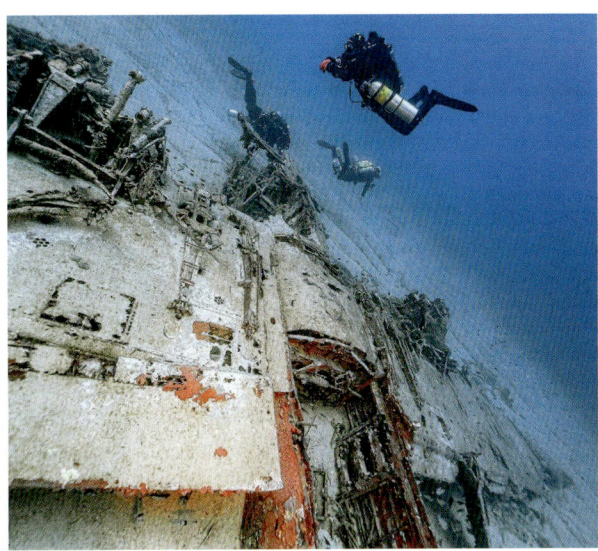

Divers over the up-turned Ju88 on the sandy sea bed at 55m.
PHOTO: JON BORG www.jonborg.com

THE DIVE The Ju88 wreckage discovered in 2009 some 4.5 miles from both St Pauls Bay and Sliema, upside down on a flat sandy sea bed at depth of 55m. well preserved with the wings still in place, the two engines lie on the sand close by. The cockpit, is upside down, with its forward machine gun. The tail section has broken off but is intact and lays some 50 metres from the main fuselage.

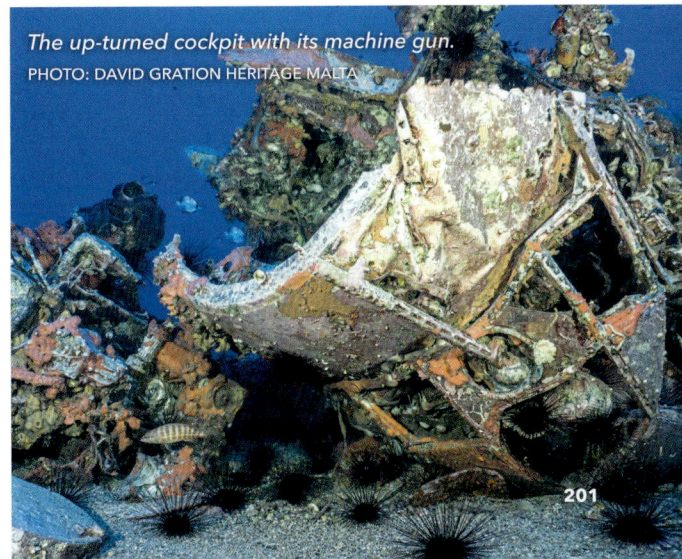

The up-turned cockpit with its machine gun.
PHOTO: DAVID GRATION HERITAGE MALTA

TECHNICAL DIVING SITES

06 - Schnellboot *S-31* War Grave

Schnellboot *S-31* was built by Lurssen in Germany part of an order of 8 boats for the Chinese National Government, but at the outbreak of WW2 they were impounded for the German Navy. They were mainly constructed of aluminum, the decking was mahogany, 33 metres in length, a 5-metre beam and weighed 100 tons. The *S31* had three Daimler Benz diesel engines, 3 propellers, a maximum speed of 38 knots with a range of 800 miles. An armament of 2 torpedo tubes 2 x 20mm guns and a crew of 24. The *S31* was launched in October 1939, commissioned in December the same year and immediately joined the 2nd Schnellboot Flotilla operating in the North Sea.

During one attack on the allies, she succeeded in seriously damaging the British Destroyer HMS *Kelly*. This incident highlighted the capabilities and danger of the Schnellboots.

In May 1940 Ostend became their base for North Sea Operations, an allied raid on their base seriously damaged a number of Schnellboots including the *S31* and their storage facilities, she was then repaired.

Early 1941 the *S-31* was handed over to the 3rd Schnellboot Flotilla the white hull was repainted blue/grey camouflage with a flying fish insignia on the side of the bridge.

After completing the Baltic operations, in September 1941 her Flotilla was assigned to the Mediterranean. This was due to the attacks from the Maltese Islands on their convoys to North Africa by British aircraft, surface vessels and submarines which had successfully disrupted Rommel's supply lines. The Schnellboots new base would be Augusta on the east coast of Sicily approximately 125 miles from Malta.

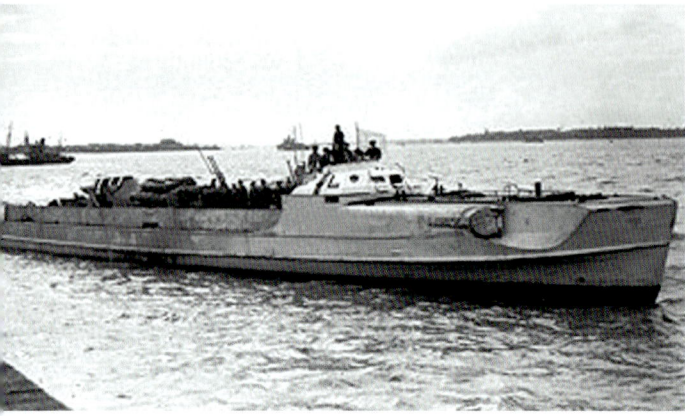

The German fast motor torpedo patrol boat.
PHOTO: UNIVERSITY OF MALTA

Below: *A torpedo still inside its launching tube.*
PHOTO: STEVEN GALICIA www.galicia.be

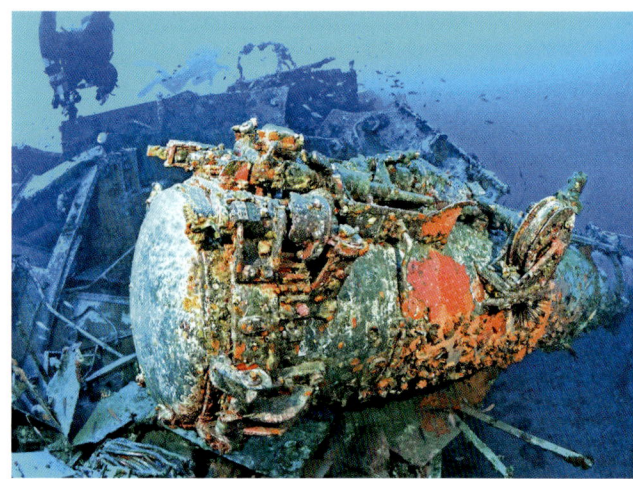

The starboard side torpedo tube still completely in tact.
PHOTOS: CATHY DELARA

Colourful coral growing on the bow of the S-31 Schnellboat.

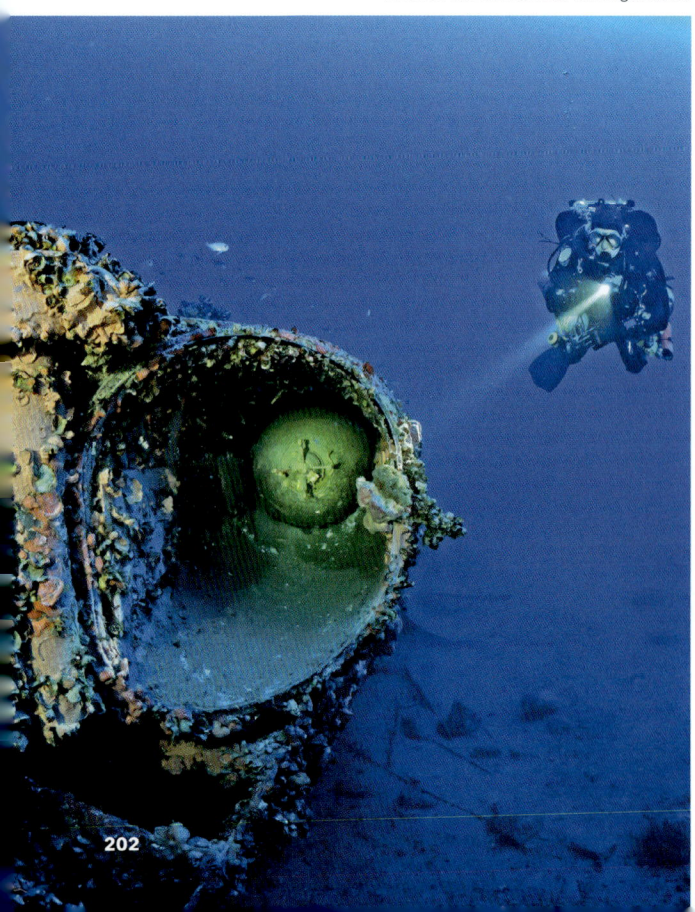

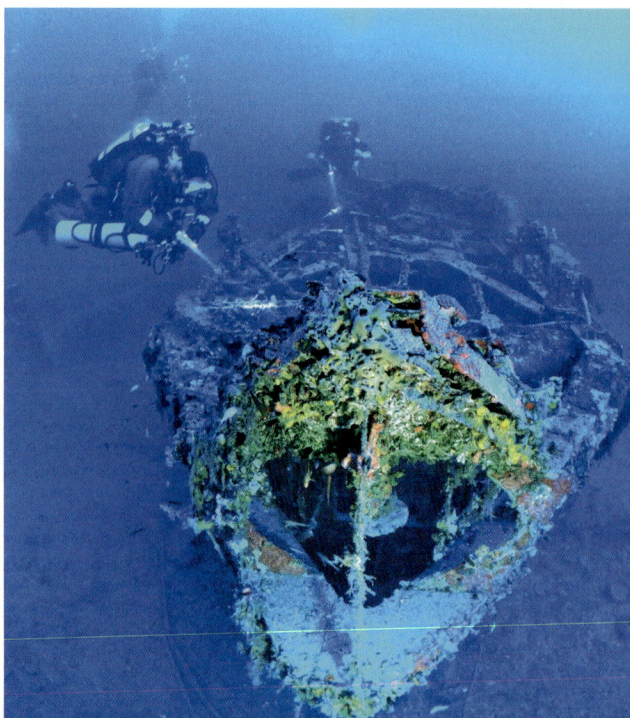

TECHNICAL DIVING SITES - SCHNELLBOOT S-31

During the afternoon of the 9th May 1942 from intelligence received, it was clear that the Luftwaffe were aware that HMS *Welshman* was making a solo run from Alexandra to Malta, carrying vital supplies to the besieged islands, and must be stopped. At 2200hrs. four Schnellboots loaded with torpedoes left Port Empedocle, Sicily to intercept HMS *Welshman*, S31 and two others left Augusta to lay mines outside the harbour entrance to Valletta.

In the early hours of the 10th May seven Schnellboots arrived on the south east coast of Malta, four would lay in wait for HMS *Welshman* and the remaining three including the *S31* began laying the minefield. This consisted of 20 contact mines, 6 explosive buoys and 2 cutting buoys, the laying of the mines was completed by 0420hrs.

The 3 Schnellboots that had been laying the mines regrouped and headed eastwards to search for the HMS *Welshman*. But suddenly after the mine laying operation had stopped, the *S-31* exploded. Possibly caused by one of her own mines which had cut loose from its moorings and rose to the surface. The Schnellboot sunk at 0438hrs and the S61 managed to save 13 survivors, including C.O. Lt. Heinrich Haag. 13 men were lost.

HMS *Welshman* made eight supply runs bringing food and essential supplies supporting the people of the Maltese Islands during the siege in WW2, before being sunk on the 1st February 1943 off Tobruk Libya, her role was featured in the UK movie The Malta Story.

THE DIVE Schnellboot *S-31* lies at around 70m depth in an upright position on a sandy silty seabed. The mahogany decking has rotted away leaving only the metal frame and panels. Apart from the explosion damage the WW2 wreck is fully intact with its original weaponry and the three engines, triple propellers and rudders, the twin torpedo tubes at the bow with torpedoes ready for launching and the anti-aircraft machine guns are still in place. A very popular dive.

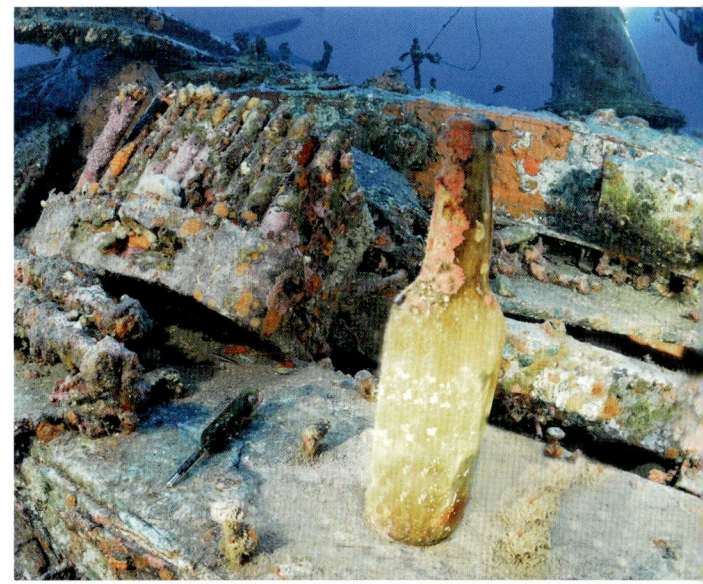
Divers find a box of ammunition and a bottle of wine!
PHOTOS: CATHY DE LARA

The open stern showing the engine, props and rudders.

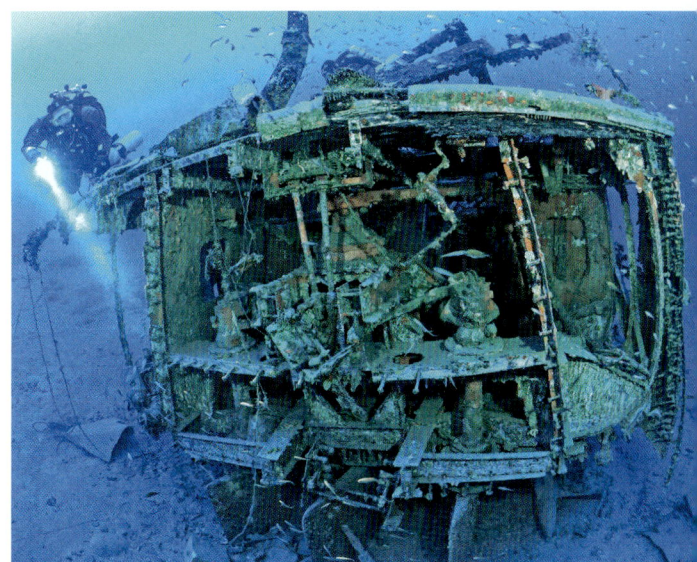

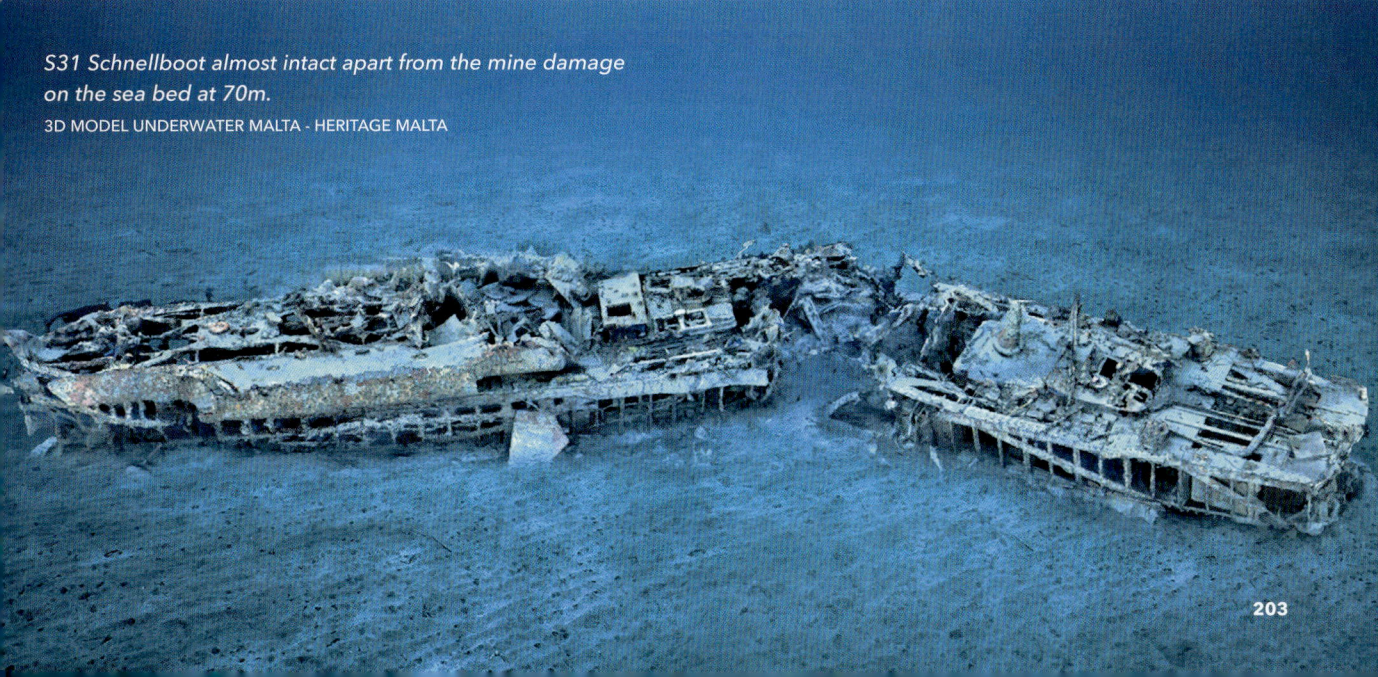
S31 Schnellboot almost intact apart from the mine damage on the sea bed at 70m.
3D MODEL UNDERWATER MALTA - HERITAGE MALTA

TECHNICAL DIVING SITES

07 - ORP *Kujawiak* L72 War Grave

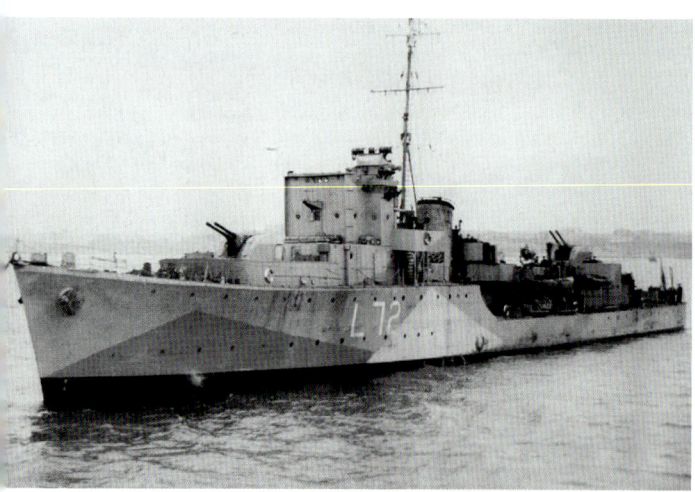

ORP Kujawiak L72 British Hunt-type II destroyer.
PHOTO: UNIVERSITY OF MALTA

HMS *Oakley* was built under the War Emergency Programme in 1939 by Vickers-Armstrong's High Walker Yard on the River Tyne England, laid down on the 22nd November 1939 with a yard number of J4145.

She was 85 metres in length, a beam of 9.5 metres and weighing 1050 tonnes. The Parsons engines have a top speed of 27 knots and a range of up to 4000 miles. Her armament was 6 x 4-inch guns on three twin turrets. 4 x 40mm, 2 x 20mm anti-aircraft guns, 6 depth charge throwers and she had crew of 160 Officers and men.

HMS *Oakley* was the sister ship to HMS *Southwold*, launched on 30th October 1940, she was transferred to the Polish Navy on 3rd April 1941 and commissioned on the 17th June 1941. She was renamed ORP *Kujawiak* meaning a type of Polish folk dance. ORP is an acronym of Okert Rzeczypospolite Polskiej which translates as "Warship of the Republic of Poland"

The ships bell, found and given to the Maritime Museum of Malta.
PHOTO: DAVE GRATION HERITAGE MALTA

The next day she was making her way to Scapa Flow for sea trials, during this journey she came under attack by a German aircraft, one of her gun turrets was hit followed an explosion and one crew member died.

ORP *Kujawiak* undertook escort and patrol duties around the British Isles before being deployed to the Mediterranean. A year later she arrived in Gibraltar for convoy duties to Malta, protecting supply ships which were defenceless against the aerial bombings of the Axis warplanes, this was a perilous task for all involved. On 14th June 1942 the convoy, known as Operation Harpoon, almost immediately they were attacked by Italian submarines and torpedo planes. Three merchant ships and one escort ship were sunk, but ORP *Kujawiak* bravely defended the convoy and succeeded in shooting down four Axis planes.

As they approached Malta on the 15th June near midnight, another ship, HMS *Badsworth*, struck a mine, ORP *Kujawiak* attempted a dangerous rescue mission and ended up hitting a mine. The Polish destroyer sunk, with the loss of 13 crew.

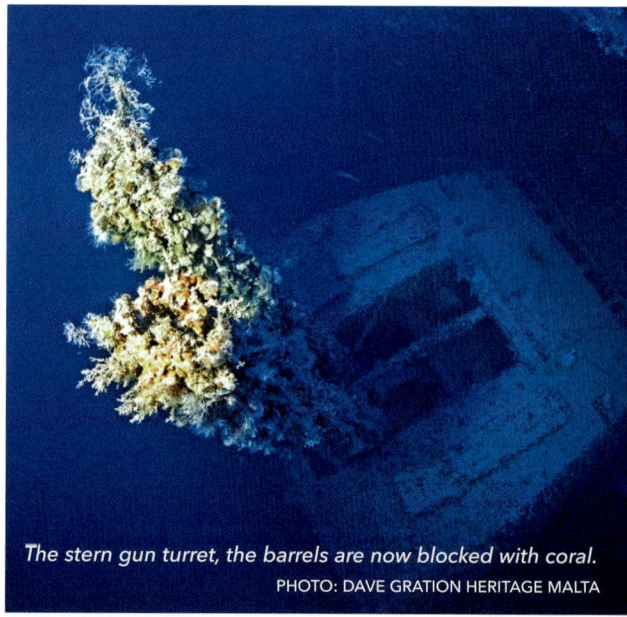

The stern gun turret, the barrels are now blocked with coral.
PHOTO: DAVE GRATION HERITAGE MALTA

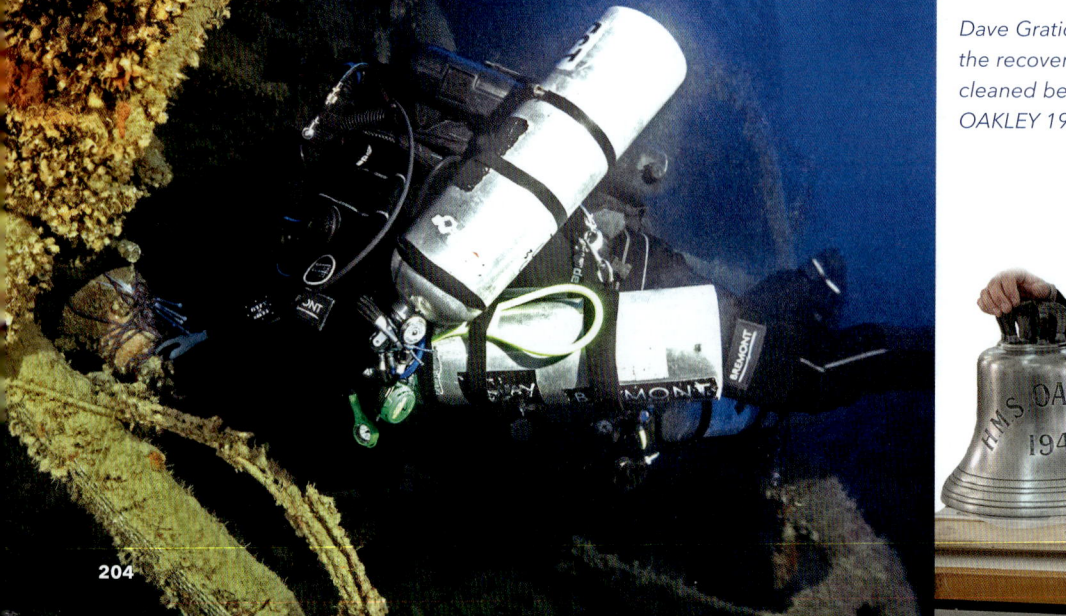

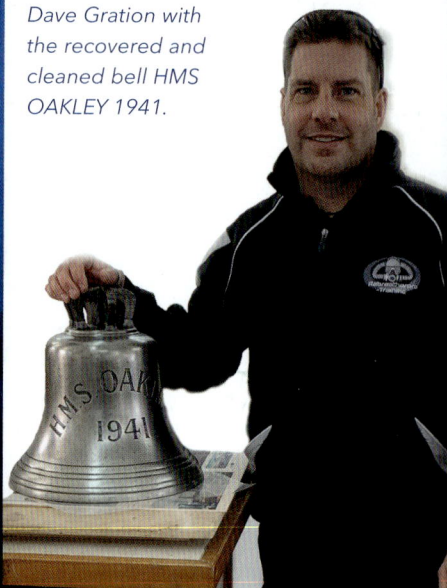

Dave Gration with the recovered and cleaned bell HMS OAKLEY 1941.

TECHNICAL DIVING SITES - ORP KUJAWIAK

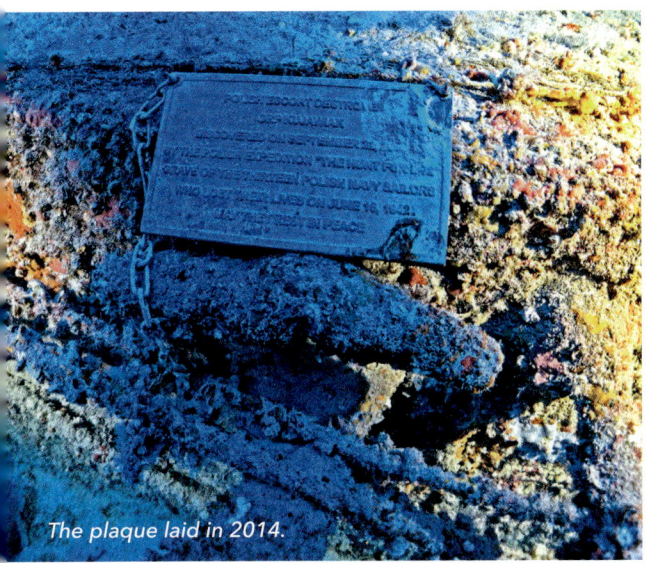

The plaque laid in 2014.

PHOTO: DAVE GRATION HERITAGE MALTA

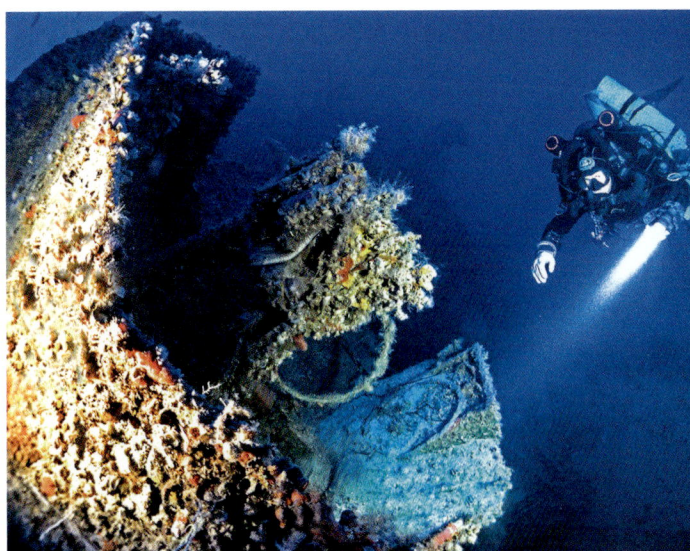

Diver above the wreckage of the compass platform.

PHOTOS: DAVE GRATION HERITAGE MALTA

Still in place one of the anti-aircraft guns.

THE DIVE After extensive research a team of Polish divers working with the University of Malta, located the wreck in September 2014, nearly 7 miles east of Valletta at a depth of 97m. Diving took place over the next three seasons and she was found to be in excellent condition, with the hull and bow in near perfect condition. Along with the forward gun turrets, with their barrels and the anti-aircraft guns. Only the ship's stern is in a bad state, as it buckled when she first hit the seabed.

During one of the dives a plaque was laid on the side of the wreck by the team. It reads: Polish Escort Destroyer ORP *Kujawiak* discovered on September 20th 2014 by the Polish Expedition "The hunt for L72" Grave of the 13 Polish Navy sailors who lost their lives on June 16th 1942. May they rest in peace.

Quotes by experienced divers "Excellent wreck". "Intact, lying on her side, a fantastic dive".

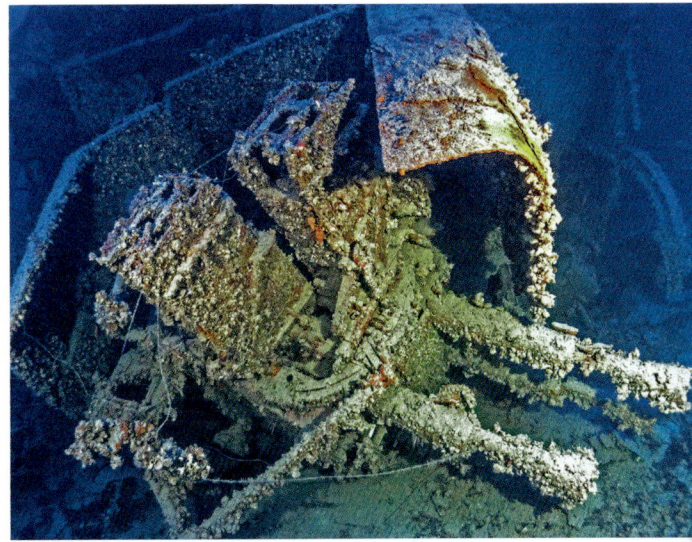

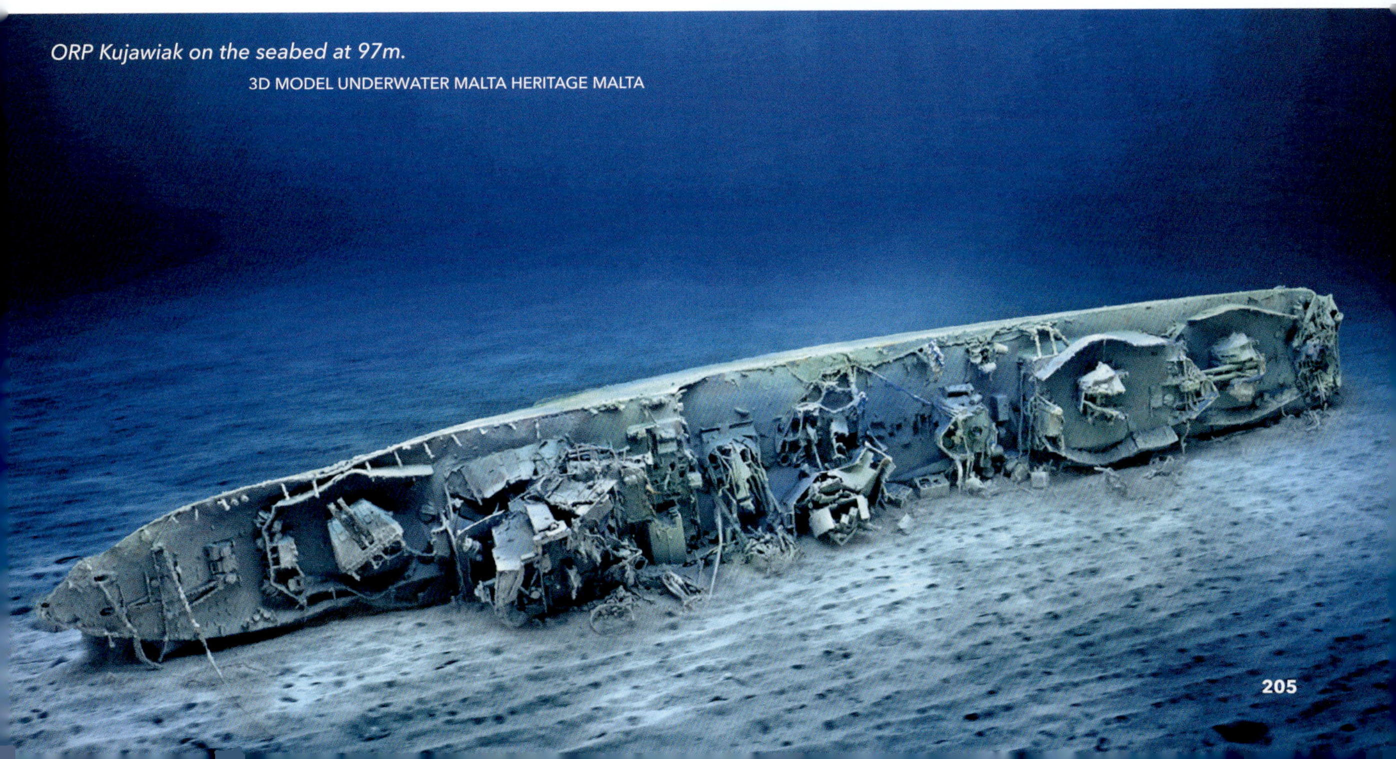

ORP Kujawiak on the seabed at 97m.

3D MODEL UNDERWATER MALTA HERITAGE MALTA

TECHNICAL DIVING SITES

08 - HMD *Trusty Star*

HMD *Trusty Star* was a Royal Naval drifter built in 1919 by Ouse Shipbuilding Ltd. Hook Nr. Goole England. The steel vessel was about 26 metres in length with a beam of 5.5 metres and had a triple expansion steam engine.

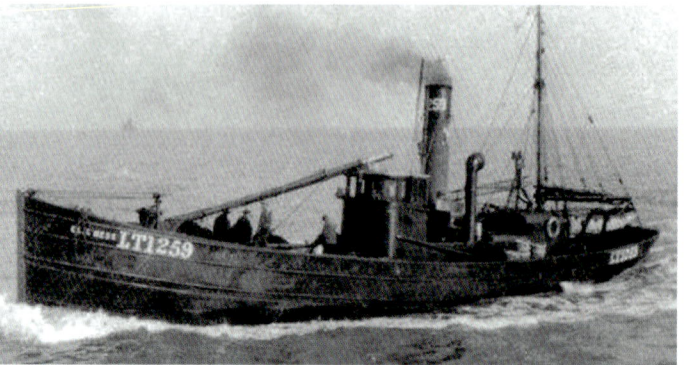

HMD Trusty Star with her fisheries number.
PHOTO: UNIVERSITY OF MALTA

Her original name was HMT *Groundswell*, she was later renamed FV *Elie Ness* by the Scottish Fisheries Board, and then sold to the Star Drift Fishing Co. Lowestoft England. In 1939 she was requisitioned by the Admiralty, renamed HMD *Trusty Star* and converted to a minesweeper and sent to Malta.

On the 10th June 1940 Italy entered WW2, now Malta found herself in the very heart of the conflict. The enemy believed that by laying sea mines, supplies could be prevented from reaching the Maltese Islands.

At the beginning of 1941 the Luftwaffe began laying magnetic and acoustic mines by parachute in both Grand and Marsamxett harbours, only drifter *Ploughboy* could deal with these mines as she was fitted with a magnetic skid sweep cable. In April, HMD *Trusty Star* and HMS *Abington* were fitted with the latest sweeping equipment. They had great success keeping the harbours open in spite of heavy mine-laying operations by the Luftwaffe.

Over the next 12 months more and more mines were laid making minesweeping more difficult and dangerous. Working in the harbour also were tugboat *St Angelo* and HMD *Eddy*. In April 1942 HMS *Abingdon* was hit by bombs near the Bighi Tower, Kalkara creek, beached, then in 1950 she was partly salvaged.

On the 10th June 1942, HMD *Trusty Star* was clearing mines outside Grand Harbour, when she hit by a mine and sank. Just one Maltese seaman was injured, the rest of the crew were rescued unhurt.

THE DIVE The wreck of *Trusty Star* is some 2 miles out from Grand Harbour Valletta, at a depth of 90m on a sandy seabed. The wreck is almost intact and in very good condition, with a list of 45-degrees on her starboard side and covered in a layer of silt.

Middle left: The bow on a sandy silty sea bed at 90m.
Bottom left: HMD Trusty Star's stern, prop and rudder.
Below: Maybe a moray lives here in the toilet.
PHOTOS: DAVE GRATION HERITAGE MALTA

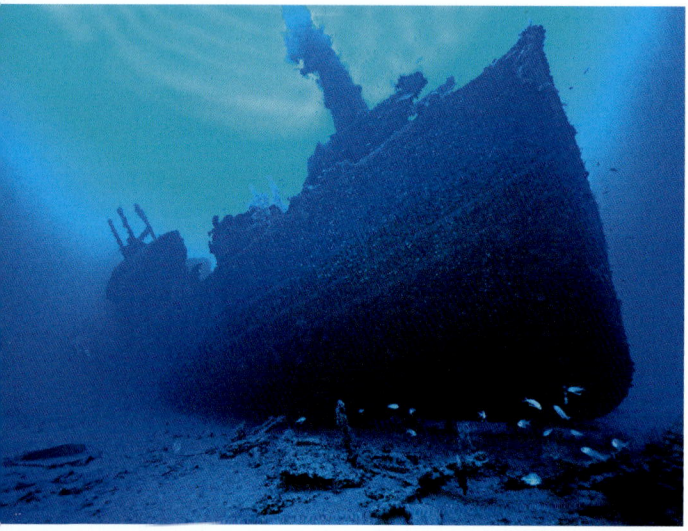

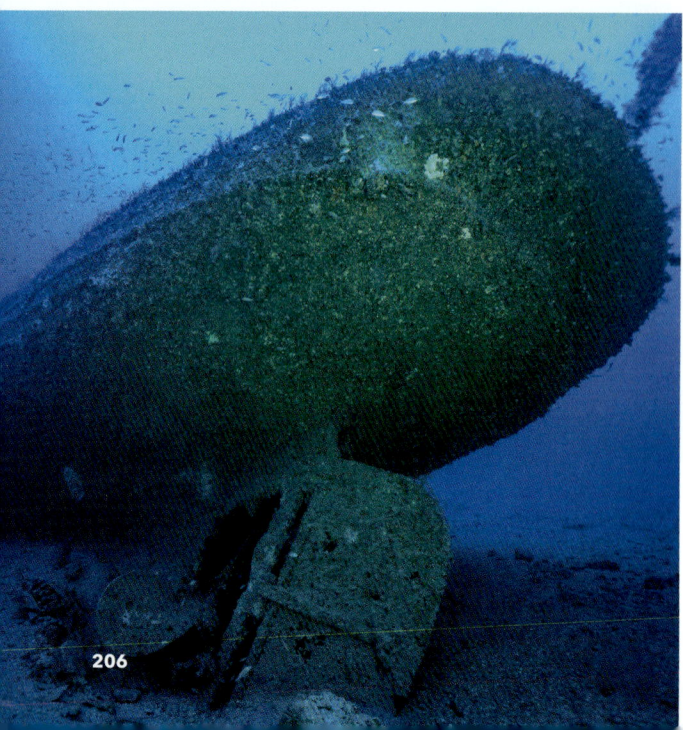

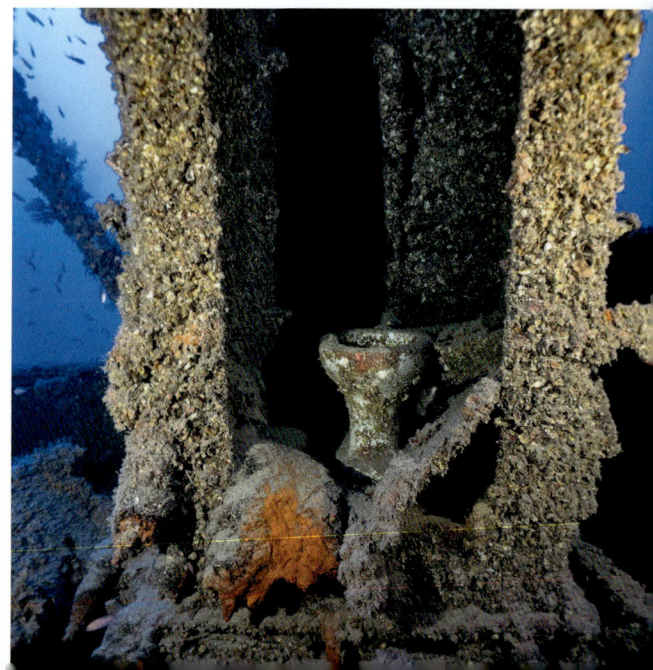

09 - HMS *Olympus* War Grave

HMS *Olympus* was a Odin-class Submarine, built by William Beardmore Co. Dalmuir Clydebank Scotland. Originally designed for the Royal Australian Navy to cope with long distance patrolling in the Pacific Ocean.

She was launched on the 11th December 1928 and commissioned in June 1930, 86 metres long, a beam of 6 metres. A displacement of 1781 tons and a surface speed of 17 knots, submerged 8 knots and a crew of 55. Her armament was 6 bow torpedo tubes and 2 at the stern, a 4-inch deck gun and two AA machine guns.

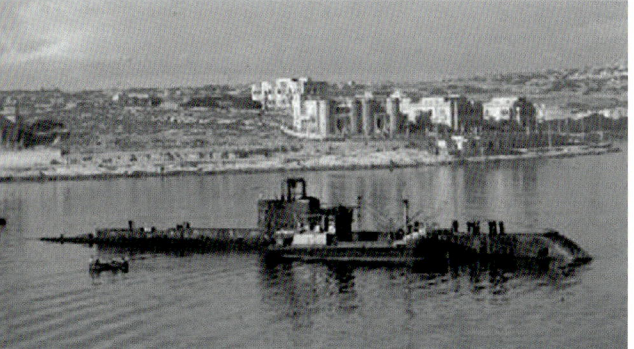

HMS Olympus moored in Marsamxett harbour, in the background Ta'Xbiex.   PHOTO: UNIVERSITY OF MALTA

During WW2 HMS *Olympus* was adopted by the city of Peterborough, the plaque is held in the Royal Navy National Museum in Portsmouth. On the 16th April 1940 she was ordered to proceed from Colombo Ceylon, now Sri Lanka, to Malta, she travelled via the Suez Canal, arriving on the 7th May. During her convoy patrols from Gibraltar to Malta on one occasion she was joined by HMS *Maori*.

On the 8th May 1942 HMS *Olympus* left Valletta for England, with some of the crew members from the three bombed submarines some nights before.

While still on the surface shortly after leaving port, she struck a mine, the crew attempted to send out distress signals and then tried to fire the deck gun to raise the alarm, but the shell got jammed and no help came, she sunk, the crew attempted a gruelling three-mile swim back to Valletta. Out of the 98 men on board, just nine survived.

THE DIVE Today HMS *Olympus* sits upright on the seabed, intact apart from the mine damage on the starboard side, 3 miles east of Valletta at a depth of 115m. She was found in 2011, using a ROV to photograph the site. Her gun is still intact, pointing upwards after failing to fire. which could have signalled her distress. The hatches are open, where the crew escaped as the submarine started taking on water.

In May 2017 a plaque was laid on HMS *Olympus* to honour the fallen men and to commemorate the 75th anniversary of this tragedy. It reads "In memory of the 89 Submariners who lost their lives when the HMS *Olympus* went down on the 8th May 1942 May they never be forgotten".

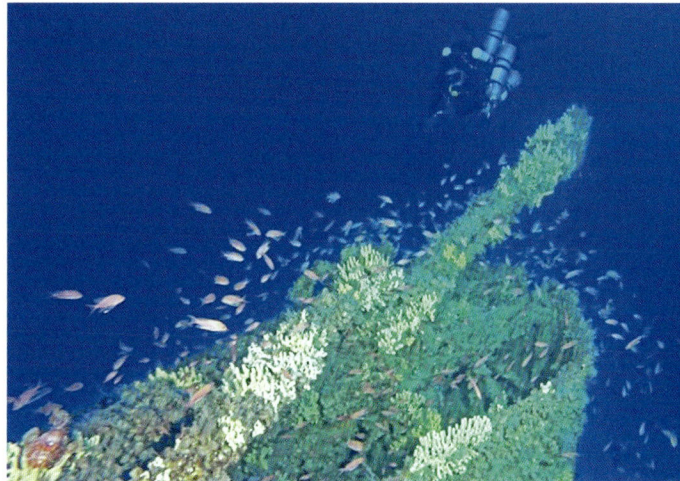

Marine life around the conning tower of this submarine.
PHOTOS: DAVE GRATION HERITAGE MALTA

Bottom left: All the escape hatches were found open.
Below: A diver checks out the plaque laid in May 2017.

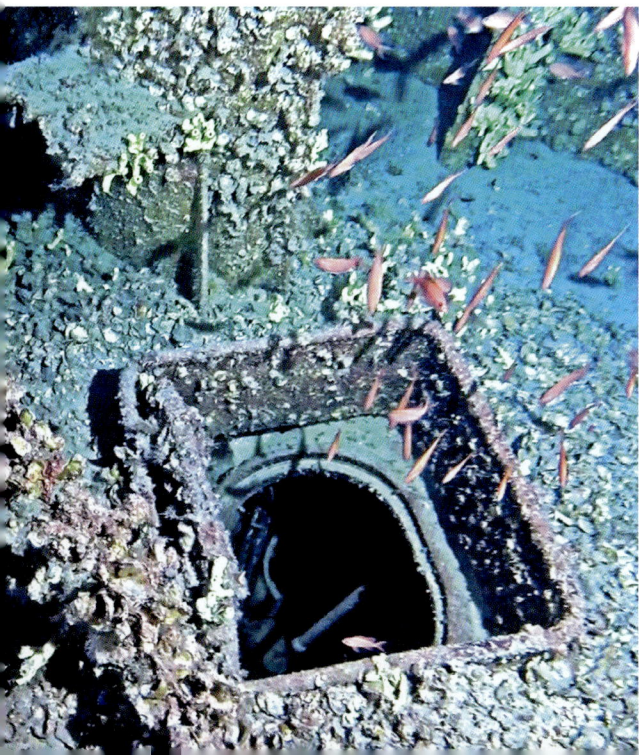

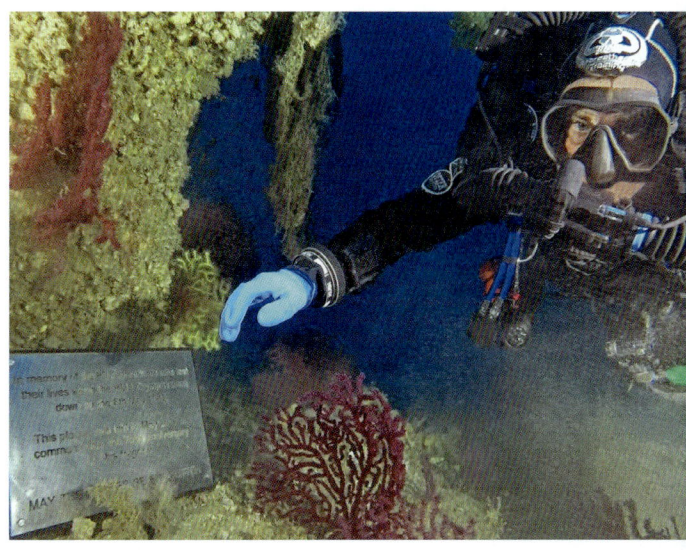

10 - HMS *Russell* War Grave

To maintain the Royal Navy's supremacy in 1889 Britain's establishment decided that our combined naval strength should match any other two countries. In response to the French and Russian ship building programmes, Sir William White was asked by the Admiralty to build a faster battleship to match the top speed of the Russian ships.

They were to be designed to be lighter, smaller and faster, when built, the Duncan-class pre-dreadnought battleships were the fastest in the world for several years.

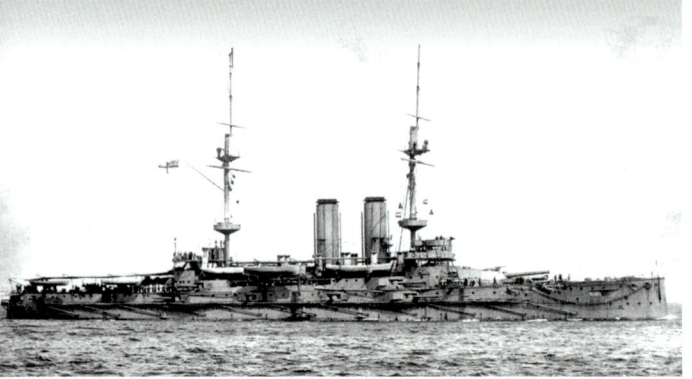

HMS Russell a Duncan-class Dreadnaught battleship.
PHOTO: UNIVERSITY OF MALTA

HMS *Russell* was built by Palmers Shipbuilding and Iron Co. at Jarrow England, March 1899, launched, 19th February 1902. She was 132 metres in length, a beam of 23 metres a draft of 8 metres and a displacement of almost 14000 tons rising to 15400 when fully loaded and painted in black and buff colours as used by the Navy in Victorian times.

Powered by a pair of 4 cylinder triple-expansion engines, with steam provided by twenty-four Belleville boilers giving her 18000 horsepower and with two propellors will give top speed of 19 knots. Able to steam for almost 7000 miles.

Her armament was 4 x 12-inch guns fore and aft, 12 x 6-inch guns, 10 x 3-inch guns and 3 x 1.9-inch guns. Battleships of that time also had 4 torpedo tubes submerged in the hull. She had a crew of 720.

Being the first of the six Duncan class battleships, she was named HMS *Russell* after Edward Russell, former Royal Navy Commander-in-Chief of the Navy in the 17th century. After being launched she sailed to Chatham Dockyard for gun-mounting, steam and sea trials, these were completed by February 1903. She was Commissioned on the 19th February 1903 and was repainted in the new grey colour scheme. Over the next few years, she served with the Mediterranean Fleet, Home Fleet, the Atlantic Fleet, visiting Canada during the Quebec Tercentenary.

On the outbreak of WW1, HMS *Russell*, with her sister ships, were assigned to the Grand Fleet. On the 6th November 1915 the Grand Fleet sailed to Gallipoli, so as to reinforce the British Squadron deployed there.

After the conclusion of the maligned Gallipoli campaign, in April 1916 she sailed for Malta, for supplies and minor dockyard repairs and to give the crew some shore leave.

On the morning of the 27th April, HMS *Russell* was some 5 miles off Valletta, when there were two separate explosions, she had struck two mines one after the other. She was badly damaged and fire broke out in the rear of the ship. After a further explosion she took on a dangerous list, and the order to abandon ship was passed. She sank slowly allowing most of the crew to escape, 27 officers and 98 ratings were lost. The mines had been laid by the German submarine U-73 the night before.

THE DIVE HMS *Russell* now lies some 5 miles east of Valletta on a flattish, sandy, seabed, at a depth of 115m. Dived for the first time in July 2003 by a British technical diving team called "Starfish Enterprise" She was found completely upside down with her stern section missing. It is believed that most of her large guns are laying around on the seabed as they were not fixed to their bases. This is a deep technical dive.

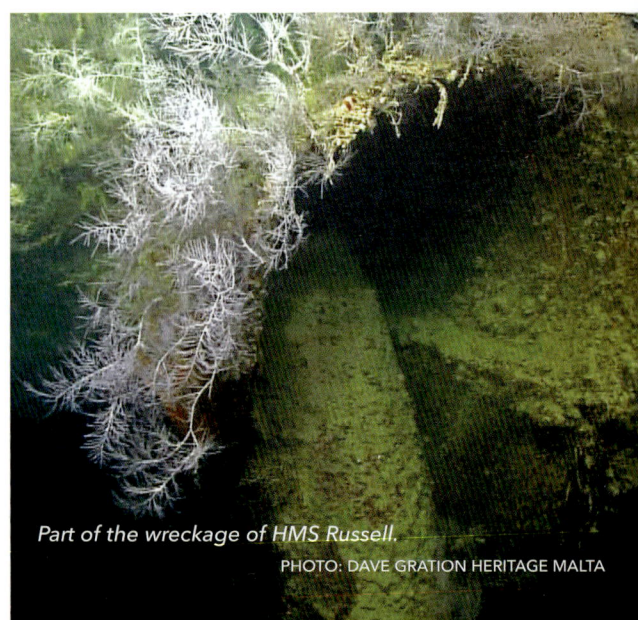

Part of the wreckage of HMS Russell.
PHOTO: DAVE GRATION HERITAGE MALTA

One of the gun turrets on this battleship.
PHOTO: DAVE GRATION HERITAGE MALTA

11 - HMS *Urge* War Grave

HMS *Urge* was a U-class submarine built by Vickers Armstrong, 49 were constructed, she was laid down on the 30th October 1939 and commissioned on 12th December 1940, only three would survive the war. These small, 630-tonne submarines were initially to be used for training, only later fitted with torpedo tubes and made operational. HMS *Urge* had an overall length of 58m, a beam of 5m and a top speed of 11 knots on the surface, submerged 10 knots. Armed with four torpedo tubes, one quick-firing 3-inch gun and an anti-aircraft gun.

HMS *Urge* was adopted by the town of Bridgend, during the war there was a nationwide campaign to raise money for the Royal Navy. Cities would adopt battleships and aircraft carriers; towns and villages would adopt cruisers, destroyers and submarine.

Under the command of Lieutenant EP Tomkinson, for most of her service, HMS *Urge* operated in the Mediterranean where she formed part of the 10th Submarine Flotilla, or the Fighting Tenth as it became known, based in Malta. The submarine had an intense twenty patrols during her service, damaging or sinking significant numbers of Axis shipping. Her most well-known achievement was the attack on the Italian battleship *Vittorio Veneto* near the Straits of Messina on 14th December 1941, the largest enemy battleship to be torpedoed at sea by the Royal Navy. On the 1st April 1942, HMS *Urge* sank the Italian cruiser *Giovanni dell Bande Nere*, with the loss of over half of its crew. These events took place during the Second Siege of Malta, a period of intensified aerial bombing. Eventually, the 10th Submarine Flotilla on Manoel Island was no longer sustainable, and the remaining submarines were to be evacuated to Alexandria, Egypt.

Outside Grand Harbour there were two minefields, HMS *Urge* left Malta Grand Harbour on the 27th April 1942, and was not heard of again, along with its 32 crew and 12 passengers including war correspondent Bernard Gray, it was thought the submarine had hit a mine.

It would remain a mystery until 2019, when the wreck of HMS *Urge* was discovered during a remote survey off the coast of Malta. Francis Dickinson, the grandson of the commanding officer, Lieutenant EP Tomkinson, was crucial in the drive to find HMS *Urge*. She was first dived in April 2021 by a Heritage Malta and University of Malta dive team; they identified the submarine as the HMS *Urge*.

A strong connection between the wreck and relatives of those who lost their lives remains, mainly driven by Mr. Dickinson. A memorial for the brave crew was placed in Fort St Elmo, Valletta, Malta, with a ceremony organized for the 80th anniversary of her loss on 27th April 2022.

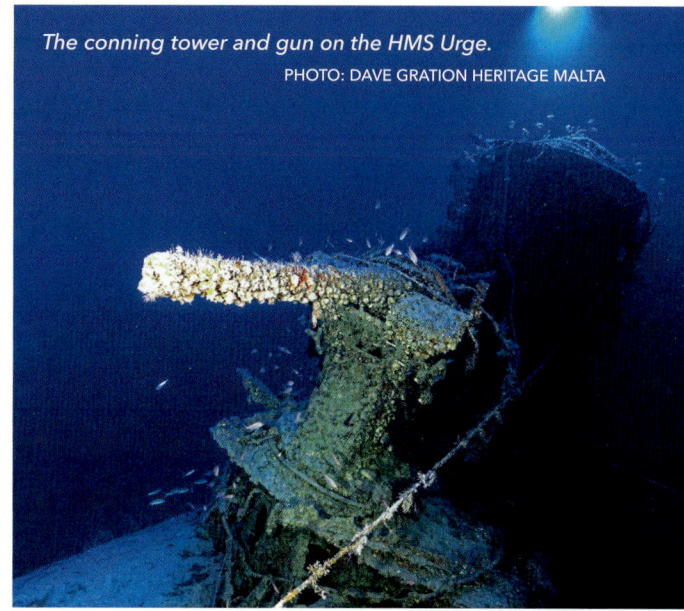

The conning tower and gun on the HMS Urge.
PHOTO: DAVE GRATION HERITAGE MALTA

THE DIVE Located some 3.2km out from Grand Harbour at a depth of 130m upright, almost intact, but heavily damaged at the bow, which is consistent with striking a mine, on a silty, sandy, rocky seabed.

The damage sustained from a mine is clearly visible, where upon impact on the seabed the hull broke just forward of the torpedo storage section.

As part of the commemoration events organized in April 2022, a Heritage Malta dive team placed a memorial plaque on the conning tower, and unfurled a Royal Navy ensign on HMS *Urge*.

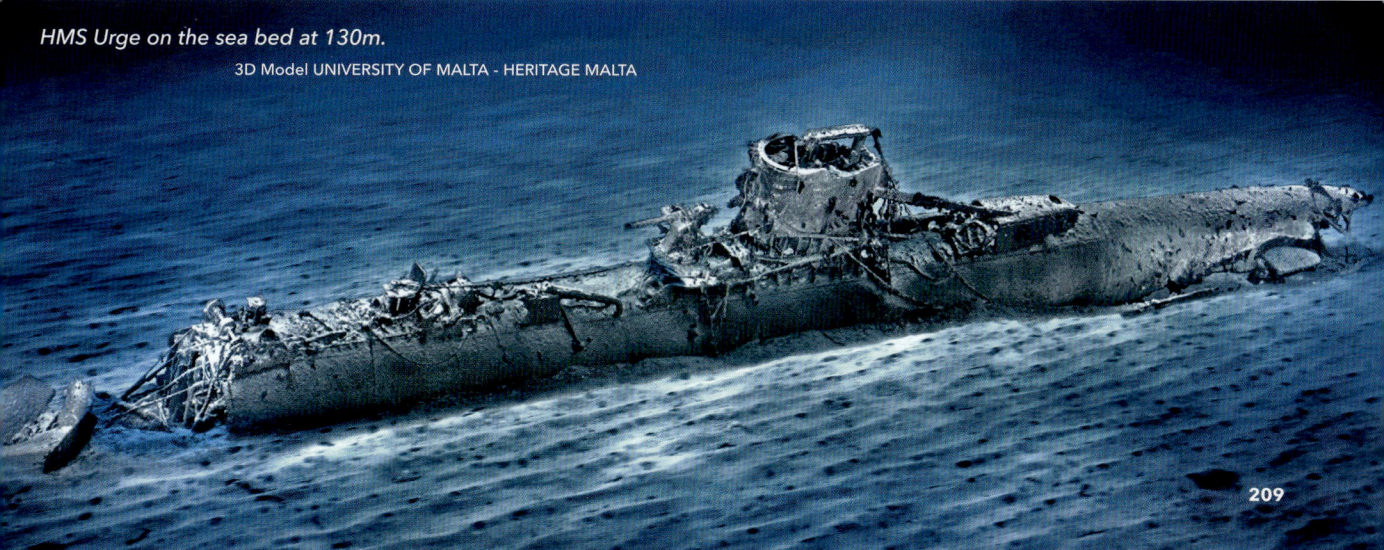

HMS Urge on the sea bed at 130m.
3D Model UNIVERSITY OF MALTA - HERITAGE MALTA

Licencing Authority

All diving centres in the Maltese Islands must be authorized by the Malta Tourism Authority, as they issue the operating licenses to diving centres, who offer Recreational Diving Services. This is defined in local legislation as training, education, accompanied diving. Diving centres are inspected by officials of the Authority at least once a year; the centres must conform to the highest standards. The legislation has been designed around the European standard for recreational diving service providers EN14467. Instructors must be officially registered to act as such through a licensed dive centre, where all training and education will be undertaken. Equipment will be issued by a licensed dive centre, where you can be assured that it has undergone regular maintenance, servicing and testing by technical qualified persons, unless of course you have brought your own.

Officials from the Enforcement section of the Authority have the executive powers which enable them to stop any activity from taking place if it is considered to be illegal. Legal action would be taken against that individual, not yourself as a consumer. If they are found to be providing illicit recreational diving services, your dive would be ordered to cease. Freelance instructors would need operate from licensed premises and therefore their operations are open to inspections, by the local government agency. This is all planned with the best interest of the consumer in mind and there are some 70 licensed diving centres to choose from around the islands.

In order to enjoy the crystal-clear waters of the Maltese Islands, make sure you take along your Certification card and your Dive Log. These will be required when you register at any of the licensed diving centres, for equipment rental, training courses, accompanied or un-accompanied dives, to confirm your qualifications and experience. Any diver who is not qualified to dive to 30m or deeper must dive in the company of a Certified Diving Instructor, who will be solely responsible for the safety of these divers.

PADI Bubble maker can be undertaken at the age of eight within an enclosed environment and must be accompanied by a parent or guardian. At the age of ten, Junior Open Water courses may be commenced. BS-AC allow minors to 'try dive' at the age of twelve and continue training to Ocean Diver. These are the regulations of PADI and BS-AC and are accepted at the majority of dive centres in the Maltese Islands.

At the dive centre you will be asked to fill in a short Registration Form with your personal details and a self-assessed medical form. If the form indicates any illnesses or conditions which may hamper the safety of your planned dive, you will be required to undergo a direct medical assessment conducted by one of the hyperbaric doctors available on the Islands. Medical checks are inexpensive and can be done within hours of registration. You may be required by the director of the dive centre to undergo a medical check to ascertain that you are medically fit to dive. The Maltese Islands have a strong and positive track record for safety in diving and all do their best to ensure that you have the safety you require

Details of the Maltese Scuba Diving Legislation may be found on the following web sites.

www.visitmalta.com

www.pdsa.org.mt

www.maltatourismauthority.com

A licenced dive centre, cylinder charging room.
PHOTO: BRIAN AZZOPARDI ATLANTIS DIVING CENTRE

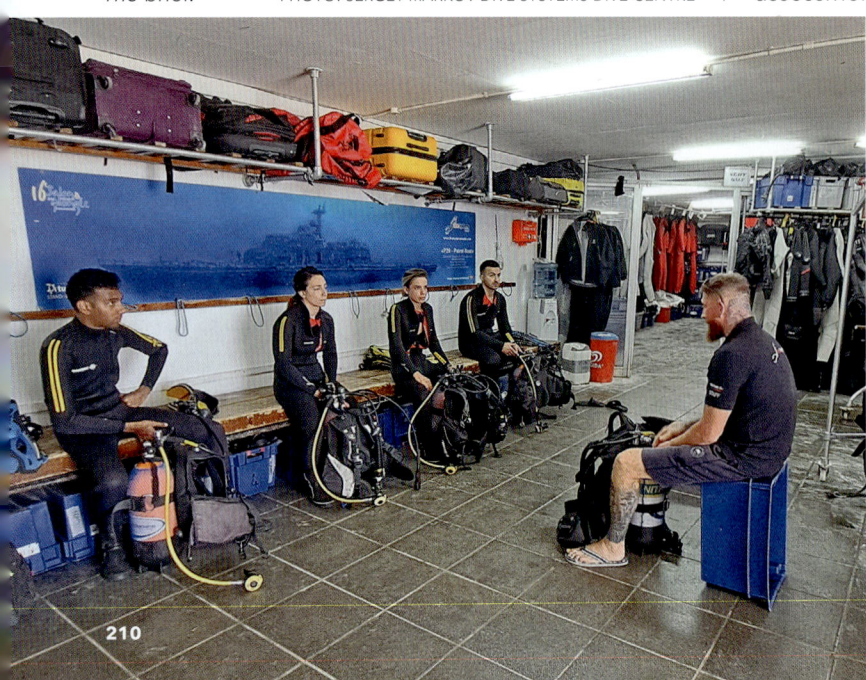

The brief. PHOTO: SERGEY MARKOV DIVE SYSTEMS DIVE CENTRE

Dive safely in Malta

Setting the standard

Look for a PDSA approved dive centre and know that you are diving with **the best** the islands have to offer.

The **Professional Diving Schools Association** of Malta, Gozo and Comino is a collective of diving professionals, all committed to a diving experience that lives up to the highest standards.

Visit **pdsa.org.mt** for more information

Dive safely and enjoyably. Dive with a PDSA member, and ensure that you get the very best out of Malta, Gozo and Comino.

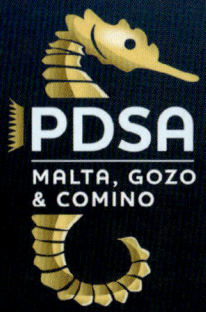

PDSA
MALTA, GOZO & COMINO

Dive Centre Locations

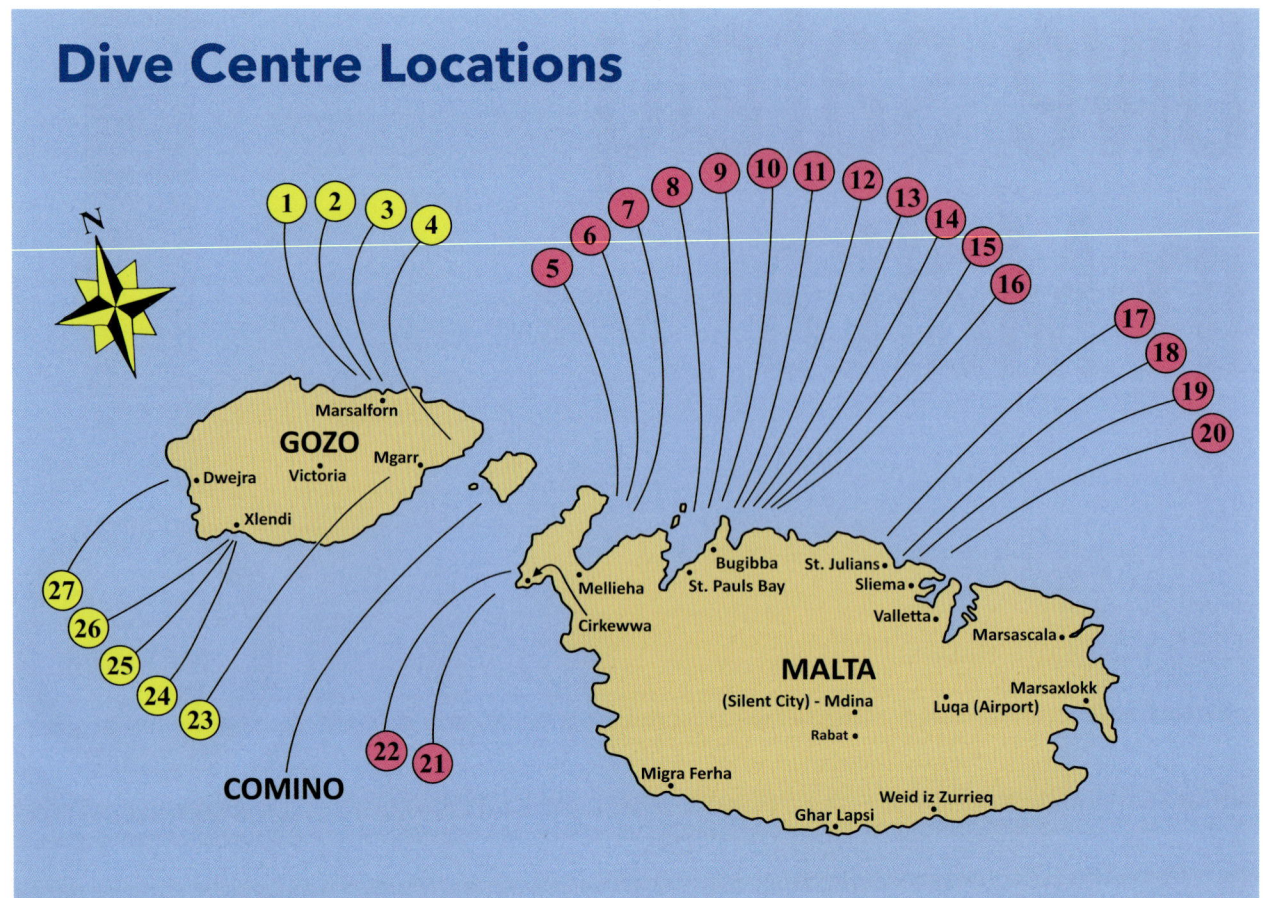

1	**Atlantis Diving Centre** - Marsalforn Gozo	Page 219	www.atlantisgozo.com
2	**Gozo Aquasports** - Marsalforn Gozo	Page 220	www.gozoaquasports.com
3	**Calypso Divers** - Marsalforn Gozo	Page 219	www.calypsodivers.com
4	**Blue Water Dive Cove** - Qala Gozo	Page 219	www.divebluewaters.com
5	**Sea Shell Dive Centre** - Mellieha Malta	Page 218	www.seashelldivingmalta.com
6	**Aquaventure Dive Centre** - Mellieha Malta	Page 213	www.aquaventuremalta.com
7	**Dune - Malta** - Pergola Hotel Mellieha Malta	Page 215	https://dune-world.com
8	**Octopus Garden** - St. Pauls Bay Malta	Page 216	www.octopus-garden.net
9	**Aquatica Scuba Diving** - St. Pauls Bay Malta	Page 213	www.aquaticadives.com
10	**Maltaqua Diving Centre** - St. Pauls Bay Malta	Page 216	www.maltaqua.com
11	**Subatech Diving Centre** - St. Pauls Bay Malta	Page 217	www.scubatech.info
12	**Buddies Dive Cove** - Pioneer Rd. Bugibba Malta	Page 213	www.buddiesmalta.com
13	**Dive Deep Blue** - Annanija St. Bugibba Malta	Page 214	www.divedeepblue.com
14	**Dawn Diving** - Triq Il-Maskli Qawra Malta	Page 214	www.dawndiving.com
15	**Mad Shark Diving** - Qwara Malta	Page 216	www.madsharkmalta.com
16	**Waterworld** - Sunny Coast Resort Qwara Malta	Page 218	www.waterworldmalta.com
17	**Starfish** - Marina Hotel, St. Julians Malta	Page 218	www.starfishdiving.com
18	**Divewise** - Dragunara Point St. Julians Malta	Page 215	www.divewise.com.mt
19	**Dive Systems Tec** - Tower Road Sliema Malta	Page 215	www.divesystemsmalta.com
20	**Diveshack** - Qui-Si-Sana Seafront Sliema Malta	Page 214	www.divemalta.com
21	**Paradise Diving** - Paradise Bay Cirkewwa Malta	Page 217	www.paradisebayresortmalta.com
22	**OrangeShark** - Ramla Bay Resort Mellieha Malta	Page 217	www.orangeshark.eu
23	**Gozo Diving** - Mgarr Rd. Xewkija Gozo	Page 220	www.gozodiving.com
24	**Ritual Dive Gozo** - Trig il-Gostra Xlendi Gozo	Page 221	www.ritualdive.com
25	**St. Andrews** - Xlendi Bay Gozo	Page 221	www.gozodive.com
26	**Utina Diving** - Rabat Road Xlendi Gozo	Page 221	www.utinadiving.com
27	**Dwejra Divers** - Inland Sea Dwejra Gozo	Page 220	www.dwejradive.com

Malta Dive Centres

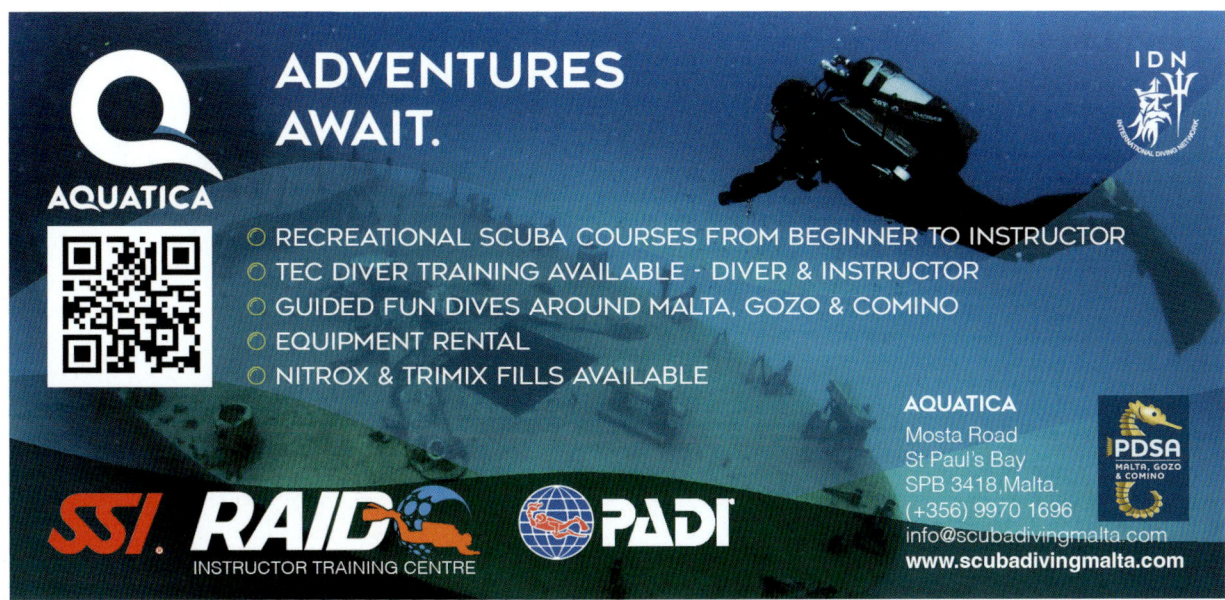

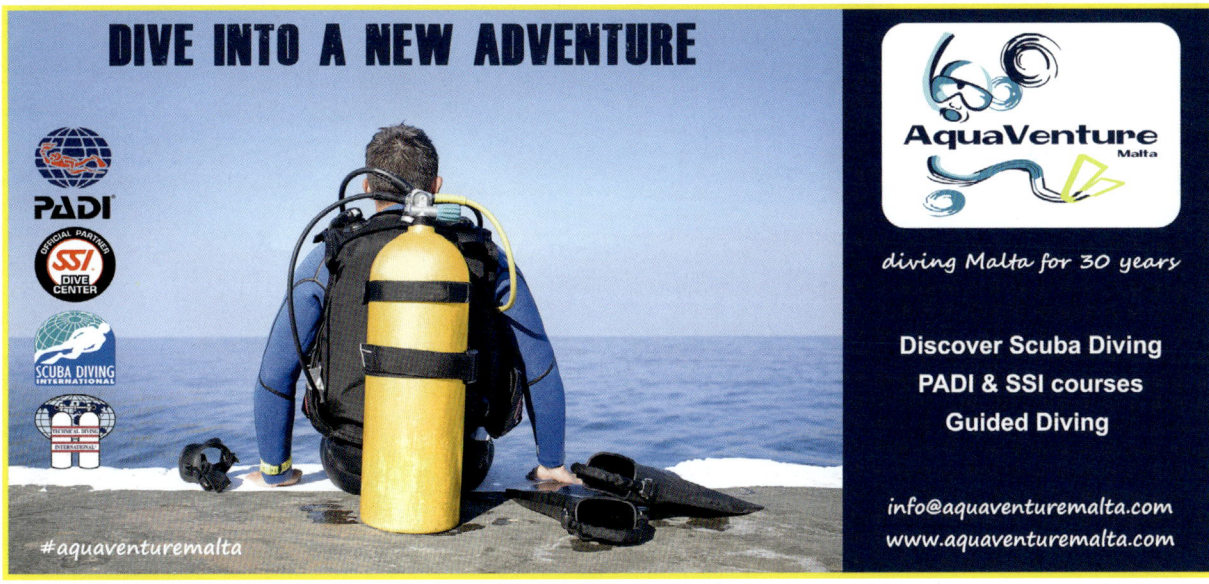

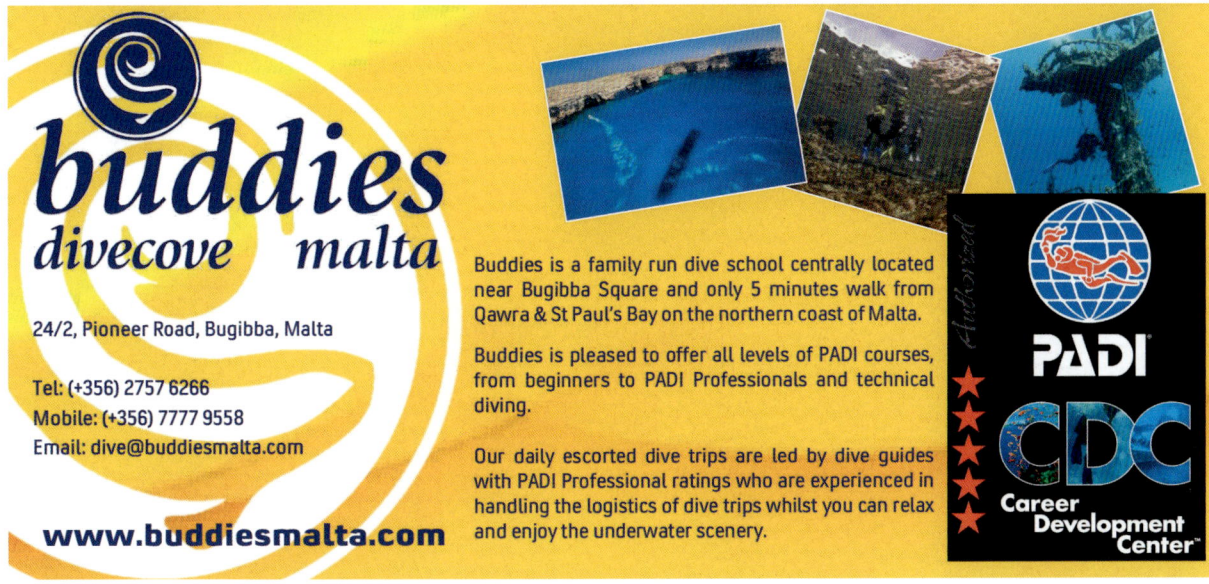

Malta Dive Centres

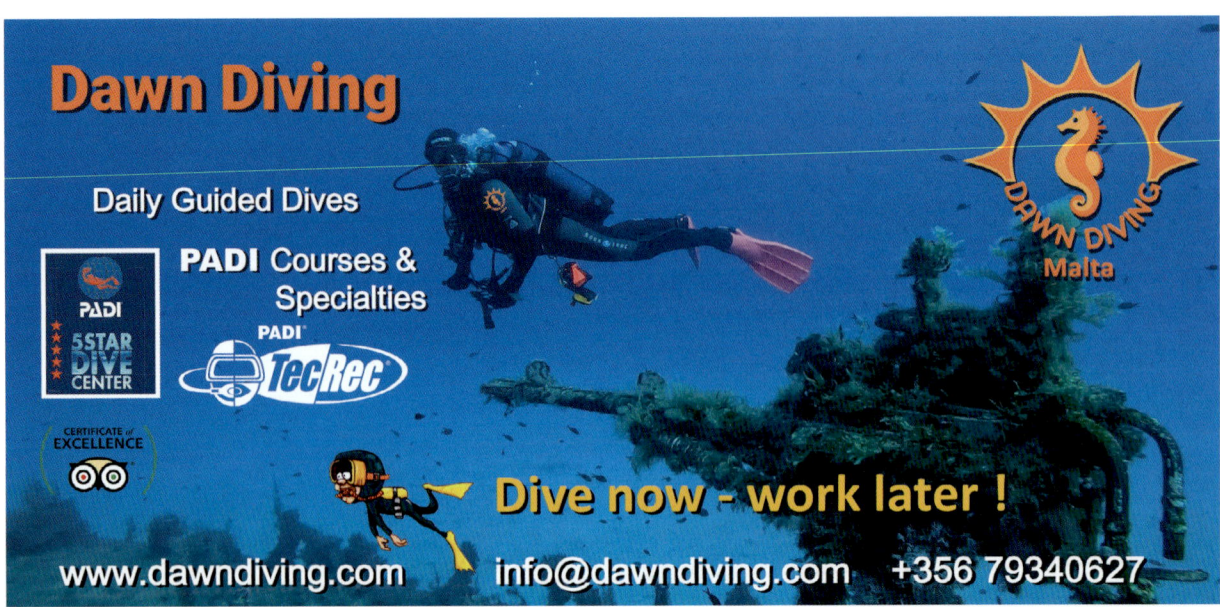

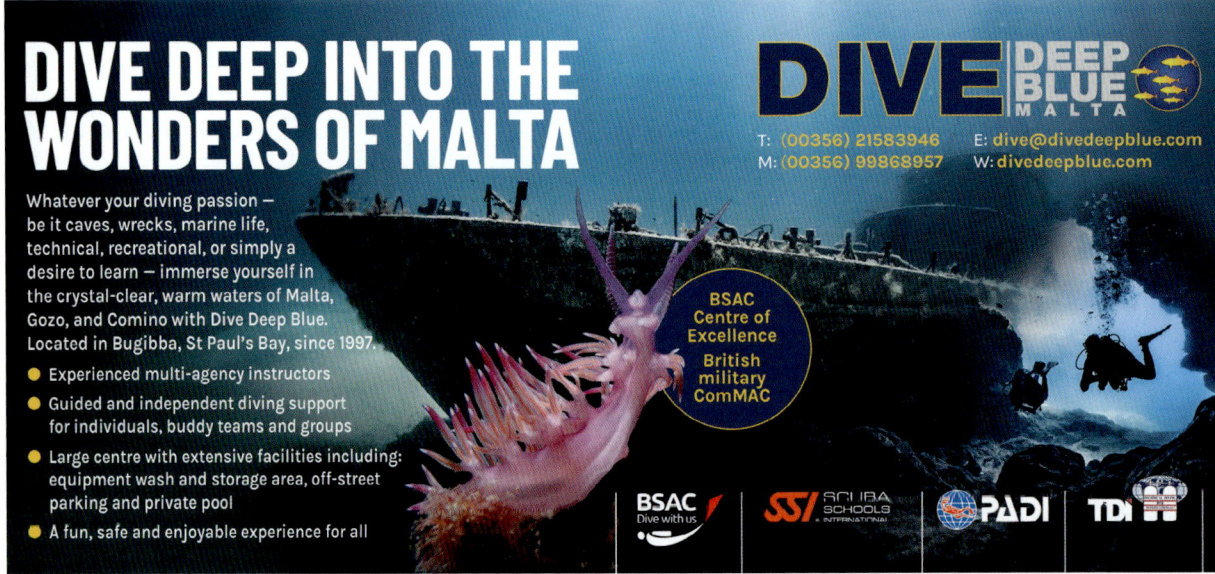

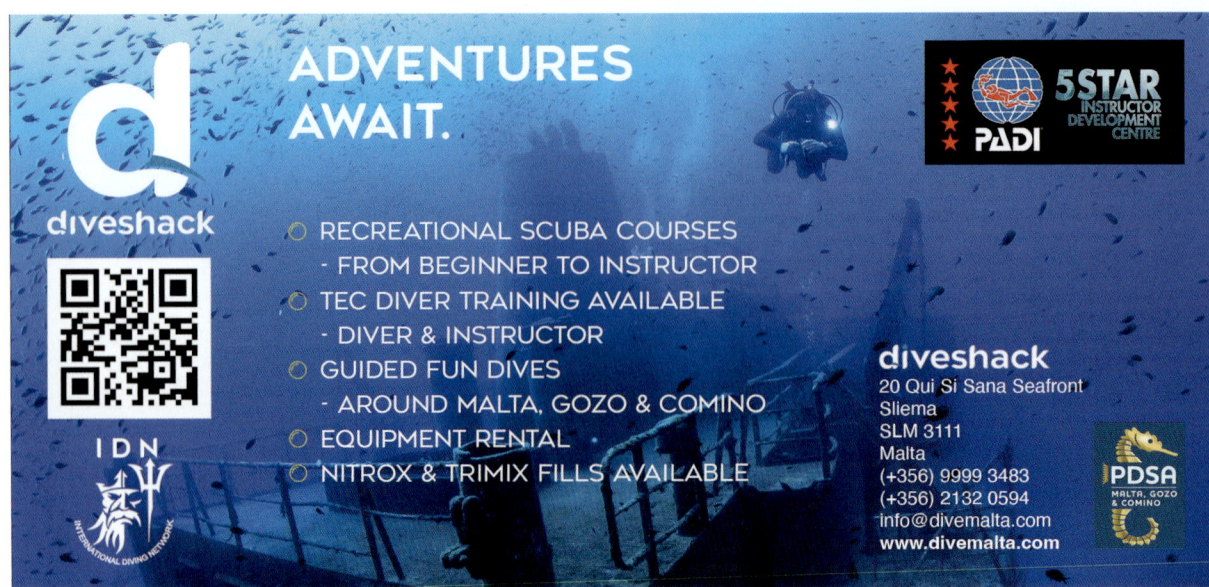

Malta Dive Centres

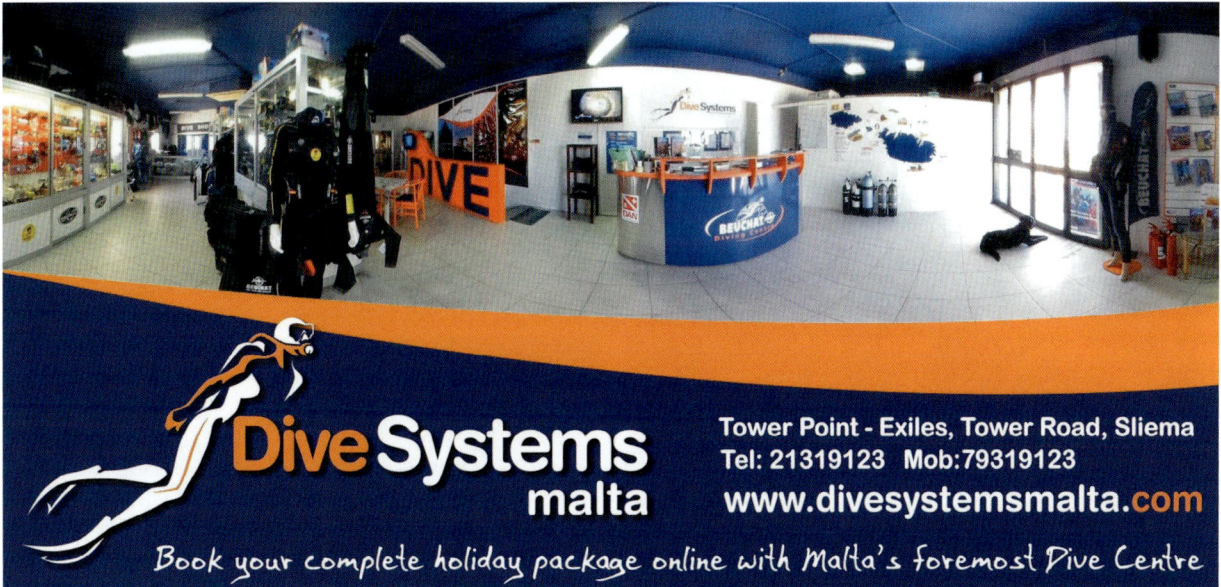

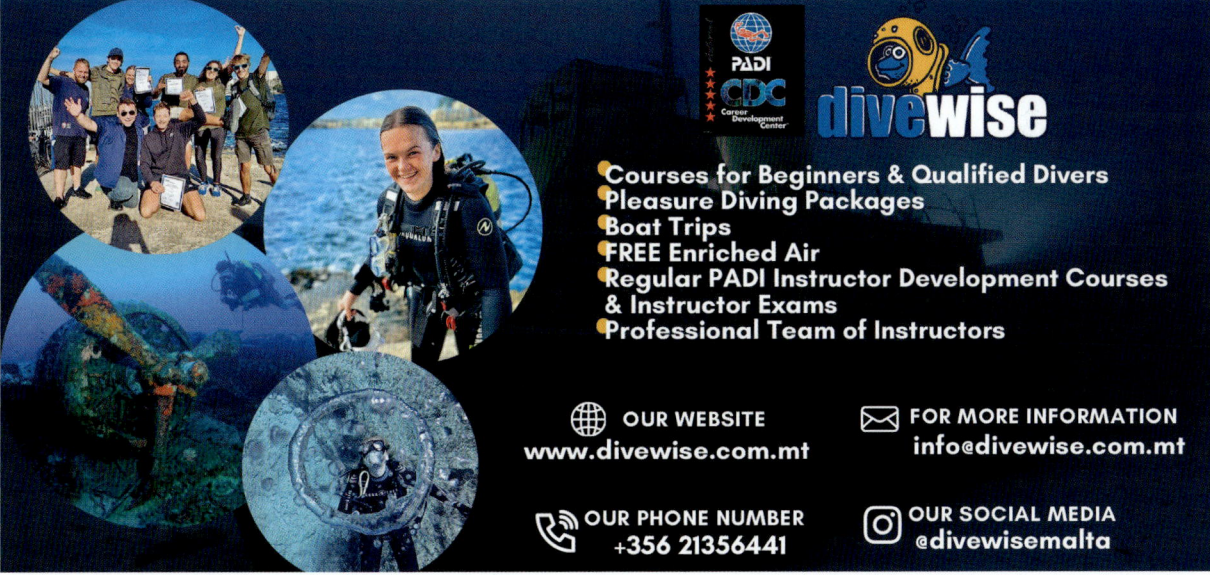

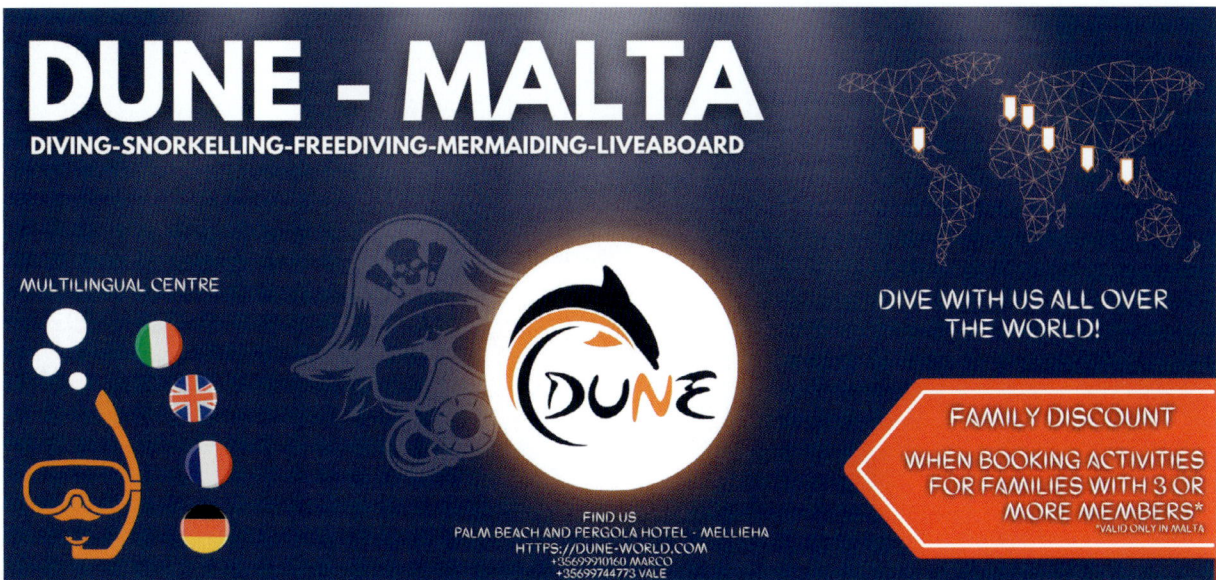

Malta Dive Centres

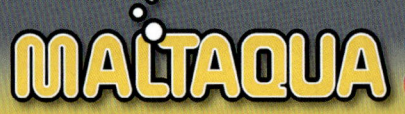

Providing the highest standards in diver training since 1969

Mosta Road, St. Paul's Bay
t: 00356 21 571 111 m: 00356 99 571 111
dive@maltaqua.com   www.maltaqua.com

Dive Shop
- Snorkeling & Diving Gear Sales & Rental
- Servicing of Dive Equipment
- Scuba Wear
- PADI Materials
- Air, Nitrox & Trimix Fills

Dive School
- Try Dives
- Kids Courses
- Beginner Courses
- Continued Training
- Technical Courses: Open & Closed Circuit

Adventure Dives
- Escorted Dives Daily
- Cave, Wreck, Night and Boat Dives around the Islands of Malta, Gozo & Comino

Holiday Services
- Accommodation
- Airport Transfers
- Car Hire
- Boat Charter
- Classroom Hire

UK Ministry of Defence ComMAC Accredited Centre

BSAC Dive with us — Dive Centre of Excellence

PADI 5STAR Instructor Development Centre

BSAC Technical Centre

TecRec DSAT

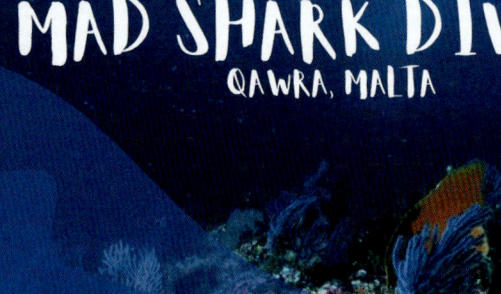

SAFETY, FUN, DYNAMIC
WWW.MADSHARKMALTA.COM
+356 7711 1767
info@madsharkmalta.com
facebook.com/madsharkmalta

MAD SHARK DIVING
QAWRA, MALTA

Dive courses Rec and Tec
Guided dives - Malta and Gozo
Small groups, focus on safety

English, Nederlands, Deutsch, Français, Español

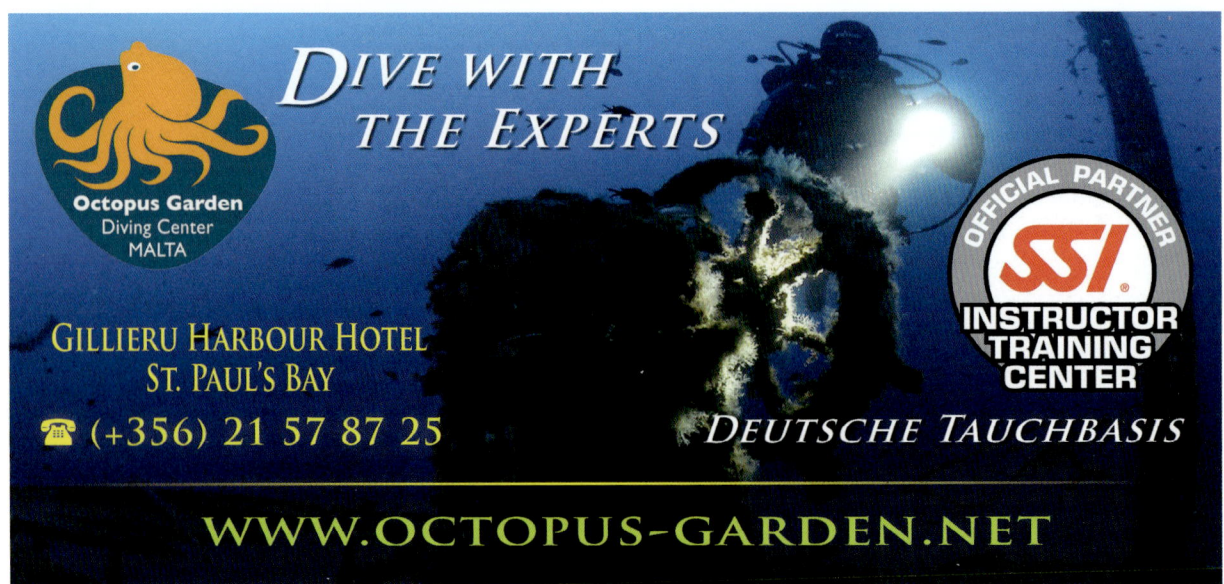

DIVE WITH THE EXPERTS

Octopus Garden Diving Center MALTA

GILLIERU HARBOUR HOTEL
ST. PAUL'S BAY
☎ (+356) 21 57 87 25

OFFICIAL PARTNER SSI INSTRUCTOR TRAINING CENTER

DEUTSCHE TAUCHBASIS

WWW.OCTOPUS-GARDEN.NET

Malta Dive Centres

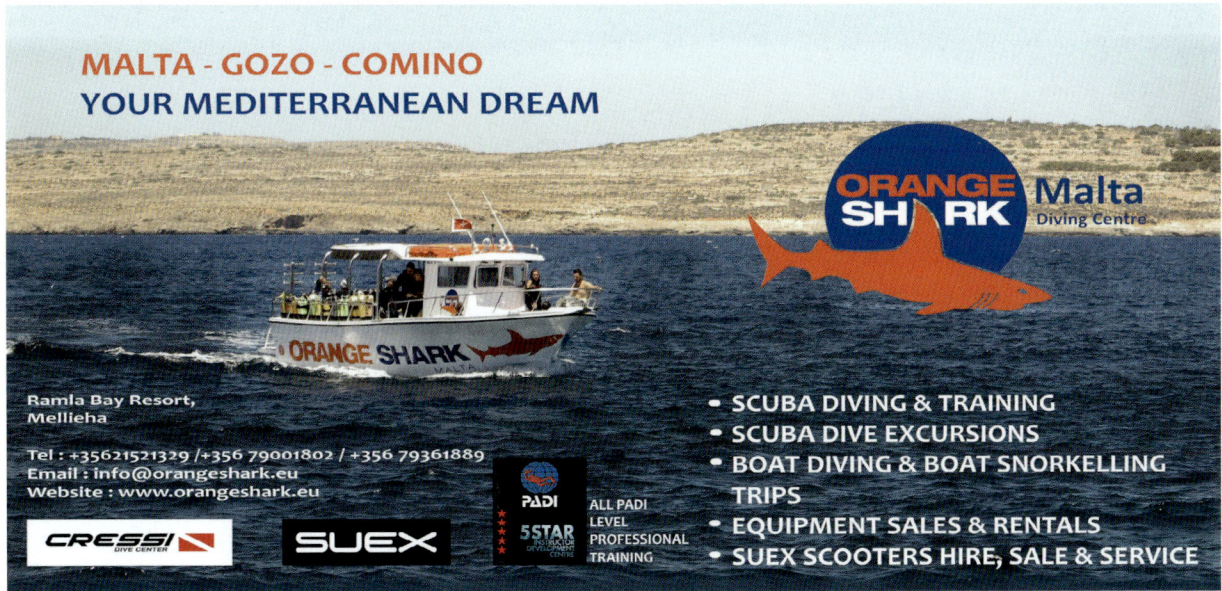
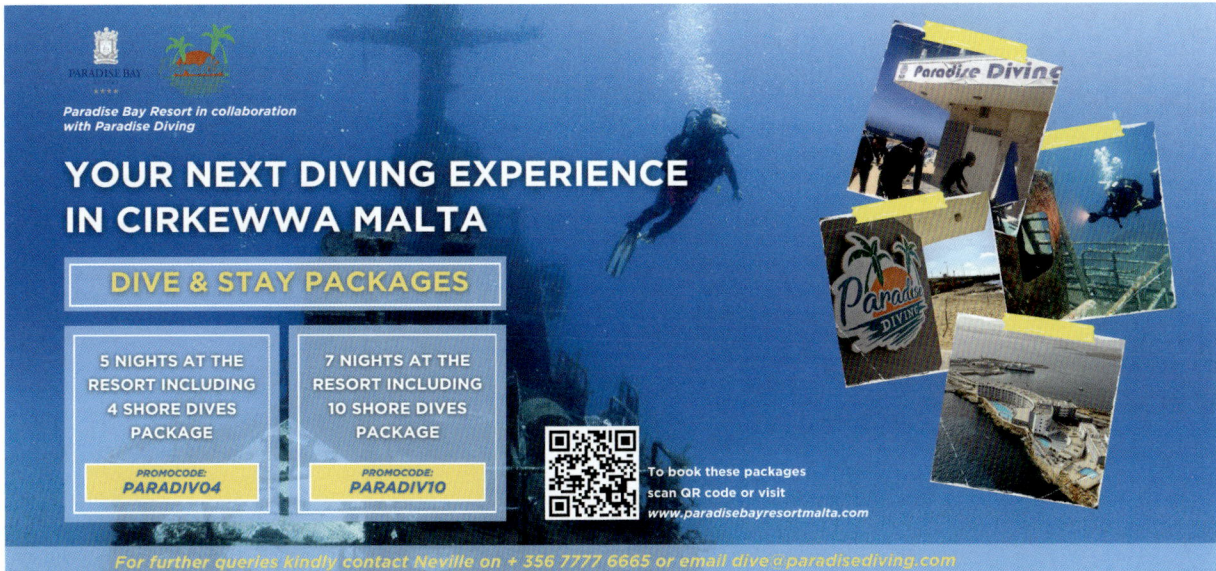
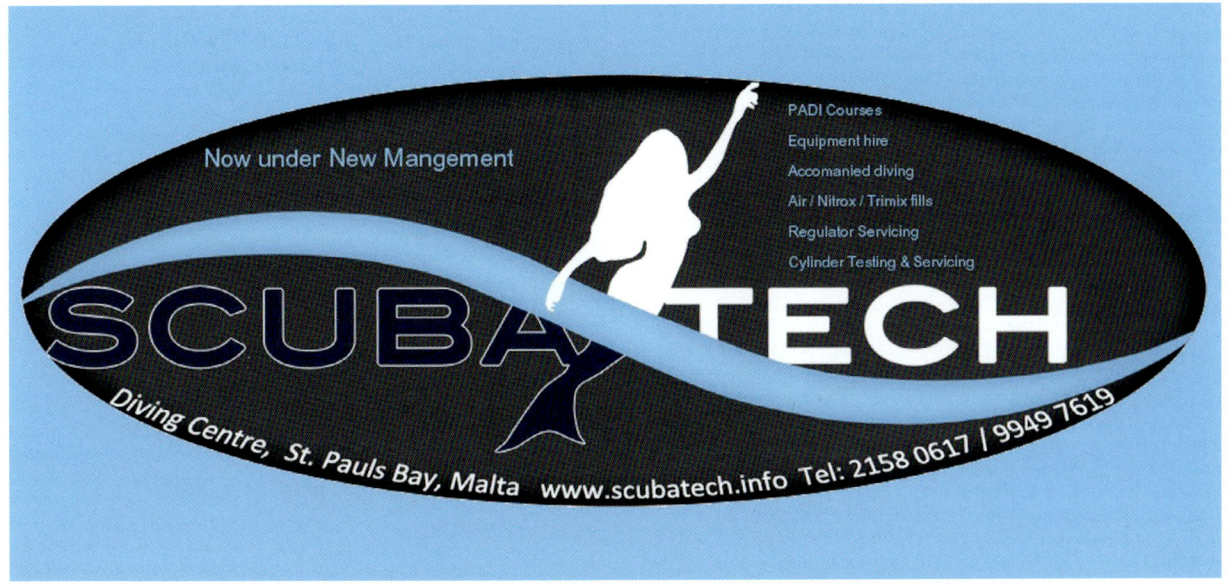

Malta Dive Centres

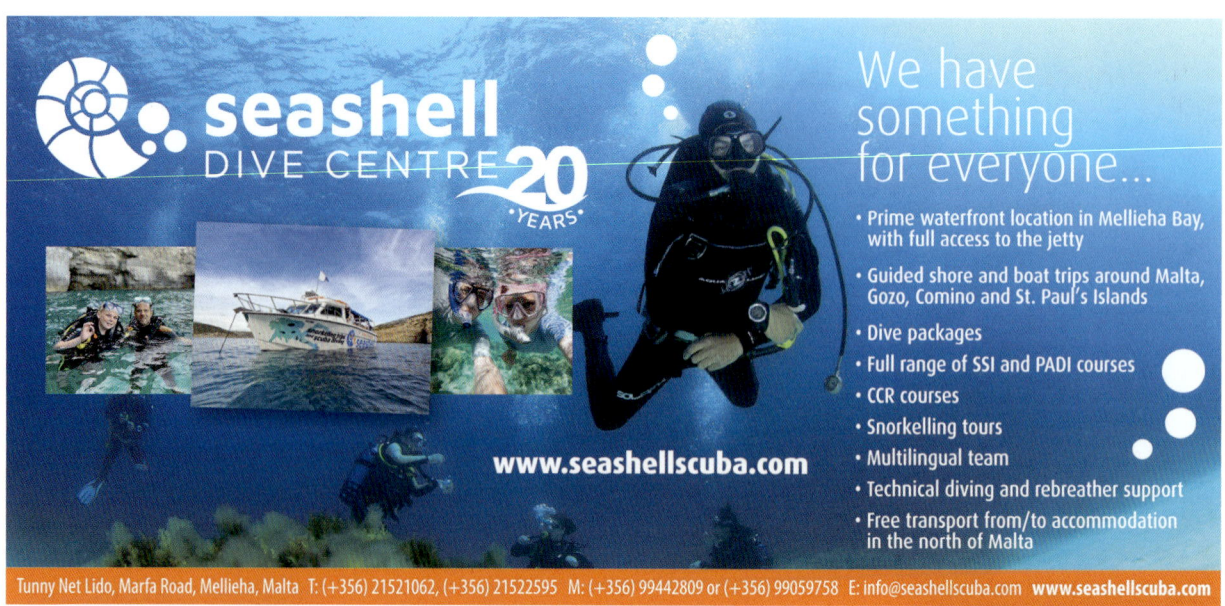
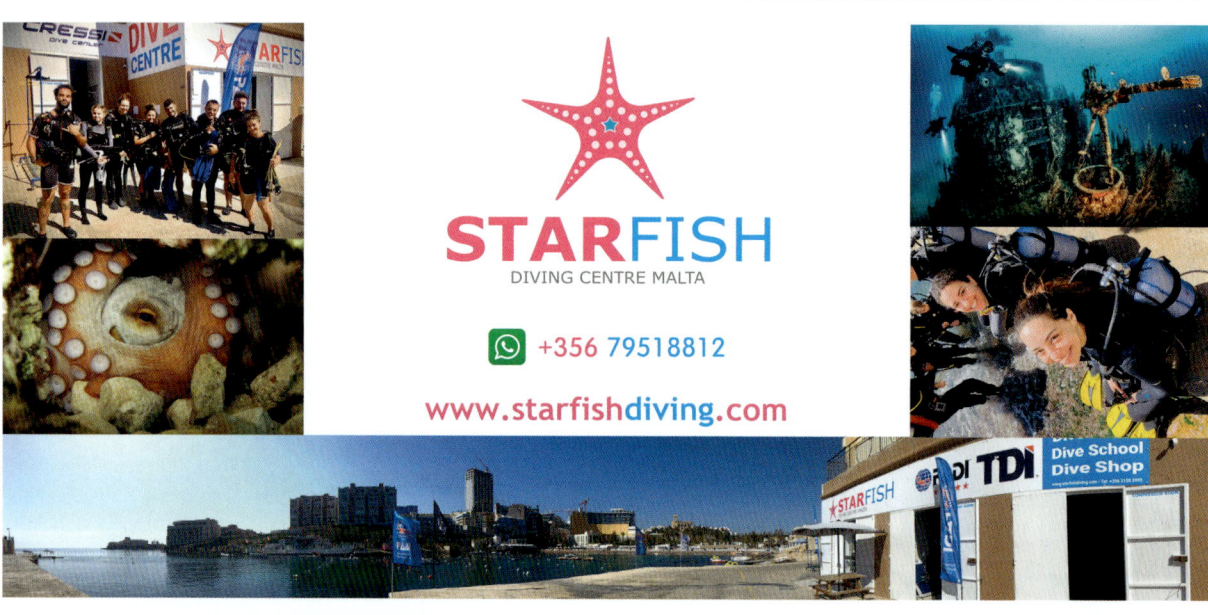
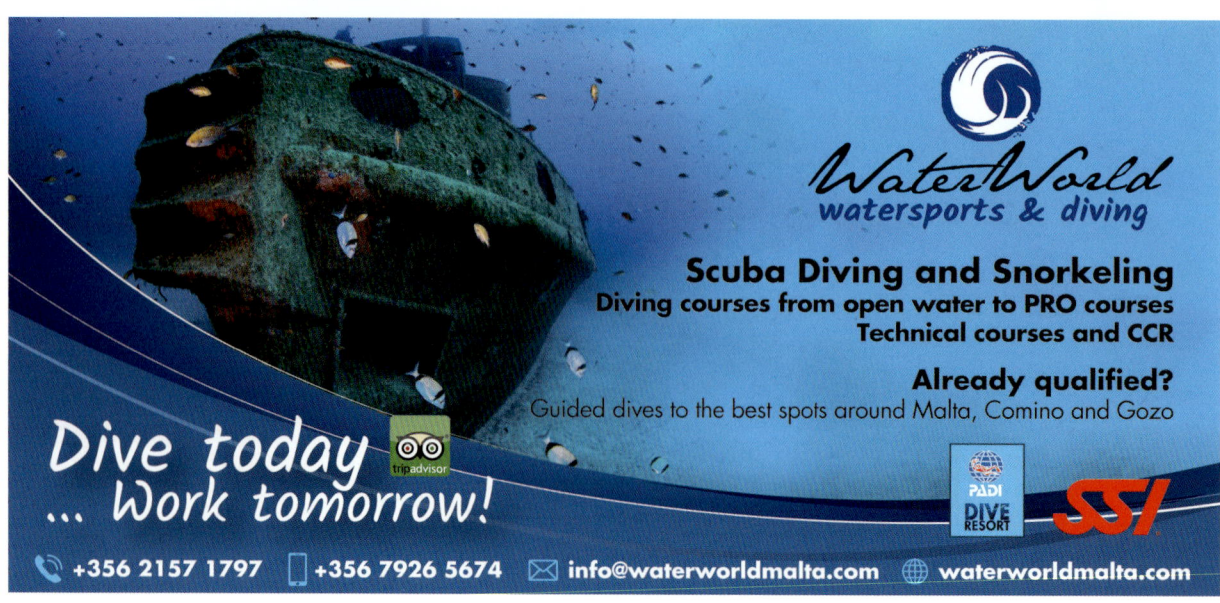

Gozo Dive Centres

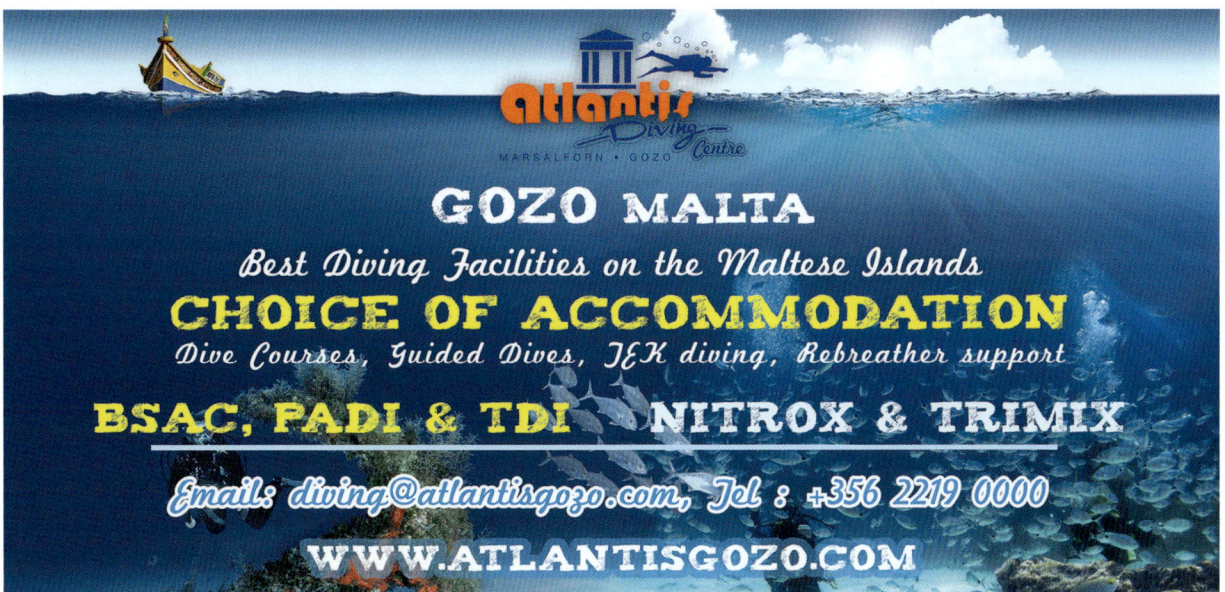

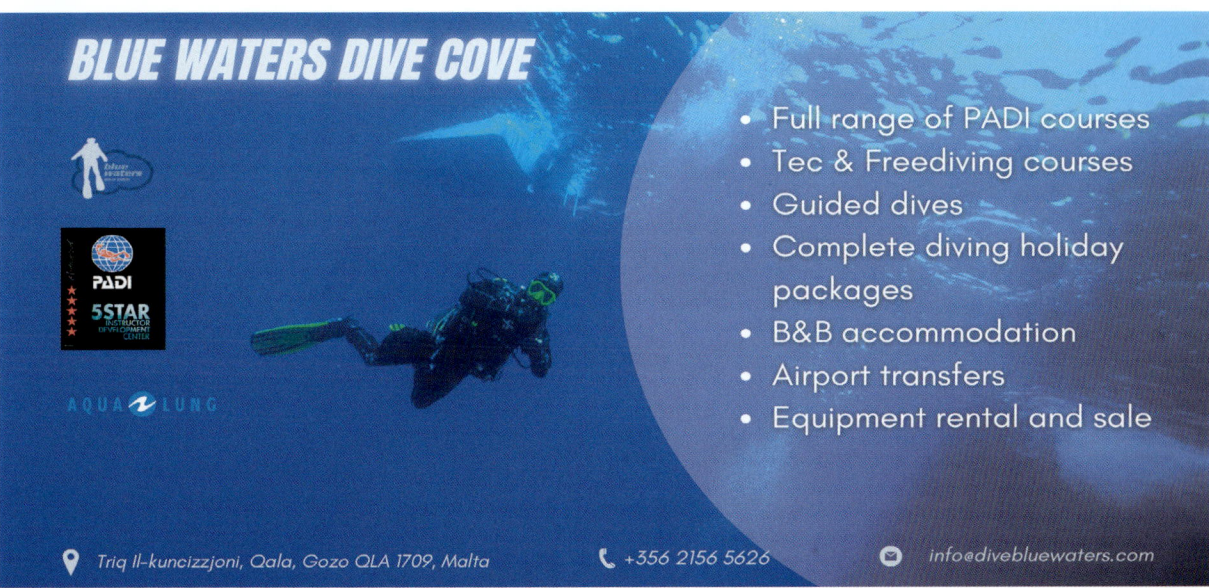

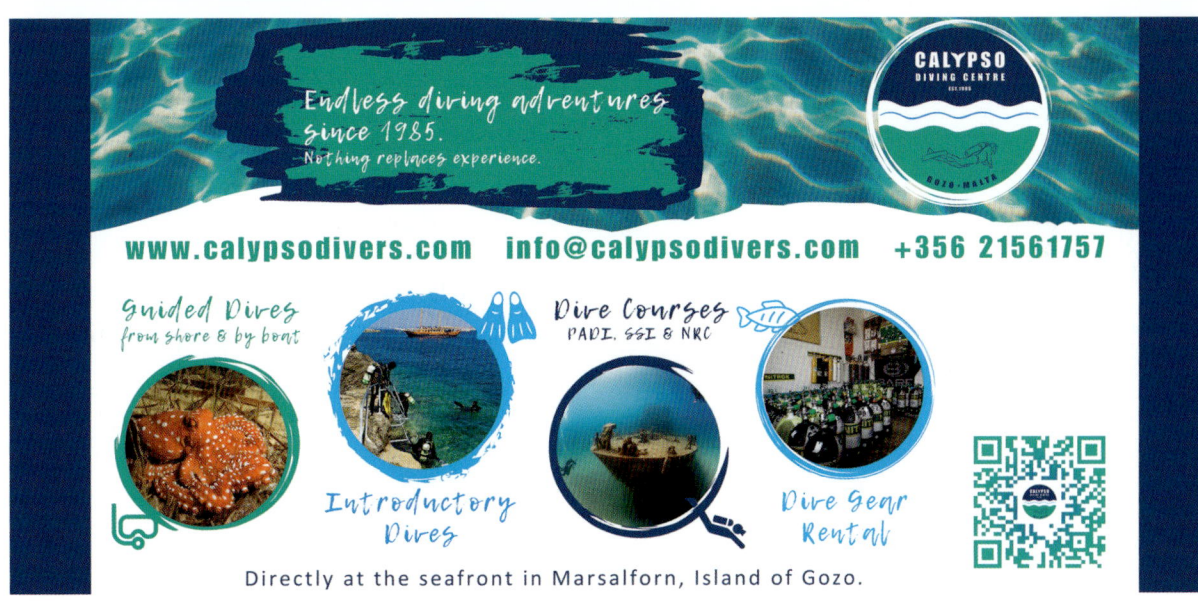

Gozo Dive Centres

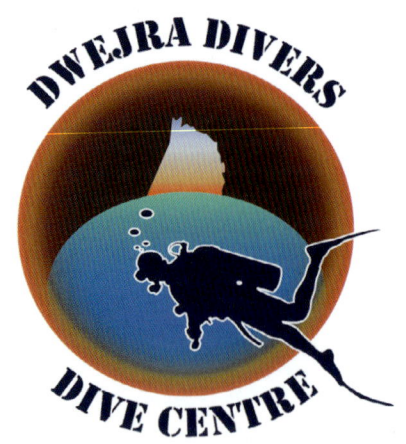

DWEJRA DIVERS
INLAND SEA - GOZO ISLAND
www.dwejradive.com

Diving is our passion and we strive to provide the best experience to our customers. Individual attention guaranteed.

Services: Air & Nitrox diving, boat diving, accompanied & unaccompanied diving

As a PSS & ISDA Dive Center we offer beginner dives & dive training from Open Water Diver up to Instructor, as well as a variety of specialty courses

 dwejradivers@gmail.com +356 21564888 +356 79564888

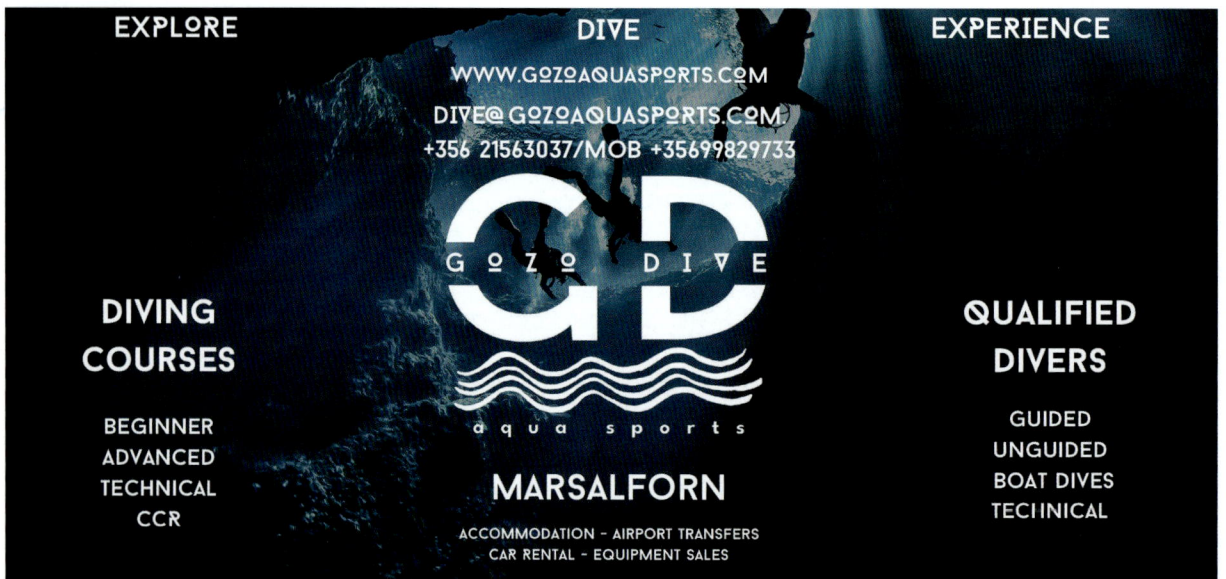

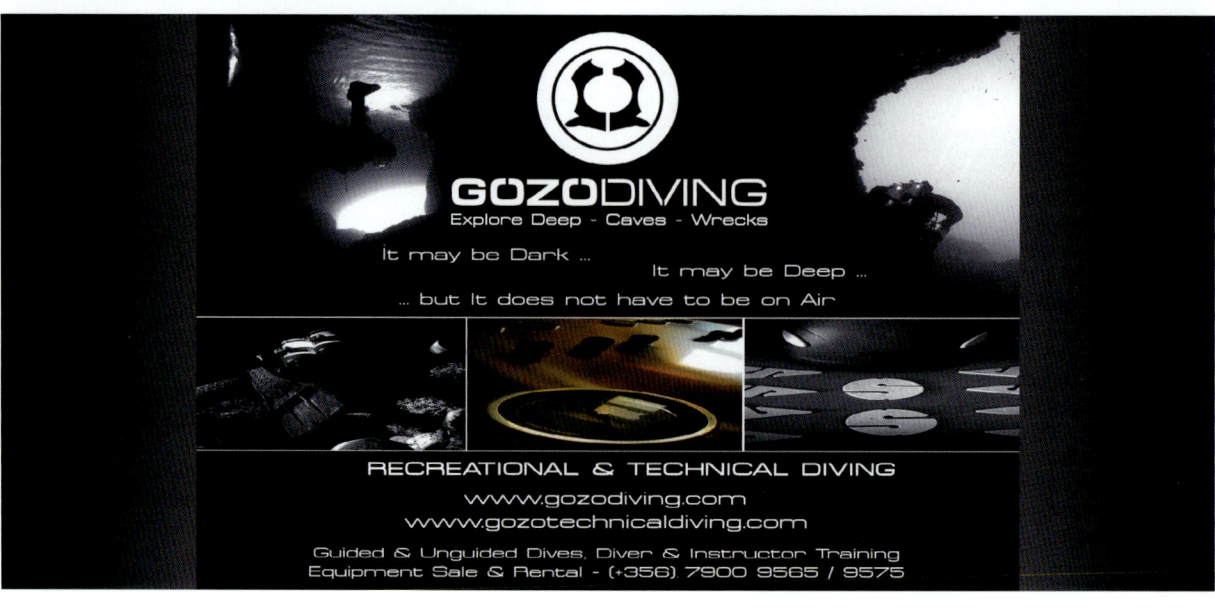

Gozo Dive Centres

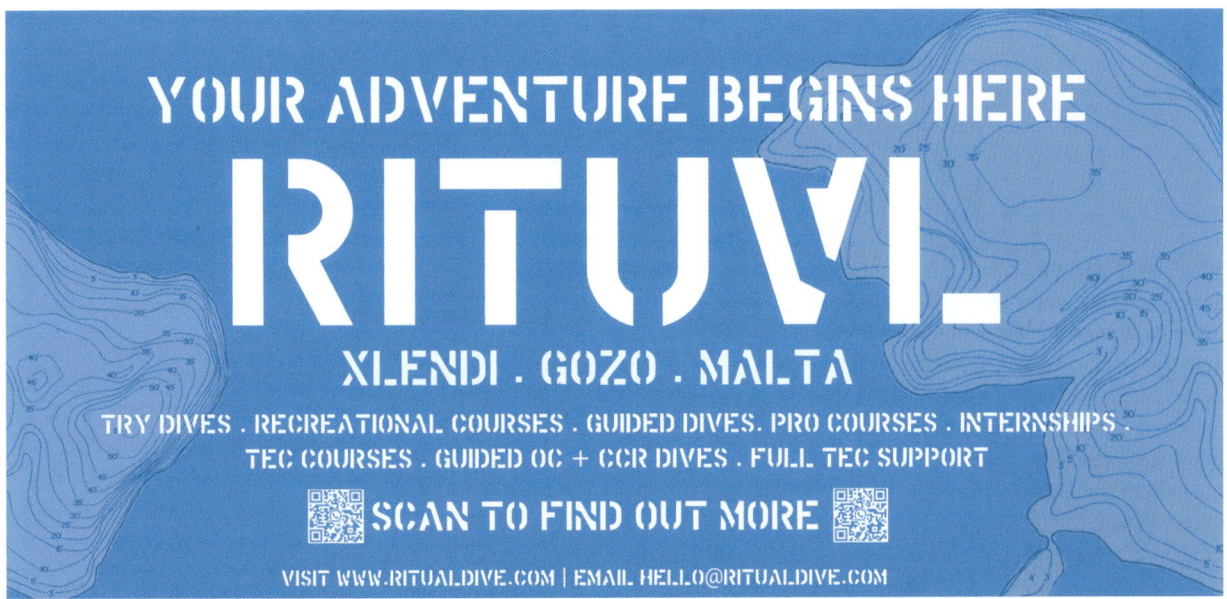
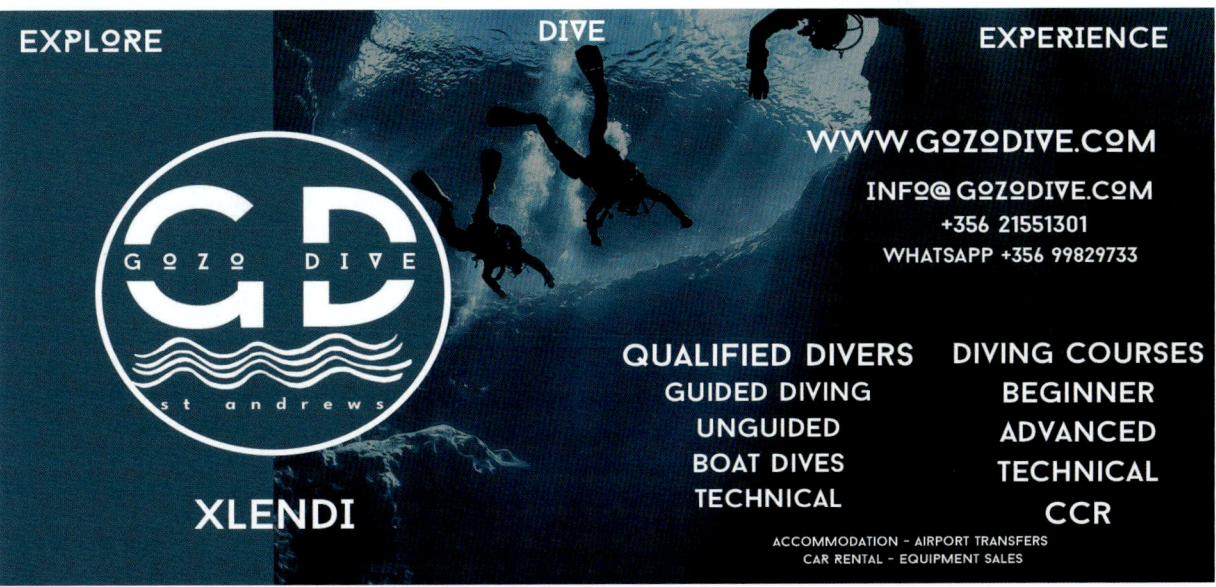
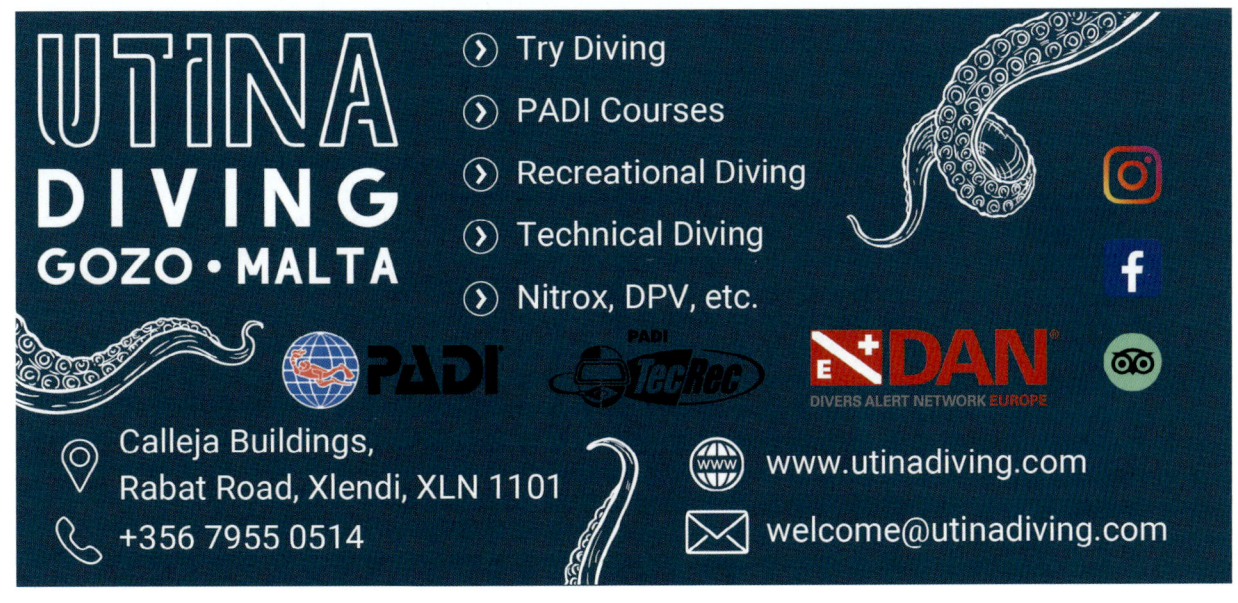

Acknowledgements

I would like to thank every one who has assisted me in producing this diving guide, without your help it would not have been possible.

Heritage Malta Underwater Malta - Dr. Timmy Gambin - Maja Sausmekat thank you for all your help and support with the new Technical section in this book.

Minister for Tourism.

Maltese Tourism Authority.

Sean King - SMK Design for his neverending, patience, advice and help.

Wade Carmichael - for updating all the original illustrations within this book.

Max and Paola Valli and instructors at Orange Shark Dive Centre, thank you for all your never ending help with the diving guide, photos, information and meetings.

Brian and Stephania Azzopardi and Atlantis Dive Centre - Thank you for your help and hospitaity both during my visits to Gozo and my calls from the UK for information.

Michael Vella De Fremeaux - Joseph Borg - Clive Perini - Miller Distributors Ltd. Malta.

Sharon & Ian Forder - for web design - underwater photographers and good friends.

Joe (Retired AFM Officer / pilot) and Tess Abdilla - for their hospitality and friendship.

Paul & Mariella Mizzi - The Foto Grafer - original Aerial Photographs.

Arkadiusz Srebnik - Polanddivingphoto - A new friend and great underwater photographer.

Lee Jellyman - Ritual Dive Centre - Excellent underwater photos of Gozo and Comino.

Jon Borg - www.jonborg.com - A variety of fantastic underwater photos.

Steven Galicia - www.galicia.be - Excellent photos of the Deep Technical Wrecks.

Per Eide Studio - www.pereide.no - Amazing aerial photos of the Gozo coastline.

Dave Gration - www.rebreathepro-training.com - Great photos of Deep Technical Wrecks.

Bent and Marthese Matusiak - Bent a very good friend and patient dive buddy. Marthese for help with Maltese literature, both for their hospitality and friendship.

Chris Gray - a friend and dive buddy, who had the original idea to produce a book.

Simone Brinch-Iversen - Maltaqua Dive Centre - Agnes Mike and Anna

Martin Stanhope and instuctors at Buddies Dive Centre for their help and information.

Simone and Claude Sciberras - and staff at Dive Systems - a special mention for Sergey Markov for his assistance and photos.

Jonathan Thomas - Dive Deep Blue for photos and helpful advice.

Divewise Dive Centre - For photos and information.

Members of BS-AC Mid Herts Divers for their support with my diving guide.

Hubert Borg - Sea Shell Dive Cove - Photo help and information.

Pam and David Mason for information on research and Sharklab.

Ivan Consiglio a friend that keeps us in touch with the Maltese Islands.

Mark Busuttil St Andrews Dive Cove - Photo help and information.

Joe Wadsworth Malta Blue Diving assisting me with your local dive site plan.

Martin Hall Neptunes Diving Malta always available for help and information.

Lina Fabri - Debbie Adams - Dave Whitlam - David Agius - Patrick Schembri - Leli Scerri - thank you all for your help and support.

David Mallard - for his painstaking research on the X 127 Lighter.

Charlie Scicluna (retired) - Malta Maritime for his help in the early days of research.

All members of the Zibel (NGO) volunteer team.

Photography

Joe Abdilla & Paul Gauci - Aerial Photos
Arkadiusz Srebnik - Polanddivingphoto
Lee Jellyman - Ritual Dive Centre
Jon Borg - www.jonborg.com
Sharon & Ian Forder - Spyder Design
Dave Gration - www.rebreatherpro-training.com
Steven Galicia - www.galicia.be
Per Eide - www.pereide.no
Max Valli Orange Shark Dive Centre
Janex Kranjc & Ivana Orlovic
Veronica Busuttil
Cathy & John De Lara
Joe Formosa - Atlam BS-AC
Sergey Markov - Dive Systems
David Agius - Calypso BS-AC
John Wood - Heritage Malta
Jurijs Bickins - Dive Med Dive Centre
Patrick Schembri - Walrus Diving Club
Wilfred Pirotta - Atlam BS-AC
Victor Fabri - Atlam BS-AC
Leli Scerri - Calypso BS-AC
Luca Paparella - Italian Air Force
Marcello Francesco - DAN
Debbie Adams
Joseph Caruana - Maritime Museum
Mark Baluci
Charlie Scicluna
Joseph Bonnici - Author
Pam Mason - Sharklab
Alfred Azzopardi - AFM
Joseph Tonna - AFM
David P. Attard - AFM
J.P. Bresser - Dive Deep Blue
Pete Bullen - St Andrews Dive Cove
Alex Duncan - Isle of Wight
Fredrick Galea - Air Museum
Gavin Anderson
Dmitry Vinogradov
Bettina Rohbrecht - Hamburg
Kevin Debattista
Anthony Chetcuti - Pilot Officer
George Zammit Briffa

I would like to thank all the people who have donated their photos to me to use in my dive guide publications, the copyright remains with the photographer.

Photos with no credit copyright remains with Peter G. Lemon

Photograph Index

Alex's Cave	187, 188
Amberjack	50, 178
Anchor Bay	17, 69
Anchor Bay Cave	70, 71
Anchor Reef Cominotto	188, 189
Anchor Reef Gozo	153, 156, 157
Aquarium	18
Arrowhead Rock	44
Azure Reef	139, 146, 147
Barracuda	90, 140, 178
Beaufighter	164
Bell Cave Zurreiq	51
Ben's Arch Cirkewwa	86
Billinghurst Cave	159, 160
Blenheim Bomber	166, 167
B24 Liberator	199, 200
Blue Dome	161, 162, 163
Blue Hole	139, 143, 144, 145, 147
Blue Lagoon	184, 191
Bogue	52, 84
Buses	13
Calypso Tunnel Cave	181
Cannons historic site	16
Cardinal fish	52, 65
Cathedral Cave	161, 162, 163
Chimney Comino	182
Chimney Dwejra	145, 147
Churches/Chapels	14, 179
Cirkewwa Marine Park	72, 73, 76, 82
Cirkewwa Anchor	76
Cirkewwa Arch	17, 74, 75
Comino	6, 182, 183, 184, 187, 191
Comino Caves	189, 190, 191
Conger	32, 101
Coral	90, 130, 177
Coral Gardens Dwejra	142, 144
Coral Gardens Sliema	110, 111
Crab	59
Crocodile Rock	138, 140, 141
Crystal Lagoon	184, 191
Cuttlefish	176, 186
Damsel fish	77, 78
Dawra Tas-Sanap	176
Delimara	40, 41, 43, 45
De Water Joffer	168
Dive boats	89, 155, 174, 189
Dive centre	110
Diver groups	12, 19, 113
Dockyard Creek	14
Double Arch	153, 154
Dwejra	14, 138, 139
Exiles	99, 102, 103, 104, 105
Fan Worm	180
Festa	14
Filfla Island	168
Fireworm	20, 42
Fish Feeding	78, 190
Flying gurnard	184
Fortizza Reef	107, 108, 109, 110
Fort St Elmo	28, 29
Fra Ben Cave	95
Fungus Rock Dwejra	130, 176, 177
Ghar Lapsi	56, 57
Ghar Lapsi Black John	57, 58, 59
Ghar Lapsi Crib & Cave	61, 63
Ghar Lapsi Finger Reef	60, 61, 63
Ghasri Valley	161, 162
Goby	95
Golden zoanthid	58
Gozo Ferry	13
Grouper	42, 73, 76, 83, 102, 181
Hannah's Reef Cirkewwa	81
HMS *Eddy*	165
HMS *Hellespont*	165
HMS *Maori*	24
HMS *Nasturtium*	194, 195
HMS *Olympus*	207
HMS *Russell*	208
HMS *Southwold*	196, 197, 198
HMS *St Angelo*	166
HMS *Stubborn*	170, 171
HMS *Talbot Base*	115
HMD *Trusty Star*	206
HMS *Urge*	209
Inland Sea	138, 139, 148, 150, 151
Jellyfish	2, 54, 58, 150, 176
John Dory	42, 52
Junker Ju88 fighter plane	201
Kalkara Creek	14
L'Ahrax	88, 89, 91
L'Ahrax Tunnel	88, 89, 90, 91
Lantern Point	6, 182, 183
Lobster	86, 183
Luzzu	14, 168, 224
Madonna Cirkewwa	80, 81
Manoel Island	107, 112, 113, 115
Marsalforn	152, 153
Marsascala	35, 36
Marsaxlokk	40
Mdina	164
Meagre	86, 103
Mercanti Reef	99, 100, 101
Mgarr Harbour	72
Mgarr ix-Xini	15, 131, 132, 133
Migra Ferha	64, 65, 66, 67
Middle Finger	127, 128, 129, 130
Moray	73, 100, 180
MV *Cominoland*	116, 122, 123
MV *Hephaestus*	125, 174, 175
MV *Imperial Eagle*	172, 173
MV *Karwela*	21, 116, 120, 121, 123
MV *Um el Faroud*	11, 17, 47
MV *Xlendi*	116, 117, 118, 119
Nudibranch	34, 66, 96, 142, 179
Octopus	28, 42, 103, 128
Old Mans Nose Cirkewwa	82
ORP *Kujawiak*	204, 205
Painted comber	98, 163
Paradise Bay	86, 87, The Anchor 82
Parrotfish	140
Pilot fish	44
Pope John Paul	173
Popeye Village	68, 69
P29 Patrol Boat	72, 82, 83, 84, 85, 211
P31 Patrol Boat	184, 185, 186, 187
P33 Patrol Boat	35, 37, 39
Qawra Point	94, 95, 96, 97, 98
Rainbow wrasse	101
Ras il-Hobz	126, Anchor 128, 129
Ras ir-Raheb	168
Ray	37
Red Bay	116, 124, 125
Red gurnard	136
Red mullet	118
Reqqa Point	153, 158, 159, 160
Ribbed helmet shell	58
Salema fish	58, 108, 127, 142
Salps	52
San Dimitri Point	178, 179
Santa Marija Reef	189
Schnellboot S31	202, 203
Scorpionfish	90, 124
Scotscraig Barge	169
Seabream	132, 190
Seahare	96
Seahorse	132
Sharklab	19
Sharpsnout	54, 132
Slugs Bay	88, 92, 93
Sponges	98
SS *Le Polynesien*	192, 193
SS *Margit*	30, 31, 32, 33, 34
Statue of Christ	173
Stoney Path Cirkewwa	76, 81
Sugar Loaf Cirkewwa	76, 80, 81
Susies Pool Cirkewwa	12, 73, 76, 80
Swimthrough Cirkewwa	76
Ta Camma - Gudja Cave - Gozo	179
The Ledge Cirkewwa	82
Tompot blenny	69
Triton shell	178
Tugboat *Rozi*	21, 72, 77, 78, 79
Tugboat *St Michael*	35, 36, 38, 39
Tugboat "10"	36, 37
Turbot	92
Turtles	18, 52
Wied il-Mielah	180
Wied iz-Zurrieq	3, 46, 47, 53, 55
Wrasse	50
Xatt L-Ahmar	116, 117, 119, 125
Xlendi	134, 137
Xlendi Tunnel	134, 135, 136, 137
X127 Water Lighter	112, 113, 115
Xwejni Bay	153, 154, 155
Zibel (NGO) Voluntary Group	19
Zorro's swimthrough	189
Zurzieb Cavern & Reef - Gozo	177

Page Index

The West Reef at Wied iz-Zurrieq	1
Copyright	2
Contents	3
Shore Diving Locations - map	4
Shore Diving Locations - index	5
Boat Diving Locations - map	6
Boat Diving Locations - index	7
Technical Dive Sites - map	8
Technical Dive Sites - index	9
Foreword	10
A note from the Author	11
Introduction	12
Travelling Information	13
To the Maltese Islands	13
Passport & Visa regulations	13
Ferry Service - Malta Gozo	13
Public Transport - buses	13
Car Hire & traffic laws	13
The Maltese Islands	14
The People	14
Language	15
Weather and Weather Chart	15
Religion	15
Medical Care	15
Shopping	15
Currency	15
Electricity	15
Drinking Water	15
Islands for Divers	16
Government Diving Regulations	16
Seas around the Maltese Islands	17
Dive Centres & Schools	17
Marine life	18
Nature Trust Malta Gozo	18
Sharklab Malta	19
Zibel Malta for cleaner seas	19
Dive Centres and Diving Clubs	20
Diving for the disabled	20
Underwater photography	20
Night diving	20
Key to Symbols	21
Special Diving Notes	21
Atlam Sub Aqua Club - BSAC	22
Calypso Sub Aqua Club - BSAC	22
Shore Diving Malta	23
My family in the Maltese Islands	106
Shore Diving Gozo	116
Malta Boat Dive Sites	168
Gozo Boat Dive Sites	174
Comino Boat Dive Sites	182
Technical Dive Sites	192
Dive Centre License Authority	210
Professional Diving Schools Ass.	211
Dive Centre Locations - map	212
Malta Dive Centres information	213
Gozo Dive Centres information	218
Acknowledgements	221
Photograph index	222
Page index	224

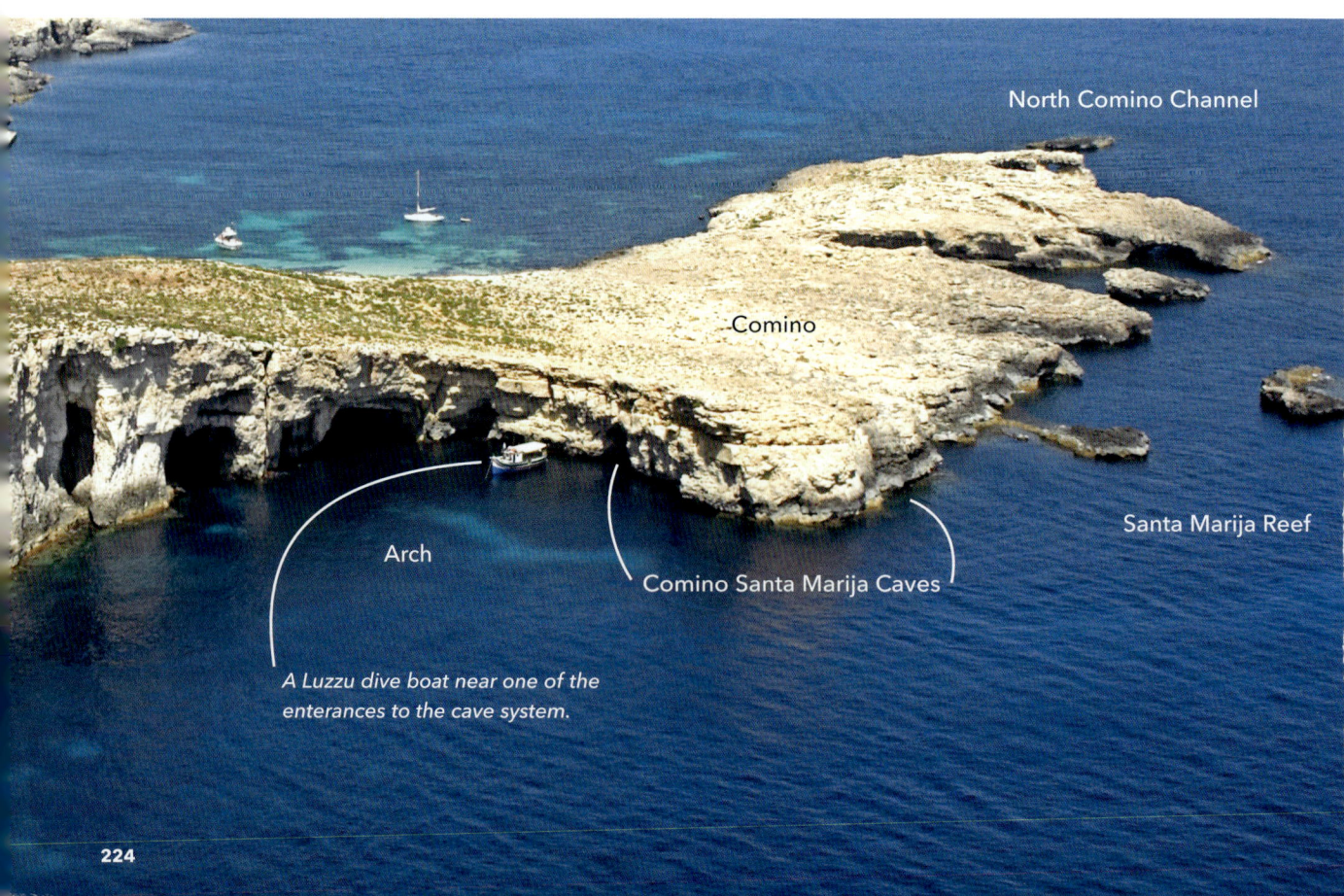

A Luzzu dive boat near one of the enterances to the cave system.

Labels: North Comino Channel, Comino, Santa Marija Reef, Arch, Comino Santa Marija Caves